SOCIALIZED MEDICINE IN ENGLAND AND WALES

The National Health Service, 1948-1961

SOCIALIZED MEDICINE

IN

ENGLAND AND WALES

The National Health Service, 1948-1961

By

ALMONT LINDSEY

Chapel Hill

THE UNIVERSITY OF NORTH CAROLINA PRESS

LONDON   OXFORD UNIVERSITY PRESS

To my wife, Irene

Preface

THE AUTHOR became interested in the British Health Service many years ago, and during a six-month visit to England in 1954 he observed the scheme at first hand. He was able to travel extensively and interrogate hundreds of people, among them medical students, nurses, pharmacists, doctors, specialists, and patients from all walks of life. Conferences were arranged with officials of hospitals, Executive Councils, local health authorities, and various other agencies and organizations associated with the Health Service. After his return home, correspondence was maintained with many of the individuals with whom he had talked, and from others additional information was sought.

Any study of the National Health Service would, of course, require far more than six months of travel in England with interviews and inspection tours. There is no substitute for a methodical analysis of the literature on the subject, and to that monumental task the author applied himself for several years. Integrating and evaluating this material also proved a task of major proportions. The subject is not one that easily lends itself to an impartial treatment, but if the author succeeds in giving the reader a reasonably unbiased understanding of the British approach to one of the more challenging problems of our age, he will feel amply rewarded for his labors.

There are actually three separate health systems in the United Kingdom, all very much alike but having certain slight variations to fit the peculiarities of each of the geographic units involved. Only in the history of the country can the explanation be found for there being a scheme for Ulster Ireland, another for Scotland, and another for England and Wales. Without minimizing the importance of the northern portions of the United Kingdom, the author decided at the outset to concentrate on England and Wales, since this area embraces about 90 per cent of the total population of the United Kingdom.

It is doubtful whether a survey of the National Health Service in Scotland or Ulster would lead to conclusions any different from those that resulted from the author's study of the Service as it operates in England and Wales.

The latter territories have a total population of forty-five millions crowded into an area of 58,825 square miles—in surface slightly larger than Illinois but little more than one-third the size of California. Great Britain is industrialized and urbanized, her people are self-disciplined, and her government, although highly centralized, is no less democratic for being so. Her Parliament, which represents the will of the people, is the source of all power, and what functions the counties and cities exercise, they do by virtue of the authority of that deliberative body.

The Health Service Law was enacted in 1946, and the scheme itself began to function in July, 1948. Such an elaborate and daring attack upon an urgent national problem aroused the interest of the world, and numerous laymen and medical experts descended on England for a quick look at this "remarkable experiment." Obviously the mere adoption of the law could not provide more nurses or hospital beds or alter much the pattern of general medical practice, but many of the hostile critics saw only what had previously existed—overcrowded doctors' offices, hospital waiting lists, and other serious deficiencies—and rashly laid such shortcomings at the feet of the new health service. These weaknesses may have been exacerbated by the initial rush of people for free medical care, but in ascribing them to the new program these critics were blind to the conditions which had prevailed prior to 1948. Dire predictions were voiced about the future of British medicine and the health of the people. The American press devoured such reports with pleasure, largely ignoring the few observers who tried to view the National Health Service with perspective and balanced judgment. From the outset the climate in the United States was unfriendly toward this British venture.

Although any comparison between the English and American approach to the problem of medical care has been excluded from this study, it should be noted that many of the same difficulties have confronted these two nations and to a greater or lesser degree have as stubbornly resisted solution in both. Many of the trends ascribed to the National Health Service had their beginnings years before and were the result of the changing pattern of medicine. How to finance the hospitals and the medical care demanded by the people and to make the facilities available to all according to need became the crux of the problem in both countries. With resources far more limited than those of the United States, Great Britain tackled the matter wholeheartedly and in a manner that deserves the most careful scrutiny.

No longer is the National Health Service in its infancy. More than a decade has elapsed since its inauguration. The time has arrived to appraise what has been accomplished, to see how well or poorly the British have dealt with the problem.

In studying the National Health Service one is impressed by the great divergence of opinion about the value of the program. A measure of unanimity could be found in Harley Street or among the members of the Fellowship For Freedom in Medicine, but this group represents the hard core of a minority of doctors who have much to say about the "evils" of the Health Service. In contrast, the Medical Practitioners' Union, the Socialist Medical Association, and the British Medical Association all accept the Health Program, subject to varying reservations and modifications. Among these organizations, as elsewhere, can be found many shades of opinions. It is not easy to measure medical opinion, since doctors as a group are quite individualistic. While the great majority of them are seldom heard from, disgruntled practitioners are quick to voice their grievances. The vocal minority could very easily give the foreigner an altogether false impression of what most doctors think of the scheme.

The National Health Service can be understood only as an institution which is the product of evolution, with roots reaching back to the first decade of the twentieth century and even earlier. Had the new service been built from scratch, a more integrated system would surely have been conceived, but such a way of doing things would have been un-English. The British move from precedent to precedent, and so the new program came to represent an expansion of the National Health Insurance, and the general superstructure of the new system came to rest upon the old health foundations, local and otherwise, which had grown out of the past. True, there were sharp changes, but where earlier institutions and practices could possibly be utilized, they were incorporated in the new program.

It is not possible to dissociate the Health Service from the British economy. Largely conceived during the throes of a global war and born at the close of that exhausting struggle, the new scheme was handicapped at the outset by bombed-out hospitals, stringent rationing, serious shortages of building materials, lack of capital, and other crippling difficulties, some of which seemed to persist for years. The unfavorable trade balance, the monetary crisis which plagued Great Britain in the postwar years, and finally the Cold War, which necessitated an expensive program of rearmament, left the nation in a straitened financial position. That position obviously had its impact upon the new service, which needed so many things, especially hospitals. In any evaluation of the Health Service, all of this background must be kept in mind.

Today rationing, which was abandoned years ago, is only a memory. The armament program has been trimmed (though the Berlin crisis may bring about a reversion), and even taxes have been somewhat reduced. Never has the British economy been so prosperous, and never has the average Englishman enjoyed living standards so high. This certainly is the foremost impression which tourists carry away from that country. But the urgent necessity to check inflation, foster exports, and restrain domestic consumption remains the dominant policy of the Exchequer. Budgets remain tight, although more money is now available in a hospital building program; but funds are still not sufficient to make the National Health Service what the founders intended it to be.

Health, like education, is vital to any economy, and the British believe that both should be made available to all without financial barriers. But the government soon learned that so comprehensive and so popular a scheme as the new health service was costly and with inflation would become even more expensive—and so certain small charges were imposed which, however, constituted no more than a fraction of the cost of the Service. All but a small proportion of the money has come from the government. The Health Service has remained essentially free, but whether Great Britain can afford such a "luxurious necessity" is another matter. The English people feel very strongly that the benefits far outweigh the cost and that their economy could not afford to be without the Health Service.

To the foreign observer many obvious questions arise about the workings of the National Health Service. How has it affected the quality of medical or dental care and the doctor-patient relationship? How do the hospitals function under the system? Has centralized administration encouraged a dangerous bureaucracy, and do politics militate against the best performance of the Service? Has clinical freedom in any way suffered? How has medical research fared? What are the major weaknesses and can they be remedied? What benefits have flowed to the patient, and what is his appraisal of the Service? In general, how efficient is it?

Answers to such questions can be found only by a meticulous examination of the vast amount of literature, mostly reports, that exists on all phases of the program. Commissions are constantly being set up to conduct inquiries into some aspect of it; the British themselves are only too conscious of the fact that there is room for improving and strengthening the program. But, all things considered,

careful study makes it clear that the British people have done in-
credibly well.

With realism and toughness of spirit, they have forged ahead
on many fronts, exploding the myth that their country is living in the
past or that the social reforms have undermined initiative and otherwise crippled their progress. Statistics prepared by the Information
Division of the British Treasury in 1958 revealed that during the
preceding ten years, which represented the first decade of the National
Health Service, production in Great Britain increased by a third, and
her exports rose to twice the prewar level. Sterling continued to
finance about half the world's trade and payments. The amount
the British were investing overseas represented a higher total per
capita than that of any other nation. Among her allies, only the
United States had carried a heavier defense burden. Per capita,
Great Britain was the world's largest producer and the world's largest
market. In such fields of technology as commercial nuclear power
and turbo-jet airliners, she led the world; and in such areas as
electronics, chemicals, and petrochemicals, radar, plastics, antibiotics,
diesel engines, cars, tractors, scientific instruments, radio, and oil
refining, she achieved extraordinary success. These and other comparable facts do not bespeak the spirit of a dying nation, but rather
the spirit of a nation in which hope and hard work and resilience augur
well for the future.

It is important to keep all this in mind when one is confronted by
the darker aspects of the British economy. The effect of two world
wars upon her overseas investments, the large foreign and domestic
debt, the perennial problem of trade balances, and the difficult adjustment necessitated by a constantly shrinking empire have left their
indelible stamp upon present-day England. The British way of life,
influenced equally by the traditions of the past and the imperatives
of the modern age, has sought to answer as many needs of the people
as the available resources have permitted. This is the motivation
which explains Great Britain's somewhat revolutionary attack upon
her social problems. And of the reforms instituted, the most ambitious was the National Health Service.

For simplicity, all British money is quoted in dollars and cents at
the following rate of exchange: 1 pound–$2.80; 1 shilling–14 cents;
I guinea–$2.94; 1 pence–slightly over 1 cent. In comparing money
values it is well to remember that the pound has greater buying power
in England than an equivalent amount of money would have in the
United States. British incomes are smaller and living standards are
lower, but money will go further in the purchase of such essentials as

housing, food, and clothing. Wages, for example, are roughly one-third of the American level but will buy one-half as much.

Many persons have contributed helpful suggestions in the preparation of this book, and for that assistance the author wishes to express his appreciation. Some of the chapters were read by Philip J. Allen, James H. Croushore, Oscar H. Darter, William W. Griffith, Robert Leroy Hilldrup, and Carol H. Quenzel—members of the faculty at Mary Washington College of the University of Virginia. All or most of the manuscript was carefully scrutinized by Dr. Frederick J. Spencer, now Regional Director of the State Health Department in Virginia and formerly a medical practitioner in the National Health Service; Eveline M. Burns, professor at the New York School of Social Work of Columbia University and at one time administrative assistant, British Ministry of Labor; and Richard M. Titmuss, Head of the Department of Social Science and Administration, London School of Economics and Political Science, who has written extensively on phases of the British Health Program.

In providing or interpreting documents and data, the following organizations gave invaluable aid: British Information Service, Essex and London Executive Councils, British United Provident Association, Social Surveys, Executive Councils' Association, Acton Society Trust, Ministry of Pensions and National Insurance, Joint Committee of Ophthalmic Opticians, Nuffield Provincial Hospitals Trust, King Edward's Hospital Fund For London, Fellowship For Freedom in Medicine, Medical Practitioners' Union, Socialist Medical Association, British Medical Association, British Dental Association, and the Ministry of Health. To the many Health Service officials, doctors, and others who so kindly gave their time in helping the author reach a better understanding of the operation of the Health Service, he desires to express his profound gratitude.

He is also indebted to the Congressional Library and the National Medical Library for their help in making vital materials available to him. He wishes to acknowledge careful secretarial assistance from Elsie di Cicco and methodical and perceptive advice in matters of style and rhetoric from his wife. Grateful recognition must likewise be given to the Research Council of the University Center in Virginia for financing a substantial part of the research.

Finally, the author desires to record his appreciation of the excellent co-operation and the careful assistance he has received from the staff of The University of North Carolina Press. Their great interest in the manuscript and the painstaking effort they devoted to its preparation for publication deserve special recognition.

ALMONT LINDSEY

Contents

SOCIALIZED MEDICINE IN ENGLAND AND WALES

The National Health Service, 1948-1961

CHAPTER I

Antecedents of the National Health Service

THE QUEST for health and economic security has dominated the history of mankind during the modern era, and particularly in the last century. Thanks to medical and technical progress, the Western World has made tremendous inroads upon the twin enemies, poverty and disease. In Great Britain, as elsewhere, the fight has not always been waged with intelligence or good planning. Her social history, and notably the hodgepodge of legislation of the past one hundred years, tells the somewhat confused story of a people groping toward a better future for the common man. It is a story of trade unionism, the rise of the Labor Party, and the growing influence of the lower classes. The ballot became their major weapon and social justice their goal. The government had little choice but to bow to the new forces. Slowly, through a succession of laws, Great Britain evolved into a social democracy. Shortly after World War II, with the Labor Party in power, Parliament enacted a series of laws, capstones in the social edifice, designed to help end poverty and insure health to all. Among these was the National Health Service Act.

On July 5, 1948, the day when the new Health Service began to operate, the pro-Labor *Daily Herald* reviewed the achievements of the past hundred years. The newspaper alluded to the investigation in 1831 by the Committee on Factory Child Labor, during which the following dialogue took place as the chairman interrogated one Elizabeth Bentley:

"What age are you?"
"Twenty-three," replied the woman.
"What time did you first begin to work?"
"When I was six years old."
"You are considerably deformed in your person in consequence of this labour?"
"Yes, I am."

"Were you perfectly straight and healthy before you worked at the mill?"

"Yes, I was as straight a little girl as ever went up and down town."

"At what time did it come on?

"I was about 13 years old. . . . it has got worse ever since."

The *Daily Herald* then proceeded to list a few of the major milestones in the long struggle to improve living conditions. In 1836, the General Register Office was created to provide statistics on health. The pens of Charles Dickens and Charles Kingsley proved potent weapons in helping to awaken the slumbering social consciousness of England. The Crimean War provided Florence Nightingale with the opportunity to revolutionize the military and civilian hospital nursing service. In 1875, the Disraeli-sponsored Public Health Act supplied the basis for such local health services as sanitation, drainage, and water supply. Sidney and Beatrice Webb, with others, waged through the years a gallant and indefatigable fight against poverty. In 1906, Parliament gave the local authorities the right to furnish meals to impoverished children, and from this legislation was to evolve the School Medical Service. A non-contributory pension for people of seventy or over was adopted in 1908. Within three years a National Health Insurance plan was enacted which more than any other measure was to furnish the basis for the comprehensive health scheme that was to receive the royal signature thirty-five years later. In 1919, the Ministry of Health was created; and in 1929 the Poor Law infirmaries and workhouses of infamous history were turned over to the county and county-borough councils for a more respectable and useful future. Gone forever were the Guardians of the Poor and the hateful stigma which this charity imposed upon its recipients, and there dawned a new era for municipal hospitals. In 1935, the milk program for schools was started. Then in 1942 came the Beveridge Report.

Much of the legislation and many of the protests cited above were directed against the poverty which haunted the working people in the nineteenth century and took its toll in the depression years of the twentieth century. Unemployment and illness were the disasters that struck with greatest frequency. The National Health Insurance improved the picture somewhat, but only in a matter of degree, especially because only the worker was insured and not his dependents. The wages of the average male prior to 1940 were £3 ($8.40) per week—little more than enough to support a family on an austerity basis. In illness the worker could claim for himself free medical care, but the additional weekly cash benefit to which he was entitled averaged little more than 14 shillings ($2). Should members of the family become sick, there was the expense of medical advice and drugs; and if orange juice, milk, and eggs were recommended as part of the diet, how could the worker possibly afford them? To meet the barest expenses of the kind, he was usually compelled to seek charity, often Poor Law relief.[1]

Mass unemployment and the dole in the 1930's left an indelible imprint upon the mind of the worker. In seeking recruits for the army, recruiting sergeants used as a common inducement, "You get meat every day." The staple diet for many families up to the outbreak of World War II consisted of tea, margarine, and bread. It is questionable whether before 1945 many manual workers throughout their entire lives "had more than a week's wages between themselves and the dole."[2] Unquestionably the social legislation of the mid-1940's was largely influenced by recollections of the "hungry thirties."

For the wife and children of the insured worker, medical care was an expense to be avoided unless the seriousness of the illness left no alternative. Recourse was had to nostrums from the drug store or to homemade remedies, and when the doctor was summoned, it was sometimes too late. How much suffering was borne in silence by mothers and wives and even children prior to the National Health Service will never be known, but a study made by a privately endowed health center at Peckham in South London gives some idea. Within a given radius of the center, membership could be had for the entire family at the nominal charge of one shilling (14 cents) per week, and one of the benefits included a complete annual health examination. Of the members of the twelve hundred or more families, mainly artisan, that received this examination, only 10 per cent were free of any discernible disorder; 25 per cent were found to be afflicted with some disease, and only a third of this group was being treated.[3]

Low incomes among the great mass of people precluded the payment of little more than nominal fees to general practitioners; and in the case of hospitals, charity was often the rule. There were privately sponsored contributory schemes which eased the situation in a rather ineffectual way. Some doctors organized family clubs for their more destitute patients, under which a few pennies a week were collected by an agent on a commission basis. More important were the Friendly Societies, some of which had come into existence before the beginning of the twentieth century. Membership costs were low, and the subscriber was entitled to the services of a doctor who had contracted to treat member patients. The remuneration, paid on a capitation basis, was exceedingly small, but it was an assured income.[4]

Under the Health Insurance Act of 1911, virtually all low-income workers were compulsorily insured and in the event of illness were guaranteed for themselves, but not their dependents, free drugs and the care of a physician. At first only those with annual incomes of not more than £160 ($448) were eligible, but by 1942 the maximum had been lifted to £420 ($1,176). At the outset the total weekly contribution for health insurance was 3 or 4 cents, but by the early 1940's it had risen to 10d (11 cents), of which the employee paid 8½d (9 cents). The state made up the difference, which was about one-sixth of the total. By the mid-1940's there were about 21 million persons, or almost one-half of the population in Great Britain, thus insured between the ages of sixteen and sixty-five, and for those insured, medical benefits would continue until death.[5]

The doctors were free to participate or not, and eventually over two-thirds of those in practice did so. In industrial regions the percentage was closer to 100. There was no interference with private practice, but the backbone of income for most doctors remained the annual capitation fee, which eventually rose to 9 shillings ($1.26) for every person on the practitioner's "panel," irrespective of whether the individual claimed medical treatment or not. Rural doctors received mileage allowance and additional payment for dispensing drugs. The maximum number of patients permitted on a panel was 2,500, but only 14 per cent of the general practitioners had lists of more than 2,000, while 35 per cent had lists of 600 or less.[6] The rate of pay was determined by negotiation between the medical profession and the government, although occasionally it was settled by arbitration. The basis of payment was largely predetermined by the capitation system in use by the Friendly Societies when the Health Insurance Act was conceived.

All the available information points to the fact that the net income of the medical profession was much too low. Some few doctors with a private practice in favored areas did very well, but the majority of English physicians had incomes that were relatively low. While it is not known precisely what proportion of the average doctor's income came from the National Health Insurance, the most accurate estimate would indicate that it was about one-third.[7] The best working years of a general practitioner are those between 40 and 55, and his earning power should then be at its peak. Yet in 1936-38 a survey showed that over 40 per cent of general practitioners in this age group had an annual net income of less than £1,000 ($2,800). In commenting on this startling fact, the so-called Spens Report on the Remuneration of General Medical Practitioners declared, "We are unanimous in holding that the percentages of low income are too high. . . . we are clear also that the proportion of practitioners able to reach a net income of £1,300 ($3,640) or over is too low. We consider that unless conditions are substantially improved in both respects . . . the social and economic status and the recruitment of general medicine could not, in the long run, be maintained."[8]

Since the capitation payment was small, most doctors preferred private patients, but the dependents of insured persons, although in this category, were a poor source of income even though many of these dependents belonged to voluntary "sick clubs." Middle-class urban communities thus tended to attract proportionately more general practitioners than industrial-mining regions where there was normally already an acute doctor shortage. In the late 1930's there were thus one-half as many doctors per capita in South Wales as in London, and only one-fourth as many per capita in the industrial midlands as in the coastal resort city of Bournemouth.

The distribution of doctors was further distorted by the established policy of buying and selling practices. The recognized method of entering general practice was by way of partnership or through the purchase of the "good will" of a retiring doctor; this latter practice usually involved, in addition, the purchase of his residence, which contained the office and reception rooms. The price for the practice depended primarily upon the number of panel and private patients. In buying a practice the young doctor heavily mortgaged his future.[9]

The National Health Insurance endeavored to maintain complete freedom in the doctor-patient relationship, while seeking also to prevent abuses. General practitioners who were willing to treat panel patients had the right to accept or reject any; and for the patients there was complete freedom of choice among panel doctors. An insured person could change doctors immediately if the practitioner granted permission; otherwise, the transfer could be made only at the end of each quarter by filing one month's advance notice with the insurance committee.

Whether panel patients received the same treatment as private patients is not clear, although the Royal Commission in its investigation of the National Health Insurance in 1926 found no evidence to support the charge that insured patients received inferior service. Indeed, the Commission felt that there was a growing tendency for doctors to be more careful to avoid offending panel patients, since they had recourse to machinery under the law for the investigation of complaints. The Ministry of Health in the annual report for 1938-39 commented on the "high standard of service" by referring to the small number of general practitioners who had been subject to disciplinary action in that year. But the disciplinary machine was unwieldy, and its application could hardly have been an accurate measure of negligence or inferior treatment. There were doctors who resorted to the "bottle-of-medicine" technique because they were overworked or because their sense of duty had been dulled, but there were some who did so because they could not possibly prescribe to their patients the kind of life necessary to insure recovery.[10]

Health Insurance increased the volume of work for many physicians, whose reception rooms became increasingly crowded. A general survey in 1938-39 covering 6,000 doctors showed that, for all those persons listed on panels, office calls during the year averaged about four per individual and domiciliary visits slightly over one for each patient, making a total of approximately five attendances per insured person.[11] The number of services required for a large list thus commanded a substantial part of a doctor's time.

There was a growing tendency among physicians to refer patients to the outpatient departments of hospitals that would accept such patients. The London hospitals in particular suffered from an enormous increase in the number of outpatients, and in the opinion of some staff members many of these patients could have been competently handled by the general practitioners.[12] There was, of course, no way of knowing in how many of these cases the doctor was not certain of his diagnosis and needed the confirmation and advice of a specialist. It was becoming evident that a major factor in the overcrowded outpatient departments was the increasing specialization in medicine and the high cost of diagnostic equipment which the general practitioner had neither the money to pay for nor the skill to use. This trend toward specialization and expensive therapeutic treatment created a new pattern in medicine which made the cost to many patients almost prohibitive and hastened the need for the National Health Service.

The practitioner was not always able to keep pace with the latest medical developments. In many cases he practiced medicine alone and worked in isolation, having little or no time for reading medical books and journals or taking postgraduate courses. His office and equipment were frequently obsolete, and his reception rooms were not always hygienic. He was often overworked because he could not afford or obtain secretarial and nursing help.[13]

The National Health Insurance was deficient in many ways. The small trader and many other independent workers, whose income and economic security were often no greater than those of factory employees, were among those excluded. Half the population had no protection, and those who did were denied access to many of the services of modern medicine. There was no provision for hospitalization, nursing after-care, X-ray diagnosis and treatment, or physiotherapy. The services of the specialist were not available to panel patients. No provision under this program was made for treating tuberculosis or furnishing orthopedic appliances or artificial limbs.[14] Beyond supplying drugs and the services of a general practitioner for the insured the statutory provisions did not go, and the Approved Societies eased the situation only slightly by their "additional benefits."

In spite of the limitations of the Health Insurance, the British Medical Association with reservations eventually accepted it as a workable plan that met a real need and by 1929 even supported a broadening of the scheme to include the dependents of the insured. But it was otherwise at the outset, when the Association greeted the proposal with grave misgivings. Doctors had long recognized the need for some kind of action and had even demanded state medicine prior to 1911, but the profession seemed to favor a public medical service organized and administered by itself for the benefit of the lower levels of the working class. In this way private practice would be preserved for all except those least able to pay.

When in 1911 the government proposed the National Health Insurance, the British Medical Association showed little enthusiasm, and, seeking to protect itself, demanded the acceptance of several cardinal principles. Agreement was finally reached on most of them, but the medical profession failed to get all that it wanted. The scheme was to begin operation on January 15, 1913, and as the deadline approached the British Medical Association became increasingly reluctant to co-operate. The financial arrangements and the income limit for participation in the plan had not been settled to the satisfaction of the profession. The fear of too much government control and interference, too little remuneration, and the loss of professional freedom dominated the thinking of many. A referendum on the issue among members resulted in an overwhelming vote against participation, and at a meeting on December 23, 1912, the Association decided not to accept service under the act on the terms offered by the government and ordered all members to support this decision.[15] But as the days slipped by there were defections in the ranks. Disregarding the advice of their leaders, more and more members accepted service on the panels. The pressure of economics and the desire to gain patients were factors. The strategy of the Association therefore failed, and on January 17, 1913, a special meeting, hastily called, revoked the ban which indeed had already become ineffectual.[16]

The Health Insurance scheme seemed revolutionary and was not at all popular with conservative-minded people. Whereas the Old Age Pension Act of 1908 was non-contributory and affected only the aged, the National Insurance proposal provided compulsory unemployment and health insurance for a large segment of the population; that insurance was jointly to be financed by the employer, the employee, and the government. The innovation of insurance cards and stamps ensuring free medical treatment for millions of people was something quite new in a country that for decades had stood by the doctrine of economic liberalism, personal thrift, and the need for each person to meet the hazards of life in his own way and without interference or assistance from the government. But the old order was crumbling; dynamic forces were at work, and Parliament was swept forward on the crest of the new wave. In hammering out the law, the government was greatly influenced by the Friendly Societies, trade unions, and insurance companies, which zealously fought to protect and extend their interests under the new scheme. The report of the Royal Commission on the Poor Laws, 1909, played a major role in effecting passage of the bill. Enlightened public opinion was in full agreement that the Poor Law approach to poverty and disease was bad and should be superseded by a dignified system of compulsory sickness insurance with cash benefits in no way contingent upon Poor relief.[17]

Administration of the scheme was entrusted to Approved Societies, which themselves were subject to government supervision. In 1940, they numbered about 800, but many had branches that functioned as separate financial units, and these ran into several thousand. A large proportion were Friendly Societies. These were completely autonomous, though some were sponsored by and related to industrial insurance companies, trade unions, and even business concerns that had made superannuation provision for their employees. The law required that all Approved Societies operate on a non-profit and democratic basis, but owing to apathy on the part of the members and to the general nature of the organizations, actual control tended to remain in the hands of an inner group. In addition to administering this national unemployment and health insurance, many of the societies offered burial benefits and life and endowment insurance. Thousands of agents were employed to collect and distribute insurance cards and to accept and pay benefit claims. In the case of the societies affiliated with the insurance companies, the same agents often served both associations, never losing an opportunity to solicit business for the profit-making parent organization. Trade unions, whose primary concern was to seek better terms and working conditions for their members, were perhaps the least qualified of all to venture into the field of sickness insurance and death benefits.[18]

Competition for members was keen and the agents were very active, but the absence of integration and co-ordination among the thousands of participating units made the scheme expensive, inefficient, and unwieldy. The cost of administration in relation to benefits was high. Some societies were more or less local, and if a member moved elsewhere it was difficult to maintain contact with the proper agents or get prompt service in the settlement of a claim. It is amazing that such a heterogeneous empire of societies was able to function as well as it did and to avoid any major scandal.

The Minister of Health, upon the establishment of his office after World War I, became the chief administrative official of the National Health Insurance in England and Wales. He was assisted by various committees. The National Insurance Audit Department kept a careful check on the receipt and disbursement of all funds managed by the Approved Societies. Substantial sums of money were handled by the post office, which sold the insurance stamps and which also retained the deposits of those who elected to join no society and paid them their benefits.[19] In every county and county-borough there was an Insurance Committee. Consisting of between 20 and 40 members, these Insurance Committees, the great majority of which were supposed to represent insured persons, more often were agents or deputies of the Approved Societies. Some of the members were appointed by the local authority, but only four had to be doctors. That so few doctors served on Committees concerned almost exclusively with medical matters was a source of resentment to the British Medical Association. The Insurance Committees made arrangements for medical treatment and the supply of drugs, maintained lists of participating druggists and panel practitioners, together with lists of all insured workers, supervised the payment of benefits, investigated complaints, and reported on health conditions.[20]

Free drugs were as much a statutory benefit for the insured as the services of a general practitioner. The doctor was privileged to prescribe any medicines deemed necessary, regardless of price, but the rising costs of the pharmaceutical benefits caused the government to scrutinize prescriptions carefully. Preparations were classified, and those listed as non-drugs were not to be prescribed. Appliances such as dressings, splints, and ice bags were prescriptible, but not artificial limbs, trusses, dentures, spectacles, and crutches. If some doubt arose about the classification of a drug or appliance, the matter was referred to a local panel committee and could be appealed to a body of referees selected by the Minister of Health. Excessive prescription was subject to disciplinary action, but few such cases arose. Each prescription was priced by officials appointed by the Insurance Committees, and the druggist was paid the wholesale price plus a percentage for overhead expenses and profits.[21]

Additional benefits were available on a somewhat irregular basis, depending upon the financial status of the Approved Society. The fact that some Societies were unable to grant extra benefits caused resentment among their members and was a major criticism leveled against the whole idea of private associations administering sickness insurance. Every five years the assets of each society were carefully appraised, and if, after allowing for an adequate reserve, there was sufficient surplus, then additional benefits could be provided. In 1938 over 80 per cent of the insured were entitled to some such additional benefits, but in such categories as convalescent homes, medical and surgical appliances, hospitalization, and nursing these extra benefits were negligible. Only in the dental and optical fields were the additional benefits of any substance. Perhaps 50 per cent of the insured workers were eligible for eye treatment and spectacles—the whole or a part of the cost being met by some of the Approved Societies.[22]

The results from the dental program were less encouraging. Only a small fraction of those eligible for dental benefits ever applied for treatment. They were privileged to visit any dentist willing to render treatment under the conditions and fees prescribed centrally by the scheme. Like most doctors, the majority of dentists were willing to accept insured patients while continuing their private practice. One-half or more of the cost of treatment normally had to be borne by the insured workers, and that may have been a deterring factor. In an expensive operation, the dentist might be denied extra payment by the Society; and in any event, the dental benefit was often hedged by the requirement that the insured individual first make application for it and then undergo an examination by a Regional Dental Officer.[23]

In all respects the dental picture was gloomy. Extractions were the rule and conservation the exception. The dental benefits when available were normally used to help meet the cost of wholesale extraction of teeth and the purchase of dentures. A letter to the editor of *The Spectator* in 1942 declared, "Many things in our land which cry out for improvement are being lost sight of, and one of the most important of these is the people's teeth, which none of our ardent reformers seem to think about at all. . . . In this village, which, I have no doubt, is like many others in this respect, the young people start losing their teeth before they are twenty, and it is an exceptional thing to find anyone of forty without false teeth."[24] The accuracy of this statement was borne out in the same year by a dental survey conducted in three Royal ordnance factories in England and Wales. Only 1 per cent of the workers were found, in respect to their natural teeth, to be dentally fit. Although the average age of the employees was less than forty-five years, 34 per cent already had both upper and lower dentures, but some of these fitted imperfectly, and over three-fourths of all employees needed new dentures or remakes or other dental work.[25]

The dental treatment offered to expectant and nursing mothers, and children under five, in the local clinics was no more adequate than that supplied by the school dental service. Too few dentists and the lack of funds enfeebled these services to the extent that only a small proportion of women and children received dental treatment, and when they did it consisted usually of extractions. Statistics showed that for every 100 mothers treated in the local clinics during 1945, 36 teeth were filled and 316 were extracted, and with children the ratio for those treated was something like two extractions for every conservation.[26]

Many reasons were offered to explain these conditions. Most important was a complete lack of knowledge among the people concerning the vital importance of dental health, although, as compared with the preceding decade or so, there was some slight evidence of an improvement in the care of teeth, particularly among children. No serious attempt was made to show the public the relationship between diseased teeth and such ailments as dyspepsia, general malaise, and rheumatism. The dental profession had only shortly before established standards that could command popular respect. Prior to 1921 there was no register of qualified dentists, but thereafter no dentist was admitted to the register without taking a prescribed course of study and passing certain rigid examinations. Those, however, who had been practicing prior to 1921 were admitted to the register, and some of them were poorly qualified.

The picture was further darkened by a tragic shortage of dentists. Few could be found in the rural areas, and they were often not competent to do first-class conservative work. The time and expense involved in going to a city to have such work done would normally preclude the preservation of teeth for low-income groups, even if they realized the importance of dental health. The dental schools simply failed to attract enough students. If the dental profession was unattractive, low incomes may have been a decisive factor. The Spens Report on the Remuneration of General Dental Practitioners disclosed that city dentists in the highest earning age group of all, thirty-five to fifty-four, were poorly compensated. Twenty-five per cent had annual net incomes under £450 ($1,260), and 50 per cent received less than £700 ($1,960). Only 10 per cent were in the £1,600 ($4,480)-and-above bracket.[27]

Certainly the most deplorable aspect of the Health Insurance was its failure to make provision for hospital and specialist care and its consequent contribution to a deterioration that had been going on for

years. The growing complexity of medicine, with its emphasis on
teamwork among general practitioners, hospitals, and consultants,
was completely at variance with the whole conception of the Health
Insurance scheme. Denied free access for his insured patients to
hospital facilities, the practitioner labored under a serious handicap.
And the specialists were too few and badly distributed. But the
hospitals were themselves largely unco-ordinated and were plagued
with obsolescence and financial difficulties. There were several types
of hospitals, including voluntary, municipal, public assistance, cottage,
and specialized, and the quality of service which they offered ranged
from the inexcusably bad to the exemplary. Many were deficient in
plant facilities, equipment, and personnel, but some compared favorably with the best to be found in the medical world. The over-all
picture was depressing, and the need for a new approach had become
urgent.

The voluntary hospitals were non-profit, charitable institutions
primarily designed to serve the sick poor. The majority of them were
founded in the eighteenth and nineteenth centuries, but a few like
St. Thomas's and St. Bartholomew's could trace their origin back to
monasteries or religious foundations of a much earlier period. They
were endowed by local citizens and depended heavily upon gifts,
charity appeals, and legacies, but patients were expected to pay
according to their means. Almoners, whose primary function should
have been to render social assistance to the patients, were often used
as assessment officers to help recover the cost of maintenance. These
hospitals varied greatly. Some, large and powerful, were served by a
staff of eminent specialists, while the majority had less than 100 beds
and were attended mostly by general practitioners. A few were highly
specialized, concentrating on specific types of diseases, while others
were little better than local nursing homes. The majority of them
were general, all-purpose institutions. Each hospital functioned as
a separate unit, having its own constitution and governing body,
which entrusted management to the House Governor in conjunction
with the House Committee. The medical care of the patients was the
responsibility of the surgeons and physicians who composed the medical staff and served in an advisory capacity to the trustees.[28]

The perennial problem facing these hospitals was financial. The
receipts from donations, legacies and voluntary subscriptions did not
keep pace with the mounting costs. Between 1913 and 1920 the
contribution from charity increased 67 per cent, but hospital expenditures rose 138 per cent and the deficit of all voluntary hospitals in
Great Britain then stood at £1,000,000 ($2,800,000). The Cave
Committee, investigating the plight of voluntary hospitals, reported

in 1921 that only state assistance could save the voluntary system and recommended a temporary Exchequer grant of an amount equivalent to the hospital deficit. Parliament came through with only one-half the sum requested. In 1925, the Voluntary Hospitals' Commission stressed the urgent need for government assistance. Parliament voted no money, but empowered the local authorities to make direct grants to voluntary hospitals, and in some cases this was done.[29]

What staved off disaster, however, was the fortuitous rise of hospital contributory schemes in the late 1920's. Multiplying rapidly and taking various forms, they were able by 1948 to recruit around seven million members, including dependents. They were managed by voluntary, non-profit associations. Some of these were sponsored by individual hospitals and served only those institutions, while others operated on a much broader basis. The members contributed weekly between two and four cents, and collection was often facilitated by the assistance of the employer through a payroll deduction plan. Hospital treatment was the chief benefit provided, but in some cases ambulance and nursing service were included. By the early 1940's, the contributory schemes were supplying about 50 per cent of the total receipts of the voluntary hospitals,[30] but they did not by any means solve the fiscal problem.

Voluntary hospitals were served gratuitously by specialists and consultants who looked to private patients for their incomes. Attached to the staff of a large city hospital, the specialist was in a position to build up a reputation, establish contacts, and otherwise lay the foundation for a lucrative private practice. The teaching hospitals, in particular, with their emphasis on experimental medicine and surgery, furnished the best opportunity to a rising specialist. His early years were difficult ones, but the financial rewards were substantial when he became successfully established. It was the policy for the specialists to perform many operations and administer to numerous outpatients without charge, but to seek reimbursement through large fees from well-to-do patients. The system tended to restrict the surgeons and consultants to large hospitals and urban communities that had a fair share of affluent patients. London never lacked specialists, but in the outlying areas and away from the great metropolitan centers they rarely took up residence and were seldom available.[31] In the hospital surveys of 1945 the shortage or non-availability of specialists was a fact mentioned again and again. To quote from the report on the North-Eastern Area: "The dearth of consultants is particularly noticeable in gynecology and obstetrics, pediatrics, dermatology, nervous diseases and psychiatry, while in medicine, if we exclude those who live in Newcastle, there are only two physicians whose practice is purely consultative in the whole region—one in Sunderland and one in Middlesborough. More consultants in every branch are required."[32]

But new forces were at work undermining the old system. The growing burden of taxation, the rising cost of medicine, and the expense of private education for their children had the effect of reducing the number of middle-class patients that could afford heavy medical fees. The need for more consultants as well as a better distribution of their services rendered imperative a new method of remuneration. Charity had to be replaced by payment for all work done. Already municipal hospitals were engaging the services of specialists on a part-time or whole-time sessional salary basis, a method which seemed to offer the only practical solution to the problem.

The voluntary hospitals were primarily interested in short-stay medical cases, acute illness, and surgery, but not in the chronic sick. There was also a lively interest in the outpatient service, and it was in the voluntary hospitals rather than in the municipal hospitals that most of the outpatients were treated. Only the larger voluntary hospitals were able to accommodate many of these patients, and their facilities were not sufficient to meet the growing demand. Overcrowded outpatient departments and overworked specialists had become the fixed pattern for years prior to 1948. Long hours of waiting discouraged many patients from using the service, and there were those too proud to claim charity and too poor to pay the fees.[33]

With the growth of specialization and the increased emphasis on experimental medicine, the consultants and specialists were becoming a distinct group, separated by a widening gulf from the general practitioner who more and more was excluded from the teaching and other larger hospitals. Elaborate methods of treatment required skills which the ordinary doctor did not possess. Only in the smaller voluntary and municipal hospitals, where specialists had not yet made an effective penetration, were the general practitioners still able to get their cases readily admitted, but here the standards were usually poor. The exclusion of the general practitioner from many of the lesser hospitals was only a matter of time, and this trend, which had begun in the closing years of the nineteenth century, was well advanced before the days of the National Health Service.[34]

The largest proportion of beds were to be found in the municipal and public assistance hospitals whose origin stemmed from the workhouses and Poor Law institutions. Intended primarily at first as penitentiaries for the improvident poor, the workhouses slowly changed into almshouses for the aged, impotent, and sick poor. The special sick ward developed into the Poor Law infirmary intended principally for the chronic sick and senile cases. The accommodations were dreary and unattractive, and the quality of service was flagrantly substandard. But a new concept of the institutional treatment of the aged sick began to emerge. In 1929, Parliament proceeded to abolish the Boards of Guardians and to transfer their authority to the county and county-borough councils. The local authorities were granted the power to provide general hospitals by utilizing the Poor Law infirmaries and by erecting new buildings. Municipal hospitals began to come into being, with the Poor Law stigma erased and with skilled staffs that compared well with those of the better voluntary hospitals. Much was accomplished, especially by the wealthier and more progressive counties, but the process was far from complete by 1948, a year which saw many Poor Law or public assistance hospitals still in existence. The picture was further complicated by the specialized local hospitals and sanatoria for infectious diseases and tuberculosis and the institutions for the insane and those mentally defective.[35]

The county and county-borough councils, as the elected representative bodies, exercised ultimate control in the management of the local authority hospitals, but administrative jurisdiction was delegated to the Medical Officer of Health. Responsible to him was the Medical Superintendent who was placed in charge of the actual operation of a particular municipal hospital. The service was financed by local taxes, with some assistance from the central government, and, with the exception of patients with infectious diseases, by those who had the means to pay. Here, too, the contributory schemes eased the financial plight of many persons.

There was much unfriendly rivalry between the municipal and voluntary hospitals. In the absence of any over-all planning, no effort was made to integrate the facilities and develop them in a manner best calculated to serve the needs of the people. Some of the municipal hospitals aspired to specialize in acute cases and resented having to accept chronic cases transferred from voluntary hospitals. Some of the hospitals were overdeveloped in certain specialties and woefully deficient in others. In the field of pathology, many general practitioners and smaller hospitals were obliged to send specimens by post to some distant laboratory. The lesser hospitals often possessed neither the equipment nor personnel to render such a vital service. Local authority hospitals would normally serve only their own residents and would refuse admission to patients who lived nearby but just over the county line, even when there were empty beds. Such patients might have to tolerate many miles of travel and endless delay in gaining admission to a similar hospital with a long waiting list. Even more chaotic was the ambulance service. The delay and confusion was attributable to the fact that so many agencies—individual hospitals, local authorities, the police, the Red Cross Society, the St. John Ambulance Brigade, private persons, and factories—operated ambulances.[36] The evidence from the Hospital Surveys of 1945 emphasized the compelling need to co-ordinate the hospital services within much larger geographic areas.

The most glaring deficiency in the hospital service was the shortage of beds. Convalescent accommodations were limited to a few homes here and there, and some of these did not belong to the hospitals but were made accessible through the co-operation of some welfare society. The shortage of maternity accommodations was a cause of growing complaint among women, who increasingly preferred hospital to domiciliary confinement. There was a dearth of private beds for those who were able to pay the full cost of hospital treatment. Insufficient accommodations existed for cancer patients. In the majority of hospitals, but particularly the larger ones, waiting lists were discouragingly long. Emergency cases were readily admitted, but for many disabilities, some distressingly painful, there were months of delay. General practitioners complained frequently about the long intervals between diagnosis and hospital treatment.[37]

For years there had been a serious shortage of trained nurses and midwives. An understaffed nursing force meant fewer hospital beds. Although the supply of nurses was expanding, it did not keep pace with demand. The loss of student nurses was high.[38] The long hours, hard work, and comparatively unattractive pay doubtlessly contributed to the large amount of wastage in the nursing profession.

England and Wales were divided into ten areas for the hospital survey of 1941-45, and the hospitals in each area were methodically investigated by a special team of experts. Sponsored by the Ministry of Health and the Nuffield Provincial Hospitals Trust, the study produced a large amount of statistical data and critical analysis of the actual condition of the hospitals. The picture was depressing. A substantial proportion of the buildings were over fifty years old, and many had stood for more than a century. Some could be modernized, but quite a few were beyond all hope and should have been demolished. Only the acute shortage of accommodations stood in the way of such action. The London Area Survey found that the "general conclusion . . . can only be that either in quantity or quality deficiencies in all types of accommodation were widespread in 1938."[39] It was the opinion of the Survey of South Wales that "roughly one-half of the hospital accommodations, expressed in terms of hospital

beds, is structurally ill-adapted for the purpose for which it is used."[40]
Said the report on the Sheffield and East Midlands area: "We have
seen far too many examples of dark, overcrowded, ill-equipped infirmary blocks in which the chronic sick drag out the last days of their
existence with few of the amenities of civilized life."[41]

The outbreak of World War II found the hospitals financially
unable to cope with the new conditions or to render the type of
service that became so urgent. The central government met the crisis
by establishing a wartime Emergency Hospital Scheme with large
financial grants from the Exchequer. In a sense the hospitals were
temporarily nationalized. New buildings were erected and old ones
renovated. Specialized treatment centers were established for rehabilitation, treatment of neurosis, chest disorders, and fractures, brain
surgery, and other comparable purposes. The X-ray, surgical, and
other medical facilities were improved; convalescent homes were
provided; and at least 50,000 beds were added to the hospital service.
The ambulance system was improved, and in general a measure of
co-ordination among the hospitals was achieved. The emergency
scheme expired at the end of the war but succeeded in raising the
level of hospital standards and, even more important, demonstrated
what the central government could accomplish through planning and
financial assistance.[42]

There were, indeed, many problems which Great Britain faced
in the 1940's, but none was more distressing than the plight of the
aged chronic sick. Despite the increasing proportion of elderly persons in the population, there seemed to be little social awareness of
the treatment that the aged sick received in the public assistance
hospitals. Neither the voluntary nor municipal hospitals were interested in chronic illness, and so the decrepit, the incapacitated, and
the chronic sick were usually herded into the former Poor Law hospitals. Most of the buildings were orginially workhouses for the pau-
pers, and although improvements had been made, many remained
"ill-designed, deficient in sanitation, often isolated, bare, bleak and
soulless." The standard of medical treatment was usually poor.
These hospitals were often without a resident medical staff or the
services of specialists. The diagnosis of chronic cases tended to be
cursory, and where patients were curable or disabilities could be
ameliorated, remedial measures were usually unavailable or ineffec-
tually administered.[43]

Caring for the chronic ill was only one of many duties within
the purview of the local authorities. In general, their functions were
in the field of preventive medicine. Some were mandatory, others
were optional, but it was the growing interest in public health that

inspired the local authorities to develop many of the new services, the most important of which was maternal and child welfare. The high death rate of infants at the turn of the century fostered a real concern with the problem. The doctor's fee discouraged mothers from seeking medical advice or treatment for minor disorders, and the limited offerings of the National Health Insurance prevented the development of a true family doctor service. Moreover, many practitioners seemed slow to appreciate the importance of public health education or preventive work in the sphere of medicine. The need for free clinics became apparent first to voluntary hospitals and welfare organizations and then to local authorities, who quickly established prenatal and postnatal clinics and child welfare centers. Here free advice and treatment for minor ailments were available to the young child and mother. Throughout England and Wales these tax-supported clinics enjoyed great popularity, but doctors resented them as an encroachment upon their professional domain. As a consequence, there was little co-operation between these clinics and the general practitioner.[44]

Other related activities further improved maternity conditions and child welfare. A domiciliary midwifery service served the expectant mother who chose to have her baby at home. Several thousand district nurses and health visitors were employed by the local governments to visit the sick and advise mothers and others on health matters. Local authorities had the power to make home nursing available for expectant or nursing mothers and small children who needed such care, but achievement in this field was not very significant. Home nursing remained much more the concern of voluntary organizations, as did the domestic help service. Local authorities made some provision for domestic help as a part of the child welfare and maternity program and during the war could even extend it to the sick and infirm, but the inception of the National Health Service found only a small nucleus of such employees on the payrolls of local governments.[45]

Provision was made for the welfare of school children, but the services set up were not fully implemented. Medical inspection was required in both elementary and secondary schools. In the former there was also medical treatment varying in scope—in some localities dealing only with teeth, ears, throat, eyes, nose, and minor ailments, but in others extending to rheumatic and orthopedic cases. Dental inspection and treatment were furnished in varying degrees, but more comprehensive was the ophthalmic service, which included treatment by specialists. In spite of shortcomings, the local educational authorities supervised what probably was the best integrated program in preventive and therapeutic medicine that existed prior to the National Health Service.

The local authorities had other major functions, including the treatment and care of persons afflicted with mental disorders. They were also entrusted with the provision of sanatoria for the treatment of tuberculosis, the operation of infectious disease hospitals, the provision of free diagnosis and treatment at clinics for venereal diseases, and the maintenance of diagnostic centers and treatment facilities for cancer. The last of these was not provided for by law before 1939, and because of the war little had been done about it when the new Health Service took shape.[46]

Impressive as were these services, they looked better on paper than in actual operation. The multiplicity of government units and the division of authority were major sources of weakness. Within the counties were political subdivisions known as districts which were responsible for the control of infectious diseases, and sometimes public health nursing and maternity and child welfare. In the administration of these functions there were no less than 400 administrative units, some of which were too small in size and limited in resources to accomplish much. And between these units there was little cohesion. Within a single area, for instance, the home nurse might be employed by the voluntary nursing association, the health visitor by the district, and the midwife by the county. There might also be no co-ordination between the midwifery and the domestic help services. The divided control over the ambulance service merely added to the confusion. It was further compounded by the unco-ordinated hospital service, the friction between the general practitioner and the clinics, and the crippling limitations imposed by the National Health Insurance scheme itself.

In evaluating the progress made by British medicine there are two sides to the picture: what had been and what might have been accomplished. Both are nebulous and neither can be reduced to a precise formula. But the vital statistics are incontrovertible. The death rate per year per 1,000 live births in 1850 stood at 153; in 1948, at 34. Between those years the mortality rates for the same number of persons declined from 22.4 to 11, and life expectancy at birth increased from 42 to over 65 years. The sweep of that century also saw the 65-and-over age group treble in size in proportion to the total population. And finally the mortality rate for many dread diseases fell sharply or almost reached the vanishing point.[47]

The fact that a few other nations had done as well in no way detracted from the British record. The march of medical progress, together with improved living standards, had made its contribution.

No less important was the long list of health enactments. Divergent
and fragmentary though they often were, their total effect on the
physical well-being of the people was of the greatest importance. But
there is no way of knowing what results could have been achieved
by a more co-ordinated attack upon the problem of disease and ill
health.

The picture was thus one of many facets, complicated, confused,
and sometimes dark, but certainly not without its brighter aspects.
Critics there were who could see only omissions and limitations and
who thundered against all the ills in the socio-medical pattern. The
cost of illness was a popular theme to exploit, and much was made
of it. In 1937 some 200 experts and authorities assisted the Political
and Economic Service—an independent non-political group—in preparing a report on the British health services. The conclusions were
startling. Exclusive of illness lasting less than four days, over thirty
million working weeks were annually lost in Great Britain from sickness. The economic cost to the nation traceable to illness represented
a figure which, to many Englishmen, was appallingly and needlessly
high. It was believed that a substantial amount of disease and mortality was preventable and that the government should seriously address itself to the problem.[48]

Editorially *The Lancet* in 1942 gave voice to the growing spirit
of dissatisfaction over current conditions:

Even before the war, there were voices crying in the wilderness that all
was not well with the medical services. The burden of their cries was that
preventable diseases were not being prevented; that the chances of avoiding
death in infancy, in childbirth from tuberculosis, and from rheumantic
carditis were much greater among the rich than among the poor; that for
most of the population such financial burdens were added to the burdens
of ill health as to discourage early treatment; that the standards of treatment available in different places and institutions, and among different
social classes, varied enormously; and that the annual income of those who
cared for the sick ranged from £40 [$112] plus keep and laundry paid to
the probationer nurse to the £40,000 [$112,000] earned by the successful
surgeon.[49]

CHAPTER II

The Emergence of a New
Health Policy

THE CREATION of the National Health Service was viewed by some as a revolutionary policy, hasty and ill-advised, which sought to accomplish at one stroke what should have been realized gradually. These critics held that the Service was the product of insufficient planning and deliberation and that Great Britain was not ready for it. While it is true that England's postwar economy labored under serious economic handicaps and was perhaps not ideally suited for the launching of such a bold program, the evidence would indicate that the scheme, the result of more than two decades of planning and thinking, was evolutionary rather than revolutionary. Psychologically and politically the British people could not have been more receptive to the new program than they were in 1948. Popular demand was overwhelming, and support came from all political parties. British thought had very definitely crystallized on the subject.

What were the factors that produced the National Health Service and fostered so much enthusiasm for it? The ordeal of the war, with its leveling effect and somber overtones, certainly helped to create the proper climate for parliamentary action. The drab and grim pattern of life was made more bearable by the expectation of a brighter and more secure future for all. In subways and other bomb shelters, and wherever the war-weary people gathered, there was much talk about the Beveridge Report and other manifestations of the new spirit that would govern the postwar era. The fruits of victory would include real security against disability, unemployment, sickness, and old age. Protection against these hazards of life was registered as a solemn pledge by a three-party coalition government headed by Sir Winston Churchill who, although a Conservative, was no less committed to such a program than were the socialist labor leaders. Speaking as Prime Minister in the spring of 1944, he affirmed that it was the policy of the government to establish a National Health Service which would make accessible to all, irrespective of social class or means, adequate and modern medical care.[1]

While serving as a powerful catalyst, the war did not spawn the basic ideas which underlay the National Health Service or create the overwhelming need for action by the government. Two mighty forces had long been at work in England. One was the discontent with inadequate medical services and facilities and the increasing tendency of the community to assume responsibility for providing them itself. The other, not so apparent at first, was the assumption by the central government of an increasingly important role in the administration and supervision of health matters. The arrangement which often granted the smallest units of government jurisdiction over some of the health services was not satisfactory.[2] The growing complexity of society and the changing pattern of medicine made central administration inevitable. The National Health Insurance laid the basis for the final emergence of the National Health Service.

The cost of specialist and hospital care had reached the point at which it was beyond the means of a large proportion of the population. Charity, the contributory schemes, Health Insurance, and self-help had all failed to meet the need. The progress of medicine was "not an arithmetical but a geometrical progression." Hospitals that once required a few general practitioners and a small nursing and administrative staff now demanded the services of a small army of nurses and auxiliaries in addition to laboratory technicians, dietitians, occupational therapists, radiographers, physiotherapists, orthopedists, clinical photographers, psychiatric social workers, hospital physicists, and many other specialists.

Medical discoveries followed one another in rapid succession, and each tended to find a broader and more expensive application. For instance, X-rays, which originally served as a means of detecting foreign bodies and fractures, became useful in the detection and treatment of a long list of diseases. In a well-known provincial hospital there were fewer than 600 X-ray examinations in 1918, but by the end of the 1940's nearly 20,000 were annually required, and each one recorded usually involved others for the same patient. During the twenty-year period ending in 1947, the same hospital saw the annual number of pathological examinations multiply 33 times and blood counts 50 times. Nor do these figures take into consideration the greater complexity of these examinations. Hospital costs mounted steadily. The cost of each X-ray examination in 1947 was three times higher than in 1930; and in the same provincial hospital the weekly cost per inpatient increased from £1 12s ($4.48) in 1906 to £8 4s ($22.96) in 1947. In 1900, the voluntary hospitals in

England and Wales spent £500,000 ($1,400,000); in 1947 the total was 640 times greater.[3]   Whereas the growth of a business concern usually leads to a greater earning capacity, the expansion of the hospital service could mean only a growth in spending capacity.

During the six-year period between the Beveridge Report and the commencement of the National Health Service, medical discoveries seemed to reach flood tide.   This era saw the improvement or introduction of many lifesaving antibiotics, the treatment of cerebral and cardiac thrombosis with anti-coagulants, the discovery of cortisone, and the medical application of nuclear physics.   Thanks to antibiotics, the general practitioner was now able to cure many diseases that formerly required hospitalization, but drugs were expensive and his dependence upon specialists, laboratory technicians, and other trained experts had become even greater.   Although life was more secure and even greater security was in prospect, cost was the great barrier.   It was this factor more than any other which rendered inevitable the creation of a state medical service.   If the government could find in unemployment, education, and old age a valid reason for action, why should it not also concern itself with health, which was certainly no less important?   This was the very essence of democracy—so British leadership felt.   And many of England's most eminent doctors believed the government had little choice in the matter.   Sir Lionel Whitby in his presidential address to the British Medical Association, June, 1948, put it in this fashion:

> With an illness no more serious than a pyrexia of unknown origin which, in due course, might cure itself, the cost of establishing the diagnosis, of determining whether the cause is amenable to modern chemotherapeutic methods of treatment, or of establishing that the fever is not due to something which is a public menace may amount to as much as £50 [$140].   A single patient with pulmonary tuberculosis for whom a thoracoplasty operation is required may call for the expenditure of more than £1000 [$2,800] from the time of admission to hospital to the time of discharge some months later.   And all will be familiar with the primary cost of penicillin or streptomycin, amounting at the outset to hundreds of pounds for a single case.   Yet, in the interest of humanity, such treatment cannot be withheld on economic grounds.   It would be a travesty of justice were such treatment to be available to only the few rich people whom successive Chancellors of the Exchequer have permitted to survive in Great Britain.[4]

Between the two wars a series of important reports on the coordination and improvement of the medical facilities was prepared by a number of expert commissions.   In these surveys can be found most of the basic ideas that were to shape the framework of the

National Health Service. Some of the bodies were official and others were voluntary, but, significantly, the medical profession played the most enlightened role of all in many of its proposals. The British Medical Association reports of 1938 and 1942 were classic examples of impartiality, constituting the high-water mark of progressive thought for that organization.

Only a few of the most pertinent reports need be examined in order to appreciate the methodical and careful spade work which preceded the creation of the National Health Service. Shortly after the establishment of the Ministry of Health in 1919, a commission was appointed under the chairmanship of Lord Dawson for the purpose of proposing what might be done to improve medical facilities. The commission found that, because of rising costs, many people were unable to afford the full range of treatment. While recognizing the need to make medical services available to all classes, the Dawson Commission was unprepared to recommend the abolition of fees, since this would have imposed too great a burden on public funds at that time. Though some of its members favored such a course, the majority believed that patients should make a contribution toward the cost of treatment and suggested insurance as a sound approach.

The Dawson Commission recommended that health centers should be established on a primary and secondary level. The former should be district hospitals staffed with general practitioners and devoted to the ordinary run of medical cases. The primary health center would include operating and radiography rooms and laboratory facilities for simple investigations and would offer community services such as child welfare and prenatal care programs and treatment for school children. Primary health centers would also offer ambulance service, a dental clinic, and a home nursing service. The secondary center or general hospital should be fully equipped and staffed by specialists to whom the more complicated cases would be referred. The specialists would make periodic visits to the primary centers and even make home visits. At none of the health centers was a whole-time salaried service envisaged for either the consultants or general practitioners, but the full co-ordination of preventive and curative medicine would be sought nevertheless. Voluntary hospitals would be sustained through grants-in-aid.[5]

In 1926, the Royal Commission on the National Health Insurance reported on the need for more effective co-ordination of the health services. The exclusion of hospital and specialist treatment from the Insurance, the non-availability of laboratory services to panel doctors, the great variation in "additional benefits" among the Approved Societies, and the denial of protection to dependents of the insured were listed among the shortcomings of the Health Insurance, which otherwise had performed a very useful service. The Royal Commission recognized that any widening of the program would have to depend upon the productive capacity of the nation to sustain the added cost. When public funds were available, then children and wives of the insured should be given protection. The Commission deplored the widespread employment of the means test, which was even used in the contributory health insurance schemes. Most significant was the judgment of the Commission that the insurance principle was not a sound method for financing medical services, and that the broader the services provided, the more difficult it would be to retain that basis. It was felt that the ultimate solution would be to finance medical benefits in the same manner as all public health activities—from public funds.[6]

The chaotic state of the hospital service was known to many before Lord Sankey's Voluntary Hospitals' Commission published its findings in 1937, but the report did much to focus public attention upon the need for co-operation between the many competing units. It was proposed that the voluntary hospitals be organized on a regional basis under the supervision of a representative voluntary council and that a central voluntary council be set up to co-ordinate the work of the regional councils. Although it was suggested that the local authorities be granted representation on the regional councils, the report was little concerned with the more numerous municipal and public assistance hospitals that stood in need of co-ordination as much as the voluntary hospitals.[7]

No group in Great Britain was more critically aware of the deficiencies in the medical service than the British Medical Association, which in two major reports candidly proposed reforms that were to have a decisive influence upon government policy in the 1940's. The first report was published in 1930 and, in revised form, reissued as the Association's statement of policy in 1938. The second report, even more ambitious, was the work of a large commission established by the British Medical Association with the co-operation of the Royal Colleges and other professional bodies. Issued in 1942 as the "Interim Report of the Medical Planning Commission," it was as significant in revealing the status of medical thinking during the war years as the contemporary Beveridge Report was in reflecting public opinion on social security.

In some respects the Interim Report was quite moderate. The Medical Association had no desire to scrap the National Health Insurance, which the Interim Report hailed as an "integral part of the social structure" and "a greater success than was anticipated either by its supporters or by its opponents." The medical profession was pleased that clinical freedom had in no way been jeopardized, that the doctors had retained a large measure of responsibility over purely professional matters, and that the Association had been freely consulted by government officials and administrators on all questions or issues of mutual concern. It was recognized that in any nationwide service, central administration was vital.

Although there was a division of sentiment in the Medical Planning Commission over the method of compensation for general practitioners, some members even advocating a salaried service, the majority of the Commission favored retention of the capitation fee by which payment varied with the number of Insurance patients on the doctor's list. It was recommended, however, that there be in addition a basic salary with some regard to length of service and other qualifications and separate fees for work not covered by the capitation payment. Remuneration would be made directly from public funds. A prescribed maximum remuneration should restrict the number of insured patients that any one doctor could serve. While the Interim Report was not prepared to advocate the immediate abolition of the purchase or sale of doctors' practices, it did contemplate that move as an eventuality. The absence of a retirement system for panel doctors was noted.[8]

No change was favored in the general method of financing the National Health Insurance. Contributions from the employee, the employer, and the government seemed a sound approach, but it was recognized that if wives and children were to be granted protection, some adjustment would have to be made in the established basis of payment. Although not oblivious to the difficulties involved in providing for the fiscal needs of the hospitals, the reports supported the old pattern of charity, fees, and contributory schemes. The last, in particular, seemed to offer the best hope as a source of revenue which, it was believed, could and should be extended. It was suggested, however, that grants-in-aid would have to be made to alleviate the plight of the voluntary hospitals. Patients should pay according to their means—pay-beds for those who could afford private care and wards for all others. It was further agreed that to increase the number and improve the distribution of specialists would necessitate a salary system, in which appointments should preferably be on a part-time basis so as not to interfere with private practice.[9]

The Interim Report of 1942 envisaged a system of medical service that would prevent disease and relieve sickness. It recognized that medical need and not economic status should determine eligibility for medical care and that the quality of treatment should not vary for the rich or poor. That many people had to visit public assistance doctors and otherwise seek treatment on a charity basis was deemed most undesirable, and so it was proposed that Health Insurance coverage be extended to include the dependents of those already insured, and all self-employed persons and others whose income did not exceed the maximum under the Health Insurance regulations. This proposal would have removed 90 per cent of the population from the private practice and almost doubled the number of panel patients. It seemed revolutionary, but experience had taught the medical profession that not more than 10 per cent of the population could actually afford the luxury of private medicine in any case. For the 90 per cent, the National Health Insurance should be broadened to include ophthalmic and dental benefits and access to the services of specialists and whatever radiological and pathological examinations were deemed necessary. Drugs for this group would be free and so would most of the other medical facilities except the hospital service, which, as before, would charge flexible fees based on the economic status of the patient.

The need for a more integrated and efficient general practitioner service led to the proposal that doctors employ a collective mode of practice. By joining with other practitioners at a single center where equipment and ancillary help could be shared, the physician could escape the stultifying influence of isolation and would also have more time to perfect a better brand of medicine. Group practice, as it was called, was promising, but even more so was the health center. It could be sponsored by the local authority, with the building and equipment furnished for the use of general practitioners, health visitors, midwives, district nurses, and others who would combine preventive and curative medicine. At the health center the practitioner would have the advantage of secretarial and other assistance, access to the pathological and X-ray service, and the opportunity to participate in child welfare, prenatal, postnatal, and school medical work. Consultants might even attend at the center, but in any event the close liaison between it and the local hospital would make specialist services accessible.

To the problem of administration, the Interim Report gave the most careful consideration. Diversity and lack of co-ordination, especially on the local level, had been the greatest obstacle to a better medical service. There were too many local units serving the cause of public health. They worked at cross purposes and without any unified design or pattern. The only solution, in the opinion of the Medical Planning Commission, was to create new and much larger areas under regional authorities or regional councils, elected or appointed, and advised by professional experts. Such representative bodies would assume responsibility for the supervision of local health services and could co-operate with their counterparts in other areas. A central authority would be concerned with the administration and co-ordination of medical service on a nationwide basis. This authority could take the form of a government department or a corporate body responsible through a minister to Parliament.

The confusion in the hospital domain was a matter of primary concern to the medical profession, and like other and earlier studies, the two British Medical Association reports recognized regional organization as the only solution. The lack of co-operation among voluntary hospitals and between voluntary and municipal hospitals could be overcome by grouping them without reference necessarily to county boundaries but in such fashion that they would have close affiliation with a large voluntary or teaching hospital. Those in the group would be largely complementary, and together they would compose a co-ordinate whole that could be effectively supervised by a representative regional council. Above the regional council, a provincial council could effect an even broader organization. While recognizing that co-operation was more vital than competition, the reports expressed the conviction that voluntary hospitals were distinctive and should retain their identity and the hope that a co-ordinated system would evolve without the necessity of nationalization.[10]

The same year that produced the highly important report of the Medical Planning Commission saw another study by some 200 younger doctors (in the forty-five-years-and-under age group) and others associated with the health services. Published in *The Lancet* as "The Medical Planning Research Interim General Report," this study in many respects paralleled the other, but there were differences, especially in emphasis. Regional organization of the hospitals was accepted as a necessity. The purchase of a practice was roundly denounced as imposing too heavy a burden on the young doctor. The needs for adequate remuneration, ample off-duty hours, refresher courses, and collaboration with other doctors were considered of paramount importance. The advocacy of the capitation fee, with a basic salary and fees for special work, showed the measure of unanimity in the medical profession over this mode of compensation. Great importance was attached to the idea of health centers where small groups of not more than twelve doctors would labor in well-equipped and -staffed buildings provided by central rather than the local authorities. Vacancies at health centers would be advertised in the medical journals and filled by small committees on which the patients of the retiring doctor would have representation.

The younger doctors believed that the central authority of the National Health Service should be a small, salaried corporate body, half lay and half medical, appointed by the Prime Minister. Administration by a department of state was rejected in favor of the corporate body, since the latter, it was felt, would remove the health service further from "day to day or even year to year inquisitions in Parliament" that tended "to discourage bold planning and initiative." The corporate body would determine the spending of health funds obtained from the Exchequer and insurance payments, and it would also build or acquire clinics, health centers, and hospitals.[11]

The idea of the corporate approach was not new and had been proposed by others, including the Medical Planning Commission, which, however, viewed it as a possible alternative to a department. Those in the medical profession that took so kindly to a corporation were perhaps more idealistic than realistic. Where large appropriations were concerned, Parliament, the watchdog of the taxpayer, would jealously safeguard its right to probe, investigate, and control and was not at all likely to accept the delegation of authority that the corporate idea implied.

Very little found its way into the National Health Service Act of 1946 that had not been recommended or discussed by the earlier reports and studies. Where the medical men left off, the politicians took over, and matters that had been largely academic now became the subject of Parliamentary debates. The doctors were perhaps most directly involved, but there were many other groups no less concerned, and towering above all of them were the labor unions and the political parties. The interests converged on Parliament, and there, under a coalition government and with Great Britain at war, the National Health Service began to take shape.

In June, 1941, it was announced in the House of Commons that a study of the various schemes of social insurance and allied services would be conducted by a committee of twelve members under the chairmanship of Sir William Beveridge. In less than a year and a half the survey was finished. It was a far-reaching attack upon want and poverty, based upon the need to cope with the loss of individual earning power that resulted from illness, disability, unemployment, and old age. A redistribution of income through a more adequate social insurance program was viewed as the most effective approach. Social studies conducted in a number of English cities showed that many persons lacked sufficient income for barest subsistence. There was an urgent need to broaden the existing schemes so as to include persons not protected, to cover risks that were excluded, and to provide greater benefits.

Sickness and disability were viewed as the most dangerous of all the hazards, and to combat these threats to Britain's well-being, the Beveridge Report favored an all-inclusive health and rehabilitation program. The proposed scheme would "ensure that for every citizen there is available whatever medical treatment he requires, in whatever form he requires it, domiciliary or institutional, general, specialist or consultant, and [would] ensure also the provision of dental, ophthalmic and surgical appliances, nursing and midwifery and rehabilitation after accidents." "Positive health," "the prevention of disease," and the "relief of sickness" were the targets. The service would be available to all on the basis of medical need and irrespective of economic status or the payment of insurance contributions. The patient would be entitled to "full preventive and curative treatment of every kind . . . without an economic barrier at any point to delay recourse to it." Thus charity and the means test, so long a part of the social pattern, no longer would be allowed to undermine the human dignity of the sick.

With sharp and daring strokes, the Beveridge Commission painted on a wide canvas the broad outlines of the new health service. Details were necessarily omitted as being beyond the scope of the investigation; and, in the description of the health program, many of the problems implied by the proposed scheme were lightly passed over. Little attention was given to financing the program. The Beveridge estimate of the total cost for the health and rehabilitation services turned out to be an absurdly low figure. Though it depended on Exchequer grants and contributory insurance payments to sustain the program, the report was not, however, averse to small charges to the patient if they did not restrict his use of the service when he was in need of treatment. But nothing should impede the duty of the state to restore a sick person to health or to remove disability.[12]

The Interim Report of the Medical Planning Commission had led the medical profession a considerable distance along the path of reform, but the Beveridge Report, with its all-inclusive provisions, aroused serious apprehensions in the British Medical Association, causing it to pause and reappraise its position. What would a total state medical service do to or for private practice? The Interim Report proposed no change in the system of private fees for the upper economic group, but the Beveridge Report would wipe out that lucrative source of income and leave the doctors without assurance that private practice in any form could survive. These doubts caused the Association to greet the Beveridge Report with a coolness quite at variance with the popular acclaim being accorded to that document.[13]

Early in 1943, the government informed the House of Commons

that it had the Beveridge Report under careful study and was now prepared to announce acceptance of its major proposals, including a comprehensive health service. The implementation of the program would depend upon the state of the national economy. There would be many competing claims upon the national resources in the postwar years—roads, agriculture, housing, education, and colonial development—but within the limits of fiscal strength, the government would seek to establish a medical scheme with a full range of services for every man, woman, and child.[14]

The Ministry of Health quietly initiated a series of conferences with the medical profession, the voluntary hospitals, the local authorities, and other interested parties in order to get their ideas about what the character of the proposed health service should be. There was a wide divergence in views, but the government went forward resolutely, using the Interim Report of the Medical Planning Commission and other documentary material gathered from many sources. The product was the White Paper of February, 1944, which set forth a provisional health plan. The release of the White Paper introduced the second phase, in which Parliament and the nation would have ample opportunity to discuss freely all aspects of the proposed scheme. Then the government would proceed to the third stage, in which the actual bill would be drawn up and submitted to Parliament for discussion, possible modification, and eventual adoption.[15] Between the first and final stages three and one-half years were to elapse.

The White Paper restated the intention of the government to establish a health program with the best medical facilities accessible to everybody without regard to the patient's ability to pay. Such a scheme was pictured simply as a further and natural stage in the steady evolution of the British health services, and the government urged that it be viewed "against the past as well as the future." "Just as people are accustomed to look to public organization for essential facilities like a clean and safe water supply or good highways . . . so they should now be able to look for proper facilities for the care of their personal health to a publicly organized service available to all who want to use it—a service for which all would be paying as taxpayers and ratepayers and contributors to some national scheme of social insurance." It was pointed out that in the past too much depended upon circumstances—financial, social, and geographic—and too many people did without medical care, were inadequately treated, or had to accept Poor Law assistance.

The disorganization of the hospital service, the inadequacy and inaccessibility of specialized medicine and surgery for many patients, and the piecemeal and unco-ordinated health services of the local authorities were identified in the White Paper as serious shortcomings in the existing health program. Such services as were offered by the general practitioner, the specialist, the hospital, the midwife, and the local clinic needed "to be related to one another and treated as many aspects of the care of one person's health."

Two possible approaches were mentioned. One was to ignore the past and the present and from the ground up to build a completely new service; the other was to utilize past experience and existing machinery, absorbing them wherever possible into the framework of the contemplated health service. The British way of life dictated the second choice, and the White Paper recommended that the new be built upon the old and that a careful sort of patchwork service be constructed.

The government was alert to the danger of too much organization and the absolute need to safeguard professional freedom and the doctor-patient relationship. The White Paper as a starting point advanced the postulate that public responsibility and a complete medical service were not incompatible with clinical freedom. The only purpose of organization was to ensure the existence of the service, and beyond that it must not go. There should be no compulsion. Doctors and patients should be free to use the service or not as they chose. But it must be there for all who needed and wished to use it, and it must cover the whole field of medical, dental, and ophthalmic care.[16]

The new service would be centrally and locally administered, with due regard for democratic processes. Central responsibility would rest with the Minister of Health, who would be advised by a group of professional experts known as the Central Health Services Council. He would be accountable to Parliament, while the county and county-borough councils, with responsibility for local administration, would be answerable directly to the local voters. The old framework thus would be largely retained. In order to facilitate a more efficient hospital and specialist service, however, the county and county-boroughs would combine into larger units under joint authorities advised by professional consultative bodies. Otherwise, the local authorities, as before, would administer within the counties and county-boroughs the local clinics and such functions as domiciliary visiting, but with greater regard to an integrated and efficient performance. And, as before, social insurance contributions, local taxes, and central funds would finance the service, but the burden falling upon the Exchequer would now be much heavier.

The proposed joint authority, having jurisdiction over a relatively large area, would be charged with the responsibility of creating a unified and balanced hospital system and an adequately distributed specialist service. The municipal hospitals would be controlled directly by the joint authority, which, through contractual arrangements, would seek to integrate the voluntary hospitals into a completely co-ordinated scheme. Though these hospitals would remain autonomous, both they and the local authority hospitals would receive financial aid from the central government and both would be periodically visited by inspectors from the Ministry of Health. Compensation would be paid for all work done by the specialists, who could serve the hospitals full time or part time.[17]

No need was expressed in the White Paper to modify greatly the character of general medical practice, which would remain a centralized service. Under the National Health Insurance, the terms and conditions of employment were determined by the Ministry of Health in negotiation with the medical profession, and that policy would continue. The employing agent would be called the Central Medical Board, which would enter into contracts with the doctors and endeavor to achieve a more suitable distribution of their services. The Insurance Committees would be abolished, and the Central Medical Board would discharge many of its day-to-day functions through other local committees. Health centers and group practice would be fostered without discouraging individual practice. A limit would be placed upon the number of Health Service patients a practitioner could serve, but this limit would in no way affect or be governed by the size of a doctor's private practice.

The government endeavored to make the White Paper as conciliatory as possible. Physicians attached to health centers would be paid by salary or an equivalent method, but negotiation would determine the method of compensation for other practitioners. They were offered a capitation fee system, a salaried service, or a combination of the two. The government would be guided by two aims: to assure the doctors an adequate income and to create a system of remuneration sufficiently flexible to reward superior qualifications and achievements. A pension system would be an integral part of health center employment, and for other doctors, a contributory superannuation system was contemplated, but the latter would be the subject of negotiation with the medical profession.

The government was particularly concerned about an efficient general-practitioner family service, with adequate emphasis upon preventive medicine. The hope was that the patient would not wait until illness struck, but under the doctor's beneficent care and advice would take the necessary precautions to stay in good health. "The doctor must try," urged the White Paper, "to become the general adviser in all matters concerned with health."[18]

Four weeks after Parliament received the White Paper, the House of Commons held a two-day debate and then approved the intentions of the government as set forth in that document. In opening the discussion, Henry Willink, Minister of Health, warned that the new health service would have to be "well fashioned and well founded," since it would be one of the main pillars of the postwar social structure. In conception and scope it would dwarf all other public health achievements, but necessity required that it be bold, for the "health of every citizen, young and old, is at the root of national vigour and national enterprise." The object of the proposed scheme, he said, would be "to fit the nation for its great responsibilities, to free its members, so far as it is humanly possible to free them, from the anxieties, the burdens and the pains of ill-health." Among the anxieties Willink mentioned was the worry of paying medical bills and getting good medical advice. There would "be no charge to those who use the service when they use it or because they use it," but he questioned the appropriateness of the word "free," since everyone would have to pay for the service through taxes and social insurance. Four fundamental principles, he emphasized, underlay the proposed plan. It would be comprehensive, with the whole range of medical care available to all. There would be complete freedom for doctors to enter and patients to use the service. The principle of democratic responsibility would be safeguarded, with Parliament and the local government answerable to the voters for the efficient operation of the program. Finally, expert and professional guidance would be employed to insure the best performance by the new service.[19] It should be noted that this ardent, even eloquent, defense of the White Paper was made by a Conservative, speaking as a member of Churchill's coalition government.

In appraising the White Paper, several factors should be kept in mind. The government may have been overly sanguine about future medical prospects and imbued with too much crusading zeal, but the primary purpose behind the document was to provoke discussion and fire the popular imagination. In many respects, the proposed plan was very realistic, being careful not to ignore local interests or prerogatives and seeking to utilize existing procedures and machinery. The White Paper reflected much of the medical thought that had found expression in the reports of the British Medical Association. The conciliatory and flexible approach to some of the more controversial issues seemed to indicate a real disposition on the part of the government to win the co-operation of the medical profession as well as all other interested parties. The success of the document as a blueprint for the National Health Service can be measured by the relatively few major changes that were deemed necessary in the plan it set forth. Under the new law, the voluntary hospitals were nationalized, the joint authority boards were not established, the local authorities lost all jurisdiction over the hospital and specialist service, and the sale of practices was abolished for all National Health Service doctors. Aside from these, only minor modifications were made.

There was little enthusiasm for the White Paper in medical circles. To test the reaction to the document, the British Medical Association sent a questionnaire to its members, only one-half of whom took the trouble to reply. With regard to compensation, the feeling was that a salaried service, whether in health centers or individual practice, should be resisted. The majority of those who replied favored capitation fees as the only method of remuneration for individual practices; for health centers, the vote was evenly divided between straight capitation fees on the one hand and a small basic salary plus capitation fees on the other.[20] Despite the disclaimer in the White Paper and subsequent disavowals by government officials, the fear of a salaried service for all practitioners was to haunt the medical profession for years.

On some vital aspects there was an embarrassing absence of unanimity in the medical profession. A majority of general practitioners, for example, supported as reasonable the power of the Central Medical Board to regulate the flow of doctors into over-doctored areas, but the *British Medical Journal* could only see in this "more than a hint . . . of authoritarianism." Very significant was the strong support of individual doctors (60 per cent) for a universal health service. This was contrary to the position of the Representative Meeting of the British Medical Association, which in September, 1943, and December, 1944, ratified by a substantial margin the recommendation for a coverage of 90 per cent that had been made by the Medical Planning Commission. The *British Medical Journal* had some misgivings about the abolition of the sale of good will in the health centers. The general practitioners were evenly divided on this issue, but they favored by a good margin the termination of the sale of good will for all individual practices.[21]

In principle, at least, there was complete harmony between the government and the medical profession on the need for health centers. The Interim Report of the Medical Planning Commission and the White Paper had strongly advocated them, and sentiment among the doctors was overwhelmingly favorable. Yet the *British Medical Journal,* sensing undue haste in the policy of the government, favored a go-slow, experimental approach toward health centers. There apparently were no reservations about the proposal that hospital and consultant service should be free to every person in the general wards. The doctors advocated this point by an almost three-to-one vote.[22]

So emphatically did the doctors react against the White Paper as a whole or to certain of the proposals in it that stormy weather seemed to lie ahead in the efforts to establish a National Health Service. On the issue of the medical service being controlled by local authorities, there was an 80 per cent negative vote among doctors. Such decisive opposition subsequently caused the government to alter its position and to favor removing all hospitals from local control and placing them under regional hospital boards. The Medical Planning Commission and other groups had recognized the imperative need for effective central administration, and the White Paper had endeavored through the Ministry of Health and the Central Health Services Council to accomplish that objective, but, strangely enough, only one-third of the doctors who voted found the proposed central administrative structure satisfactory. Most surprising of all was the large proportion of general practitioners (62 per cent) whose general impression of the White Paper was unfavorable. A 60 per cent majority even declared that they would not regard medicine as an attractive career for their children if the National Health Service, as contemplated by the White Paper, were established. An even larger proportion of general practitioners felt that under such a scheme private practice could not possibly survive.

The consultants and specialists exhibited a much less conservative attitude on many of the issues than did the general practitioners. This may have been due to the fact that, working within the framework of a hospital, they were accustomed to committee assignments, controls, and organization. While some were paid for their work, many served in the voluntary hospitals gratuitously, but under the proposed plan all would receive full compensation for their services. Whatever the factors, the specialists seemed more receptive to the White Paper than other doctors. Among general practitioners, the younger group displayed the least opposition. Many of them were with the armed forces, and apparently this government service did not interfere with clinical freedom or leave them with a bias against "organization" or compensation by salary. At any rate, the young doctors displayed far greater enthusiasm for a salaried service, health centers, and a wholly free service and revealed much less fear of many other aspects of the proposed scheme than did their older colleagues.[23]

An analysis of the questionnaire raises this important question: why was there so much support for many of the specific reforms proposed but such strong opposition to the White Paper as a whole? Since most of the negative votes were cast on administrative matters, it would seem that there was a profound fear of public direction and organization. The doctors quite understood the need for a free hospital and medical service for all, but shrank from the implications involved in the administration of such a service. The overwhelming vote against control of the medical service by local authority illustrates the point very well. The Medical Officer of Health and his associates were regarded as salaried bureaucrats and were not at all popular with general practitioners. Many of the municipal and most of the public assistance hospitals had low standards and inferior plants, and there was a consequent reflection on the local authorities that gave them a bad reputation in the eyes of many doctors. This suspicion of local control was unconsciously transferred to the proposed central administration, which hardly merited such treatment since it was similar in form to that which for so many years and without much criticism had served the National Health Insurance. Basically the issue was "bureaucratic" control, which was viewed as a threat to clinical freedom, financial security, and the traditional privacy of the doctor-patient relationship.

The role of the Medical Association at this juncture bears examination. Although not a trade union, it was impelled by a desire to protect the economic and professional interests of its members. Financial considerations were often the mainspring behind its policy. It favored, for example, maternity clinics and a school medical program for examination and educational purposes but not for therapy. The inclusion of medical treatment would obviously diminish the opportunities for private practice. But the economic factor was not the only one. The fear that the freedom of medicine would be imperiled by onerous controls created on occasions at Tavistock Square what was almost hysteria.

The Association at times seemed to be the arch enemy of liberal forces, and again it appeared in the more satisfying role of the champion of reform. During the inception of the National Health Insurance, the British Medical Association was in an angry and fighting mood, dragging its feet and demanding modification in the terms and conditions of that program. Concessions were granted and peaceful relations came to prevail between the government and the medical profession. Full acceptance of and then a desire to expand the National Health Insurance placed the Association at the head of the forces demanding a more progressive program. The Interim Report of 1942, as we have seen, climaxed twelve years of liberal medical leadership, but with the Beveridge Report the Medical Association lost its passion for reform and returned to a role variously described as "conservative" and "reactionary."

Since the White Paper was a serious attempt to implement the Report of the Medical Planning Commission and reflected much of its spirit, why did the leadership of the British Medical Association develop such an animus toward the new scheme? To be sure, the White Paper went beyond the Interim Report in some respects, but that hardly explains why the Association chose to sabotage proposals which its rank and file heartily endorsed. A good majority of doctors favored health centers, a free service for all, the abolition of the sale of practices, and a central board with power to exclude doctors from over-doctored areas. Yet the British Medical Association supported health centers only on an experimental basis and viewed control of the distribution of doctors as despotic. The other two measures were condemned without reservation. In view of this somewhat anomalous situation, it is reasonable to wonder how accurately the policies of the Association represented the opinions of the ordinary doctor, who was often too busy to read the *British Medical Journal,* much less to think in terms of ever becoming a delegate to the annual congress of the Association?

Since the medical profession had made a complete adjustment to the National Health Insurance as a workable necessity, it is difficult to understand the logic behind the sudden hysteria over the alleged threat to the freedom of medicine. Neither the British Medical Association report of 1938 nor that of 1942 raised the issue. Indeed, the latter report expressed pleasure that the independence of the medical profession had not been impaired by the Health Insurance. Serious shortcomings there were in the National Health Insurance, but no complaint was registered about the status of the doctor in relation to the patient or the government. For thirty years one-half of the population had had free practitioner service, and there was no apparent feeling that the doctor was any the worse for the experiment. If the Association was not disturbed about professional freedom in the spring of 1942, when it favored 90 per cent free coverage, why should it become so agitated in 1944 simply because a universal service was proposed?

The New Statesman and Nation, a publication noted for its frankness, charged in 1946, when the National Health Service bill was pending, that the real reason for professional criticism of the proposed law was monetary. The critics, it was claimed, were willing enough to accept as unavoidable a more comprehensive free medical service for patients unable to pay, but wanted an income limit so as to preserve for private practice all those with incomes above that level. Declared the editorial: "As soon as the government made clear its intention of providing an all-round service for all comers, this section of medical opinion became irreconcilable; it would have picked every possible hole in any 'universal' scheme."[24]

Historically, the doctors had favored reforms, but when the test came in the mid-1940's they were afflicted by doubts concerning the proper course of action. The fact that medicine was so highly competitive made it difficult for the doctors to agree on details. Dissension left the profession without a positive program, and their leaders took negative positions on issues that once appeared to have wide support. It was only on the issue of remuneration that the doctors were able to achieve a large degree of solidarity. As in 1911, they believed that a general policy of opposition to the proposals of the government offered the best hope for good financial terms.

With public opinion solidly behind the White Paper, the coalition government went steadily forward in working out the details of the new health program. Then came the general election of July, 1945, and the sweeping victory of the Labor Party. Clement Atlee succeeded Sir Winston Churchill as Prime Minister, and Aneurin Bevan replaced Henry Willink as Minister of Health. In the matter of health legislation there was no break in the continuity of preparation, since the White Paper was a coalition expression and the National Health Service was a bipartisan affair.

The new Minister of Health was a Welshman who, by dint of hard work and a commanding personality, had climbed from his beginnings as a coal miner to a position of influence in the Labor Party. Clever in debate and a master of repartee, he handled himself well on the floor of Parliament, though he sometimes showed little skill in diplomacy or conciliation. The workers admired his courage and strong socialistic leanings, but the medical profession came to detest him because of his militant defense of the new Health Service.

In working out the details of the law, the new Minister of Health was careful to consult frequently the medical profession, nurses, midwives, dentists, local authorities, voluntary hospitals, pharmacists, opticians, and insurance committees. Discussions were conducted on a wide front. Bevan himself presided over twenty conferences and his associates over thirteen. Consultation rather than negotiation characterized his method. To Parliament he later explained, "I had no negotiations, because once you negotiate with outside bodies two things happen. They are made aware of the nature of the proposals before the House of Commons itself; and furthermore the minister puts himself into an impossible position, because, if he has agreed with somebody outside he is bound to resist amendments from members in the House.   Otherwise he does not play fair with them."[25]

Although Aneurin Bevan had strong convictions on the subject of a national health service, he was politician enough to yield when such a course seemed imperative.   He and the majority of the Labor members in Parliament would have preferred a salaried service and no pay beds in the hospitals.   The medical profession, however, demanded a small quota of private beds in the National Health Service hospitals and the capitation fee system of compensation, and to these demands Bevan agreed, but he held out for a small basic salary in order to give a measure of security to the beginning doctor.   In the abolition of the sale of good will, the Minister of Health would make no concession beyond agreeing to compensation for the value of the practices destroyed.   In this policy he had the support of rank-and-file doctors, but the bitter opposition of the Medical Association.   To Bevan the sale of a practice was "tantamount to the sale and purchase of patients."   He felt it was a denial of "freedom of choice," since patients passed from the old practitioner to the new one.

The Minister of Health took cognizance of professional opposition to local authority control of the medical service and supported regional hospital boards and executive councils as an arrangement that would be mutually satisfactory to the Medical Association and the government.   Bevan favored giving the doctors a substantial voice in the administration of the health program, but in order to avoid the danger of syndicalism he felt it was necessary to subordinate them to lay control.   He had no desire, however, to make civil servants out of the doctors, as some charged, and he was confident that the new scheme had adequate safeguards against this danger.[26]

Few men in public life recognized more clearly the need for a broad and adequate health program than did Aneurin Bevan.   He was later to set forth his views in a book, *In Place of Fear.*   He clearly perceived that endowment and private charity, although useful at one time, no longer could meet the needs of society.   In his opinion there was no adequate substitute for a comprehensive, state-financed program.   The insurance basis was unsatisfactory.   If of the personal contributory type, the insurance required a qualifying period and offered a limited range of benefits, and those who did not qualify and could not otherwise afford treatment either did without or had to take the means test and accept charity.   Group insurance was expensive because of dividends and administrative costs.   Benefits were less than adequate and coverage was usually restricted to a particular segment of the population.   In Bevan's judgment this type of insurance was "the most expensive, the least scientific, and the clumsiest way of mobilizing collective security for the individual good." Industrial insurance also was subject to serious limitations, since it was usually too narrow to meet the full medical needs of the worker and his family. The varying range of benefits provided by the Approved Societies was partly due to the variation in the incidence of sickness among areas and industries.

The British experience with these various approaches had proved to Bevan that only the state could cope satisfactorily with the problem, and it would have to assume ultimate financial responsibility for the solution. The service offered by the government should be universal; anything less would make "the worst of all worlds." Imposing an income limit would, Bevan believed, create "a two-standard health service, one below and above the salt. It is merely the old British Poor Law system over again. Even if the service given is the same in both categories, there will always be the suspicion in the mind of the patient that it is not so, and this again is not a healthy mental state." With the creation of a full, adequate service, he affirmed, "society becomes more wholesome, more serene, and spiritually healthier, if it knows that its citizens have at the back of their consciousness the knowledge that not only themselves, but all their fellows, have access, when ill, to the best that medical skill can provide."²⁷

The National Health Service Bill for England and Wales was called up before the House of Commons for its second reading on April 30, 1946, at which time the Minister of Health explained at some length the more essential and controversial provisions. The primary purpose of the law, he stressed, was to make medical assistance accessible to all who required it—and, at a time when the individual needed most to be free from financial worry, without charge. Instead of the insured workers only, all would now be protected, and a full medical and allied service would become available. He commented upon the deficiencies of the existing hospital facilities and the shortage of nurses and dentists, while acknowledging that "it will be some time before the Bill can fructify fully in effective universal service." He deplored the fact that the condition of British teeth was a "national reproach" and that deafness had been largely neglected. The failure to deal adequately with mental health would also be remedied under the new bill.

The hospitals, explained the Minister of Health, would be "the vertebrae of the health system." The voluntary hospitals had performed well, but they had usually been founded "by the caprice of charity" and bore little relationship to each other. Unfortunately, endowments were often left to hospitals in communities where the well-to-do live, leaving the industrial areas with a great shortage of beds. Bevan particularly lamented the dependence of hospitals upon charity: "I believe it is repugnant to a civilized community for hospitals to have to rely upon private charity. . . . I have always felt a shudder of repulsion when I see nurses and sisters who ought to be at their work, and students who ought to be at their work, going about the streets collecting money for the hospitals." Such solicitation would not be necessary under the new law. He acknowledged that the nationalization of the voluntary hospitals had aroused some resentment, but explained that his primary concern was with the people who would be served by these institutions. The hospitals, he pledged, would be systematically grouped and improved. Specialists would not only be accessible in the hospitals but would also be available for visits to the homes.[28]

The bill passed the second reading by a better than two-to-one vote, and on July 26 it was presented for the third reading. Very little change had occurred in it; nothing had transpired to weaken the confidence of the government in the essential soundness of its provisions. The Parliamentary Secretary to the Minister of Health, Charles W. Key, undertook to answer the objections raised by the opposition. To the charge that the bill discouraged voluntary effort and association, he pointed out that, on the contrary, the opportunity for such initiative was even greater than before, since the regional boards, management committees, and house committees for the hospitals would all be based on voluntary service. The allegation that the bill dangerously increased ministerial power and patronage was denied by Key, who explained that the appointments to the various boards and committees would be made by the Minister in consultation with professional and other interested groups. The regional boards and management committees, he reminded the House of Commons, would select virtually all the hospital staff, so here there could be no question of ministerial patronage. In the distribution of doctors, the Minister of Health could exercise only a negative control over the Medical Practices Committee. In this matter the Minister would have virtually the same power that his office had enjoyed for over thirty years under the National Health Insurance.

Of all the charges, the one that the Parliamentary Secretary considered most unjust was the alleged loss of independence and freedom of the medical profession. Doctors, he said, were free to join the service or not and to accept or reject patients. If they received a salaried post in a hospital, they would no more lose their freedom than had the Medical Officer of Health, who serves the local government. As a matter of fact, Key emphasized, "no body of public or private employees has ever had the same freedom as the medical profession will have under this Bill." He revealed that half the members of the local Executive Council would be professionals selected by the professions themselves and that the Medical Practices Committee, the real employer of the general practitioners, would consist almost wholly of doctors, a majority of whom would be engaged in active practice.[29]

The third reading witnessed the passage of the bill in the House of Commons by an even greater margin than did the second reading. Approval by the Lords followed, and on November 6, 1946, the royal signature was affixed and the bill became law. The new service, however, was not actually to be launched until July 5, 1948. The long delay was deemed essential in order to set up the necessary machinery, prepare regulations, and reach agreements about terms and conditions of employment with the various professional groups concerned. The transition from a restricted service to one free and universal would have been difficult enough had the hospital service been adequate and the other services in good condition. But there were the frightful shortages and deficiencies—and an atmosphere that was, because of some members of the medical professions, charged with tension.

The Medical Association proceeded to poll its membership on this question: "Shall we or shall we not enter into any discussions on the framework to be created within the limitations of that act?" So great was the concern in England and Wales that 90 per cent of the doctors replied, and their answer was a resounding "no." The general practitioners registered a negative vote of 64 per cent, but among the specialists and consultants it was only 55 per cent. Among the younger consultants and among doctors on whole-time salaries, however, the vote favored negotiation. The younger general practitioners showed a much greater disposition to approve the continuation of negotiation than the older ones. The Council of the British Medical Association lost no time in resolving that the profession completely break off all discussion with the Ministry of Health. A Special Representative Meeting of the Association ratified the resolution by a vote of 252 to 17.[30] Thus within a matter of weeks following the final enactment of the new law the Medical Association opened hostilities against the government, and the weapons chosen were propaganda and non-co-operation. The offending provisions of the new law would have to be eliminated or drastically modified or the medical profession would remain aloof from the new service.

Aneurin Bevan seemed to accept the situation rather calmly. Upon hearing of the Council's proposal to discontinue negotiation, he expressed the hope that before any final decision was reached "wiser counsels will have prevailed." He felt certain that the medical profession would "take no steps which would make it difficult for them to take part in the comprehensive health service which the people of this country so ardently desire." In any event, he believed his duty to Parliament under the law was clear and did not feel able to delay any longer the consultations necessary in getting the administrative machinery set up. He announced his determination to negotiate with all other groups concerned, and, as for the medical profession, he would consider what should be done to give it "the opportunity of assisting to shape, and of playing its part in the new service."[31]

CHAPTER III

The New Program as a Controversial Issue

THE CONFLICT between the British Medical Association and the government reached a climax and was resolved during the first five months of 1948. Opposition to the White Paper of 1944 had been determined, but even more militant was the resistance to the National Health Service Act of 1946. Driven by a fear that fed upon a sharp distrust of the Ministry of Health and the Labor Party, the leadership of the medical profession resorted to techniques that at times approached the level of demagogism. The absolute need the Association felt for solidarity among its membership may explain the rabid appeals and provocative allegations that characterized some of the editorials of the *British Medical Journal* and speeches of the officials from Tavistock Square. Sinister meanings were ascribed to provisions of the new law, and dangerous implications were read into some of its terminology. Some doctors appeared to fear that an unfriendly Minister of Health might interpret the law to the detriment of the medical profession. These apprehensions may have been genuine enough, but for the most part they were little justified in the light of the National Health Insurance experience or subsequent developments.

The course of Aneurin Bevan during this critical period was unfortunately marred by occasional brusqueness and some intemperate remarks, which served only to exacerbate the already intense feeling. As the "appointed day" for the implementation of the Service approached however, he seemed to display more patience in the negotiations and a greater willingness to alleviate the fears that had so aroused the medical profession. With Parliament and public opinion solidly behind the new law, the medical profession stood isolated—a factor of considerable significance to many doctors. The solidarity of the medical profession was first breached when the consultants and specialists decided to enter the Health Service. Then the unity of the rank and file began to disintegrate. This shift was reflected in a new, less intransigent spirit in the leadership. Final acceptance of the National Health Service law by the Association came within less than six weeks of the inauguration of the new program.

The decision of the British Medical Association in December, 1946, not to continue negotiation with the Ministry of Health was soon reversed. In a conciliatory reply to a joint letter from the Presidents of the Royal Colleges, Aneurin Bevan in January, 1947, gave assurance on a number of controversial points and expressed a desire for advice and help from the medical profession. With the understanding that discussions would cover a broad area and that additional legislation might be considered, the Negotiating Committee of the Medical Association resumed its meetings with the Ministry of Health. Subcommittees were organized and protracted discussions were held throughout the summer of 1947.[1] So "microscopic" were the conferences in which Bevan participated that he later complained that he was "almost weary of the issues because they have been so much investigated." In December he met the Negotiating Committee for a two-day discussion and was presented with a printed circular which opposed so many provisions in the law that to Bevan it was equivalent to a rejection of the whole program.[2] An unbridgeable gulf seemed to separate the medical profession and the Ministry of Health, with little hope that a common meeting ground could be reached. This appearance was strengthened in January, 1948, when a Representative Meeting of the Medical Association declared that the National Health Service Act in its present form was "so grossly at variance with the essential principles of our profession that it should be rejected absolutely by all practitioners."[3]

This blunt rejection of the law sparked an all-out campaign by the leadership of the Association to build up a solid phalanx of resistance. The *British Medical Journal* was already active in maligning the new program by catchword phrases and innuendos and in otherwise putting the worst possible construction on the Act. In an editorial on January 3, designed to rally all consultants behind the policy of the Association, the journal referred to the new program as "a state medical service"—a term which to the medical mind had a very bad connotation. The law was called "Mr. Aneurin Bevan's Act," a term that, in view of his great unpopularity among doctors, was calculated to create an emotional bias against the scheme. Reference was made to the "danger of too much planning, of too much government." The editorial observed, "We live in times where deeds and traditions are at a discount and when the cynic may too easily prove his case that principles may be dissolved in gold." Medical men throughout the world, it proclaimed, "are all sorely perplexed by the growing tendency of the state machine to thrust itself between the individual doctor and the individual patient. They see this intervention of the state as something harmful to medicine, and they look to this country for a lead and are anxiously awaiting the outcome of the present struggle."[4]

No longer did the Association oppose the idea of a universally free service. Official acceptance of this policy had come even before the adoption of the National Health Service Act. Among some doctors, however, especially the more affluent ones, its universality was one of the most repugnant aspects of the law. If a doctor derived his income almost completely from public funds, it was averred, he might feel that "he has surrendered both his present status and his opportunities for enterprise," that "he could no longer play Robin Hood (as so many have done to the benefit of their poorer patients)," and that "his livelihood and even his manner of practice would depend on central decisions." An indeterminable number of practitioners, unprepared to accept the necessity of a comprehensive free service for all, deeply resented the anticipated loss of fees from middle-class patients. These doctors fought the law wherever such action seemed feasible with the hope that it could be emasculated or somehow destroyed, even as they voiced support for a health service of the "right sort."

There was a multiplicity of issues, real and imaginary, and for a time they drew many shades of medical opinion together. Dr. H. Guy Dain, Chairman of the Council of the British Medical Association and Dr. Charles Hill, the Secretary, were among the most effective spokesmen in marshaling arguments, crystallizing medical sentiment, and ferreting out hidden clauses in the new law that could possibly be viewed as a threat to the future integrity and well-being of the profession. Not all doctors, however, were willing to accept as realistic or valid the charges and representations which flowed from the headquarters of the Association. *The Lancet,* an independent medical journal that had no partisan cause to argue, approached the controversy in an impartial spirit. Its editorials attained a high measure of objectivity; its primary purpose was to heal the rift between the government and the medical profession and to bring about the creation of an effective health service. In seeking to clear the atmosphere, *The Lancet* addressed a number of questions to the Minister of Health during the latter part of January, 1948. The answers contributed to a better understanding of the real intent of the government on many matters, though they had little immediate effect in reassuring the Medical Association.[5]

The most disquieting aspect of the new program seemed to be the uncertainty about how doctors would be paid. The White Paper and various government officials had endeavored to assure the medical profession that capitation fees would constitute the primary method of compensation for general practitioners, but there was no statutory guarantee of this pledge. Since the matter would be subject to regulation, what would prevent some future government from introducing a full-time salaried service? In 1943 the Labor Party Conference had endorsed such a policy, and in 1946 Bevan in discussing the matter said: "There is all the difference in the world between plucking fruit when it is ripe and plucking it when it is green."[6] There was thus a reasonable doubt about the ultimate intention of the Labor Government, although Bevan, both in piloting the act through Parliament and afterwards, opposed a full-time salaried service as being impracticable. He favored a small basic salary of £300 ($840) plus a capitation fee for each patient on the doctor's list. Such a scheme would give the beginning practitioner an assured income while he was acquiring patients and would be useful in helping to sustain doctors in sparsely populated regions.

The dread of a salaried service became almost an obsession with the British Medical Association. Many doctors believed that a salaried service would reduce them to civil servants and destroy their incentive for high professional standards. The new law was interpreted by some as "the first fulfillment of the government's policy to introduce a whole-time salaried state medical service" in which "the doctor can call neither his practice nor his soul his own."[7] Dr. Dain charged that "with a salary as small as £300 ($840) we shall begin to experience control, and there is nothing in the act to prevent the Minister by regulation changing it into a full-time salary."[8]

The Lancet, in a much more detached vein, reminded the doctors that in 1911 their profession labored under a great fear that the National Health Insurance would lead to a state salaried service, but that after 37 years the capitation fee method had remained intact. Nor was there any provision in the National Insurance Law prohibiting full-salary remuneration. While recognizing that the risk did exist and was real, this journal did not believe that a salaried service would be imposed as long as the capitation fee system worked.[9]

The proposed remuneration rates also caused uneasiness, but they were adjustable and did not trouble the Medical Association at this time nearly so much as the loss of the right to buy and sell the good will of a practice. To the leaders at Tavistock Square, this was an essential right which should be vigorously defended, although the questionnaire of 1944 indicated that a good majority of general practitioners did not think so.   One of the high officials of the Association even went so far as to equate good will with freedom by warning that in surrendering this right the doctor "will therefore lose the plot of ground which in a free society enables him to preserve his freedom as an individual."[10]   *The Lancet* took quite a different view of the matter, describing it as one of the less pleasant features of medicine. This journal even charged that the buying and selling of practices increased "the difficulty of correcting maldistribution of medical resources."   "Its defenders," affirmed the editorial, "must sometimes find it hard to speak in the same breath about the sacredness of the doctor-patient relationship."[11]

The Minister of Health was somewhat perplexed over the adamant stand of the medical leadership on this issue.   To him, the sale of good will was the negation of freedom.   "How can it reasonably be argued," he queried, "that there is an effective free choice of doctor when the doctors negotiate the terms between themselves and the patient knows nothing at all about it?"   Under the existing system, he explained, a young doctor could enter general practice by becoming an assistant or he could buy a practice "by borrowing sums of money and, therefore, for the first 15 to 20 years of his professional life, loading himself with debt, so that when he is approaching his patient, he is not in the state of mind in which a doctor ought to be."[12]

The act outlawed the sale of medical practices for those who entered the National Health Service and by threat of fine and imprisonment sought to prevent circumvention of the law through a disguised contractual agreement.   But all doctors who entered the service on or before the appointed day (later extended sixty days) and who suffered loss from the abolition of the right to sell their practice would receive compensation at the time of their retirement or death.   The sum of £66,000,000 ($184,800,000) would be allocated for this purpose.   The amount was calculated by actuaries on the basis of 1938 values plus an additional 16 per cent to allow for inflation.[13]   Yet to Dr. Dain the compensation was too low, and there would, he warned, be a long delay before the doctors would get their money.   He took a dim view of this attempt to right what he considered a great wrong.[14]

The government believed that the sale of good will was incompatible with an equitable distribution of general practitioners and primarily for this reason decreed its abolition in the National Health Service.   Doctors who entered the scheme would be privileged to practice where they wished, subject to the approval of the Medical Practices Committee.   Only where there was excessive competition would permission be denied, but few areas would be affected in this manner. Since the Committee would consist mostly of doctors in active practice, the Ministry of Health felt that the system would protect the interests of the medical profession while gradually effecting a better balance between the under-doctored and over-doctored areas. The vote in the referendum of 1944 approved such negative controls, but to the leaders of the British Medical Association this approach constituted a dangerous interference in the freedom of movement for general practitioners.[15]

The threat to professional freedom seemed to come from many quarters—so the medical profession believed—but the most serious source of all was the alleged absence of adequate safeguards against unjust dismissal from the National Health Service. If a doctor's name were struck off the National Health Service lists, the Association seemed to believe that he would almost have to emigrate to make a living. Anticipating this objection, the government planned to set up a special tribunal composed of one layman, one doctor, and one lawyer for the purpose of determining whether a practitioner whom an Executive Council had found guilty of unprofessional conduct should be expelled from the Service. The Executive Council, it was expected, would proceed cautiously in initiating disciplinary action, since one-half of its membership came from the professions. If the tribunal decided in favor of the accused, his name would remain on the roster and no further action could be taken; but if dismissal were ordered, the defendant could then appeal to the Minister, who had the right to overrule the tribunal.[16] Under the National Health Insurance there was no such protective machinery, the Minister having the power arbitrarily to eliminate doctors from the service, but the medical profession seemed little disturbed about any threat to professional freedom during all those years. Now, however, the Medical Association was aroused over the "inadequate" protection available under the new scheme.

The Association demanded that practitioners be granted the right of appeal to a high court from any decision of the Executive Council or the Minister. Bevan flatly denied the request, contending that if a doctor were unlawfully discharged, like anybody else he had the right to seek justice in the courts, but that no other group had the right, nor should the doctors have it, to go to the courts to reverse the lawful termination of a contract. The lawyer on the tribunal, he stated, would be a distinguished person appointed by the Lord Chancellor, and the deliberations of this body would be privately held unless the doctor desired otherwise. In the courts, however, there could be no secrecy, and the doctor's reputation might suffer irreparably.[17]

On the status of partnership agreements, the Medical Association was in some doubt as to what effect the law might have. The Minister of Health was advised that partners were adequately protected, while the medical profession, receiving different legal advice, insisted upon the need for clarification. The usual procedure, Bevan pointed out, was to first let the courts construe the law, but he agreed, with the co-operation of the Lord Chancellor and Attorney General, to appoint a legal committee to see if the law adversely affected partnerships. If so, he promised to seek an amendment to the act.[18]

The nationalization of the hospitals was viewed as a move to create a "hospital monopoly." Although it was announced that 200 nursing homes were not to be appropriated by the government, there was fear that even these might subsequently be taken over by the state, leaving private medicine with little access to hospitals. Bevan endeavored to assure the medical profession that it was unlikely that these nursing homes would ever be nationalized since, once disclaimed, their subsequent acquisition would require outright purchase. Where circumstances permitted, he promised that a proportion of the available private beds in National Health Service hospitals would not be subject to any prescribed maximum charges governing doctors' fees. Bevan's refusal, however, to incorporate into an amendment his assurances left the Medical Association dubious about future hospital policy. Dr. Hill voiced regret that the profession had not earlier taken a stronger stand on the issue of nationalization when it might have done some good. Now it was too late.[19]

The broad issue of freedom was exploited in every possible way. The right to join or not to join the National Health Service was interpreted as the right to accept service with the government or starve. To live, doctors would be dependent upon state payment; and if they did not become civil servants, they would, the Association warned, be subject to control by civil servants, which would be worse. Practitioners with a full list would be terribly overworked. The National Health Service proposals, declared the *British Medical Journal,* conflicted with "the traditions and standards of a great profession." The proposals were "part and parcel of the levelling down process to which this country is being subjected by the present Government on the curiously unbiological thesis that all men are equal."[20]

The Minister of Health was unable to see how the new law could possibly jeopardize the doctor-patient relationship. He explained that if there were any interference, he would be the first to take remedial action. Looking at the National Health Insurance, he could observe no threat there to the relationship, nor had the doctors registered any such complaint. He insisted that the responsibility of the doctor to his patients would not be impaired under the new service, either. In Parliament he sharply denied that he would send "a snooper into every consulting room in the country to see whether the doctor is subordinating the interests of the state to those of his patient."[21]

The leaders of the British Medical Association left nothing undone to prepare the membership for a referendum to be held early in February. Declared Dr. Dain to a large gathering of doctors: "I see no reason why we should not have practically 100 per cent disapprovals. . . . I as chairman of the council must be the spearhead of the association in this matter. I say that the new service as propounded in its present form is entirely unsuitable, entirely improper for us to accept, and we should endeavor to persuade our colleagues to vote against accepting any service under the act in its present form. The B.M.A., so far as I have any influence, and the Representative Meeting will most certainly stand firm on that position." The officials at Tavistock Square were determined to avoid the unfortunate division which occurred in the ranks of the Association during the fight against the National Health Insurance in 1912-13. The risk of such a split in 1948, however, did not seem to trouble Dain, who confidently asserted, "we have better organization now, and we will jolly well see it does not happen this time."[22]

The story of the group pressure applied in local meetings all over England during this period is yet to be told. One general practitioner informed the author that so inflamed was the feeling in his local medical group that, had any doctor dared to defend the National Health Service, he would have invited ostracism, if not physical ejection from the room. The doctors were reminded by the *British Medical Journal* of their right to refuse service under the new law. If the plebiscite went against the government, then the Association would urge the general practitioners to continue administering to the needs of their patients without having any part of the new scheme.[23]

The Lancet urged moderation. In a leading article, it endeavored to show that there was another side to the National Health Service that was being ignored by the medical profession in the heat of battle. The journal analyzed the issues one by one and found that there was a great deal to be said for the position of the government. Much had been made about the "excessive concentration of power in the hands of the Minister," but to *The Lancet* it was undeniable that "responsibility and therefore power" had to be lodged in some person answerable to an elected representative body. The many voluntary administrative boards and committees, however, were specifically designed as a decentralizing influence to check the tendency toward too much central authority. In the opinion of this journal, the medical profession had no right to denounce an "administrative structure to which it has suggested no preferable or practicable alternative."

Bevan's handling of negotiations was scrutinized by *The Lancet,* which recognized that, despite allegations to the contrary, he had made substantial concessions, as indeed had all groups concerned, including the local authorities and the voluntary hospitals as well as the medical profession. In permitting private practice to all National Health Service doctors and private beds in the public hospitals and in accepting capitation fees as the principal method of compensation for general practitioners, the Minister of Health had departed from socialist doctrine. To those who felt that he could have yielded more on non-essentials, his reply was that he was no oriental bargainer and that the major concessions were already a part of the law. On the matter of partnership, he did recognize the possible need for an amendment. The act itself, declared the editorial, was a co-operative achievement.

If we remove the picture from the beam of light in which the B.M.A. is now presenting it we see that, whatever its faults of composition, it is certainly not a study in scarlet. Actually it is a composite picture containing plenty of green, blue, and yellow touches recalling the work, among others, of Lloyd George, the Royal Commission on National Health Insurance, Lord Dawson, the British Medical Association, the Medical Planning Research and the Coalition. And if it did not happen to be signed 'Aneurin Bevan' it might perhaps be more justly praised.[24]

If this appeal to reason had any effect upon the inflamed spirit of the medical profession, it was not evident. The columns of the *British Medical Journal* during January and February, 1948, overflowed with correspondence from angry doctors pouring acid comments upon the new health scheme. Within a period of three weeks this journal received at least 75,000 words in letters, and with few exceptions the letters railed against Aneurin Bevan and the new act, while urging an uncompromising defense of the principles of the Association. Only a selected few could be published, and these were given such provocative captions as "Resist Now," "Censorship," "The Fight for Freedom," "The Moral Issue," "Years of Conscription," "Doctors and Dictators," "Liberty of Patient," "Intimidation," "State Medical Servant," "The Act or Liberty," "No Confidence in Minister," "The Paternal State," "A Warning," "Economic Persuasion," and "Defiance of Dictatorship."

On February 9, Aneurin Bevan complained in the House of Commons about the personal abuse to which he had been subjected from a small group of medical spokesmen who, he charged, "have consistently misled the great profession to which they belong." He drew a distinction between "the hard working doctors" and "the small body of raucous voiced people who are alleged to represent the profession as a whole." It had been, he said, "this small body of politically poisoned people" who from the beginning had fought the Health Act and had stirred up as much emotion as possible. In one of the irate letters that a doctor had written for publication, Bevan noted these unflattering words about himself: "In brigand-like fashion this would-be Fuehrer points an economic pistol at the doctor's head and blandly exclaims 'yours is a free choice—to enter the service or not to enter.' "

The Minister of Health reminded the House of Commons of the long history behind the National Health Service Act and of the great labor on the part of so many that helped to shape the new program. The White Paper, he noted, required 32 days of deliberation in the Commons and 10 days in the Lords. He explained that, although he himself seemed to be the target, the criticism was not in reality directed at his "personal deficiencies" but at the act that some wished to destroy. His predecessors had not escaped the displeasure of the British Medical Association. Mr. Brown, a Liberal, was "abominable," and Mr. Willink, a Conservative, was "intolerable." It had never been possible, he observed, to find a Minister of Health acceptable to the medical profession. Bevan said that failure to reach agreement with the Negotiating Committee did not occur because of any unwillingness on his part to engage in discussion, but rather because of the intransigence of a "body organizing wholesale resistance to the implementation of an Act of Parliament." "In fact," he said, "the whole thing begins to look more like a squalid political conspiracy than the representations of an honored and learned profession and, I say this deliberately, when the bulk of doctors in the country learn the extent to which their interests have been misrepresented by some of their spokesmen, they will turn on those spokesmen."[25]

The returns from the February questionnaire revealed more clearly than words the temper of the medical mind. In an 84 per cent poll, 90 per cent of the doctors expressed disapproval of the National Health Service Law as it then existed, and 88 per cent declared themselves not in favor of accepting service under the act. By a six-to-one vote the general practitioners agreed to abide by the majority decision and to refuse service under the law. Fewer than 4,000 doctors in all categories indicated they would accept service no matter how the vote went.[26] Obviously, with such a small number of doctors the program could not possibly work. The victory for the leadership of the British Medical Association could scarcely have been more conclusive.

The *British Medical Journal* was jubilant over the results, which, it said, showed "Mr. Bevan how completely he has misjudged the thoughts and feelings of the medical men and women of this country, and how ill-timed, inept and untrue were his vicious remarks about raucous-voiced and politically poisoned people." "There are compelling reasons," admonished a leading editorial, "for keeping medicine independent of the state. If, however, the people of this country through Parliament . . . pursue with success the idea that a paternal state should provide every kind of medical service, then the medical profession must at least see that within the state framework the maximum amount of freedom and independence of the medical man is made secure."[27]

The referendum caused considerable apprehension in the press. The *Manchester Guardian* could see a stage "perfectly set for a trial of strength which would be a disaster." The pro-labor *Daily Herald* viewed the referendum as having only "propaganda value." The Medical Association was accused of having "spared no effort to whip up anti-Health Service, anti-Bevan, and anti-Labour emotion," but the editorial confidently asserted the "real test of the doctors' sanity and loyalty will come in April when they have to sign or refuse to sign their contracts with the Minister. And on July 5, as appointed by Parliament, the National Health Service will start."

The *Daily Telegraph and Morning Post*, conscious of its political leanings, took the opportunity to attack Bevan. "The situation," it was admitted, "is a nationally unpleasant one, but should no change for the better prove possible, the responsibility for the tactics, or absence of them, which have brought it about must be placed squarely on Mr. Bevan's shoulders." The *Daily Express* could see in the mutual antipathy between Bevan and the British Medical Association a cause for the deadlock.[28] The *Observer* believed the roots of the difficulty went deeper. It could observe a great difference between the nationalization of an industry and the nationalization of a "profession with a long and valued tradition of independence." Establishing an effective National Health Service under existing conditions, with all the shortages, would, the editorial asserted, "be a long term enterprise." The new service should therefore be achieved by gradual stages.[29]

The Times (London) noted four basic issues that divided the Medical Association and the government. Each was briefly evaluated. To the "right of appeal" there were serious objections. The sale of good will appeared to rest upon the misconception that the retention of it "would somehow guarantee the flourishing survival of private practice." But it will survive, asserted the editorial, only if it should prove superior to public practice. The newspaper recognized the need to regulate the distribution of practitioners and could see in the Medical Practices Committee a group of doctors that would in no way sacrifice or harm the interest of the medical profession. While the basic salary of £300 ($840) was essential for young doctors and others in special areas, it was not necessary for all practitioners, and so *The Times* (London) suggested that, as a conciliatory gesture, the government should abandon it, providing the "B.M.A. to which so much has already been conceded, should make in return the concession of calling off hostilities and using the great opportunities presented by the service to work for its perfection from within instead of denouncing it from without."[30]

Not all who wrote to the *British Medical Journal* applauded the policy of the Association. Dr. Aleck Bourne, an eminent consultant, wondered to what extent the referendum reflected the real opinions of the doctors. Quite obviously, he observed, nobody could approve of the entire act, since it was a compromise measure, and so the Medical Association might have assumed an overwhelming negative vote without bothering to poll the profession. The critical query, he indicated, was the one seeking to ascertain the solidarity of the rank and file. Many who answered affirmatively did so, he said, "under a mistaken sense of loyalty . . . and in some cases under a moral duress." "The question," he pointed out, "has been put at a time when the profession has been goaded into a state of emotion, heat and anger, and I submit that the majority is quite worthless as an indication of what even a substantial number of doctors will be ready to do on July 5." Dr. Bourne insisted that it was not the time for "emotion, heat, battle-cries, and the metaphors of war. . . . We need a cold re-examination of the points of dispute. . . . If the B.M.A. attempts to lead the profession into conflict on July 5 by continued refusal to accept the Minister's offer to re-examine the four unacceptable provisions of the Act it must fail because no sectional resistance can prevail against the wish of the community."

Dr. Stephen Taylor, a member of the House of Commons and of the Labor Party, openly defended the new act as the collective will of all political parties. He warned that "any attempt to frustrate the law by extra-parliamentary means is bound to end in failure." He explained that on such issues as the sale of good will and the right of appeal there was complete unanimity in Parliament, and on the question of negative direction the British Medical Association could expect only lukewarm support from the Conservatives. On the issue of a salaried service, the government had repeatedly disclaimed any intent to employ this mode of remuneration, and its future use would be determined solely by need. In defense of Bevan, Taylor declared

that if it had not been for him there "might have been no private practice for all general practitioners and no private wards in the hospitals. . . . no tribunal between the executive councils and the Minister,
and no participation of doctors in the executive side of the service.
And strangely enough, but for him we might well have had a whole-
time salaried service." Taylor predicted that the present course of the
Association would end in ultimate defeat. He assured the medical
profession that the law offered "a fuller freedom than in the past."
"Labour people," he concluded, "are just as keen on liberty as you
are. They do not want a servile tribe of doctors, but a strong free
profession with whom they can join in the battle for health."[31]

No man was more adamant in uncompromising opposition to the
new law than Lord Horder, a member of the Council and an eminent
doctor. In addressing the Special Representative Meeting of the
Medical Association on March 17, he hailed the results of the referendum as an expression of complete confidence by the profession in the
policy of the Association. "We believe," he continued, "that the association regards the points at issue as we regard them, not bargaining
points but signs of the doctor being a free man, free to practice his
science and art in his patient's best interest." He conceded that they
could lose by "arguing as to which of these principles we should yield
to the Minister first or last." "That way," he warned, "madness lies."
"We must not yield," he pleaded, "on any of the points which collectively or individually spell the doctor's freedom. I have watched
the Negotiating Committee cut the joint to the bone. There is nothing
left to go, except our freedom, and that we dare not give."

On this occasion the spirit of unity in the Special Representative
Meeting seemed a real and enduring force, and there was no hint
of the rift that was soon to come. There was no talk of compromise
or conciliation. For over eight hours, with two short intervals, the
meeting remained in session. Lord Horder requested a motion in
refutation of the "mendacious" charge in Parliament and the press
that the Association was not a constitutional democratic body and
that the Negotiating Committee was a small group of elderly doctors
dictating to all the others. This resolution was carried, as was also
another notifying the government that only by making the concessions
demanded could it expect co-operation from the medical profession.[32]

The Medical Association could see in the tactics of the trade
unions and the government a deliberate attempt to employ propaganda and pressure as a means to force the doctors to join the National
Health Service. A practitioner in Cambridge, for example, received
a letter from the Secretary of the Transport and General Workers'
Union requesting information about whether he expected to join the

new service. The letter ended thus: "Should your decision be a negative one we think it only fair that we should know this in order that
we should be in a position to take such steps as may be open to us
for the protection of our members."   Since other physicians were
receiving similar communications, it appeared that there existed a
systematic program of coercion under the "guidance of a central
hand."

On March 15 a circular was issued by the Ministry of Health to
local authorities suggesting that they give wide publicity to the details
of the new service and arrange to handle all personal inquiries. The
Central Office of Information for the Ministry, it was revealed, had
prepared a leaflet which would be available for distribution about the
middle of April, the substance of which was conveyed in this excerpt:
"Choose your doctor now. If one doctor cannot accept you, ask
another, or ask to be put in touch with one by the new Executive
Council which has been set up in your area."   The Representative
Meeting deplored such techniques and resolutely condemned "as
grossly improper the bringing to bear of pressure for political purposes upon individual doctors."   The *British Medical Journal* charged
that by "the use of films, posters and pamphlets they [the government]
are preparing a huge publicity campaign to induce the public to bring
pressure upon the medical profession. The trade unions, the Government's masters, are aiding and abetting this campaign."   But the
editorial "did not believe that the public wish to be treated by doctors
bullied and threatened into a service they do not like, and we do not
believe that medical men and women will allow themselves to be so
coerced."[33]

With little more than three months left before the new service
was scheduled to start, it was imperative that the deadlock be broken
quickly. No one felt the urgency to eliminate misunderstanding more
acutely than the Minister of Health. His performance in Parliament
on February 9 had served only to intensify resistance. The referendum demonstrated a unity in the medical profession which Bevan did
not question. Other tactics would have to be employed. More
clarification, more assurances, and if necessary, an amendment in-
corporating some of the concessions. On February 19, he announced
to Parliament that he was "always ready to listen to any fresh representations that may be made."[34]

On April 7, Bevan disclosed in the Commons a new policy of
conciliation, which further emerged in his answers to a number of
questions submitted to him by the British Medical Association. It
was the spirit more than the substance of his concessions that reversed
the whole trend of belligerence between the Ministry of Health and

the medical profession. In order to banish the greatest fear of all, the Minister of Health agreed to sponsor a statutory provision prohibiting a full-time salaried service. The universal basic salary would be abandoned, and most doctors would be paid solely by capitation fees. A fixed annual payment would supplement capitation fees for young doctors entering practice and others who might need or desire this mode of remuneration, and the details of this supplementary payment would be worked out in discussion between the medical profession and the Minister of Health.

The conciliation was in nearly everything else a matter of reassuring the medical profession and not of any real modification of policy. There would be complete freedom in clinical matters, as well as freedom of speech and publication about the administration and organization of the service. Approval of place of practice by the Medical Practices Committee would be automatic except in areas where there was an excess of doctors. Hospital appointments for consultants and specialists would in most cases be part time. Private doctors would be able to obtain free hospital and specialist benefits for their patients. In selecting medically trained men for membership in administrative and advisory bodies, the Minister of Health would consult with the professional associations.

Bevan announced that an expert legal committee was being set up to investigate the effect of the act upon partnership agreements. This was in fulfillment of a pledge given earlier. On the hotly contested issues involving appeal to the courts, negative direction, and the sale of good will, the Minister refused to surrender. He did agree that at the end of two years there could be a special review of the machinery to insure an equitable distribution of general practitioners, but he tactfully rejected as too restrictive the stipulation that the chairman of the tribunal should be a high court judge instead of a lawyer. As a curb on the power of the Minister of Health to make National Health Service regulations, it had been suggested that they should be subject to some more limiting procedure. This demand was unacceptable, since all regulations had to be submitted to a special committee of Parliament for review as the law already stood, and this, Bevan believed, operated as restraint enough on the authority of the Minister. The specially compiled local roster of obstetricians the law provided for was objectionable to the Medical Association, but the Minister deemed such a list useful. And finally, no absolute assurance could be given that nursing homes would not some day be nationalized.[35] In refusing to yield on these matters, Bevan couched his replies in such a friendly and sympathetic manner that a cursory glance at them left the impression he had given away much.

Although impressed with what had been gained, the Council of the British Medical Association did not feel that the freedoms of the profession were adequately protected yet. It did believe, however, that enough had been conceded to justify another referendum. The recalcitrant attitude of the leadership was changing to one of moderation. The results of the questionnaire, published early in May, showed the medical profession still opposed to the National Health Service, but less strongly than before. In a 77 per cent poll, two-thirds of the general practitioners voted disapproval of the act. Only a slender majority of them, however, were now opposed to serving under the law. In all of Great Britain fewer than 10,000 general practitioners were unwilling to accept service, and that number fell considerably short of the 13,000 deemed necessary by the Representative Body to make resistance effective.[36]

The unity of the rank and file had begun to dissolve. Dr. Alfred Cox, medical secretary of the British Medical Association in 1911, advised the Association to approve the National Health Service and avoid the unpleasantness experienced in the struggle against the National Health Insurance. While the Representative Body in December, 1912, was denouncing the law as unworkable, thousands of doctors were "flocking to the panel." Influenced by "some eloquent diehards," the Association continued to ignore reality until it was too late, and then a humiliating retreat had to be executed quickly by an embarrassed leadership. All of this was vivid in the mind of the former secretary, who now advised the Association "to accept the verdict of the plebiscite ungrudgingly" and to give "wholehearted support" to those who joined the new service.[37]

All eyes now turned to the Special Representative Assembly. Eager for a favorable response from that body, the Minister of Health sent a letter to the Association seeking to further dispel the "old" fears which had so prejudiced the medical mind against the National Health Service. There was little new in the communication, which merely confirmed that an amending bill would be passed to clarify the position of partnerships, prohibit a whole-time salaried service for general practitioners, permit the Executive Council to choose its own chairman, and make the professional member of the tribunal an *ad hoc* representative from a panel of the appropriate profession.[38]

The Special Representative Assembly which met in the Great Hall of the B.M.A. House on May 28 was faced by the necessity of reaching a decision for which it had little enthusiasm. The referendum had shown that further resistance would be futile, and the Council, led by its chairman, Dr. Guy Dain, favored acceptance of the National Health Service as the only practicable course open. A strong minority, however, was prepared to oppose that decision. The group from Marylebone led by Lord Horder spearheaded the attack upon the Council. Even before Dain could open the discussion, it moved that the Council resign, and 38 per cent of the delegates supported that motion. The right of the Council to hold the April plebiscite was sharply challenged. It was this questionnaire, the opposition declared, that had spread confusion in the rank and file and "split the profession far more effectively than Mr. Bevan could have dreamed of doing." A good majority of the delegates condemned the referendum as premature.

In defending the policy of the Council, the Chairman sought to balance the demands that were granted against those that were not, and he found that the Association had won notable concessions and assurances which were sufficient to protect the freedoms of the medical profession. He reminded the delegates that for thirty years under the National Health Insurance the Ministry of Health had dealt fairly with the profession and had always consulted it about regulations. He recognized failure on the issue of good will and appeal to the courts, but insisted that "on practically every other matter we have succeeded either in getting rid by agreement of the difficulties which confronted us or modifying them in such a way that they will be practically non-existent." He reminded the delegates of the unexpected split in 1912-13. There were at present, he said, all shades of opinion in the Association. Some doctors opposed the Act because they resented a national health service and would not take part in it under any conditions. Others opposed the law but desired a comprehensive health service. The latter group, he averred, had now been placated, and a cleavage of opinion had developed in the Council and among the membership as a result. Rejection of the new scheme, he warned, would leave the profession divided and weak. It was only by remaining strong and united, he emphasized, that the Association would be able "to determine the conditions of service for those of us who are here today and those who follow after for many years to come."

Lord Horder spoke in hot anger, condemning the Council and what he considered was its policy of betrayal. Only if all the conditions were met, without deviation or compromise, should the National Health Service be accepted. This was the strategy of the Council and the Association, he explained, when the membership stood together as an invincible force. What happened, he wondered, to this "vaunted" unity? "Where did the rot set in? Was too much attention paid to the stragglers and deserters so that some of the generals on the other side said to each other: 'We are going to be left—let's go home?' What was this 'resounding' victory which had been achieved? It was the assurance of the Minister that they would not lose their liberty all at once. The Minister was demonstrating the age old truth that no man or no state lost his liberty all at once." Vainly Lord Horder urged the Representative Assembly "to arouse itself and resume the fight." "Resistance will grow," he promised, "and, like all resistance movements against defeatism, it will eventually succeed."

Others felt as Lord Horder did. One doctor, a member of the Council, referred to the debate as the "El Alamein of British medicine, for what they did today would decide the course of medical practice for a hundred or more years to come." He could not believe that the concessions which they were unable to win as free men they would obtain as state servants. The Association, he said, was being offered its "last chance of fighting back."

However "tragic" the meeting or strong the "smell of appeasement," the majority of delegates recognized realities. Resistance was no longer expedient. Dr. Dain was convinced that, in compelling the government to accept an amendment to the law, the Association had won a great victory. Actually, this point was debatable, but not so was the rush of doctors to accept service in the new program. Already more than one-fourth of the general practitioners had joined, and many more had indicated they would do so. Time had run out. The resolution of the Council to accept the National Health Service was sustained, and one of the most dramatic sessions in medical annals passed into history.[39]

A new spirit seemed to prevail at Tavistock Square. The *British Medical Journal* opined that the ordeal of the past six years had brought new strength and prestige to the Association, which, through negotiation, had so modified the Health Service that it was now "possible for the medical profession to take a foremost and active part in moulding it according to the highest traditions of a learned society."[40] In a letter to *The Times* (London), the Chairman of the Council reassuringly wrote, "I believe I speak for the overwhelming majority of the medical profession when I say that there will be no shortage of good will on the part of the profession and that it will seek to make the new public service the best which is humanly possible under present circumstances."[41]

As the appointed day approached, the *British Medical Journal,* in a leading article called "Retrospect and Prospect," hailed the National Health Service as "the most ambitious scheme yet launched." The need was acknowledged for such a comprehensive health plan even for the middle class. The increasing expense of medical care placed such a heavy burden upon the family that it was only logical that the cost should be borne by the entire community. "The price Britain will have to pay for this new service is high," it was admitted, "but the fact that the country is prepared to pay this high price shows that it is well aware that on the crude economic level an efficient medical service will pay a good dividend in health, happiness, and efficiency in work."   There were dangers in a state medical service, but there was also "the opportunity to mould the new service in a real partnership of enterprise . . . with the Ministry of Health."   Mistakes would be made, it was predicted, and there would be "much trial and error before anything like a perfect medical service comes into being."[42]

The Lancet was hopeful about the new era that was dawning, but its optimism was tempered by the limitations in the existing medical facilities.   In greeting the new service, this journal stressed the benefits that would be conferred on "medicine by lessening the commercial element in its practice."   "Now that everyone is entitled to full medical care," it was observed, "the doctor can provide that care without thinking of his own profit or his patient's loss and can allocate his efforts more according to medical priority."   In conclusion the editorial cautioned that the National Health Service must be thought of not as a "state service" but as "our service," and then only would it become an increasing success.[43]

The reaction of the ordinary doctor must have been mixed.   One effect of a free health service would be the elimination of charity patients, and one doctor at least viewed this with regret.   Writing in one of the more specialized medical journals, he mentioned that there was a deep satisfaction in administering to poorer clergy and other patients who could not pay, "whose unsolicited thanks" brought him pleasant recollections.   "Those of us," he wrote, "who worked at Moorfields on Mondays and Thursdays in the early years of this century will recall how Sir Arnold Lawson's desk was usually piled high with bunches of flowers, a tribute alike to his professional ability and kindness of heart.   We fear that in the future these floral tributes will largely disappear along with much of the competition and friendly rivalry of the past."[44]

In appraising the conflict which occurred in the British Medical Association over the acceptance of the National Health Service and the subsequent division in sentiment toward the program, it must be remembered that doctors varied in their clientele, character of work, economic status, and location, and that these factors often determined their medico-political philosophy.   The practitioners who served the working class and who looked to panel patients for a substantial proportion of their remuneration were more receptive and could more easily make the adjustment to the new service than the resort and suburban physicians whose income was derived much more from fee-paying middle- and upper-class patients. From this latter group came the most concentrated opposition. Eminent specialists and physicians, who were able to command substantial fees, naturally resented a free hospital and outpatient service. But the less affluent and younger consultants reacted more favorably to sessional work in the hospitals that carried adequate salaried remuneration.

To what extent the more affluent and more conservative doctors controlled the policy of the British Medical Association cannot easily be determined, but they had the leisure and money to afford the luxury of medico-politics. They were over-represented in the Assembly and the Council, whereas the average practitioner in the industrial and rural areas could seldom afford and rarely had the time for such activity. He was badly represented. It was not until 1956 that elected representatives to centrally arranged meetings were finally granted a subsistence allowance.[45] While the conservative element may have exerted proportionately more influence at Tavistock Square than any other group, it is also true that the Association was responsive to rank-and-file demands, if they were sufficiently vocal. The leadership fought vigorously for better terms and greater remuneration and in other ways tried to protect the interests of the average member. If the Association, in its policy toward the National Health Service, did not always reflect the sentiment of the majority, that did not matter so much. What really counted was the fact that the leadership was able to steer a course which, despite sharp differences of opinion, prevented a split in 1948. Indeed, the organization grew in strength and unity, and by 1960 an all-time high enrollment of over 73,000 was reached, with 79 per cent of the working profession having membership.[46]

Acceptance of the National Health Service by the Association did not diminish the deep resentment shared by hundreds of doctors, who, under the leadership of Lord Horder, formed the Fellowship For Freedom in Medicine, a militant organization designed primarily to protect private medicine. Although seventy-eight years old, Lord Horder accepted the chairmanship so he could continue the fight which he had lost as a member of the Council and of the Representative Assembly of the British Medical Association. He had acquired a reputation as a distinguished Harley Street consultant and became even better known in medico-politics, for his flair for pungent speech-making won him considerable publicity. To Lord Horder, no greater misfortune could have befallen British medicine than nationalization, which he had warned would be as disastrous as church domination during the medieval era, or even worse, because "at least the church was cultured." He predicted that the progress of medicine would be set back one hundred years.[47]

Two things, he affirmed, were vital to a doctor: satisfaction in his work and a feeling of economic security, and both would be lost under "state medicine." He charged that the doctors had surrendered "like a rabble" and that the weakness of the profession was partly responsible for the National Health Service being "born in dishonor." "We let ourselves be used as pawns in the game instead of masterpieces," he lamented, with the result that "the living power of medicine" has been lost to the "dead machinery of the bureau." For all of his gloomy utterances, he was hopeful that the medical profession could recapture its freedom, and it was to that end that the Fellowship For Freedom in Medicine was dedicated.[48]

In response to a letter which he published in the *British Medical Journal* and *The Lancet,* he received hundreds of replies from doctors who were concerned about the future of medicine. Fortified by such an outpouring of feeling, Lord Horder called a meeting in the fall of 1948, and the new organization was born. In no way an opposition body to the British Medical Association, it sought rather to influence the policy of the medical profession. The Fellowship was not set up with any permanence in mind. Once its principles were adopted by the British Medical Association or otherwise achieved, it was pledged to dissolve. Its purpose was to reform the National Health Service so that private medicine would not be stifled or in any way restricted. Among its specific objectives were free drugs and grants-in-aid for private patients and the restoration of the sale of good will; among its broader goals were the "preservation of the ethical and professional freedom of the individual doctor" and the maintenance of "the highest standards of medical practice."[49] Its bulletins and printed memoranda vigorously publicized its views. No opportunity was lost to exploit any apparent weakness in the new service.

The membership grew until it reached a peak in 1951 of over 3,000 doctors; thereafter the number declined, until by 1958 it had approached 2,000, a figure which showed little variation during the next two years.[50] If the organization drew its strength primarily from "elderly doctors and diehards," as alleged, then the failure to offset the deaths and resignations of old members by new recruits could be expected to produce a progressive reduction in size and influence. But if waning membership had any effect upon the Fellowship's spirit of resistance, it was not apparent in the publications of the organization, nor did the death of Lord Horder during the summer of 1955 diminish in any way its determination to press home its attacks upon the National Health Service.

If the Service had hostile critics, it also had its advocates. Among them was the Socialist Medical Association. Founded in 1930, this organization was committed to the creation of a nationalized health service and toward that end directed most of its energies. In 1933, the Socialist Medical Association became affiliated with the Labor movement, thereby acquiring a substantial number of associate members. The active paid membership, however, was never very large, the number in 1957 being about 2,000, of whom perhaps not more than one-fourth were medical men.[51] Among the honorary vice-presidents have been many labor leaders, including Aneurin Bevan. Through the Labor Party, the Socialist Medical Association had a part in shaping the National Health Service, and it later claimed credit for much of the "conception and theoretical development" of the new law. The Socialist Medical Association viewed the new program as a great achievement, but deplored the absence of a salaried service and the subsequent failure to give sufficient emphasis to preventive medicine or to carry out the original program of health centers and an absolutely free service.[52]

As liberal but less doctrinaire was the Medical Practitioners' Union, an organization founded largely as a protest against the policy of the British Medical Association in the National Health Insurance dispute of 1912-13. Although registered as a trade union and affiliated with the powerful Trades Union Congress, this group followed a strictly non-political course. Membership remained fairly stable at about 5,000 doctors. The Practitioners' Union has two publications, the *Medical World* for members, and the *Medical World Newsletter* for distribution to all practitioners in the Health Service. In addition, the Practitioners' Union provided its members with advice on insurance, legal, and other matters and sought for them satisfactory terms and conditions of work. Since the inception of the National Health Service, its relations with the British Medical Association have been harmonious, and the two organizations have co-operated on all matters of mutual interest involving negotiations with the government.

As a friendly critic of the new program, the Medical Practitioners' Union had little patience with those who sought to exploit the "temporary difficulties and frustrations of the service." While recognizing that the new scheme deserved much credit for "the very great improvement in the health of the people," the Union contended that the program could be made more effective through health centers, a salaried service, abolition of all charges, and greater integration among the three administrative divisions. Private practice, it felt, should be permitted but not encouraged, "for fear a dual standard of service" would be established. Because it often advanced new concepts, the

Medical Practitioners' Union won the reputation of being "left" in its views; actually its policy has been quite flexible and geared to no ideological pattern.[53]

It is no exaggeration to say that the new service was born in travail and conflict, nor were the years to follow placid ones. Too many interests were involved to expect tranquil conception of a program which, although evolutionary, in many respects represented a rather sharp departure from the past. In addition to the medical group, there were dental, pharmaceutical, and ophthalmic interests. Separate agreements had to be reached with these and separate regulations prepared for them. Only with the opticians did negotiations move smoothly. They welcomed the National Health Service, established harmonious relations from the outset with the Ministry of Health, and continued to give loyal and friendly support to the new service.[54] The dental and pharmaceutical groups, on the other hand, disgruntled and resentful, resisted the overtures of the government for weeks after the British Medical Association had put down its cudgels.

The Pharmaceutical Journal greeted the adoption of the National Health Service Act with the rueful observation that whether "we like it or not our future as pharmacists in shops and hospitals has become subject to state control and dictation, and the nature of our work and the size of our income will be matters in which the state will have a dominating voice."[55] Here, as in the case of the medical profession, the issues of freedom and economic security loomed large. The failure of the pharmacists to get an additional representative on the Executive Council was a grievance, but more serious was the difficulty of reaching mutually satisfactory terms of service. Although the National Pharmaceutical Union did not advise its members to resist the scheme, there was little enthusiasm for the terms offered, and an unwillingness to accept service in the new program was general. As the appointed day approached, however, the pharmacists reluctantly agreed to sign the contract for inclusion in the pharmaceutical lists, subject to any revision in remuneration which might be granted as a result of their application for a higher rate of pay.[56]

The dental profession had the doubtful distinction of being the last group to accept the National Health Service, the one least pleased with the Act or the terms of service, and the one destined to suffer most from a feeling of frustration. The tragic condition of British teeth, the acute shortage of dentists, and the absence of popular appreciation of the need for dental health may have been conditioning factors, but no less important was the lack of unity in the profession. There were three dental organizations, the largest of which was the British Dental Association, with a membership of approximately two-thirds of all practicing dentists. Although a Consultative Committee was set up to represent the three groups in dealing with the Ministry of Health, there was no certainty of solidarity, as indeed was to be proved when the British Dental Association was deserted by the other two within fourteen days of the start of the new service.[57] Amalgamation later eliminated the two smaller organizations, but other weaknesses were to persist.

While accepting the broad principles underlying the new act, the dental profession was apprehensive over the absence of certain guarantees. Not one of the major amendments proposed by the dental organizations was accepted for enactment into law.[58] Early in 1948 the profession pressed the government for assurances and statutory protection, but with little success. Economic considerations and the issue of professional freedom dominated the approach of the Consultative Committee in its negotiations with the Minister of Health. During the first part of June, a very important conference was held in which Bevan agreed that there would be no whole-time salaried dental service in private offices, but rejected the demand for a prohibitive amendment. Nor would he accede to the request for a system of grants-in-aid under which the government would pay a portion of the fees for services rendered to patients. This method, Bevan insisted, was incompatible with a free service. The profession was afraid that its freedom would be threatened by the requirement of prior approval by the government of estimates for treatment and asked that this condition be restricted to dentures. Here also the Minister would accept no modification, but gave a general pledge that clinical freedom would be protected in every way consonant with the best interests of the Service. A few other assurances were given, with the promise of an amending bill for certain matters, but on the major issues the profession felt rebuffed. There was uncertainty about remuneration even after a subsequent announcement that the scale of fees would be reviewed within a year.

By a tremendous majority, the Extraordinary Meeting of the British Dental Association in June sustained the recommendation of the Representative Board that members be advised not to serve under the new law.[59] When the Board met in October to appraise the situation, it was faced by the disturbing fact that the defection of the members to the new scheme had been overwhelming; but it still preferred to persist in its policy of non-recognition and nonco-operation, characterizing the National Health Service as "detrimental to the welfare of the public and to the profession." The Dental Association would continue the fight for revision of the law and more satisfactory conditions of service.[60]

Despite anxieties and forebodings, there was no delay in the commencement of the National Health Service. July 5 was a day of special importance, signaling the fruition of years of legislative and administrative planning. In a broader sense, July 5 was the climax of forty years of social history. The National Health Service was only a part of the new social security program ushered in on the appointed day. There was the Industrial Injuries Act, which set up a new social service for those injured or incapacitated while at work. Financial aid was provided by the National Assistance Act to those whose income was otherwise insufficient. Most important was the National Insurance Act, which granted cash benefits during widowhood, injury, sickness, and unemployment, furnished pensions for the aged and those industrially disabled, and provided payments at childbirth and death. National Insurance benefits were available only to contributors and their families, whereas the National Health Service was accessible to everybody, whether insured or not.

When it came, the appointed day was hailed in the press and at meetings all over the country. Mingled with pride there was the sobering recognition that these benefits were expensive and would have to be paid for out of the productive resources of the British economy. This point was stressed in a nationwide broadcast by the Prime Minister on July 4. In an impressive advertisement in *The Times* (London), the government paid tribute to July 5 under the heading, "This Day Makes History." While acknowledging the various pieces of social legislation as "great landmarks," the government explained that "if we are to have these new benefits and all the goods we want . . . we've got to make more goods. And we ought to find that the freedoms from anxiety that insurance will give and the better health resulting from the health service will help us to answer the call for more and more production." The benefits drawn by the ill, and the old, and the unemployed, it was emphasized, represented their claim on a portion of the nation's production, even though they could add nothing to that production themselves.

There was no illusion about the inadequacies of the medical services then in existence, and a word of caution was given to the public about expecting too much. The Prime Minister commented upon the fact that the war had produced great lags in the hospital and other health facilities. The Minister of Health warned that no overnight miracle would remove the serious shortages of doctors and nurses, but he hopefully pointed out that the medical schools were full and the resources of the nation could now be used more effectively.[61] The *Daily Express* reminded its readers that the scheme could not "begin at anything like maximum efficiency" and urged them to exercise retraint in utilizing the services. The *Manchester Guardian* was not too much perturbed about the lack of adequate facilities, since the law created something solid on which to build. The hospital services were viewed as resting upon a "sound and rational basis." "One must think of the health service," declared the editorial, "as a huge natural organism in process of growth, and not as a creature of magic, called out of the void by the wand of the Minister of Health."

The removal of the financial barrier received special emphasis. The *News Chronicle* recognized that to "care for the sick and lighten the financial anxiety which ill health brings are no ignoble purposes of political action." Said the Minister of Health, "I believe that in a few years' time we shall look back with astonishment on the days when people had to face bills at the same time as they struggled with illness and misfortune. This scheme will be of special value to many families of the middle and professional classes so often hit cruelly hard by heavy surgical and medical fees which have a habit of coming at the wrong moment." The elimination of fees, he felt, would greatly improve the doctor-patient relationship and would remove an aspect of practice which many practitioners found disagreeable.[62] The *Times* (London) observed that the doctor would now become more of a social servant, partly because fee-paying would no longer determine medical care, but even more because it was becoming difficult for a practitioner to remain aloof from the general social services that protected the family.

In a letter published by *The Lancet,* the Minister of Health disclosed to the medical profession the picture which he had always visualized: "one, not of 'panel doctoring' for the less well-off, nor of anything charitable or demeaning, but rather of a nation deciding to make health-care easier and more effective by pooling its resources— each sharing the cost as he can through regular taxation and otherwise while he is well, and each able to use the resulting resources if and when he is ill." He remarked that the doctors would play an important role in the administration of the new service and pledged vigilance in seeing that their scientific and intellectual freedom would in no way suffer. "In this comprehensive scheme," he declared, "— quite the most ambitious adventure in the care of national health that any country has seen—it will inevitably be you, and the other professions with you, on whom everything depends. My job is to give you all the facilities, resources, apparatus and help I can, and then to leave you alone as professional men and women to use your skill and judgement without hindrance."[63]

CHAPTER IV

Administration of the National Health Service

POPULAR RESPONSE to the National Health Service was overwhelmingly favorable. When the appointed day arrived, at least three-fourths of the population had been accepted by Health Service doctors, and subsequently the total reached 97 per cent, where it leveled off. No less impressive was the record of the professions, which rallied almost as promptly to accept service in the scheme. Within three months, about 80 per cent of the dentists and an even larger proportion of the general medical practitioners had joined, and when the service became stabilized not more than 6 per cent of the dentists, 2 per cent of the family doctors, and even fewer pharmacists elected to remain out of the program. The number of practitioners refusing to serve as National Health Service doctors dwindled to an estimated 600.[1] In recognition of the almost universal acceptance of the new service, an article in one of England's more liberal journals declared:

A year is a brief span in the life of such a scheme. Indeed, even the well-wishers of the Service can marvel with the Select Committee on Estimates that "the scheme is settling down with surprisingly little friction." That certainly would not have been expected from the blusterings of the B.M.A. a year ago. Then it looked as though the scheme would be frustrated by the reluctance of the family doctors, resentful at being corralled. There was a misgiving that the public would be slow to join the scheme and that, in any event, the middle-class would boycott it. How differently things have turned out! . . . To make the scheme work the Minister had to recruit 19,000 family doctors. He got 20,600, or 86 per cent, of the country's total. So well did the "Doctors' Rebellion" advertise the Appointed Day—July 5, 1948—that 95 per cent of the population registered from the inception.[2]

The *British Medical Journal* had predicted "endless confusion in the administration" of the new service and great popular disappointment.[3] Neither of these conditions characterized the first or any subsequent year of the program. But there were hospital waiting lists, overcrowded doctors' offices, and shortages in personnel and equipment that hampered the Service without crippling or demoralizing it. These deficiencies were not new. The National Health Insurance had long been similarly afflicted; the National Health Service inherited the deficiencies and, since its scope was much larger, found the strain on its medical resources greater as well.

The new scheme was inaugurated at a time when Great Britain had not recovered from the war. She was still handicapped by rationing and lacked sufficient resources to remove the defects that had been accumulating for years. The tripartite character of the National Health Service machinery blocked the most efficient utilization of all the facilities. The nationalization of such a great array of hospitals posed a major difficulty in modernization and expansion. Notwithstanding all this, the Service quietly accomplished an incalculable amount of good in relieving human misery and dispelling financial worry—and, what is more, promised an increasingly greater realization of its potentialities.

For the most part the new service started smoothly, something the British Medical Association was quick to acknowledge, but there were problems and misunderstandings that aroused comment in Parliament and the press. There were, for instance, doctors, perhaps only a small minority, who by pressure or persuasion endeavored to prevent patients who could afford to pay private fees from getting on the National Health Service list. Some practitioners refused to serve such patients except on a fee-paying basis or informed them that only by remaining private patients could they expect "to get the consideration, care and attention to which they had been accustomed." Doctors in select residential areas had depended almost wholly on private fees, and for some of them the transition to a capitation basis meant a financial loss. It was disquieting and even depressing for such physicians to see their private patients seek free service.

When a number of such cases were paraded before the House of Commons, the Minister of Health expressed the conviction that responsible medical opinion condemned these misrepresentations and circumventions. The British Medical Association did disapprove of any discrimination against patients because of financial status or because, as children or old people, treating them involved more time and effort, but the Association was careful to point out that "free choice works both ways" and that doctors had a perfect right to choose their patients. There were two misapprehensions that the medical profession desired to clear up: first, that everybody was required to be on a National Health Service list, and second, that private practice was no longer lawful. Both were incorrect.[4]

The *British Medical Journal* could see advantages and disadvantages in the new service. Junior hospital posts paid higher salaries than formerly. A newly qualified doctor stood a good chance of getting a house appointment, if not in a teaching hospital then in one of the associated regional hospitals. Although many registrars were gloomy about the prospects of becoming consultants, the National Health Service had made hospital work more attractive while making competition keener. The *Journal* even found entrance into general practice to be much easier, now that the purchase of a practice was no longer permitted. The Association, however, was disturbed about the volume of work that burdened some of the practitioners.[5]

In appraising the first year of the National Health Service, Aneurin Bevan admitted that in some parts of the country family physicians were overworked and that it would take time for the scheme to make proper adjustments. While recognizing this shortcoming and others, he denied that they were the "result of intrinsic defects," and insisted that they occurred as a result of the "overwhelming volume of need" which the new program had disclosed. In the past there had been a tremendous amount of "silent suffering and preventable pain." He observed that present facilities were not adequate and that until more could be provided there would necessarily be difficulties. Although there was evidence of some abuse, the great majority of the professional people were devoted and conscientious, he felt, performing their work in exemplary fashion. He pictured the year as having begun in an atmosphere of doubt, controversy, friction, and great hope. During the year there were, he acknowledged, shortages, gratitude to the Service, relief at its method of operation, friction here and there, and "much silent good work," but on the whole he believed the results had been exceptionally good.[6]

The Practitioner, a magazine that recognized no politics and was the spokesman for no organization or group, undertook an impartial survey of the initial year of the Health Service. A number of experts in various fields were invited to contribute to the project. In order to encourage absolute objectivity, all articles, whether individual or joint efforts, were published anonymously in a special edition of the journal. The coverage was broad, including almost every professional phase of the new service.

In summarizing the evidence, *The Practitioner* acknowledged that a year was too little time to enable the Service to be viewed with true perspective. Some people had expected too much. Obviously an act of Parliament could not suddenly increase the number of nurses, practitioners, or available hospital beds, and since most doctors had been working to the full extent of their capacity before the inception of the Service, they could not do much more. In the hospital picture, little change could or did occur in so far as inpatient treatment was concerned. Owing to the shortage of nurses, there was little or no increase in the number of beds, but the waiting lists, if anything, had grown larger. The outpatient departments, however, served far more patients—the increase in some metropolitan hospitals was 40 per cent. *The Practitioner* expressed the hope that health centers would in due time ease the increasing burden on the hospitals. For almoners the new law had proved a boon. They could now devote their full time to social work, because they no longer had to appraise the financial ability of patients to pay hospital bills.

The administration of the hospital service had begun with a minimum of difficulty. The selection of hospital boards had been "made with wisdom and breadth of vision." The integration of hospitals on a regional basis was being accomplished with the full support and co-operation of the medical profession. The availability of specialists to outlying hospitals through a system of rational planning was one of the most promising aspects of the scheme. No longer would people in remote areas have to make laborious journeys to metropolitan hospitals for specialist services. Another significant and hopeful development that impressed *The Practitioner* was the establishment of special geriatric clinics in several hospitals (formerly public assistance institutions). No aspect of medicine had been more neglected than the care of the aged.

The family doctor situation was less encouraging than many other aspects of the new service. Here *The Practitioner* could see both difficulties and advantages. In spite of the fears about the regulation of the distribution of doctors, the Medical Practices Committee had performed satisfactorily, giving no offense to the medical profession. In some districts the National Health Service had brought a greater measure of co-operation among physicians. The old spirit of rivalry was yielding to a friendlier frame of mind that had resulted in rota arrangements that gave participating practitioners more leisure. The new bill of amendment had eased professional fears on the issue of partnership and other vital problems. But in such matters as pressure of work and financial security, the new scheme had not proved an unmixed blessing. Practitioners in crowded areas, with large lists, benefited financially, while also being relieved of the bother of dispensing drugs; but in sparsely settled areas the doctors traveled long distances, dispensed their own drugs, and could less easily refer patients to hospitals. And with small lists, their economic position had grown worse. Where numbers counted, the conscientious physician was at a disadvantage as compared to the "practitioner who was quick but not so thorough."[7]

A very revealing article in *The New Statesman and Nation* placed in perspective the successes and failures of the first year. The most conspicuous weaknesses were in the ancillary services—dental and ophthalmic—where demand had completely overwhelmed the limited facilities and had skyrocketed costs above all expectation. But in all branches of the National Health Service, the evidence pointed to difficulty in preserving professional standards and rendering prompt treatment. There was a pressing need for many more doctors, opticians, nurses, and dentists; and there was an equally great need for health centers where doctors would be able to "work their rotas, get proper rest. . . . and take those refresher courses for which the scheme provides." An overworked doctor was not an efficient one, and a thorough diagnosis was not compatible "with a waiting queue and a ticking clock." In spite of all the shortages and cramped facilities, however, the scheme was justifying itself and the public was appreciative.[8]

How the people responded to the new service was not subject to statistical analysis, but in millions of British homes there was deep gratitude that seldom found expression except in a quiet determination that the new scheme was good and must live. Criticisms of the program were freely voiced, but the almost universal acceptance of the new service did not require testimonials or affirmations; it was there, deep and abiding, well known to the politicans of all parties.

The reaction of one family during the first and most trying year of the program was set forth in the special 1949 edition of *The Practitioner*. When their old physician, who lived five miles distant, refused to serve them as National Health Service patients, they found a practitioner nearer home who gladly accepted them on his list. For this family, rising costs had made private medical care an "increasingly expensive burden." It was the freedom from worry over the expenses of childbirth and any catastrophic illness in the family that made the head of this household, a business executive, appreciate the new service even though, as he well knew, the cost would have to be borne by the nation. With several employees on his staff, he more than paid his share in taxes and social security contributions. He described their new doctor as one whose "conscientiousness is beyond praise." Concerning the birth of his fourth child, he wrote:

Our fourth child was born in May of this year. The whole pregnancy and birth were 'on the State.' My wife attended an antenatal clinic at specified intervals in a nearby town; she saw the obstetrician once. In the evening of Friday, May 13, her labours, and my superstitions, began. I summoned the ambulance, went with her to the Maternity Unit, where she courageously held on until the dangers of the date were over. The baby was born safely and without difficulty early on May 14. At the maternity unit every care and attention was given my wife and the baby; far more care and kindliness than in the local nursing home where for 12 guineas ($35.28) per week, my wife had had our third child two years before. That this time she had a private room on the ground floor was, perhaps luck, but nothing else was left to chance. I think it is fair to say that probably the efficiency and general air of kindness was due more to the personality of the matron and the staff than to the NHS itself.[9]

The editor of *The Practitioner,* Sir Heneage Ogilvie, did not view the National Health Service as "perfect or even very good," but he did resent distortion of facts, and when some foreigners in a quick look at the program painted a picture that had little resemblance to reality, his anger was aroused. One of the worst offenders was a well-known American politician who, after a hurried trip to England, published in a widely read magazine in the United States an article entitled "Granny is Gone." In *The Spectator,* Sir Heneage Ogilvie analyzed the deceptive use of facts made by this American. "Granny," a lady of 62, died in London from lobar pneumonia seven months after the inception of the National Health Service. The Emergency Bed Service had failed to obtain hospital space for her. The incident was publicized in the papers and gave the American the theme for his devastating attack upon the new service. Whether a hospital bed would have saved "Granny's" life will never be known, but the incidence of illness was high at the time and the "dislocation inevitable in the change-over" to the National Health Service was probably at its worst. That there was a bed shortage was undeniable, but whether the new service was responsible for it was another matter.

The American observer claimed that a hernia operation in London required a year of waiting, that the volume of surgery was decreasing, and that Londoners were "getting less than they once did and at a higher cost." Ogilvie replied that these statements "would be good propaganda if they were true." The allegation that since 1948 there was a slight decline in the number of medical students would, he insisted, be of interest to the deans of medical schools, who "were trying to cope with the most fantastic rush of applications in history." In trying to show a jump in Britain's death rate, the American had selected statistics from two quarters in which seasonal fluctuations were reflected and which were therefore not at all representative of the declining over-all mortality rate. He preferred to ignore the infant death rate, which was less subject to seasonal variation and which as a consequence put the National Health Service in a more favorable light in the kind of comparison he made. "Every Briton who knows the United States," declared Ogilvie, "has the greatest admiration for the American medical profession. He admires its independence, its courage, its fertility in new ideas. He cannot but be perturbed by the wave of socialized-medical hysteria which is clouding its usually clear out-look at the present time, and demanding this sort of dishonest rubbish to allay its fears."[10]

Far more persuasive was a study of British general practice by Joseph S. Collings, a New Zealand doctor (Australian trained), who at the time of publication was a research fellow at the Harvard School of Public Health. When he conducted his survey, the National Health Service was less than a year and one-half old, which hardly allowed sufficient time for the old order to be greatly modified by the new. He visited 55 practices, but supported his conclusions with detailed reference to eight.

In the practices that came under his observation, Collings found little that was commendable. Rural practices were largely anachronistic, although much pleasanter for the physicians than those in the industrial areas. The urban-residential practices had superior equipment to work with but functionally were almost as unsatisfactory as their counterparts that served factory workers. His description of industrial practices was grim and depressing. Most of the waiting rooms were "too small, cold and generally inhospitable," and from the point of view of equipment, the consulting rooms "ranged from satisfactory to dangerously poor—with too many approaching this last category." The ability as a "snap diagnostician" seemed to be an essential requirement in these practices. Collings' general conclusion was that conditions in the Service "tend to reduce the work of both good and bad doctors to a common level. . . . The over-all state of general practice is bad and still deteriorating."

Collings observed among family physicians a feeling of "futility and insecurity." They "are having little share in determining their own destiny or professional future, and this is leading to a demoralization which can only accelerate the decline and fall of general practice." The emphasis on specialities and the exclusion of the family doctor from the hospital staff were deplored as indirect effects of the National Health Service. For the most part, however, Collings did not condemn the new law except as it failed to change the *status quo* of general practice. If there was abuse by patients, Collings blamed the doctor who failed to exercise proper disciplinary influence. His quarrel, then, was not so much with the new act at it was with long-term trends and conditions;[11] but to unfriendly critics of the Health Service, his observations were grist for the mill.

Subsequent studies and surveys, which will be reviewed later, convincingly disproved in large part Collings' bleak observations. The practices which he described were characteristic of only a very small minority of doctors. In trying to prove a thesis, he was given to exaggeration and sweeping generalizations. It would seem that "Dr. Collings fell among thieves more often than he would have done had he worked on a random sample."

In the administration of the new program, the most critical test came in the dental and ophthalmic services. The government had prepared estimates of probable demand, but it completely misjudged the pent-up need that would have to be met in a free service. A survey in 1948 at Wolverhampton showed that one-third of all old men and women had inadequate teeth and one-tenth were without any kind of teeth and ate with their bare gums. Nearly one-third had badly adjusted spectacles, many of them obtained from chain stores which did not provide vision-testing services.[12] With the inauguration of the new service, there was a rush for dentures and glasses that soon reached major proportions. Some people, perhaps only a small minority, through careless use of their spectacles or dentures made replacements necessary. Bevan's exhortation to use these services "prudently, intelligently and morally" was not always heeded. But it was legitimate need rather than abuse that accounted for the soaring cost of the two services. Once the initial demand was met, the volume subsided to a more normal level.

There were other problems, such as the increasing cost of drugs and the pressing need for new hospitals, that admitted of no easy solution. The resources of Great Britain at no time had been adequate to permit the full flowering of the National Health Service. The cold war, trade deficits, and the inflationary threat took precedence in budgetary calculations. The policy of the government involved rigid economy and retrenchment, the postponement of this or that hospital building, and the virtual suspension of the grandiose program for health centers, which was to have been the cornerstone of the new health scheme.

Neither fiscal difficulties nor deficiencies, however, could undermine the new service, to which all parties had promised full support. In so far as the National Health Service was concerned, it mattered little which party dominated the government. Sir Winston Churchill told a political gathering of the Conservative Party at Plymouth early in 1950 that his party was determined to make the National Health Service "work efficiently, fully and humanely." The Conservative

Party Manifesto of the same year declared, "We pledge ourselves to maintain and improve the Health Service. . . . Administrative efficiency and economy and correct priorities throughout the whole service must be assured, so that a proper balance is maintained and the hardest needs are met first."[13] When this party came to power in the fall of 1951, the National Health Service went on as before, unchanged except for the imposition of additional charges that merely continued the policy of the Labor Government that some small payments by the patients were necessary as a temporary expedient to raise revenue and to encourage a more frugal and judicious use of the Service. Significantly, the first two of the amending acts to the National Health Service Law, passed in 1949 and 1951, were sponsored by the Labor Government, while the third one, passed in 1952, was initiated by the Conservatives. None of them made any fundamental alteration in the law.

The Amendment Act of 1949 was in redemption of a pledge to the medical profession. Its chief purposes were to prohibit a full-time salaried service for general medical and dental practitioners and to validate all medical partnership agreements in existence on July 5, 1948, regardless of the abolition of the sale of good will. Provision was made, however, for equitable alternative settlements; should a partner claim to have suffered hardship by virtue of the Act of 1946, he could refer the matter to arbitration. The Amendment Act further established that whole-time hospital employment of all specialists could not be established by Service regulation. The government was granted the authority to make charges for pharmaceutical services and could require payment from foreigners for any medical or hospital services they might receive. The chairmanship of the Executive Council was made elective. Finally, the professional member of the tribunal to which the Council referred recommendations of dismissal from the Service was to be chosen from one of six panels (of six members each) in order to insure that a qualified representative from his own profession would sit on the tribunal judging the person whose conduct was in question.[14]

In defending before Parliament the amendment bill of 1951, the Minister of Health explained that the rising cost of the National Health Service made imperative greater economy and the raising of revenue within the Service. In considering where the charges could most wisely be imposed, the government was guided by four desiderata: to insure the maintenance of all essential phases of the Service, to burden as little as possible those who were seriously ill, to keep collection costs low, and to deter abuses. He explained that the advisability of levying a "hotel charge" on hospital inpatients was considered but that this proposal was abandoned, since "all the patients in the hospital are sick and ill and unable to earn, and the vast majority have lost their wages and receive only sickness benefits."

In surveying all factors, the government decided that appliances and not treatment or services should bear the charge. An assessment on dentures and spectacles, defraying only a part of the actual cost, would raise several million pounds and encourage a more prudent use of these appliances. Generally, neglect of the teeth created a need for dentures, and by imposing a charge upon them the government hoped to encourage individual conservation of teeth. Another purpose of the Act was to accelerate the fight against tuberculosis. The bill provided that individuals suffering from respiratory tuberculosis would be treated outside Great Britain, where climatic conditions were more favorable for recovery. The proposed assessments, it was noted, need not be regarded as permanent and could be revoked or modified by the cabinet through an Order in Council. It was evident from the debate that many members in Parliament entertained grave misgivings about the charges, but the measure passed.[15]

Budgetary considerations prompted the government in 1952 to seek authority to levy charges on prescriptions, certain drug store appliances, and dental treatment. But there would be broad exemptions. Hospital inpatients, students, and all persons under 16 years of age were excluded from some or all of these charges; those charged who were financially unable to pay could recover the amount from the National Assistance Service. Expectant and nursing mothers, and individuals under twenty-one years would not be subject to any dental charge for conservative work.[16] Although the proposed charges were relatively small and in the case of prescriptions even nominal, the Conservative government encountered heated opposition from the Labor Party, which henceforth committed itself to the elimination of all charges. The 1952 bill passed by a narrow margin.[17]

Neither political party was able or willing to use the amending process to correct what was perhaps the major defect in the administrative machinery—the lack of effective co-operation between the three major divisions. Instead of creating a unified system, with all parts completely co-ordinated under central jurisdiction, the National Health Service Law recognized three types of statutory agencies, more or less independent of each other. The hospital or specialist service was directly responsible, through the regional hospital boards, to the Ministry of Health. The local health authorities, however, being elected by the ratepayers, were less amenable to the will of the Ministry, although still subject to its influence. Conterminous with the local health authorities were the Executive Councils, which, predominantly elective, were semi-autonomous but still not free of supervisory controls.

The local health authority, which in reality was the county or county-borough council, performed essentially the same role in the National Health Service as before, except that it had lost jurisdiction over the hospitals. It was responsible for such services as ambulance, health visiting, domestic help, home nursing, vaccination and immunization, maternity and child welfare, and after-care. Under the new law it was assigned the task of operating health centers. The Executive Council was responsible for the pharmaceutical, dental, and medical practitioner services and had temporary control over the supplementary eye service. The remaining class of agency, the regional hospital board, constituted the third leg of the tripod which supported the new program. Mutually dependent, the three divisions should have been brought under more centralized control. As matters stood, they were given no statutory liaison, and such co-operation as existed was largely voluntary or had been achieved through the interlocking membership of some of the boards and committees.

In the evolutionary character of the National Health Service can be found the primary reason for the tripartite arrangement. The local health authorities were in a sense a vested interest and could not very easily be deprived of their long-established role in administering certain health services, nor was such a policy deemed advisable in view of the consensus favoring a decentralized program. The old Insurance Committees, having proved their usefulness, were reorganized under the new title of Executive Councils. Since the medical profession demanded and public opinion endorsed the integration of the hospitals on a regional basis, a new and radical approach was required. Here the new service was to achieve its greatest triumph.

The National Health Service Act of 1946 imposed upon the Minister of Health the duty "to promote the establishment in England and Wales of a comprehensive health service designed to secure improvement in the physical and mental health of the people . . . and the prevention, diagnosis and treatment of illness." In order to carry out this assignment, the Minister of Health was granted a vast amount of legal power, especially in his relationship with the hospitals. He was specifically directed "to meet all reasonable requirements" for hospital and specialist services, and through his management of hospital finance and by virtue of his appointive power, he was able to wield a large measure of control. In dealing with local health authorities and Executive Councils his authority was more circumscribed.[18]

In shaping the Service, the government had desired to avoid the danger of too much centralization and so provided for the exercise of considerable authority at the periphery of the Service by voluntary boards, committees, and councils. The delegation of some of the power, however, was discretionary with the Minister, who, because of his own reponsibility to Parliament, naturally hesitated to relinquish it. This was particularly true of finance. Hospital boards, while exercising considerable autonomy in non-financial matters, suffered at times from a feeling of frustration because of the tight grip the Minister of Health kept on expenditures. The increasing cost of the hospital service forced upon the government stringent financial controls, which were exercised by the Minister through his supervision of the budget for each regional board.[19]

The law made provision for an advisory body of 41 members, the Central Health Services Council, which was predominantly professional. Aside from the six heads of medical bodies, who served on the Council ex officio, all other professional members were appointed by the Minister of Health in consultation with the appropriate professional bodies. While all major professional groups were represented, the medical practitioners, with fifteen members, constituted the largest category. In addition to the nine standing advisory committees of the Council, *ad hoc* committees were set up whenever the occasion required special reports. Meeting quarterly, the Central Health Services Council prepared memoranda for the Minister and once a year published a report that was laid before Parliament.[20]

No difficulty was experienced in putting the ophthalmic, pharmaceutical, and practitioner services into operation. The Executive Councils, which replaced the Insurance Committees, continued to perform about the same administrative functions, though their volume of work more than doubled and additional office space and personnel had to be obtained. In no other area was the continuity between the National Health Insurance and the National Health Service greater. When the appointed day arrived, it was little more than a matter of hanging out a new shingle and broadening operations. Since the doctors would not be civil servants or local government officers and since they preferred to serve the public under contract on a capitation-fee basis, the old system continued in force, except that the contracts were now with the Executive Councils.

As before, the work of these Councils was mostly routine, consisting of registration and the maintenance of records and lists. Elaborate cross-reference files were kept of all practitioners and their patients. In the London Executive Council, to cite one example, maps with small flags pinpointed the location of every doctor. Upon receipt of a phone call, the record card of the patient and his doctor could be produced in a moment. The Executive Council and its committees heard complaints, handled disciplinary cases in their initial stages, supervised the enforcement of regulations, and saw that the practitioner service functioned efficiently. The Council was little concerned with shaping policy, a function that was reserved mostly for the Ministry of Health, which, through frequent memoranda, guided local administration. The Council's clerical employees were not civil servants; the terms of their employment, including remuneration, were determined, as were those of the professional groups, on a nationwide basis, either through the so-called Whitley Councils or by direct negotiation.[21]

The Ministry of Health had originally favored amalgamating the Executive Council areas, but decided to leave them conterminous with the local governments except in eight instances. These eight Executive Councils each represented two counties or county-boroughs. There were thus 138 Executive Councils in England and Wales, compared with 146 local health authorities. The reason for preserving the local orientation of the Councils was primarily to facilitate close co-operation between the practitioner and the domiciliary health team. Each Executive Council comprised 25 members, eight selected by the local health authority, seven by the local medical committee, three by the local dental committee, two by the local pharamaceutical committee, and five by the Minister of Health. The Council elected its own chairman after 1949, but previously he was appointed by the Minister, who then chose only four remaining members of the Council. The appointees did not receive compensation, but they were allowed traveling and subsistence expenses. Numerous committees, some appointed by the Council itself and others chosen by local professionals, expedited the Council's work.[22]

The volume of the work and the size of the staffs of the Executive Councils varied greatly. The London Executive Council, one of the largest, served close to 3,250,000 people. Its administrative and clerical staff in 1960 was about 270, and on its lists were nearly 6,000 doctors, dentists, pharmacists, and opticians.[23] Among the Executive Councils, as elsewhere, economy was practiced; there was a 17 per cent reduction in clerical and administrative personnel during the five-year period ending in 1954.

There was some delay in setting up the Executive Councils during the spring and early summer of 1948, owing to the belated decision of the professions to participate, and there was shortage of office space. Aside from these temporary hindrances, there were no complications.[24] Even before the National Health Service began to function, an Association of Executive Councils was organized to share experiences and to promote the general interests of this phase of the

Service. Judging by the roster of Council members for London, individuals of wide experience and broad affiliations were selected for this voluntary work. Of the agencies that were a part of the National Health Service, the Executive Councils seemed to operate with the least difficulty and to earn the greatest commendation. Among the witnesses who testified before the Guillebaud Committee, there was general agreement that the Executive Councils had functioned well, and the Committee itself applauded the Executive Councils for their efficient performance.[25]

It was in the establishment of the hospital service that the most sweeping changes occurred. The government nationalized 1,143 voluntary hospitals with some 90,000 beds, and 1,545 municipal hospitals with approximately 390,000 beds.[26] The sharp divergence in standards, together with the great variation in administrative controls, posed a complicated problem. Since the hospitals were strong in their local attachment, their co-ordination on a regional basis was an achievement of almost revolutionary proportions. Necessity required central direction, but there was a vigorous impulse toward decentralization. The law gave the Minister extraordinary power over the hospital service, but it also turned the administration of hospitals over to voluntary bodies. In a sense, a partnership was created between the Minister and these appointive groups, and had it not been for financial controls, perhaps that partnership would have emerged more fully. Even so, the boards and management committees influenced policy and performed a vital administrative role.

England and Wales were divided at first into fourteen and then later into fifteen hospital regions, each of which was associated with a university having one or more medical schools. Within each area all hospitals, except those used for the training of doctors and dentists, were gathered under the control of a regional board whose primary task was to develop and co-ordinate the hospital and specialist services. Actual hospital administration was delegated to management committees, which supervised the operation of a group of hospitals or in some cases only a single hospital, such as a large mental or mental deficiency institution. Particular types of hospitals, such as sanatoria, were sometimes brought together for administrative purposes, but normally a group included the hospitals within a given area—sometimes a town and its surrounding area or a group of neighboring towns—the purpose being to create a more or less self-contained unit that would supply most of the medical needs of the people within each district.

There were originally 388 management committees, members of which were chosen by the regional hospital boards, members of which in turn were selected by the Minister of Health. In making these appointments, the Minister was required to consult the local health authorities, the associated university, the medical profession within the area, and other interested organizations; in making its appointments, every regional board was under obligation to seek the advice of the Executive Councils, the local health authorities, the senior hospital medical and dental staffs, and others within the area in which the management committee would exercise its authority. The membership of the boards and committees varied in size, according to need as determined by the size of the region or district. Appointments were for a three-year term and could be renewed, but to insure continuity, only one-third of them expired each year. Members received no money except to cover expenses and loss of earnings.[27]

The teaching hospitals (26 in London and 10 in the provinces) were administered separately by boards of governors. These bodies performed the combined functions of the regional hospital boards and the management committees, were subject to the same controls, and were equally responsible to the Ministry of Health. There was some modification, however, in the method of selection of members of the boards of governors. The Minister's appointive power was restricted by the requirement that one-fifth of the members were to be nominated by the associated regional hospital board, one-fifth by the dentists and doctors who were teaching in the hospital, and one-fifth by the university with which the board was associated. The teaching hospitals endeavored to furnish hospital and specialist services of a type best suited for research and the training of dental and medical students.[28]

Despite the revolutionary aspect of the hospital machinery, there was no dislocation in the service during the transitional period. A feeling of uncertainty nevertheless prevailed among the staff, since there had been no opportunity to arrange contracts prior to July 5, but the work went on and subsequently interim contracts became available. Toward the end of 1948 the regional hospital boards were instructed to set up committees of eminent specialists for the purpose of reviewing the status of individuals and of working out a scheme for the future staffing of hospitals. The Ministry of Health remained aloof from the assessment of the medical staffs, but encouraged interregional meetings between these special committees in order to develop a uniform policy. To the public, July 5, 1948, brought no visible change in the hospital picture, except busier outpatient departments and in some cases longer waiting lists. Some difficulties were experienced, the handling of emergency cases in London during the winter of 1948-49 among them, but in general the hospital service was "adequately maintained and improved in some ways" during the first year,[29] and what was more important, the groundwork was laid for future progress.

The law required that the local health authorities prepare plans for implementing such services as were required of them and that these plans be submitted to the Minister of Health for approval. During 1947, many schemes were proposed and amended, the total reaching one thousand. The first year witnessed little change in the tempo or character of domiciliary midwifery, health visiting, maternity and child welfare, and immunization. Vaccination of infants suffered somewhat because of the failure of local authorities and the Ministry of Health to reach an agreement on terms. Except for tuberculosis, the care and after-care of the sick in the homes remained in the early stage of development. The domestic help service was expanded. There was a tremendous increase in demand for the ambulance service, with the mileage in some areas doubling during the first quarter. Few schemes were proposed for health centers because of uncertainty and the advisability of awaiting authoritative guidance from the Central Health Services Council.[30]

It was quite natural that the National Health Service should utilize the Whitley Council machinery in determining rates of pay and conditions of service, since it had long been used in the civil service and in many other non-industrial fields. The Whitley Council procedure for conciliation was proposed in 1916 by a Parliamentary committee under the chairmanship of J. H. Whitley, was applied to industry, and was subsequently extended to other areas. The Insurance Committees, the local health authorities, and the voluntary hospitals had not availed themselves of this machinery, with the result that there was among them great diversity in staff grades, scales of pay, and working conditions. Only a few of the grades, among them nurses, had nationally established rates of pay. Recognizing the need to institute uniform remuneration scales and terms of service in the National Health Service, the Ministry of Health at the outset sponsored meetings between the professional associations and representative trade unions on one hand and the employing authorities on the other. These meetings led to the creation of ten Whitley Councils, one general and nine functional, serving nearly every category of staff employed in the Health Service.

The Whitley Council, in the simplest terms, was a joint negotiating body representing the employee and the employer. Each of the nine functional councils was the bargaining agency for the management side and for the staff side of one division of the Service—medical, dental, optical, pharmaceutical, nursing and midwifery, ancillary, administrative and clerical, and so forth. The general council, drawn from the functional councils, dealt with matters of common interest—holidays, maternity leave, point of entry to salary scales, and procedure for settling differences about conditions of service. The functional councils were principally concerned with rates of pay and other terms of employment, and once agreement in the functional councils was reached and approved, it was applied on a national basis. The management sides of the functional councils might include the hospital authorities (management committees and regional boards), the health departments (English and Scottish, and the Welsh Board of Health), the local authority associations, and the Executive Councils. The staff sides included trade unions, professional associations, and other organizations representing the grades or staff concerned.

In a Whitley Council negotiation, any agreement the two sides reached required ministerial approval, which almost invariably was given. In the National Health Service there was no special tribunal for arbitration, but by mutual consent a dispute could be referred to the Industrial Court, and the decision of the Court was accepted as if it had been a Whitley decision. In practice, the staff side of the ancillary council (representing the domestic workers, tradesmen, and craftsmen) could by unilateral action refer a dispute to the Industrial Disputes Tribunal, and its judgment was just as binding as a Whitley agreement. During the first five years of the Health Service, 23 awards were rendered by the Industrial Court and 40 by the Industrial Disputes Tribunal.[31]

Prior to 1957 every Whitley Council award was approved by the Ministry of Health, but in the fall of that year it refused to accept a 3 per cent wage increase for some 40,000 Health Service workers as recommended by the Whitley Council for Clerical and Administrative Staff. This unprecedented action created quite a furor among the aggrieved employees, who charged the Minister with a breach of faith and who for several weeks retaliated by enforcing a ban on overtime work. The Minister defended his policy on the grounds that acceptance of the award would contribute to inflation. In the House of Commons, however, and throughout the nation there was sharp criticism of government policy in the matter. During the summer of 1958, the controversy was finally resolved after both sides decided to refer the whole question of remuneration to arbitration. The application of a new grading structure was involved, and precisely how the new salary scales should be introduced was left to the Industrial Court. Its decision resulted in immediate pay increases of substantially more than the award of the Whitley Council which had been vetoed by the Minister of Health.[32]

In accepting the Whitley Council method of settling disputes, the medical profession demanded and more or less obtained a position of virtual independence within the general Whitley structure. In practice, matters involving terms and conditions of employment were handled by direct negotiation between the Ministry of Health and the General Medical Services Committee of the British Medical Association. There was no provision for compulsory adjudication, and it was only by the consent of both parties that a dispute could be referred to arbitration, which would be *ad hoc* in nature.[33] The Whitley system functioned least satisfactorily for the doctors, owing to the absence of any acceptable method for resolving a controversy over remuneration after negotiations with the government had collapsed. In 1960, provision was made for machinery which promised to solve this deficiency in the Health Service.

Despite the lack of flexibility in the Whitley Council procedure, it provided on most occasions a reasonably satisfactory mode of adjusting differences for the great majority of Health Service employees. Bitter disputes over wages, hours, and working conditions were usually avoided, and in general the *esprit de corps* among the staff personnel remained good. In case of a grievance other than dismissal or any disciplinary action, the necessary machinery existed, with the right of appeal, to insure a fair hearing and justice.

Although not always successful in negotiation, the professions were in a position to make their views known and their influence felt. So true was this of the doctors that some critics charged there was too much "medical syndicalism" in the administration of the Service. Including the ex-officio members, the medical men normally had a majority in the Central Health Services Council. The Medical Practices Committee, which restricted the admission of new doctors into areas in which there existed a disproportionate number already, consisted of nine members, of whom seven were practitioners appointed by the Minister after consultation with the medical profession. The terms of service and other regulations affecting general practitioners in the Health Service were mostly the result of discussion between the Ministry of Health and the British Medical Association. In commenting on the great number of such regulations, the Minister of Health in 1956 said that "they represented years of patient scrutiny and improvement by the General Medical Services Committee, and, long before that, by the Insurance Acts Committee under the old National Health Insurance scheme, who had met together periodically with officers of his department. They were monuments to an enormous amount of painstaking day-to-day work which had been put in by generations of general practitioners in slowly improving and building up the service they had today."[34]

On the local and regional levels, the professional interests were equally well protected. One-half of the members of each Executive Council were professional, and of this number seven were elected by the local medical committee. Each Executive Council had a medical service committee, to which disciplinary cases were first referred. It was composed of six members, one-half of whom were physicians selected by the local medical committee. Although the members of the hospital boards and management committees were appointed, the medical profession was consulted, and in practice many doctors were selected. In 1959, they represented a little over one-fourth of the membership of the hospital boards and a slightly smaller percentage of membership of the management committees. During the earlier years, the proportion was somewhat larger. In setting up the hospital service, doctors played a major role, serving on medical advisory committees and subcommittees.[35]

Influential as the doctors were, the original policy of keeping them subordinate to lay administration continued to prevail. In professional matters and issues involving clinical freedom, the medical profession was most sensitive, but here the government wisely refrained from encroachment. Clinically the doctors remained as free as ever. It would seem that lay control of the National Health Service administration was largely accepted by the medical profession except in the hospitals, where two sharply differing schools of thought existed. Many doctors insisted that their profession should have the right to elect or at least nominate a definite proportion of the members of the hospital boards and management committees, and they strongly opposed the subordination of hospital medical and nursing personnel to lay administrators, but the Ministry of Health consistently took the position that the members were appointed as individuals and not as representatives of any group or section. Some doctors agreed and saw no objection to lay control, providing the medical staff was in a strong advisory position and enjoyed complete clinical freedom. Their position was graphically set forth by T. F. Fox, editor of *The Lancet,* who pointed out that the hospitals and their equipment belonged to the public and that a host of nonmedical persons worked in the hospitals. Since lay administration prior to 1948 had worked well in the voluntary hospitals, he could see little reason why doctors should administer such institutions. Knowledge of medicine, he insisted, was not a qualification for the administration of a public service. He accepted as sound the "general principle in the N.H.S. . . .

that executive power rest with laymen, advised by doctors and others."[36]

Bureaucracy and politics as they affected the National Health Service were perennial topics for discussion in medical circles. An institution as large as the Health Service could not very well escape criticism, even if appointments were free of political influence and waste had largely been eliminated. The hospital service alone ranked third in size among the nationalized industries, surpassed only by the National Coal Board and the British Transport Commission. The hospital service employed half a million persons and accounted for the largest part of the funds spent by the Health Service. The regional hospital boards and the boards of governors required the services of several hundred appointed voluntary workers. In addition, there were the Executive Councils, each with 25 voluntary members, of whom five were appointed by the Minister of Health. Quite obviously, with so much appointive power in his hands, the Minister of Health, who was a politician, could have been guided by political considerations. These appointments, however, were hardly "political plums," since they carried no salaries and involved much hard work. And, as explained, the Minister's appointive power in the hospital field was somewhat circumscribed by the need to consult with others before making the appointments.[37]

To what extent there was political trafficking in appointments is a matter that does not lend itself to statistical demonstration. It is significant, however, that in the vast amount of literature on British hospitals there are virtually no important allegations about abuse in this matter and there is certainly no suggestion of the need for an investigation. In 1951, an impartial, non-governmental study was made of the voluntary service in the hospitals. The report spoke highly of the original appointees as being individuals of experience in the field, who had previously served on hospital boards. In subsequent appointments, however, there was some evidence of deviation in the direction of political favoritism. In some cases the consultations required by law were apparently merely a gesture, and recommendations made by regional boards were ignored. But it did not appear that this deviation constituted any serious threat to the integrity of the voluntary hospital service. While there very likely would always be some political appointees, such persons, it was felt, might "well prove to be useful members of the Boards."[38]

All of the hospital authorities who testified before the Guillebaud Committee were of the opinion that the system of appointments was "working satisfactorily and calls for no radical change." With this the Guillebaud Report was in agreement, but expressed the view that medical representation on the regional hospital boards and management committees was too high and should not exceed 25 per cent.[39] The Ministry of Health accepted the recommendation in this matter and notified the hospital boards that they were also to comply with this policy in the appointments to management committees.[40]

The Ministry of Health made extensive use of circulars. They were informative and instructive, ranging from policy and regulations to general information. During the interim between the passage of the law and the appointed day, the Ministry was a beehive of activity, establishing machinery and otherwise laying the groundwork for the Service. As the peripheral administrative structure began to take shape, it was inevitable that a large number of documents should emerge from Savile Row to guide the actions of the local and regional authorities. In writing about these busy months, one official referred to the "endless inquiries on points of detail requiring elaboration in correspondence, at conferences, in personal discussions and sometimes in further amending memorandum." The inception of the Service was the occasion for more circulars, and they seemed to flow in a steady stream. Some were statutory instruments, which first had to lie on the table of the House of Commons for a prescribed period; the great majority, however, required no sanction by Parliament. During the two-year period ending in June, 1950, the Ministry of Health issued 29 statutory instruments and 263 ordinary circulars to the regional hospital boards and management committees.[41] To critics of the National Health Service, the issuance of all these circulars was unnecessary and bureaucratic and was the evidence of over-centralization.

The Guillebaud Committee received complaints on this score, and in investigating the matter, learned that possibly a third of the circulars issued between 1950 and 1953 concerned rates of pay and conditions of service as determined by the Whitley Council. The rest pertained to other agreements centrally negotiated or to matters of national interest, or were for guidance in answer to inquiries from the hospital authorities. When the Service was being organized, the circulars were often issued without taking into consideration the opinions of the hospital bodies; but as conditions began to stabilize, it became the practice of the Ministry of Health to engage in regular consultations with the chairmen and officers of the hospital boards, who in turn conferred with their management committees. This policy, together with the steady fall in the number of circulars, should, declared the Guillebaud Committee, prevent much of the irritation which the system of ministerial circulars had occasioned.[42]

To what extent, if at all, the efficiency of the National Health

Service was impaired by political control is difficult to determine. There was no misappropriation of funds, or any scandal, or any evidence that the Service did not function with reasonable competence. Brian Abel-Smith and R. M. Titmuss in their painstaking research found nothing that was the least incriminating in the financial conduct of the Service; indeed, the picture painted was one of prudence if not frugality. And the Guillebaud Report gave the Health Service a clean bill of health. One member of Parliament, a doctor, complained early in 1957 that it was not a question of taking medicine out of politics, because that had already been done. He explained that during his eighteen months in the House of Commons there had been only one full day's debate on the Health Service. He insisted that the need was to bring it back into politics, with more medical men in Parliament.[43]

The fact that the National Health Service was a bipartisan achievement and had the unwavering support of all parties did not mean that individual members of Parliament were happy about the shortcomings or difficulties that cropped up from time to time. In the question and answer period, members often directed inquiries to the Minister of Health. Some may have seemed rather insignificant for an airing in the House of Commons, but they showed a watchdog attitude on the part of the members toward the Health Service. Politics may have prompted some of these queries, but they kept the Minister of Health alert and always conscious of his responsibility to Parliament for the successful operation of the Service. As an example, in April, 1957, a member asked the Minister if he was aware that, due to overcrowding at the Birmingham Accident Hospital, a woman was compelled to remain in the casualty ward seventeen days and there developed a condition that hastened her death. The Minister replied that he had requested a report about the matter. The member thereupon inquired whether the Minister would examine the evidence submitted by a specialist at this hospital. The specialist, the member said, stated that things like this occurred more frequently than was brought to the notice of the public. The Minister answered that he had received medical reports which showed the very opposite, and that was why he thought it advisable to secure a full report on this incident.[44]

In certain circles there was strong feeling about the urgency to take medicine out of politics. Most active in this respect was the Fellowship For Freedom in Medicine, whose chairman in 1952 trenchantly announced, "We have to lift this business of the health services of the nation right out of the political field. The administrator is essential to our purpose; the politician is not only not essential, he is an incubus."[45]   The Representative Assembly of the British Medical Association in 1955 requested that the Council take whatever action was necessary in order to remove the Health Service from "the political arena."[46]   In 1956 the Social Surveys disclosed that, in a 40 per cent response from 1,250 general medical practitioners, 58 per cent replied that they felt the National Health Service had "brought 'politics' into medicine by excessive 'bureaucracy' on the part of the local Executive Councils and other authorities."

It would seem that the medical profession was most militantly conscious of the need to take politics out of medicine when there was a controversy over remuneration.   During the first and last few years of the fifties a crisis over pay developed, and the extreme reluctance of the Ministry of Health to make an acceptable adjustment led to accusations of bad faith and political intransigence.   Once the Danckwerts award was made in 1952, medical unrest subsided and the atmosphere was largely cleared of suspicion and resentment.   By 1957, however, the monetary gains previously achieved had been wiped out by inflation, and the unwillingness of the government to arbitrate the issue of remuneration created anew a spirit of anger and frustration that found expression in sharp criticism of the National Health Service.   Fearful that arbitration might prove costly to the Exchequer, as indeed it did in 1952, the government belatedly and by unilateral action set up a Royal Commission to investigate all phases of the matter—a course which at first infuriated the British Medical Association.[47]

In 1957, the *British Medical Journal,* in an article reminiscent of the acrid editorials of 1948, referred to the "parlous position in which it [the medical profession] finds itself as a nationalized profession controlled in the details of its employment by party politicians."   And another leading article declared, "No one denies that there is much that is of value in the present N.H.S.   What bedevils it is party politics. . . .   What we need is the minimum of interference with the individual practitioner of medicine, and the maximum responsibility for the individual hospital in the management of its affairs.   Medicine in its growing enforced subservience to the State machine is in real danger of becoming static, frozen in a series of servile attitudes.   Medicine needs to be freed from much that is inhibiting in the present scene if it is once more to become free and dynamic in its responses to challenge."[48]

Some and perhaps much of this can be dismissed as pure rhetoric, as can some of the caustic comments from individual members that appeared in the *Journal.*   "Doctors had lost their prestige.   They were dictated to by politicians from the Prime Minister to every

Councillor on the Executive Council"; or, "the hospital staffs should not be the technical assistants of the employing authority but should be free and unfettered professional people"; or "there was no safeguard for doctors improving their ancient traditions or even maintaining them if they were tied to the strings of politics."[49] Significantly, such charges and allegations largely disappeared when the government in 1960, acting upon the Pilkington Report, reached a satisfactory financial agreement with the medical profession.

Quite obviously, any actions taken by the Ministry of Health or Parliament, good or bad, that were not in accord with the views of some doctors would by them be viewed as the sinister machinations of politicians. The imposition of charges for appliances and services, the refusal to restore the sale of good will, the denial of free drugs to private patients, and strict ministerial control over hospital expenditures were attributed by one group or another to political considerations and cited as evidence justifying the need to separate medicine from politics.

Much was made of the decision of the government in 1955 to ban the prescription of heroin. The British Medical Association and other groups sharply denounced the action as a dangerous example of political interference with medicine, "aimed at curtailing the freedom of a registered medical practitioner to prescribe." Reference was made to the black market that such a policy had fostered in the United States. Apparently the Minister of Health had acted upon the advice of the Medical Advisory Committee and the Central Health Services Council when he recommended the prohibition of the manufacture or sale of heroin. In the face of medical pressure, however, the Minister reversed his original position and rescinded the proposed ban.[50]

Another incident that caused resentment was the failure of the Ministry of Health in 1956 to give the medical profession advance notice of its policy on poliomyelitis vaccination. A new vaccine had been devised by British medical research which was considered absolutely safe and effective in reducing the danger of paralytic poliomyelitis, but since the amount available was quite limited, the Ministry decided to carry out the first immunization only through the local health authorities. The Minister recognized that it would take some time to get the technical information to the practitioners and believed that a public announcement should be released immediately. The announcement was made to the extreme chagrin of the doctors, who were soon besieged by patients desiring more information. The Representative Meeting of the British Medical Association adopted a motion censuring the policy of the Minister on this occasion. The

General Medical Services Committee, however, acquiesced in the immunization program of the government, with the understanding that when the vaccine became more plentiful general practitioners would take an active part in the vaccination program. Had the Minister consulted the negotiating committee of the British Medical Association in advance, as was his usual custom, this embarrassing incident would have been avoided.[51]

Whether the foregoing evidence, if such it may be called, could constitute an effective case against ministerial control of the Health Service would presumably depend upon one's medico-political philosophy. The public and the press seemed little disturbed by the allegations; nor did the sampling of medical people with whom the author conferred during his visit to England reveal any apprehensions over the "threat" of political interference with their practice of medicine. There seems to be little confirming evidence that the Health Service was, as one consultant surgeon warned, "a colossal vote-catcher and unless properly buffered from party politics is liable to be used at the hustings."[52] The various studies on the operation of the program, which will be treated later, by no means establish the thesis that the doctor in ministering to his patients and otherwise fulfilling his role as a clinician suffered any real loss of freedom as a result of administrative controls or the impact of politics.

Prior to the inauguration of the Health Service, there was considerable sentiment for control by an independent national board or corporation, and among some medical men sentiment in favor of such control has persisted. The feeling was that a specially constituted organization with corporate status would remove the Health Service from the "baleful" influence of politics and give the medical profession a more dominant role in the administration of the Service. The British Transport Commission and the National Coal Board have enjoyed corporate freedom but, being revenue earning, they differ drastically from the National Health Service, which is almost entirely financed by the state. This factor alone would have rendered corporate status meaningless for the Health Service, which, because of the expenditure of large public funds, would still have been held accountable to Parliament for its stewardship.[53] In explaining this consideration to the Fellowship For Freedom in Medicine in 1957, Dr. Donald Johnson, a member of Parliament, referred to the whole idea as a "mirage which has to be dispelled."[54] The Council and the Representative Assembly of the British Medical Association in 1956 openly acknowledged the fact that it was "impossible to divorce the Health Service . . . from Parliamentary control."[55] And the Guillebaud Report in the same year dismissed the suggestion of a national board or corporation with the comment that a service costing so much money must be "accountable, through a responsible minister," to Parliament.[56]

Sentiment in general was favorable toward the administrative framework of the Health Service. Few responsible critics believed that the imperfections and deficiencies evident in the everyday operation of the program justified or would be materially reduced by any drastic modification of the machinery. Such shortcomings, it was believed, could be handled in other ways. None of the surveys attacked any major aspect of the administrative structure, which, in the opinion of the Cohen Report, had "revealed no fundamental defects" and which represented "a successful evolution from the system of administration which was used in the National Health Insurance Scheme before 1948."[57] "We believe," declared the Guillebaud Committee, "that the structure of the National Health Service . . . was framed broadly on sound lines, having regard to the historical pattern of the medical and social services of this country."[58]

However nostalgic some of the doctors may have been for the "golden age of voluntary hospital committees and the dominance of private practice," those things were gone forever. The great majority of medical practitioners were to condition their thinking to the new order, and among the young recruits to the profession there was little real opposition, since fee-paying patients and the sale of good will were more or less foreign to their experience. But few doctors were to view the National Health Service as being without defects. Even among the least critical members of the profession, the Health Service was viewed not as something static, but as an evolving organism that would undergo changes and modification with experience.

In commenting on the early period of the Health Service, Arthur Howard, a member of the Central Health Services Council as well as of Parliament, observed "that despite personal and professional anxieties persisting through a prolonged period, doctors, nurses, and thousands of other workers, professional and lay, paid and unpaid, have continued over an enormous range to provide the public with continuous personal services of a very high and where possible even an improved character. Such a record would not have been capable of achievement had there not been throughout the service . . . a widespread will to cooperate."[59]

CHAPTER V

Cost of the National Health Service

AMONG THE FORCES shaping the National Health Service, none was more decisive than finance. During the very period that the Service was struggling to get on its feet, it was severely hampered by financial restrictions and adverse economic conditions.

When the program was in the blueprint stage, it was not possible to determine accurately its cost. With the limited offerings of the National Health Insurance as a guide, statistics were projected which served to guide the Ministry of Health in launching the Service. The government viewed the inadequacies of the health facilities as more or less temporary, to be eliminated systematically through the erection of health centers and new laboratories and hospitals. A full complement of doctors, dentists, and nurses would be trained so that preventive medicine, as well as curative medicine, would be available to all. Once the Health Service began to function, however, the carefully prepared estimates proved much too modest and the anticipated building program impossible of attainment. Actual costs seemed to have increased alarmingly, owing partly to the unexpected popularity of a comprehensive free health service and even more to inflation.

Other factors played their part in circumscribing the ambitious plans of the National Health Service. World War II left the British economy in straitened circumstances. Great Britain needed years of peace to recover, but they were denied her with the outbreak of the cold war, which necessitated a greatly accelerated military spending program. The government was forced to trim expenses elsewhere, and the social services suffered in consequence.

Owing to the erosion of inflation, virtually every category of the budget showed sharp advances over estimates, and the National Health Service, no less than the others, spent more and more money, but it is important to note that in pounds of constant value the increase in spending for the Service was relatively small. Looking at the annual budgets, many people could only see larger and larger sums being spent on the new Health Service, and there was genuine apprehension as to whether the economy could sustain the increased expenditures.

The critics lost no time in explaining why the planners of the National Health Service had so badly misjudged the pattern of costs and why more and more funds were required to sustain the Service. The sharp increase in the cost of living was recognized as a factor, but there was a tendency to discount its importance. Some people were more inclined to put the blame on abuses—the rush for dentures, spectacles, and wigs, the improper use of the ambulance service, the over-prescribing of drugs, and the treatment of trivial ailments. It seemed almost a truism to certain observers that when a highly prized service such as medical care became free, people were bound to scramble for it. Other critics ascribed the swelling costs to bureaucracy, extravagance, faulty methods of bookkeeping, and other administrative waste. And even more important, in the opinion of some, was the failure of doctors to reduce the incidence of illness by devoting their attention to the cure rather than to the prevention of sickness.[1]

Until the Conservatives came to power in the fall of 1951, the cost of the Health Service was an issue which that party did not fail to exploit in its attack upon the Labor Government. When the Chancellor of the Exchequer asked Parliament in February, 1949, for a large supplementary appropriation to finance various civil agencies, chief of which was the Health Service, Sir Winston Churchill spoke out in apprehension against what he considered was an exorbitant demand for money.[2] The *Conservative Campaign Guide* in 1950 proclaimed that "one of the most alarming features which have come to light during the first year's operation of the Health Service has been the rising costs of the scheme."[3] Despite all these forebodings, the Conservatives, once in control of the government, were as helpless to retard the growing cost of the program as the Labor Government that had preceded them.

It was assumed by some that once the National Health Service was adequately established and able to serve fully the medical needs of all the people, the incidence of disease would decline, and with it the cost of the Service. The Beveridge Report visualized a scheme that would diminish sickness by prevention and cure—and this concept underlay the plans for the new service. If costs were high, they would have to be paid by the present generation in order to create a healthy basis for society. Posterity would be the chief beneficiary. A healthy people would strengthen the wealth-producing capacity of the nation. The benefits would indeed far outweigh the costs.

In 1952, Dr. Ffrangcon Roberts, Honorary Physician in charge of Douty X-ray Clinic, Addenbrooke's Hospital, Cambridge, published a provocative book, *The Cost of Health,* which challenged some of these established concepts concerning the future costs and expected achievements of the Health Service. He endeavored to show that the extraordinary progress in the conquest of disease during the past half century "had been accompanied by a greater demand for treatment and a greater inadequacy of supply" than ever before, and that the Health Service, however beneficial it might be, could not expect to reduce the incidence of disease. He asserted that higher living standards, improved sanitation, miracle drugs, advances in surgery, and a decline in the death rate seemed to have produced an increase instead of a decrease in the amount of illness. He pointed to the overcrowded reception rooms of the doctors and the hospital waiting lists as proof. He did not feel that Britain's limited economy could possibly support a health service which would be able to keep pace with medical progress and the growing demand for treatment.

Dr. Roberts observed that there were two major categories of disease—acute and chronic. The former, caused by traumata and microorganisms, could usually be cured or prevented by proper health measures, immunization and vaccination, and the use of powerful drugs and surgery. Chronic diseases were primarily afflictions of older people, and, while they were not curable, they could be treated, with a resulting prolongation of life. The treatment of such disorders of old age as degenerative diseases of the kidneys and heart, rheumatoid infections, and senile dementia was often very expensive. Since the proportion of aged persons was growing, chronic diseases would make an increasingly heavier claim upon the medical resources. Acute diseases were confined mostly to the younger and working segment of the population, and the cure of these patients did indeed contribute to the productive capacity of the nation, but the treatment of chronic diseases among the aged consumed national wealth with little compensation except the satisfaction of humanitarianism.

The picture painted by this physician was not encouraging, since the incidence of illness could be expected to make the Service progressively more expensive without achieving the goals set forth by the architects of the Health Service. In the opinion of Dr. Roberts, national frustration and an overtaxed economy might be the results of the ambitious program launched in 1948. Despite all the limitations, however, he was willing to concede that "by the pooling of resources and the more equitable distribution of facilities every individual can now obtain treatment which might otherwise have been beyond his means."[4]

Aneurin Bevan, who as Minister of Health guided the fortunes of the Health Service during the first two and one-half years, was aware of the inadequacies of the health facilities when the Service began to function, but he misjudged the extraordinary demand which developed for dental and medical care and did not reckon with the more subtle effects of inflation. While recognizing the need to restrain the growing expenditures, Bevan was nevertheless convinced that it was a mistake to view the cost of the program as an additional burden upon the economy. It was, he reasoned, "not so much a new expenditure as a substitute expenditure," since it was a "gigantic transfer of expense from the private pocket to the public purse." What had been spent privately was now charged against the Exchequer, but under the new scheme everybody had free access to medical treatment.[5]

The absence at first of any very complete data made it difficult to evaluate the comments concerning the finances and the performance of the Health Service. The Ministry of Health issued reports, but during the early period the statistics were somewhat fragmentary, not well co-ordinated, and difficult to interpret. The increase in expenditure was an undeniable fact, but whether it was the product of inflation, of abuses, or of legitimate growth was not known until the government set up the Guillebaud Committee to make an exhaustive study of all relevant factors. Published in 1956, its report did much to clarify matters and to counteract many of the most damaging allegations.

In preparing the initial estimates of the cost of the Health Service, there was little factual information that could be of any practical use. The National Health Insurance statistics seemed useful enough as a crude basis on which to project figures for the Service, but as events were to show, there was little from a financial standpoint that the two systems shared in common. At postwar rates the government had been spending annually £60 million ($168 million) on the old health program, but whether twice this amount would suffice for a free comprehensive scheme was purely conjectural. In view of the breadth of its proposals, the Beveridge Committee refrained from preparing a detailed financial plan for a new health scheme, but in the Appendix to the report of the Committee, the Government Actuary gave £170 million ($476 million) as the estimated annual gross cost for Great Britain. The financial memorandum for the National Health Service Bill, 1946, reckoned the gross cost per year in England and Wales at approximately £152 million ($425 million), the net or Exchequer part of the total being £110 million ($308 million). At the end of 1947, £27 million ($75 million) was added to the earlier estimate,[6] but this figure also was to prove unrealistic.

Once the Service began to function, the magnitude of the miscalculation became apparent, and as the years passed the costs rose higher and higher. Original appropriations had to be supplemented, despite every effort to enforce the most rigorous economy. The first full year of the program saw the gross cost reach £402 million ($1,125 million), of which the Exchequer paid £305 million ($855 million). The following year the figures were even higher.[7]

Most unexpected was the demand for dentures and glasses, which greatly overtaxed the resources of the services concerned and pushed costs to what were considered entirely unreasonable heights. The White Paper of 1944 assumed that several years might elapse before the cost of the ophthalmic service would reach £1 million ($2,800,000) and the dental service £10 million ($28 million). Yet during the first full fiscal year of the Health Service the government spent £22 million ($61 million) on the eye service and £43 million ($120 million) on the dental service.[8] The great need for spectacles among the elderly people and the neglect of teeth among all segments of the population explain the popularity of these services. Once the backlog in demand had been met, these services were to settle down to a more normal pattern of performance. In the meantime, dentists and opticians worked overtime, earning large incomes. Disturbed by what he considered were excessive fees, the Minister of Health adopted a rather drastic policy of fee reduction, which in 1949 and 1950 lowered the income of the optical profession at least 15 per cent[9] and that of the dental profession approximately 30 per cent.[10] In determining subsequent charges, the government was to pursue an even more rigorous policy, but it should be noted that these two services in 1949-50 accounted for only 16 per cent of the total gross cost of the Health Service. In later years the proportion was to fall to less than 10 per cent.

The pharmaceutical service was to pose a much more serious fiscal issue than either the eye or dental services, and neither charges nor investigations were to resolve the problem satisfactorily. Within three months following the inception of the Health Service, Aneurin Bevan was so impressed with the phenomenal rate at which prescriptions were being dispensed that he predicted an annual total of 50 million of them. The volume for 1949 actually exceeded that estimate by a good margin, and two years later reached 227 million prescriptions. Because of rising costs, attributable largely to new and more expensive drugs, the average price per prescription rose from 32/42d (37 cents) in 1948 to 43/91d (51 cents) in 1951.[11]

Disturbed by the trend of rising expenditures, Bevan endeavored to impress upon the doctors that over-prescribing was as bad as under-prescribing and that it was not "a good thing to evoke merely psychological response by prescribing too expensive drugs."[12] When the Service was barely a year old, the Central and Scottish Health Services Council appointed a Joint Committee on Prescribing to classify proprietary preparations according to therapeutic value and price in comparison with the less expensive standard preparations. But Bevan was no more successful than were his successors in halting the growing cost of the drug bill. Although a strong opponent of prescription charges or any measure that would interfere with the freedom of doctors to prescribe, he nevertheless recognized that free prescriptions were susceptible to abuse. "Now that we have got the National Health Service based on free prescriptions," he observed on one occasion, "I shudder to think of the ceaseless cascade of medicine which is pouring down British throats at the present time. I wish I could believe that its efficacy was equal to the credulity with which it is being swallowed."[13]

The worsening of economic conditions caused the Chancellor of the Exchequer, Sir Stafford Cripps, in March, 1950, to impose a ceiling on the amount of money available from the national treasury for the Health Service. The estimate for 1950-51 was recognized as the maximum that could be appropriated by Parliament, which for England and Wales was in the neighborhood of £358 million ($1,000 million).[14] The ceiling was accepted as binding by the Conservative Party when it took over the reins of government toward the end of 1951. Until the 1954-55 fiscal year, Parliamentary spending on the Health Service pretty well stayed within the prescribed limits, except for the 1952-53 supplementary grant, which provided additional remuneration to general practitioners.[15] This budgetary feat was accomplished, despite rising costs, by rigid economy and by imposing certain charges. These charges were designed to discourage abuses while raising revenue. Provision was always made for hardship cases, and, to insure unhampered use of the most vital services by such groups as students, children, and pregnant and nursing women, further exemptions were granted. In spite of the charges, the Health Service was to remain essentially free.

What were the sources of revenue prior to the imposition of charges in 1951 and 1952? Using the 1949-50 budget as an example, the national treasury furnished 76 per cent of the funds; the local authorities 3.5 per cent; the National Insurance Fund, which comprised contributions from employers and workers, 9 per cent; superannuation contributions, 5 per cent; and other sources, including payments from persons using certain of the facilities, 6.5 per cent.[16] It should be noted that there were charges at the outset for such services as the replacement of dentures and the repair or renewal of glasses if carelessness had been the cause of the damage or loss. More expensive spectacles, dental treatment, and artificial limbs than were deemed clinically necessary required payment for the extra cost. In the case of hospitals, there were private beds available, the full cost of which had to be paid by the users. Those who desired privacy, but whose condition did not require it, could obtain an amenity bed for a small payment, but there was no charge for maintenance or cost of treatment in this instance. Such charges affected comparatively few inpatients.

Until 1959, the local health service was financed equally by local rates and by central funds. Thereafter, the Exchequer contribution to the local health authorities was absorbed into the new general grant to the local governments. As in the other categories of the Health Service, local health spending increased steadily, but the ratio which it bore to the total gross costs of the entire Service remained fairly constant at about 8 or 9 per cent. Except for domestic help, and in certain cases the provision of bedding, nursing requisites, and meals as a residential accommodation, there were no charges prior to 1952. Then an additional charge for day nurseries was permitted, but this, as with the other fees, was required only of those who could pay. The revenue realized from the charges constituted only a very small part of the gross cost of the local health authority services. The great bulk of the local health services, including midwifery, health visiting, ambulance, mental health, home nursing, vaccination and immunization, pre- and postnatal and child welfare clinics, and dental care for expectant and nursing mothers and young children, remained free.[17]

Superannuation contributions, another source of finance, were collected under the National Health Service retirement plan from individuals, but the government contributed an even larger proportion of the superannuation funds. The National Insurance Fund was based upon regular payments from the employees and employers. Administered by the Ministry of National Insurance, the money was used primarily to finance a comprehensive program of unemployment benefits, retirement pensions, widows' benefits, sickness and maternity benefits, family and guardians' allowances, and death grants. Only a small part of the weekly insurance payments was allocated to the National Health Service. From the outset, many people labored under the mistaken idea that the National Insurance Fund largely financed the Health Service, and there were some who utilized its facilities on the slightest pretext, believing that the weekly insurance contribution paid for their right to do so. Beginning with Aneurin Bevan, the various Ministers of Health endeavored to correct this erroneus notion, but with little success.

As early as April, 1949, Sir Stafford Cripps, in introducing the budget, said there were valid reasons for levying some Health Service charges as a source of finance and to impress upon the people that the Service, while almost entirely free to individuals, was not without its ultimate cost.   Sentiment seemed to grow in certain governmental circles that the patient should pay a part of the cost of the medicine, possibly a shilling (14 cents) for each prescription. But when Bevan was approached on the matter he flatly opposed it, on the grounds that if the charge were nominal it would amount to very little, and if it were large enough to produce sufficient revenue it might work a hardship on the patient and restrict the usefulness of the Service.[18] While the popular response to a prescription charge was unfavorable, the prescription clause was not eliminated from the Amendment Bill of 1949.   Yet the government refrained from imposing this charge during the next three years.

Growing apprehension over alleged abuses and rising expenditures, however, induced the Labor Government in the spring of 1951 to amend further the National Health Service Act so as to permit charges on spectacles and dentures.   The necessary Service regulation followed, and, effective May 21, 1951, glasses and false teeth were no longer free.   In the case of the former, the amount required from the patient was £1 ($2.80) per pair, plus the actual cost of the frame.   Students and all children under 16 years of age were exempted from the payment on spectacles.   The charge on false teeth, roughly half the cost, ranged up to a maximum of £4 5s ($11.90) for full upper and lower dentures.   Those unable to pay could obtain help from the National Assistance Fund.   With a ceiling established on future expenditures, the only alternative to charges appeared to be a progressive curtailment of the Health Service, a course which no responsible politician could accept.   What the government did in the matter seemed to be necessary, but it evoked no enthusiasm and much resistance in Parliament.   In protest, Aneurin Bevan resigned as Minister of Health.[19]

Within a year, additional charges were imposed by the Conservative Party, which had come into power.   In the face of strenuous opposition from the Labor Party, no longer in favor of such a policy, the new government secured the passage of the National Health Service Act of 1952 and by June of that year was collecting revenue on a number of new items.   Invoking the Amendment Law of 1949, the government imposed a shilling (14 cents) assessment on each prescription form, to be paid to the pharmacist or the general practitioner, depending on who did the dispensing of drugs. Under the Act of 1952, dental treatment was made subject to a charge of £1 ($2.80) for a course of treatment or the actual cost if it were less than that amount. Elastic hosiery, wigs, surgical footwear and surgical abdominal supports likewise became subject to charges. The local health authorities were authorized to levy a fee for the use of day nurseries. Except for the prescription charge, all students regardless of age and all children under sixteen years were exempted from the new payments. Nursing and expectant mothers and all persons under twenty-one years of age could still claim free dental treatment, which, however, in the general dental service did not include the supply or the relining of dentures, for which there was the usual charge. Such groups as hospital patients, pensioners suffering from war disabilities, persons afflicted with veneral diseases, hardship cases, and those receiving National Assistance were either reimbursed or excused from some or all of the charges.[20]

Professional and popular reaction to the charges of 1952 was unfavorable. Most vehement was *The New Statesman and Nation,* which saw a serious threat to the two basic principles on which the Health Service had been founded—"its universality and the deployment of medical resources in accordance with medical need." It was further averred that the increased emphasis on preventive medicine would be largely destroyed and that "once again, as before 1948, the undiagnosed pain will be allowed to go untended until one more working-class family is stricken with grave and perhaps permanent sickness." The dental charges, it was alleged, would undermine the dental service, since most wage earners would be compelled to delay conservative treatment until extractions again became the standard remedy.[21]

The British Medical Association concentrated its fire on the prescription charge, as did the Pharmaceutical Society, while the British Dental Association was more concerned over the dental payments and the ophthalmic profession was disturbed about the fees imposed upon spectacles. In measuring the effect of the charges upon its membership, each profession could see either a loss of earnings from a possible curtailment of the Service or a cause of friction and annoyance with few compensating advantages.

Both doctors and pharmacists viewed the levy on prescriptions as burdensome to administer and as a barrier to medical treatment. It was alleged that the shilling fee bore heavily on families afflicted with considerable illness. Although there may have been some truth in these allegations, the Guillebaud Committee could find no convincing evidence that the charge hindered "the proper use of the service by at least the great majority of its potential users." So far as prescribing was concerned, it was recognized, however, that the fee may have caused some doctors to prescribe more items on each prescription and possibly to prescribe larger quantities.　While opposed in principle to charges, the Guillebaud Report did not believe that the removal of the charge on prescriptions would necessarily improve the operation of the Health Service.[22]

Approximately 12 per cent of the general practitioners were obliged to do their own dispensing because of the rural character of their practice, and they found the collection of the shilling charge a nuisance.　Often the patient did not have the money at the time and later forgot to make payment.　Collections per patient by these physicians averaged considerably less than those of the pharmacists.　The efforts of the Ministry of Health to improve the rate of general practitioner collection were not very successful because the individual doctors did not always co-operate and the local medical committees were reluctant to take disciplinary action against such practitioners.[23]

It was assumed by the Ministry of Health that a charge would operate as a deterrent to what was considered an extravagant issuance of prescriptions.　To what extent practitioners made excessive use of prescriptions could not easily be measured, but many patients, having great faith in the bottle-of-medicine remedy, demanded drugs regardless of their real need.　Unwilling to offend their patients, some doctors had a tendency to prescribe too freely.　No less objectionable was the practice of prescribing proprietary medicines when pharmaceutical formulae, therapeutically as good and much cheaper, could be used.　Both patients and doctors were influenced by the high-pressure advertisements of the drug companies, and trade names were used increasingly on prescriptions when their equivalents could be compounded by pharmacists at lower cost.

The rising cost of drugs was a worldwide phenomenon and was by no means peculiar to England.　The Hinchliffe Committee, which was appointed to investigate the cost of prescriptions, confirmed in its Interim Report of 1958 that "the increase in the total cost of drugs to the National Health Service is proportionately less than in other countries of Europe and the Commonwealth which have similar (but usually more restricted) systems of insurance."　While other costs in England continued to climb at an accelerated pace, wholesale drug prices by 1958 had increased only 6.6 per cent over the 1949 level.[24]

The effect of the prescription levy was disappointing.　Although at first the number of prescriptions declined rather sharply, the trend was soon reversed.　In 1956 the total reached the record figure of 229 million, or 13 per cent more than in 1949.　Nor did the shilling charge seem to deter the steadily advancing cost per prescription.

The charge, however, was something that the Exchequer had no desire to relinquish, since the revenue from this source represented about 13 per cent of the pharmaceutical costs. But the prescription levy did not prevent drugs from absorbing a larger proportion of the gross cost of the Health Service—between 1949 and 1957, a rise from 8 to more than 10 per cent.[25] Exhortation, education, investigation, and disciplinary action seemed to prove ineffectual. Perhaps the rise in drug costs was not unreasonable in view of the inflationary spiral and the increasingly important role of such expensive preparations as cortisone and hydrocortisone. Yet, to an economy-minded government the need to check the mounting expense of drugs was urgent.

During the latter part of 1956, the government pursued a more stringent policy in the matter of prescription charges. Instead of requiring a shilling for each prescription form, the Exchequer was now authorized to collect that charge on every item. Since the levy was viewed as a budgetary matter, the government did not bother to consult any of the professional associations. Effective December 1, 1956, the new prescription assessment was expected to raise an amount sufficient to boost the payments for drugs and appliances to almost one-fifth of the total pharmaceutical costs. The usual provision was made for hardship cases and National Assistance recipients, with reimbursements to be more quickly expedited. To ease the effect of the new charge on low-income groups, the Ministry of Health decided that for composite or multiple packs, "two or more mixtures of the same type or two or more packages of the same proprietary," the charge would be only one shilling. Nor did the government have objection to the prescribing of larger quantities of drugs at one time for patients who would need them.[26]

Sharp protests greeted the new prescription charge. Neither *The Times* (London) nor the *Manchester Guardian* viewed it as fair to patients requiring many drugs, and both of these journals felt that a more equitable approach would be to raise the levy on each prescription form to one and a half or two shillings instead of charging for each item. *The Pharmaceutical Journal* was disturbed about the effect the charge would have not only upon the patient relationship but upon druggists who would be confronted by a heavier work load.[27] The British Medical Association, no less critical of the new charge, pointed out that it would work a special hardship on chronic patients, such as those afflicted with epilepsy, pernicious anaemia, diabetes, and heart disease. Such persons would often need four or five items every time they visited the doctor. Fear was expressed that those who could not afford to pay the new charge and were too proud to seek public assistance would suffer, with a resulting deterioration in the doctor-patient relationship.[28]

The charge produced less than 15 per cent of the cost of the drugs in 1959-60, which was far below what had originally been expected, and the corrective results were even less encouraging. Although the total number of prescriptions declined appreciably, reaching in 1958 a figure almost as low as that registered ten years previously, the cost of the pharmaceutical service continued to rise. In 1959, even the number of prescriptions began to move sharply up.[29]

The Committee on the Cost of Prescribing in its final report, 1959, concluded that "the deterrent effect of the shilling charge, whether per form or per item, has not been particularly marked." It was noted that both patients and doctors resented the charges as "a tax on illness and old age" and that wasteful habits had accordingly developed, such as the prescribing of larger quantities of drugs when there was no clear evidence the patient would need them. The Committee was of the opinion that the charges had not fostered the proper incentive to keep prescribing costs economical. It was hoped that ultimately the way could be cleared for the complete elimination of these charges. In the meantime, the Committee suggested that the Ministry of Health and the appropriate professions should reach an agreement concerning a limit on the quantity of drugs to be supplied on one prescription.[30]

The ophthalmic service followed a somewhat different financial pattern than that of the pharmaceutical service. The unexpectedly large demand for glasses at the outset came from those who needed them but had never had their sight tested and from those for whom a sight test was overdue. By 1951, the rush for spectacles had eased substantially. This was before the imposition of charges. The effect of the levy was to hasten the decline, with the result that sight-testing and the supplying of glasses by 1951-52 had fallen to a level at least 50 per cent below that recorded during the first year or so of the program. Beginning in 1952, however, the trend was reversed, owing to the growing need for the re-testing and replacement of spectacles, and each succeeding year showed an expanding demand for the ophthalmic service, though at no time did the figures approach those of 1949 and 1950. During the first three years the number of glasses supplied annually averaged nearly seven million pairs, whereas from 1952 to 1960 the average per year was four and one-quarter million.[31]

The optical profession was convinced that the charge, which averaged £1 10s ($4.20) for two lenses and a standard frame inflicted great harm, since it had the general effect of discouraging periodic retesting. For impecunious wage earners and aged persons who failed to qualify for National Assistance or who were too proud to accept it, the charge worked a special hardship, denying to them the visual aid which they needed.[32] The Guillebaud Committee agreed that the levy served as a barrier to the most advantageous use of the service and strongly recommended that the fee should be substantially reduced as soon as the resources of the nation permitted.[33]

Whatever may have been the deterrent effect of the charge, the evidence indicates that only a small part of the spectacle-wearing population had not made use of the ophthalmic service by 1953. By March of that year, 26 million pairs had been furnished to the 19 million persons that wore glasses. A sampling of persons who appeared for eye-tests in September of that year showed that less than 5 per cent of them had not previously received at least one pair of National Health Service glasses.[34]

In the most expensive year for the ophthalmic service, 1949-50, it absorbed a little more than 5 per cent of the gross budget of the entire Health Service, making it even then the least costly of all the services. Owing to a decline in the cost of glasses and a reduction in the scale of fees paid to opticians, prices dropped 14 per cent soon after the service was established. Falling demand, which was accelerated by the charge, further reduced the financial outlay, which in 1952-53 was 54 per cent less than the sum spent in the peak year. The eye service then absorbed only 2 per cent of the gross cost of the Health Service. Thereafter, expenditures on the ophthalmic service rose as demand for spectacles grew, but the amount never exceeded 3 per cent of the total outlay of the Health Service. Payments made by patients ranged between 35 and 39 per cent of the cost of the eye service, which was by far the highest proportion collected in any branch of the Health Service.[35]

The dental service was beset with its own peculiar difficulties. Apart from cost, the major problem was an acute shortage of dentists. From the outset, the tremendous demand for treatment overwhelmed the dental resources of the country. The priority service, which was concerned with the dental health of children and mothers, suffered grievously because of the exodus of so many dentists from the local authority clinics and the school dental service into the field of general dentistry, in which earnings were much larger. Conservative work on teeth was neglected as the dentists labored feverishly to cope with the long-accumulated demand for dentures. It became apparent that, until there was a substantial expansion of the profession, dental resources would have to be allocated where they were most vitally needed, and this could be accomplished most effectively by a system

of charges that would bear more heavily upon dentures than conservative work and would give special encouragement to priority
patients to keep their teeth in a state of fitness.

The dental charges were designed not only to encourage the best
use of the limited resources but also to ease the financial strain which
the unexpected costs imposed upon the Exchequer. As in the case
of the ophthalmic service, expenditures immediately rose to unfore-
seen heights, but once the accumulated demand had been met the
pressure began to relax. The decline in the rush for dentures was
already under way when charges were imposed, the effect of which
was to greatly quicken that trend. From a peak of about £34 million
($95 million) in 1949-50, the cost of dentures fell 74 per cent by
1953, and thereafter began gradually to rise. Whereas dentures
claimed 79 per cent of the total dental budget in 1950, they absorbed
only 27 per cent in 1960. By 1954, the priority service had made
good its losses in personnel, and each subsequent year was to show
gains in the conservation of teeth not only for children, who were the
primary beneficiaries, but adults as well.[36]

While recognizing the necessity for some charges as a temporary
expedient to protect the priority services, the Dental Association took
the position that as circumstances permitted the charges should be
reduced step by step until they were abolished. In the meantime, the
dental profession felt that some modification should be made in the
levy for conservative work. The maximum fee for any course of
treatment, regardless of the number of visits, was only £1 ($2.80),
but if the cost was less the patient paid the actual amount. The effect
of this policy, declared the British Dental Association, was to deter
patients from going regularly to the dentist for the minor work that
such periodic visits usually entailed. Instead, the tendency for the
patient was to go only when considerable work was required, since
the total charge would never exceed £1, whereas a number of regular
visits would add up to much more. The dental profession suggested
that the government should refund the fee to those who visited the dentist at least once every year for the purpose of staying dentally fit. This
proposal was endorsed by the Guillebaud Committee, which could
see in the charge on conservative work an obstacle to the most effective
use of the dental service. It was urged that the abolition of the charge
be given the highest priority as soon as additional resources became
available.[37]

The declining demand for dentures combined with a reduction in
dental remuneration and, more important, the charges to patients to
produce a sharp drop in expenditures for the dental service, which by
1953 reached a level of 34 per cent below that of 1949-50. Begin-

ning in 1954, however, the cost of the service began to rise, and by 1959 it surpassed the record level of 1950. The proportion of the Health Service budget required to finance the dental service dropped from about 10 per cent in 1950 to about 6 per cent in 1953, a percentage which rising expenditures in subsequent years did not greatly alter. In 1960, it was a little over 7 per cent. The payments contributed by the patients in that year represented nearly 18 per cent of the cost of the dental service.[38]

Although the Exchequer viewed the income from the dental, ophthalmic, and pharmaceutical charges as essential, their importance in the general financial picture was not very impressive. Such revenue at no time exceeded 4 per cent of the gross cost of the Health Service. Including all other payments from patients, such as fees for private and amenity beds in the hospitals, the total did not rise much above 5 per cent. What the patients contributed directly was thus only a fraction of the over-all budget. Yet the abolition of these payments would have cost the Exchequer much more than the immediate amount lost, since an absolutely free service would have meant greater demand and higher expenditures. It was this fact, coupled with the necessity of establishing dental priorities, that conditioned the attitude of the Guillebaud Committee. While taking a firm stand against the imposition of any additional charges, the Committee advocated the repeal of the existing ones as soon as the economy would allow.[39]

In view of the steadily rising demand for Exchequer funds, there was no evidence that the government had any intention of abandoning charges at this time. With the average prescription cost rising to 86/92d ($1.01) in 1960, the government in 1961 decided to boost the prescription charge to 2s (28 cents) per item. Prices for welfare foods were raised to cover cost. The maximum charge for a pair of full dentures was increased to £5 ($14) and for lenses to 12/6d ($1.75) each; and the maximum charge for an amenity bed was doubled. Such a bed in a single room would now cost 24s ($3.36) per day. Under the new schedule of charges, however, children and expectant and nursing mothers no longer would be subject to a charge for dentures in the general dental service.[40]

Except for the prescription fee, the general medical practitioner service was in no way provided with a charge. Important as was this service, its share in the total gross cost of the Health Program in the 1950's did not rise above 11 per cent, except for the 1952-53 fiscal year when the Danckwerts award was granted. In 1960, the proportion was not over 10 per cent. A 59 per cent rise in actual cost did occur, however, between 1950 and 1960, but this increase was moderate when compared with the increase of 100 per cent in hospital costs and 145 per cent in expenditures on drugs during the same period. The general medical service, which almost every year had required more money, sometimes substantially more, than the pharmaceutical service, cost several million dollars less in 1956-57 and during the years that immediately followed.[41]

The services administered through the Executive Councils—dental, ophthalmic, pharmaceutical, and general medical—accounted for about 30 per cent of the gross costs of the Health Service. The administrative costs of these Councils were surprisingly small, at no time exceeding 2 per cent and occasionally falling to 1.5 per cent or less of total Executive Council expenditures.[42]

The most expensive branch of the Health Service was the hospital and specialist service which, despite the most careful economy, accounted for an increasingly larger proportion of the total gross cost of the Health Service. In 1949-50, the hospital and specialist share was 53 per cent; by 1955-56, it was 57 per cent. While the proportion in 1959-60 was no higher, the cost of the hospital and specialist services in that year was £415 million ($1,160 million), which represented a rise in the amount of money actually spent.[43]

Most of these increases went to defray higher operating and maintenance costs, but possibly a third of this additional money was devoted to developments and improvements. The replacement of obsolete equipment and the modernization of old buildings took the greater part of the capital improvement funds, but the total amount available, especially during the first years, was meager. Only 3 or 4 per cent of the hospital budget, or an average of £9 million ($25 million) per year, could be used for capital expenditures at first, and even with the more liberal policy initiated after 1955 the total did not rise above 5 per cent before the 1960's. In spite of the greatest frugality, mere maintenance and operating expenses consumed most of the money, leaving little for new buildings. The postwar years were a period of comparative stagnation in hospital construction. With 45 per cent of the hospital buildings more than 60 years old, there was the most impelling need for an extensive replacement program. Plans were developed in the mid-1950's for a gradually accelerated program of hospital construction, but in medical circles and elsewhere there was disappointment over the paucity of the sums to be spent. The budget allocated £12,400,000 ($35 million) for hospital capital expenditures in 1956-57 and £17,200,000 ($48 million) in 1957-58. In 1959-60, the government provided £22 million ($62 million) for this purpose and was pledged to spend an additional £3,500,000 ($10 million) in the following fiscal year. The figure announced for 1961-62 was £31 million ($87 million).[44]

Labor unions, the British Medical Association, and various other groups urged upon Parliament the need for more and better hospital facilities. Some persons felt that the situation called for a capital spending policy of £100 million ($280 million) or more per year.[45] The editor of the *Hospital Year Book* was dismayed at the sums voted by Parliament. The £20 million ($56 million) allocation which was at first envisaged for 1957-58 and was finally set up as the maximum capital expenditure for 1958-59 was deemed much too low by the editor, who pointed out that such a sum represented only a 1 per cent replacement rate of the current value of capital assets.[46]

Wages and salaries were primarily responsible for the high cost of the hospital service. Nearly 60 per cent of hospital expenditures went for this purpose, and any increase in remuneration was reflected immediately in a bigger budget. Provisions, uniforms, drugs, and medical supplies absorbed about 17 per cent, and fuel, utilities, laundry, repairs, and the maintenance of buildings took 13 per cent. Central administrative costs, including administrative expenses of the regional boards, management committees, and boards of governors, averaged 2.5 per cent. Since hospital patients were largely exempt from charges (regular inpatients were assessed no charges at all), all but a very small proportion of the gross expenditures had to be financed by funds from the national treasury.[47]

Despite the handicaps that a niggardly fiscal policy imposed upon the hospitals, they were able to function in a manner that drew the praise of many critics. The Select Committee on Estimates, for instance, in its searching probe of the running cost of hospitals in 1957 expressed satisfaction "that there is no evidence of declining efficiency on the part of hospital authorities in spending the money allocated to them; indeed all the evidence suggests the contrary. Nor [does the Committee] believe that there is much, if any, gross inefficiency or obvious waste."[48] Numbering 2,621 in 1960 and containing over 500,000 beds, the hospitals constituted an empire in themselves.[49] The sprawling institutions of the hospital service, for all of their antiquation in plant, gave exceptional value for the money invested.

What was the over-all cost of the health program? The net cost of the National Health Service—the amount which Parliament had to raise by taxes to finance the program—averaged not less than 78 per cent of its total cost during the first nine years (1948-1957) and about 74 per cent in the next three. In 1949-50, the Exchequer grant represented about £7 ($20) per capita; in 1959-60, it was £11 ($31). During this period, the gross cost of the Health Service, including local expenditures, rose 80 per cent, while the per capita gross cost increased roughly from £9 6s ($26) to £16 ($45).

The total gross cost now exceeded £725 million ($2 billion) for England and Wales. About 10 per cent of the national budget was required to finance the Health Service.[50] For a family of four in 1960, the combined gross cost averaged somewhere near £64 ($180)—a sum which included local rates and Exchequer funds, and all fees and contributions. The total per capita gross cost was thus about 6/2d (87 cents) per week, and for that amount every person had the right to complete medical, dental, and hospital care, as well as the necessary drugs, appliances, and spectacles.

The rising cost of the Service had to be met. Early in 1957, the government decided to double the National Insurance contribution to the Health Service. The expected yield would be about £80 million ($224 million) per year, or more than twice the amount that had been received annually from the outset of the Service and that, in spite of inflation, had undergone no adjustment in the intervening years. Whereas previously all insurance payments went into one National Insurance Fund from which the Health Service received its share, now the Service would have its own separate fund into which its insurance contributions would be paid. The Ministry of Pensions and National Insurance would continue to collect the money, selling, as before, a single insurance stamp, which, however, would carry a specific reference to the part of the contribution that was destined for the Health Service.

In the face of opposition, the Minister of Health, the Chancellor of the Exchequer, and other members of the government defended the National Health Service Contributions Bill vigorously. Since the fixed purpose of Parliament under its mandate from the people was to maintain and advance the Health Service, the question was how it should be done. Rather than raise money through general taxes or new charges, the government believed it advisable to adjust the insurance contributions in accordance with the rise in costs and earnings. The National Insurance Fund, which was originally intended to pay one-fifth of the gross cost of the Health Service, at no time had contributed more than 10 per cent and by 1956 contributed only 6 per cent. Under the new scheme, the insurance payments would provide an expected 11.5 per cent of the gross cost of the Service, reducing the proportion of tax funds in the gross cost from 80 to 75 per cent. The new insurance stamp should dispel some of the confusion about how the Health Service was financed. Whereas charges for medical services imposed a tax upon the sick, insurance contributions followed the well-established principle that a health program should be financed by those who are able to work.[51]

The Labor Party vigorously attacked the Contributions Bill on the grounds that it was a part of the strategy of the Conservative Party "ultimately to finance the National Health Service from contributions by the workers and by charges on the people." The Labor opposition warned that it not only opposed a contributory system but would seek to abolish all charges. Taxes, it believed, were the better way to finance the program.

Conservatives categorically denied any intent to finance the Service wholly from contributions and charges. "Now and in the future," declared the Minister of Health, "the bulk of the expenditure will always come from general taxation." The Minister of Health in this debate and earlier ones sought to show statistically and otherwise that during the five years of Conservative leadership the National Health Service had made gratifying progress. The government was quite eager to refute the allegation that it had malevolent designs against the Health Service or, for that matter, against any of the social services. Indeed, the Minister of Pensions and National Insurance had gone to great pains to portray his party as seeking to preserve and strengthen these services by a sound economic approach.[52] The National Health Service Contributions Bill passed in June, 1957, and became effective in the early fall of that year.

The government soon discovered that the new Health Service budget necessitated a further boost in Health Insurance rates. In discussing the matter before Parliament in February, 1958, the Chancellor of the Exchequer disclosed that in the next fiscal year the total Insurance Fund for the first time would show a deficit and that the deficit could be expected to grow progressively larger. The insurance scheme, he insisted, would have to be put on a sounder financial foundation. The treasury could not assume an unlimited liability for the rising cost of the Health Service. Other resources would have to be found. Such alternatives as reducing the standards and cutting the service or increasing the charges to the sick were open, but the Chancellor of the Exchequer did not believe that the House of Commons favored either of these and was sure it preferred that "the extra burden should be carried by the fit and able-bodied rather than by those who are in trouble."

It was proposed that the weekly Health Service contribution for men be increased to 2/4d (33 cents), of which 1/10½d (26 cents) would be paid by the employee from his earnings. For women and juveniles, the rise in payments would be somewhat less. As a result of these increases, the total contribution from Health Service insurance would rise to 13 per cent of the gross cost of the Service. Contributions and charges combined would then more nearly approach the proportion that in the beginning was envisaged as the proper share for the individual to bear.[53]

The total insurance contribution for pensions, unemployment and disability benefits, the Health Service, and all other purposes would now be 18/2d ($2.55) per week, of which 3.9 per cent of his average weekly wage was paid by the worker and 3.2 per cent by the employer. This did not seem excessive in comparison with the German rates, which, it was disclosed, were 12.2 per cent for the employee and 14.9 per cent for the employer, or the French rates, which were 6 per cent and 30.2 per cent, respectively.[54]

In defending the new insurance measure, the Minister of Health, Derek Walker-Smith, assured Parliament that the contributor was "getting a better bargain than the citizen is in other countries, and he is getting a better bargain than he could have expected in the early days of the service." The great threat was inflation. "All of us, on all sides of the House," declared the Minister, "take pride in the Health Service, though we may feel at times that it requires improvement." But it should be remembered that although "the National Health Service is the object of much international admiration and even of envy, the world does not owe its continuance. We can guarantee its continuance only if we can earn it for ourselves on the basis of a sound economy." In the face of strong Labor opposition, which condemned the proposal as a burdensome levy on the poor, the proposed increases passed by the usual Conservative majority. The new Health Insurance rates became effective in July, 1958.[55]

Three years were to pass before the government again felt impelled to boost the rates. Effective July 4, 1961, the Health Insurance contribution from each male employee rose to 2/8½d (38 cents) per week, with the employer adding 7½d (9 cents) to that sum. Their combined weekly insurance payments for all social security benefits now stood at 22s ($3.08), of which the employee paid 12/2d ($1.71) and the employer the remainder.[56]

That the Conservative Government could be absolutely impartial toward the Health Service was amply demonstrated in the appointment of the Guillebaud Committee. The announcement to Parliament in the spring of 1953 that a committee of inquiry was being set up for the purpose of determining how the increasing costs could be avoided without impairing the adequacy of the Health Service was not well received by the Labor Party. The fact that this committee could suggest modifications in the organization of the Service or make any other recommendations deemed necessary to achieve more economy was viewed by Aneurin Bevan as proof that the Minister of Health, Iain Macleod, was "seeking another instrument by which he might mutilate the National Health Service." But Macleod assured the House of Commons that the enquiry would be absolutely impartial and would not in any way be linked, through the personnel of the committee, to any of the professional bodies associated with the Health Service.[57]

The Minister could have delegated the investigation to the Central Health Services Council, a body of experts on the Health Service, but he preferred to appoint a completely independent committee. Differing widely in background, the members were perhaps as well qualified for an unbiased probe as any group could have been. The chairman was Claude Guillebaud, a Cambridge economist, who was assisted by four others: J. W. Cook, a distinguished research chemist; Miss B. A. Godwin, the General Secretary of the Clerical and Administrative Workers' Union: Sir Geoffrey Vickers, a member of the National Coal Board and of the Medical Research Council; and Sir John Maude, the Permanent Secretary of the Ministry of Health during the war years.

Desirous of having a careful analysis of Service costs as a basis for the investigation, Guillebaud suggested that the National Institute for Economic and Social Research sponsor such an analysis. The task was taken up by Brian Abel-Smith, with Richard Titmuss of the London School of Economics as consultant. For two and a half years the Guillebaud Committee sifted evidence presented orally and in memoranda from more than one hundred organizations and interested groups. Its report, a voluminous document which covered the period from 1948 to 1954, was published early in 1956. There were few aspects of the Health Service that were not methodically covered in the study or had not been carefully evaluated by the commission. Some of its opinions could be and were challenged, but with regard to cost, the conclusions, based on the most carefully assembled data, were beyond question.

The report came as a surprise to the press and the nation as a whole. By critics of the National Health Service, the report had been eagerly awaited as a document that would support their allegations, but to their chagrin, its approach, generally speaking, was friendly and sympathetic toward most aspects of the Service. The Committee, of course, saw weaknesses that required corrective measures. Recommendations were freely offered, but there was no disposition to modify in any drastic way the basic features of the program. Perhaps the most significant effect of the Guillebaud Report was to reveal how grossly the economic factors of the Service had been distorted in the minds of many. The "rocketing cost" had been erroneously interpreted as evidence of excessive spending and, as well, of a long-term trend that was rapidly getting out of control. In coldly examining the facts, however, the Guillebaud Committee could see little proof of waste, mismanagement, and inefficient administration, and certainly no indication that spending was disproportionately high in terms of the benefits that accrued to the nation. If anything, the rate of expenditures was too low. Substantial improvements had been achieved in the scale and quality of the services offered, despite the fact that the amounts spent represented a declining proportion of the national income.

In 1949-50 the National Health Service cost 3.8 per cent of the gross national product, but in each of the succeeding years covered by the study the proportion diminished, reaching 3.42 per cent by 1953-54. The decline in the consumption of the national wealth during that period was thus nearly 0.4 per cent. If the Health Service had consumed the same proportion of the national wealth in 1953-54 that it had five years earlier, the gross expenditures would have been £51 million ($143 million) more, and the net cost would have been £67 million ($188 million) greater.[58]

The Guillebaud Committee could suggest no way of effecting any real savings in the operation of the Health Service or of realizing any new source of income within the framework of the program. Nor was there any apparent hope of reducing the costs without impairing the level of efficiency. More money, not less, should be made available, especially to the hospitals, which, in spite of a splendid record of economy and the judicious use of funds, stood badly in need of greater capital allocations. The Committee, however, did not feel that it could set up goals or determine standards of adequacy for the Service. Parliament would have to decide from year to year what the nation could reasonably afford. In scrutinizing the operation of the Service, the report found little that merited disapproval. "We have reached the conclusion," affirmed the committee in the summary, "that the Service's record of performance since the Appointed Day has been one of real achievement. The rising cost of the Service in real terms during the years 1948-54 was kept within narrow bounds, while many of the services provided were substantially expanded and improved during that period. Any charge that there has been widespread extravagance in the National Health Service, whether in respect of the spending of money or the use of man power, is not borne out by our evidence."[59]

Contrary to the fears expressed by Dr. Ffrangcon Roberts and others concerning the increasing cost of providing hospital and medical care for the aged, Abel-Smith and Titmuss felt that the statistical evidence available did not indicate that there was anything to worry about from this source. Forming their judgment upon a projection of current expenditures for the aged (about one-fifth of the Health Service budget) on the basis of population trends, these experts were of the opinion that the increase in cost for this group would not be disproportionately higher during the next twenty years. There were, of course, imponderables that might alter the picture, such matters as improving the standards of medical treatment for the elderly or establishing for the general practitioner a differential in remuneration so as to allow for the additional care required by older people.[60]

The very breadth of its investigation and proposals made the Guillebaud Report all the more an object of praise and censure. The Fellowship For Freedom in Medicine made no attempt to conceal its deep disappointment that the Report did not contain, as expected, a sweeping indictment of the health program. While conceding that it was not "wholly devoid of merit," the Fellowship labeled the Report as "mainly whitewash."[61] *The Times* (London) was of the opinion that the Guillebaud Committee had "argued the case with considerable thoroughness." The financial task was well done, and the findings, it was pointed out, "should bury the myth that the health services claims have been steadily growing." There was reason to believe, declared the editorial, that it "should be possible to secure a gradually improving service while keeping any increase in cost well below the increase in the national income, provided that the nation does not try to obtain 'ideal' standards of care all round very rapidly and provided that inefficiency in operation is gradually reduced."[62]

Some journals, such as *The Economist,* took a cautious view of the Report,[63] but there were others, like *The New Statesman and Nation,* that hailed the study as a vindication of "both the service and, by implication, Mr. Bevan, who as a responsible minister bore the brunt of ill-informed criticism." Instead of there being "reckless waste and inefficiency," this publication was pleased to note, "the nation had been getting an excellent service rather cheaply." There was danger, however, that the Report might induce complacency. Since it offered no opportunity for economies in the Service, *New Statesman* was afraid that no additional funds would be spent on hospital construction or other projects for improving the Health Service. "Far from being the prodigal son of the welfare state," admonished the editorial, "the service is likely to become its promising but neglected child."[64]

The *British Dental Journal* was in full accord about the position on dental charges expressed in the Report, having recommended it, and was pleased that the Guillebaud Committee had "found so little to criticise in the efficiency of the dental service."[65] The *British Medi-*

cal Journal felt that the Guillebaud Report had aired "in a judicial manner all the criticism expressed about the health service in the last seven years," had stated "the pros and cons of each proposed reform," and had given "an impartial judgment on it." "On the assumption that the state should provide a comprehensive medical service for the whole population the Report," it was acknowledged, "shows that by and large this country has not made such a bad job, which is not surprising in view of the fact that there were some four or five years of planning behind it; and the self-discipline of an established profession made a revolutionary change possible, something which cannot be put into a balance-sheet."[66]

The House of Commons received the document with unrestrained approval. The Minister of Health hailed it as a "welcome vindication of the National Health Service as it now exists." He warmly expressed the gratitude of the government to Guillebaud and his colleagues "for the very thorough and efficient way in which they tackled their terms of reference." The Minister commented at some length on the recommendations, some of which he accepted in principle, explaining that further study would be required before certain of them could be implemented. In the application of other proposals there would be obvious difficulties. The lack of ample funds was the biggest obstacle. As the debate progressed it was apparent that the area of agreement between the Ministry of Health, the Guillebaud Committee, and Parliament was quite large.[67]

The years which followed the period covered by the Guillebaud investigation showed little variation in the ratio between the cost of the Health Service and the gross national product. Until 1955, there was a slight decline in the share of the national wealth spent, a trend that was reversed during the following three years. In 1959-60 the proportion expended stood at an estimated 3.6 per cent. The earliest years of the Health Service thus had the highest ratios, but even those fell short of 4 per cent of the gross national product, which the available figures would suggest was the normal proportion spent by most industrialized countries on their health services.[68]

Any comparison with the United States should be approached with caution. The evidence nevertheless points to a much larger expenditure on health in that country per individual than in England and Wales. The *Medical World Newsletter* in October, 1961, disclosed that American health costs approximated 6.6 per cent of the national income of the United States. The annual per capita amount spent for drugs was then £9 ($25.20) in the United States but only 30s ($4.20) in Great Britain. The annual health costs for each American, it was claimed, then averaged £56 ($156.80), compared with £18 ($50.40) for every Englishman. "If our rate of expenditure," declared this British publication, "were brought up to the level of that of the United States, we should have an additional £325 million ($910 million) to spend on the NHS each year. . . . We are not spending too much on our health provisions. We are spending too little."[69]

CHAPTER VI

Remuneration in General Medical Practice

THE IMPORTANCE of general medical practice in the National Health Service was frequently emphasized by the Ministry of Health. However much specialization may have modified the activities of the general practitioner, it did not diminish his stature as the "clinical leader" or the "pivot of the whole health service."[1] The widely publicized Cohen Report of 1954 was not unique in its assertions that the "general practitioner service is an essential, not a subordinate service" and that "in a sense, the general practitioner must hold the key position in the Health Service." General practice, it was affirmed, "is fundamental to the best practice of medicine and to the best interests of the patient. It cannot be replaced by a congeries of specialisms, for only general practice can ensure that the patient is treated both as an individual and in relation to his family background and general environment."[2]

Recognition of the role which the general practitioner was to fill in the Health Service did not eliminate the difficulties which accompanied the transition from private to public practice, nor did it prevent the rise of other problems. A program of such magnitude was bound to harbor defects, foster frustration, lead to inequities, and require modification. Considering the breadth of the scheme, the amazing thing is that from the very beginning it functioned as smoothly as it did.

What were some of the irritants and difficulties that seemed to plague general practice? Doctors were unevenly distributed and patient lists varied greatly in size. Despite precautionary measures, the problem of inflated lists arose and became a source of perennial embarrassment to the government and the medical profession. For all the rosy hopes engendered by the new service, entry into general practice was not easy. Three main avenues were open to the young doctor: setting up a new practice in an under-doctored area, competing with many other applicants for the few advertised vacancies, or obtaining an assistantship with a view toward eventual partnership. The last offered him his best hope, but in that case also the number and variety of openings were limited and competition remained keen. Although abolition of the sale of good will removed a financial burden from the young doctor entering general practice, it also greatly reduced the mobility of older physicians, who were more or less frozen in their practices.

The reluctance of the government in the early 1950's to implement the Spens Report on remuneration had created a considerable resentment in medical circles. The doctors demanded an adjustment in compensation to offset inflation and the falling value of the pound. It appeared that the Service system of remuneration tended to penalize good doctoring and to deny sufficient recognition to those with long experience. The exclusion of practitioners from the hospitals, if anything, had been intensified under the new service. The paucity of practitioner hospital beds and the lack of direct access by many practitioners to the X-ray and pathological laboratories of the hospitals were subjects of frequent comment. The failure to achieve full co-operation between the general practitioner, the local authority, and the hospital service had proved a major stumbling block. In the field of preventive medicine, the contribution of the general practitioner had been disappointing. And there were the ever-present questions about the doctor-patient relationship, which some physicians believed had been adversely affected.

Some of these problems represented a heritage from the past or were the result of the evolution of modern medicine. Others were perhaps a part of the teething period of the Service or were aggravated by the lack of adequate funds. Some of the defects could be corrected, while others, more or less endemic, might very well defy effective solution. The compensation issue, a source of much illfeeling, was obviously a matter of economics and could be resolved by negotiation or arbitration. A more equitable distribution of practitioners could be effected only gradually. The medical profession as a whole recognized that time, patience, and a willingness to institute constructive reforms would be required to make general practice the sort of thing it was intended to be by the architects of the program. There were some uncompromising souls, however, who could see little hope for the practitioner in the new scheme, and they lost no opportunity to condemn it without reservation. Regardless of particular point of view toward the Service, it seemed clear to all in 1950 that a re-examination of general practice, in all of its ramifications, might well serve the best interests of British medicine.

And so, after the Health Service had been in operation two years, the British Medical Association and the Ministry of Health set up separate investigating commissions to probe all aspects of general practice and to determine what improvements or changes could be made so as to "enable general medical practitioners to provide the best possible standard of service." The committee appointed by the Council of the Medical Association comprised thirty doctors from various parts of Great Britain. Under the chairmanship of Dr. C. W. Walker, a general practitioner in Cambridge, this group conducted a postal inquiry among 13,000 general practitioners. In addition, Dr. Stephen J. Hadfield, Assistant Secretary of the Association, was assigned the responsibility of making a field survey embracing 188 practices. The research was done in 1951 and 1952, but not until the fall of 1953 were the results of the two surveys, together with the report of the Walker Commission, published. They particularly revealed what the medical mind thought about the many facets of the practitioner service. There were commendations, criticisms, suggestions, and even some forebodings, but withal the appraisal was a balanced one. Only those who preferred to believe the worst about the Health Service found the report and survey results discouraging.

The commission set up by the Central Health Services Council of the Ministry of Health in December, 1950, was placed under the chairmanship of Sir Henry Cohen, a distinguished professor of medicine at the University of Liverpool whose contributions in the field of research and health investigations later caused him to be raised to the peerage. Published in 1954, the Cohen Report did even more than the Walker Report to reaffirm public and professional faith in the inherent soundness of the National Health Service. There were, of course, weaknesses in the program, but these could be remedied, and toward that end recommendations were made, none of which would modify the basic aspects of the scheme. In the judgment of the *British Medical Journal,* the Cohen Report was the most accurate summary of the debate on the state of general medical practice since 1948.

One other survey should perhaps be mentioned as contributing at this time to a clearer understanding of the general practitioner service. Sponsored by the Nuffield Provincial Hospital Trust and conducted by Dr. Stephen Taylor, this non-statistical study was based upon thirty practices involving ninety-four doctors. Published in 1954, it gave a detailed picture of different types of rural and urban practices, with suggestions on how physicians could improve the quality and efficiency of their work. The general tenor of the report and the data upon which it was based further confirmed the opinions of those who could see in the general practitioner service much good and the prospects for an even better service in the future.

Without such surveys, the problems and workings of the practitioner service could not properly have been measured. Among these problems, the most disturbing was remuneration, which was closely related to other important aspects of the Health Service. Fostering, instead of large lists, lists medium in size and encouraging more co-operation and less competition through partnerships and group practice could not be achieved without regard to the issue of remuneration. In most matters the medical profession and the Ministry of Health were able to co-operate smoothly, not only in shaping policy but in the everyday administration of the service. On the question of compensation, however, that was not true. As paymaster and tax collector, the government was most anxious to keep expenditures at the minimum. The government's postwar years, in which it was burdened by inflation and heavy military spending, tended to harden the Exchequer against pay claims that actually deserved consideration.

When they joined the National Health Service, members of the medical profession had accepted the two Spens Reports as providing a sound basis for remuneration in the belief that there would be adjustments as money values changed and national productivity increased. Two separate committees, each under the chairmanship of Sir Will Spens, prepared the reports. The one involving specialists and consultants was published in May, 1948, while the other, which covered the medical practitioners, was completed two years earlier.

The latter report, which can be treated appropriately at this point, did not prescribe any one method of remuneration, but recognized that the capitation system was "a possible method and the most obvious method of securing such variations of income as are necessary if different degrees of ability, effort and resulting work are to be suitably remunerated." The three-year period ending in 1939 was taken as the basis for the study on practitioner income, and, as noted in an earlier chapter, the picture in that period was rather depressing. Convinced that the economic status of the practitioner would have to be improved if able young men were to be attracted to the general medical service, the report recommended a basis of remuneration deemed ample in terms of 1939 money values. To others was left the responsibility of making adjustment to changes in the value of the pound and the increased earning power general among all the professions.[3]

In full accord with the report on practitioner remuneration, the British Medical Association and the Ministry of Health had no trouble reaching an agreement on the total sum of money, in terms of the 1939 pound, that would be required to carry out its recommendations. The difficulty came in trying to adjust that sum so as to make full allowance for the inflationary trend and the economic advances of other professional groups during the decade since 1939. Failing to reach an understanding in the matter, the government proceeded to implement the Spens Report in its own way by providing an over-all increase of 70 per cent over the prewar total income of the medical practitioners. What the government considered to be generous was to the medical profession grossly unfair. No allowance in the so-called Central Pool of funds for the general practitioner service had been made for the increase of more than 1,000 general practitioners above the prewar total of 17,900. The betterment factor was deemed much too low. The flat capitation rate left many small-list doctors with meager incomes. The British Medical Association demanded that the Spens Report be implemented as it thought proper.

The Central Pool, as initiated in 1948, was based upon a capitation rate of 18s ($2.52) multiplied by that part of the population, estimated at 95 per cent, which would take advantage of the Health Service. The government's contribution to the retirement fund, 8 per cent of the net earnings of each doctor, was additional. The primary charge against the Central Pool was mileage payments due rural physicians and others whose practices covered a large area. The balance was allocated by a Distribution Committee to the Executive Councils in proportion to the number of people on doctors' lists within each area plus an additional one-third. Provision was made for payments covering the administration of anesthetics and emergency treatment and the service of temporary residents. The balance was then available for distribution among the practitioners, a portion being used for fixed annual payments and the rest for capitation payments, the average rate being between 16/6d ($2.31) and 17s ($2.38) per person on the doctors' lists.[4]

Three years were to pass before the Ministry of Health agreed to submit the issue of remuneration to arbitration. During that period there was much negotiation, which, for the most part, was fruitless, and as the months passed, feeling became intensified. The Ministry recognized the need for certain reforms, offered concessions, but would not accept the monetary claims of the medical profession and was reluctant to entrust to a neutral body the responsibility of determining the amount of money the Exchequer would have to spend on the medical service. In the early summer of 1951 a special conference of local medical committees served notice that the failure of the government to accept arbitration by September 25 would result in the mass resignation of all general practitioners from the Health Service. An impasse had been reached. The situation had so deteriorated that the only practical alternative was arbitration.

The agreement that followed provided that an independent adjudicator would determine the size of the Central Pool and that a Working Party, representing the British Medical Association and the Ministry of Health, would decide how the money should be distributed. The Working Party would be guided by the need to stimulate group practice, to facilitate the entry of new doctors into general practice, to discourage large lists while improving the financial position of practitioners with smaller lists, and, in general, "to enable the best possible medical service to be available to the public."[5]

The outcome was a settlement as gratifying to the medical profession as it was beneficial to the medical service. The adjudicator appointed by the Lord Chancellor was Justice Harold Danckwerts, who announced his decision on March 25, 1952. He ruled that the betterment factor for the Spens 1939 remuneration figures should have been 85 per cent for 1948 and for 1951 and subsequent years should be 100 per cent. Allowing 38.7 per cent of the practitioner service funds for practice expenses and using the number of general practitioners instead of the number of persons participating in the Service as the basis for his calculation, he fixed the size of the Central Pool for the fiscal year ending March 31, 1951, at 23 per cent more than the amount allocated by the government.

The claims which the medical profession had so vigorously pressed had at last been vindicated. With foresight the British Medical Association informed the Minister of Health that "in their view the award is capable of the interpretation that a varying betterment factor should be applied to future years." This the Minister promptly denied.[6] During the latter part of the decade, when remuneration was again to erupt into a burning issue, both sides were to reiterate their earlier interpretation of the Danckwerts award.

In shaping the future course of the practitioner service, the achievements of the Working Party were more significant than the increase in practitioner service funds. Published on June 5, 1952, and put into effect on April 1, 1953, its report not only sought to establish a new and fairer basis for capitation payments but to introduce certain other constructive changes. Reclassification of areas and Initial Practice Allowances will be discussed subsequently. These were of special benefit to small-list doctors and young practitioners. The redistribution of physicians was further stimulated by a reduction of 500 in the maximum number of persons the practitioner could have on his list. Under the new arrangements, the limit was 3,500

for a single doctor and 4,500 for a member of a partnership, providing the average for the partnership did not exceed 3,500. The
limit for a permanent assistant was now 2,000, or 400 fewer than
previously.

The primary purpose of the new remuneration scheme was to
increase the income derived from smaller lists, thus alleviating to some
degree the plight of the less favorably located practitioners. The
basic annual capitation fee set at 17s ($2.38) per person would be
supplemented by an additional "loading" fee of 10s ($1.40) for each
patient in excess of 500, up to 1,500 patients. Although the precise
size of the capitation fee was provisional, depending upon what prior
charges were made against the Central Pool, every effort would be
made to maintain the proposed rate. The increase in remuneration
from capitation fees was 43 per cent for a list of 1,500, but less than
20 per cent for the maximum number of patients. With large lists
earning proportionately less, the incentive to acquire more and more
patients was considerably blunted, and for many physicians smaller
lists now became more attractive.

Through financial inducements, the desire of the medical profession and the Ministry to foster group practice and partnerships was
also realized. Each year a sum of money, provisionally set at £ 88,000
($246,000) for England and Wales, would be allocated from the
Central Pool for interest-free loans to promote the establishment of
group practices. To encourage the acceptance of an assistant as a
partner, two approaches were employed. The additional patients
brought into a practice by an assistant were not counted in the
computation of loading fees, but a partner's patients, of course, were.
More important was the provision that allowed partners to be paid
on whatever basis would represent the most advantageous division of
their patients so as to yield them maximum loading benefits. For
example, if one partner had 2,000 patients and the other only 1,000,
each could be paid as though he had 1,500. This concession created
a strong financial motive for single doctors to form partnerships.[7]

Apart from remuneration, but related to it, was a pension system
that the medical profession heartily endorsed. With the exception
of those who were excused at the outset because of existing insurance
commitments, virtually all Health Service personnel were required to
enter the scheme. Although it was not the same for all groups, there
was a substantial identity among the arrangements for part-time specialists, general dental practitioners, and general medical practitioners.
As in the case of the other professionals, doctors contributed 6 per
cent of their net income to the pension fund. To this amount was
added a contribution from the government of 8 per cent of the total

net income of the doctors, a share that was later increased to 9.5 per cent. Upon reaching the age of sixty, or earlier in case of ill health, a practitioner with ten years of service to his credit could claim a pension, although sixty-five was recognized as the ordinary pensionable age or the age when contributions to the pension fund would normally stop.

The annual pension was 1.5 per cent of the total net income of the doctor for a period not to exceed forty-five years. In addition, there was a lump-sum retirement allowance—1.5 per cent of the total net income for a married man and 4.5 per cent for a single man. A widow received roughly one-third of her husband's pension.[8] Based upon the remuneration rates for 1961, the pension of a married doctor after 25 years of service would be about £970 ($2,700) per year, if his income were average. He would upon retirement also draw an additional tax-exempt lump-sum payment of £970 ($2,700). By English standards such a superannuation arrangement was generous.

It was the size of the Central Pool that determined how much the general practitioners collectively should receive. The award of 1952 provided that the amount which the Exchequer put into the Central Pool had to be sufficient when combined with other sources of income to guarantee general practitioners as a group an annual net income twice the amount received in 1938. By this method of reckoning, the total net income per doctor came to an average of £2,222 ($6,221), a figure that remained unchanged until 1957. This amount was multiplied by the number of doctors in general practice; to the resulting sum were added all practice expenses. From the grand total, however, was subtracted professional income from other sources. The balance was the amount the Exchequer was to deposit in the Central Pool for distribution in the service. These calculations were not easy to make, since practice expenses as well as all earnings of the practitioners had to be estimated. Naturally, the income from private practice could not accurately be assessed without a special inquiry, but the government was unable to reach an agreement with the medical profession about when or how this survey should be made, and so the arbitrary figure of £1 million ($2,800,000) proposed by Justice Danckwerts was used year after year.

What the practitioners received in earnings from the Executive Councils, hospitals, local health authorities, and other sources could be computed without much difficulty, but to get data on practice expenses was more complicated, requiring the assistance of the Board of Inland Revenue and, in fact, involved so much work that a full-scale inquiry was conducted only in certain years. In others a sample survey was deemed adequate. The final calculation of the Central

Pool, which was negotiated between the Ministry of Health and the General Medical Services Committee of the Medical Association, was often delayed many months after the close of the fiscal year. The practitioners, of course, received on schedule the prescribed payments, including capitation fees, but enough funds remained in the pool in some years to constitute a balance of over £3,500,000 ($10 million). This balance could be distributed only when the exact size of the pool for the year had finally been determined.[9]

Although the proportion of the Central Pool annually required for practice expenses ranged from 33 to 38 per cent, some doctors spent much more and others much less. All, however, were reimbursed on the same basis, with the size of the reimbursement prorated to the size of their lists. In some medical circles this procedure was considered manifestly unfair, since it tended to reward the doctor who spent the minimum on office facilities and ancillary help.

The *Medical World Newsletter* in 1958 cited two practices, both managed by well-trained doctors, as examples of how great the difference could be. One was a group practice of three partners, with ample nursing and clerical assistance and a combined list of 7,000 patients; the other practice, shared by two partners, was managed from separate offices (their homes), with little ancillary assistance, but had the same number of patients. The group practice, with an expense ratio of 49 per cent, yielded each partner a net annual income of £1,320 ($3,700). The amount spent on practice expenses by the two partners was only 23 per cent, which left each a net profit of £3,000 ($8,400). Since the two doctors did the same work as the other three, they deserved a larger income, but if the expense ratio had been the same for both practices, the differential in earnings would have been much less. The cost to the government of the 7,000 patients was the same in each case as far as direct expenses for the practices themselves were concerned, but there was a difference in the standard of service and therefore in the effect on the Health Service at large. In the group practice, the prescribing cost per patient was low, co-operation with the local health authority was good, the time given to each patient was sufficient, and the referral rate to the hospital outpatient department was considerably below the national average. With the two partners, the picture was almost the reverse.[10]

A high expense ratio did not necessarily mean greater efficiency, as some general practitioners demonstrated, but a practice well equipped and properly staffed was generally in a position to offer better service than one without such advantages. It was obvious enough to progressive doctors that niggardly spending in the operation of a practice was a false economy, even though the monetary gain to the individual practitioner might be larger. Since minimum spending seemed to be encouraged by the existing machinery, a plan was recommended by the Medical Practitioners' Union that would separate completely net remuneration from practice expenses by creating a second pool intended specifically to meet such expenses. Each doctor would receive an advance on expenses, but his share of the expense pool when finally calculated would be governed not by the national average but by his individual practice expenditures.[11] This proposal seemed to evoke little active support among the great body of doctors.

In opposing change in the so-called "global sum" method, Dr. S. Wand, Chairman of the Council of the British Medical Association, explained in 1958 that "there might be minor inconsistencies, but . . . if you take it over all the life of a doctor, I think you will find that throughout the years he will have had a fair crack of the whip in regard to his percentage of expenses."[12] There was no apparent enthusiasm for any revision of the global scheme on the part of the Ministry of Health, which recognized that the existing division of the pool, whatever its limitations, appeared to have the virtue of greater simplicity than a plan such as that proposed by the Medical Practitioners' Union. The need for action in the matter did not appear so urgent in view of a survey of doctors' premises made by the British Medical Association. Comparatively few of them were below acceptable standards. It was also recognized that tax exemption on practice expenditures tended to mitigate to some degree the inequity of the present expenses distribution scheme.

Since the total net income for all practitioners was fixed by agreement between the Ministry of Health and the medical profession and the purpose of the Central Pool was merely to insure payment of that amount, any change in the fees would mean that for some doctors there would be more money and for others less. Some physicians, in other words, would profit at the expense of others, and this consideration served to discourage revision. When, for example, in 1957 it was moved in the Representative Assembly of the British Medical Association that doctors who lived in London, like civil servants similarly situated, should get a higher rate of pay, the motion got a chilly reception.

The same Assembly also rejected the proposal that the greater care required for aged people should entitle doctors to a higher capitation fee for that group of patients. The motion was opposed on the grounds that, if it were adopted, higher fees would next be demanded for other chronic patients—those with tuberculosis, chronic bronchitis, and diabetes. A capitation fee, it was explained by one speaker, had to be "administered as a flat system, and what was lost on the swings would be made up on the roundabouts." The chairman of the General Medical Services Committee said that, despite his sympathy for the motion, the individual advocating it was "pleading a special cause," and if some doctors were to benefit from special causes, other practitioners would lose proportionately.[13]

Where an urgent need existed, however, a revision of fees did occur, and special fees were regarded as an equitable method of payment for unusual services. Almost three-fourths of the average practitioner's income came from capitation and loading fees, but the remaining fourth was partly, at least, made up of such special fees. The fee in 1961 for temporary residents, i.e., persons who were present in a region for less than three months, was £1 ($2.80), though in the case of a camp or institution consisting of ten or more individuals, the amount per patient was not as much. An individual who happened to be within a district for less than twenty-four hours or whose regular doctor was not available and who needed immediate treatment could go to any practitioner as an emergency patient. This service carried a fee of 8/6d ($1.19).

A few of the fees, such as the one for immunization, came from the local health authority. This payment was intended as remuneration for issuing a certificate and making a report, rather than for the actual immunization. Although the hospital service was the source of some of the fees, the greatest portion of them were financed by the Executive Councils. Assisting another practitioner in administering a general anesthetic paid as much as £1 15s ($4.90). The maternity fee in 1961 for a practitioner with recognized obstetric experience was £12 12s ($35.28); otherwise, it was only £7 7s ($20.58).[14] Other sources of income were hospital staff work, drug dispensing, sight tests in the ophthalmic service, sessional work in local clinics, and service on a medical board for a government department. I will discuss elsewhere Inducement Payments, Supplementary Annual Payments, Initial Practice Allowances and Trainee Practitioner Grants.

For many years doctors were paid on a quarterly basis, although any practitioner, by pleading hardship, could obtain payment on a semi-quarterly or even a monthly basis. Beginning in 1955, the medical profession pressed for uniform payments on a monthly basis. Since that method would involve no extra clerical expense, the Ministry of Health in 1957 yielded in the matter, and thereafter monthly advance payments on account became the standard procedure for all Executive Councils.[15]

Concerning the best way to remunerate general practitioners there was no unanimity in the medical profession, although the great majority supported the capitation system.   Thirty-five years of experience with this method of remuneration under the Health Insurance scheme made its adoption by the National Health Service almost a certainty.   There was, it will be recalled, very little choice, since the only apparent alternative, a salaried service, was objectionable to the medical profession.   Under the Health Service, all the polls indicated strong support for the capitation method of payment.   The Postal Survey of 1952 revealed a majority of 85 per cent in favor of it.[16] The Social Surveys of 1956 showed that three-fourths of the practitioners were eager to maintain it.[17]   An extensive postal questionnaire in Scotland, where medical sentiment seemed to be very much the same as in England, disclosed that two-thirds of the doctors in 1959 were in favor of the capitation fee system.   Twelve per cent preferred remuneration by salary, and 17 per cent supported payment by item of service.[18]

The capitation system, although vulnerable to criticism, seemed to work well enough.   It enjoyed great popular support and was never seriously challenged in Parliament or by the Ministry of Health once the Health Service was established.   Dissident voices, of course, were raised, principally by the Socialist Medical Association and the Fellowship For Freedom in Medicine, which favored respectively a full-time salaried service and payment for each visit or item of service. But these organizations represented two extreme positions, neither one of which seemed practicable or acceptable to the majority.   If a salaried practitioner service had ever had any chance of adoption, it was lost with the postponement or abandonment of the health center program, while the fee for service was by general consensus ill-adapted to a health service accessible to an entire population.

In seeking to strengthen private practice, the Fellowship engaged in what seemed to be a hopeless fight to win support for a plan involving payment for each service rendered.   Such a system, the Fellowship insisted, would result in less strain on the hospital outpatient departments and a more judicious use of the practitioner service.   A compulsory private insurance scheme, heavily subsidized by the state, was proposed to sustain the larger part of the fees.   Only for pensioners and any low-income groups that might be exempted from insurance payments would the capitation system be retained, and perhaps even for them remuneration by the state could be paid by a fixed-item-of-service method.[19]

The Ministry of Health was opposed to the Fellowship approach because it was "open to all kinds of abuse."   There was the fear that it would operate as a strong financial inducement for practitioners to do unnecessary work.[20]   The Medical Association was not against the idea as such, if the state would underwrite such a scheme with adequate financial support and insure a proper scale of payments. But realistically the Association recognized that the government was not likely to provide this kind of support because the cost could not be anticipated.   The leaders of the medical profession could see other objections, such as the tremendous amount of record-keeping that would be required and the elaborate machinery that would be necessary to process and price an estimated annual 250 to 300 million items of service.

There was apprehension also about the effects upon good doctoring.   In the opinion of the chairman of the General Medical Services Committee, remuneration by item of service would jeopardize continuity of treatment.   The practitioner's list, he averred, served to discourage patients from wandering from doctor to doctor, but with the fee-for-service scheme there would be no registration and no such deterrent.   In viewing the over-all picture, he expressed the belief that the capitation method had many advantages over the other schemes in a comprehensive health program that had to operate "within a ceiling of payment."[21]

On the question of a full-time salaried service, the position of the Medical Association was one of emphatic opposition, and to leave no doubt in the matter the Representative Assembly from time to time reaffirmed its stand.   There was perhaps no need for such fears, since the Amendment Act of 1949 had prohibited this method of remuneration for practitioners and there was no apparent sentiment in the Ministry of Health or Parliament to repeal the law.   Without health centers, moreover, there was not the necessary framework for a salaried service.   To those who were economy minded, it seemed obvious that the capitation system, with private ownership of premises, was much less expensive to the Exchequer than a salaried system, with government-financed health centers, would have been.   Even so, the Socialist Medical Association never lost hope that the "competitive" capitation system would some day be replaced by a "co-operative" salaried health center program.

In the medical and lay press the merits and evils of a full-time salaried service were aired periodically.   In the spring of 1958, for example, two Medical Officers of Health, both of whom were salaried but who held opposing points of view, were among those who became involved in a spirited discussion in the columns of the *Manchester Guardian*.   One of them explained that for twenty years he had enjoyed complete freedom in his work, that his initiative had not been impaired, that his relationship with the Ministry of Health had been co-operative and courteous, and that he had in no way been subject to dictation. "A salaried service," he opined, "would enable better medical care to be given to the people through co-operative action by practitioners. . . . Herein lies the pattern of the future." The other Medical Officer willingly admitted that a salaried service would not suffer by loss of efficiency, but he felt that there was a "sharp distinction between a service which is efficient alone and one which fully satisfied the sick of heart." In "a material age," he contended, "the members of the profession are human, and it is difficult to see the universal maintenance of high standards of conduct in the absence of a spiritual incentive, unless some other incentive remains. The opportunity to improve his earnings by his own individual mental and physical efforts is such an incentive."[22]

Some years before, the *Manchester Guardian* had editorialized in favor of a salaried service, even declaring that if the Health Service had been started on that basis many of the problems "might by now have been solved, at the cost of some hard feelings among the older doctors."[23] *The Economist,* however, more accurately reflected the sentiment of the medical profession when it charged that a salaried service would lower professional standards by removing "the incentive to work harder and better."[24]

If a salaried service meant health centers, better facilities, greater efficiency and more teamwork, it also involved, so the critics argued, certain disadvantages. Among these were a top-heavy administrative hierarchy, financial stultification, and the absence of allowance for individual differences in capacity for work. But that many of the arguments for a salaried service were merely opinions unsupported by any factual evidence seemed to matter little to a profession whose spokesmen solemnly warned that a full-salaried service would be a "complete disaster for medicine."[25]

Years of experience with the capitation system had revealed weaknesses that, however, seemed to be overshadowed by the advantages. The capitation method was comparatively easy to administer and in a rough way paid the doctor for the amount of labor he did. There was no need to evaluate the practitioner's work in order to determine the amount of remuneration. The financial bar between doctor and patient was swept away. If more time was spent on one patient than another, the volume of work, it was believed, tended to balance out in the long run. The government did not have to make provision for the doctor's premises. As an independent contractor, he was free to practice almost anywhere he wished and to choose his patients. Supplementary fees encouraged additional work, thus supplying the doctor with a monetary incentive to pursue his special interests and to broaden his medical activities.

There were certain features of the system that operated to the disadvantage of some doctors. Most serious was the fact that the flat rate of payment ignored both age and experience. The White Paper of 1944, which contained the blueprint of the Health Service, recognized that the method of remuneration should take into account qualifications and achievements. The system adopted failed to do so, although the loading arrangement corrected in some measure the worst features of the straight capitation fee, so that doctors with small lists, many of whom were elderly, were more equitably paid. In partnership agreements, the division of income among the partners was usually based upon the greater experience of the senior members. It was assumed that, as a practitioner acquired experience and became better established, he would obtain more patients and larger earnings, but this development did not always occur, nor could it very easily occur at all in over-doctored areas.

It was evident that if a feasible scheme of remuneration could be devised which more closely accounted for knowledge, skill, and the quality of work, it would command the support of many doctors. The Medical Practitioners' Union suggested giving physicians with experience a special additional fee. The General Practice Reform Association, a small organization of younger doctors, proposed that recognition of age and length of service could be made by giving a flat annual increment for a period of twenty years in addition to the regular payments.[26]

More publicized was the suggestion that general practitioners, like specialists, should be granted merit awards. But it seemed very doubtful that meritorious work among practitioners could with justice be measured by any known system of appraisal. In the Annual Representative Meeting of the British Medical Association in 1958, there was, however, considerable sentiment in support of some form of incentive payments, providing they differed from the merit awards already used in the consultant service and were over and above the level of remuneration demanded by the profession for all doctors. After a lively debate on the matter, the Assembly moved that it would have no objection to merit awards for general practitioners, if a "practicable scheme" could be devised and subsequently endorsed by the Representative Body.[27] In considering possible criteria that might be used in determining such merit awards, the Council subsequently expressed doubt as to whether any scheme could be devised that the profession would accept "as affording proper recognition."[28] In 1960, the Royal Commission on Doctors' and Dentists' Remuneration nevertheless recommended distinction awards for general medical practitioners, but suggested no plan for administering them.

What were other limitations from which the capitation system allegedly suffered? It seemed to foster competition and rivalry among practitioners, some of whom seemed more concerned about enlarging their lists than serving the best interests of the Health Service. To hold their patients, some physicians were inclined to prescribe, especially in borderline cases, what was demanded by the patient rather than what was needed. Payment on a capitation basis did not always supply the strongest incentive to improve the standards of practice. Too many patients, it would seem, were referred to the hospitals. Entry into practice was made no easier by this method. Not all of these disadvantages, it should be observed, were peculiar to the capitation system; they might exist, in greater or lesser measure, under other types of remuneration.

The Newsam Report was unique in its evaluation of the various methods of practitioner remuneration. Although sponsored by the British Medical Association, this Report departed in major ways from prevailing medical sentiment and was accordingly given a chilly reception by that organization. While recognizing that there was no perfect way to compensate family physicians in a comprehensive health service, Sir Frank Newsam was inclined to view remuneration by salary as the method which the medical profession might ultimately find best suited to its needs. He rejected the fixed-item-of-service method as "unsuited to a learned profession," since it offered large rewards "to any general practitioner who is prepared to keep his patients sick, and to neglect the very patients to whom he should pay most attention." Newsam seemed to be almost as critical of the capitation method of payment, whose shortcomings he did not believe could be corrected by the system of loading fees.[29]

If the capitation system was open to criticism, it was also subject to favorable comment, much of which came from the more important surveys. Stephen Taylor referred to the capitation payment as "a great social invention." "It avoids," he said, "the possible abuses of fee-for-service or salary; the one invites the doctor to do too much, and the other too little."[30] The Cohen Report was no less favorable in its appraisal: "Payment by capitation fees allows the maximum of flexibility and independence for individual practitioners and interferes as little as possible in the establishment of the right relationship between the doctor and his patient on the one hand, and between the doctor and the Executive Council on the other."[31] The Walker Report asserted that there "seems little doubt that practitioners on the whole, are happier in their relationships now that fee-charging and the rendering of accounts are almost a thing of the past . . . . the Committee firmly holds the view that where the doctor is receiving payment for each individual patient by capitation fee, as at present, the relationship is better than it would be in a salaried service."[32]

The failure of the government to adjust the remuneration of doctors in 1956 led to a major conflict with serious implications. The Danckwerts award had boosted the earnings of practitioners to a level 137 per cent above that of 1938. Based upon 1951 prices, the real income of doctors had improved 12 per cent, leaving them in an especially favorable category. This advantage, however, suffered from the attrition of inflation and was eventually wiped out. Within six years, the price index had advanced 24 per cent.

During these years, the average annual net income of practitioners remained frozen at £2,222 ($6,221), which, it should be noted, was equivalent in purchasing power in the United States to an amount 25 per cent larger. This income was net only in the sense that it was in excess of professional expenses, and it included the superannuation contributions of both the doctor and the Exchequer. When taxes were paid, the balance for a married doctor with two children was on the average not more than £1,680 ($4,700). For practitioners with small lists, the situation was even worse. But doctors were not the only victims of inflation. Civil servants, landlords, and teachers were in a particularly unhappy position. The working classes, on the other hand, had been more than able to hold their own, advancing wages to a level three and one-half times above what they earned in 1938.

Representative of many physicians were two partners in Lincolnshire, one of whom had been in practice thirty years. With more than the average number on their lists, none of them private patients, these doctors each worked about 65 hours a week. During the period from 1952 to 1956, their expenses increased 25 per cent but their earnings remained almost stationary. After superannuation and tax payments were met, each partner in 1956 had only £1,525 ($4,272) left, out of which £200 ($560) had to be set aside to replace their automobiles. The purchasing power of these practitioners during the five-year period had declined 26 per cent.[33]

In 1955, the doctors began to urge their leaders to seek a further betterment in remuneration, but official action was delayed until the following year. Citing the recommendations of the two Spens Committees as the basis for its plea, the British Medical Association in June, 1956, requested an increase in compensation of not less than 24 per cent for practitioners and hospital doctors. The Association's memorandum denied that the claim ran counter to the recent plea of the government to halt new salary and wage demands. The medical profession was asking only for the "implementation of a contractual obligation" that had been in existence since 1948.[34]

The Minister of Health promptly rejected the demand, not necessarily because it lacked merit, but because it could not be reconciled with the anti-inflationary policy of the government. If accepted, the claim would cost the Exchequer an additional £20 million ($56 million). It would mean for the doctors an income nearly three times their average prewar earnings. The Ministry denied that there was any moral or legal obligation on the part of the Exchequer to give the medical profession an automatic increase whenever prices rose. The government had accepted the Spens reports, it said, only to get the Health Service started and not as a permanent basis for the adjustment of remuneration claims. If, as the British Medical Association insisted, the Spens principle were binding for an indefinite period, then the medical profession became a privileged group, completely protected against inflation. Such a position no government could accept.[35]

The medical profession reacted angrily. The *British Medical Journal* declared that the Minister "should at least recognize the legal force of a contract. He should recognize more than this: that doctors, coming unwillingly into the N.H.S. in 1948 because Parliament, press and people bludgeoned them into it, nevertheless thought that the people through Parliament would keep their word, would honour their bond."[36]

Although not a trade union, the British Medical Association some years previously had established a subsidiary body, known as the British Medical Guild, which would enable the doctors to take measures "more familiar to workmen in other walks of life." The Guild, which had functioned in the remuneration crisis of 1950-51, was again notified to prepare for action. Local meetings would be convened. All other measures failing, the doctors, it was announced, might be called upon to withdraw from the Health Service or to restrict their activities within the Service.

The contractual implications of the Spens Reports were not clear. The fact that the Danckwerts award was based upon the Spens principle seemed to the doctors to give it a validity that the government was not prepared to recognize in any future dispute. While it was doubtful that a legally enforceable contract existed, many felt, as did the *Manchester Guardian,* that the doctors had a strong moral case.[37] *The Times* (London) was not certain that the pledge inherent in the government's acceptance of the Spens Reports was still valid. "For how long," queried this journal, "can it be regarded as binding on future governments who have no responsibility for what their prede-cessors did in the wildly optimistic days of 1946 and 1948? When will the doctors' leaders and the authorities frankly admit that the Spens reports are outmoded and that some more practical and durable method of reviewing remuneration from time to time is required?"[38]

The complete rejection of the Spens principle by the government led to a collapse of the negotiations between the General Medical Services Committee and the Ministry of Health. Even if the govern-ment had been willing to resort to arbitration, that course was not feasible, since in its view there were no clear lines on which arbitra-tion could take place. In view of the impasse, the government de-cided on a unilateral course of action. Without consulting the British Medical Association, the Prime Minister announced that the time was "opportune for a full review of medical remuneration through an independent inquiry which would take into account the position of the medical profession in relation to other professional classes in the community." A Royal Commission was accordingly set up in April, 1957, for the purpose of determining the proper level of dental and medical remuneration and of proposing machinery to keep such remuneration under review. Under the chairmanship of Sir William H. Pilkington, an industrialist, the Commission of nine members, none of whom was a doctor, proceeded to gather data and evidence on all related aspects of the subject.

The government further announced an interim increase of 10 per cent for junior members of hospital staffs, 5 per cent for senior doctors and dentists in hospitals, and 5 per cent for general medical and dental practitioners. The Central Pool was enlarged so as to boost the average net income for medical practitioners to £2,333 ($6,532). The division of money was arranged so as to give the maximum benefit to doctors with medium-sized lists.[39]

If the government expected these actions to reassure the medical profession, it completely misjudged the temper of the British Medical Association. Instead of moving "away from the atmosphere of distrust, accusations of bad faith, trial of strength, [and] non-coopera-tion in the Health Service," the government seemed to be moving into a struggle that threatened to undermine the very foundations of the Health Service. The Medical Association viewed the Royal Com-mission as a subterfuge, designed to postpone for an indefinite period the solution of a dispute that the doctors felt should be settled im-mediately. The leadership of the Association promptly proposed a policy of nonco-operation toward the Royal Commission. If the government persisted in its refusal to negotiate the remuneration claim or to submit the matter to arbitration, then the practitioners would be urged to carry out a plan for progressive withdrawal from the Health Service.

According to the strategy, which was well publicized, the British Medical Guild would collect the resignations of all practitioners, and if by October 2, 1957, the government was still unwilling to reach a satisfactory settlement, doctors in a few selected areas would resign. Such physicians would at first treat individuals on their lists on a private basis, but without any fee, after one month would make a token charge, and finally would make their regular charge. If the government remained obdurate, other areas would gradually be affected, and more and more practitioners would leave the Health Service. Doctors in the selected areas would receive financial support from a defense fund to which all practitioners were expected to contribute. There would be no interruption in medical service. The plan was designed "to get the maximum embarrassment for the Government with the minimum inconvenience to the public."

In explaining the scheme to the representatives of the regional divisions of the Association, Dr. Talbot Rogers, chairman of the General Medical Services Committee, denied that the practitioners would be going on strike; they would simply be withdrawing from the Health Service. The response of the representatives to the proposal was favorable, a "full-throated roar." "All over the room," observed one reporter, "doctors were stamping their feet, banging their chairs and slapping the backs of their neighbours."[40]

Throughout England during March and April, 1957, local meetings were called for the purpose of rallying the support of all practitioners. Judging by the vote of most of the gatherings, the support for selective withdrawal was overwhelming. But there were voices raised in protest. At the Manchester meeting, for instance, one physician labeled the plan "utter nonsense." Another insisted that if some doctors withdrew, others would take their places.[41] The absence of unanimity became more apparent as letters began to appear in the lay and medical press. In a communication to the *British Medical Journal,* a practitioner in Sheffield condemned the scheme as "unpractical." Observing that the country was in a critical financial situation, he feared that public opinion would turn against the doctors.[42] A physician in Brighton wrote to *The Lancet* that what "the association advocates, if the claim fails, really amounts to strike action," but "whether called 'strike' or 'resignation' it is really nothing but shameless blackmail, since . . . [such] action would cause a crisis." The Association would, he warned, "thus forfeit what little is left of public sympathy for the medical profession."[43]

In a letter to the *Manchester Guardian,* a practitioner raised the query: "Do these stalwart defenders of professional status charging into battle with Spens and Danckwerts emblazoned on their banner imagine that they have the general public behind them? They had better turn around and look." "I am quite unable to support the plan for withdrawal," wrote a physician, "because it will add burdens on the sick poor who are already overburdened." Another doctor, who said he would "blackleg any walk-out," explained that "whatever grievances we may have—and they are few considering the newness of the Service and the complete revolution of 'benign, bespectacled physicians' that it inevitably brought about—the fact remains an indisputable one that the Health Service has improved beyond measure the lot of the community and of every efficient, conscientious doctor in large industrial practice. To return to private practice for the working classes in the days of streptomycin and a hundred remedies outside the purchasing range of 80 percent of the population should be unthinkable to any doctor worthy of his qualification."[44]

The Lancet condemned the proposed strategy of the British Medical Association as "an alien procedure, out of keeping with the character of any profession, and especially that of medicine." It was denied that doctors could "have both the prestige of a profession, whose strength lies in the merits of its case, and the power of a trade union which is organized to apply pressure." In challenging the government, the medical profession might find resistance hardening and public opinion aroused.[45]

The Socialist Medical Association viewed the tactics of the Medical Association as a "blow not at the Government as employer but at the public." "The right of British citizens to a full health service," it was asserted, "must be preserved."[46] Although its opinion was favorable at first, the Medical Practitioners' Union soon developed misgivings about "phased withdrawal" and decided that co-operation with the Royal Commission would be the wiser course.[47] One member of Parliament, in addressing the Minister of Health, asked, "Will you convey to leading members of the medical profession that this suggestion [withdrawal of doctors from the Health Service] is in the view of most people, including those who are sympathetic to their claim, both irresponsible and ridiculous?"[48]

The New Statesman and Nation felt that the best plan was for the medical profession to abandon the Spens principle and to seek a fresh approach as a basis for negotiation. In an extraordinary burst of frankness this journal declared, "Part of the difficulty of this problem . . . is that the doctors have a peculiarly privileged position in our society. They regulate the entry, the standards, the ethics and, to a large extent, the structure of their profession. But they also deploy the monopoly power they thereby wield to strengthen their business interests. The mores of public-service and self-interests are hopelessly mixed up. That is all the more reason why the public interest requires the Royal Commission to look very carefully at the methods (as well as the amount) of paying the doctors."[49]

However irrefutable may have been their claim for more pay, the doctors nevertheless ranked as one of the highest income groups in Great Britain. Few people could become distressed over the plight of the practitioners when their demand for an additional £10 ($28) per week represented more than many persons earned altogether. A survey conducted in London and Edinburgh during spring, 1957, revealed that most individuals guessed the compensation of physicians to be less than the actual amount. When queried if a net income for doctors of £2,143 ($6,000) before taxes was reasonable, the great majority thought so, and only one in four believed it was too low. Considerably less than half the persons polled knew that practitioners earned more than members of Parliament.[50]

Even before the Special Representative Meeting of the British Medical Association gathered to deliberate the proposed strategy, rifts began to appear in the unity of the medical profession. The willingness of the Dental Association to co-operate with the Royal Commission was soon equaled by the Royal College of Physicians, whose President, Sir Russell Brain, was reassured on a number of points by the Prime Minister and the chairman of the Royal Commission. Both Harold Macmillan and Sir Harry Pilkington made it clear that the Commission would take a broad view of the problem in its investigation, accepting all relevant evidence and taking into account the Spens Reports and the income of a wide range of other professions and occupations. The Commission would seek to formulate "balanced conclusions on what should be the proper levels of remuneration" for dentists and doctors in the Health Service. Once its report was complete, the government would take no action without first entering into discussions with the professions.

Since Sir Russell Brain was joint chairman of the negotiating committee of the medical profession, his refusal to support a boycott of the Royal Commission left the General Medical Services Committee in an awkward position. And when Dr. Talbot Rogers, chairman of the Services Committee and also joint chairman of the negotiating committee, decided to support a policy of co-operation, the leadership of the British Medical Association was badly split. Feeling ran so strong that Rogers had to resign both chairmanships, but the General Medical Services Committee now decided by a narrow margin that evidence should be given to the Royal Commission.[51]

In view of the divided sentiment, the Special Representative Meeting which convened on May 1, 1957, to ratify the proposed strategy of the Association had no choice but to postpone its decision. The chairman of the Council, Dr. S. Wand, who had previously supported vigorous action, now found himself cast in the role of counseling restraint and advising co-operation with the Royal Commission. That policy, he felt, was justified by the broad terms of reference to be employed by the Royal Commission and by the interim adjustment in remuneration. Although the position of Wand was sustained by the assembly, there were bitterly angry remarks from delegates who viewed the reversal in policy as a betrayal.

One doctor referred to the conciliatory letter of the Prime Minister as a "form of words" which the Association was now swallowing just as it had swallowed "a form of words at the crucial moment in 1948." In doing so, he said, "you were delivered into a paradise where you are the door-mats of the Welfare State." "These concessions," he warned, "were not concessions at all, but phases in a carefully planned process of brainwashing. These promises were the type which had been the daily stock-in-trade of politicians since the technique had first been devised by Machiavelli." Another representative expressed the fear that the members of the Association were substituting "one phased withdrawal for another; they were preparing not for a phased withdrawal from the National Health Service, but for a phased withdrawal from their resistance to Government dictation."[52]

On June 12, in another dramatic meeting of a Special Representative Assembly, this one lasting seven hours, the British Medical Association reached the final decision to give evidence to the Royal Commission and to postpone indefinitely the withdrawal of its members from the National Health Service. The action was taken with reluctance and with the knowledge that the profession had no choice in the matter. "The decision to give evidence," remarked one member of the Council, "has now become inevitable. Had we had more unity—and I am sorry to say that our unity has been lacking—we might have come to a different decision." Another member of the Council somberly announced that "the power of the Government over the profession is very nearly complete and that is a terrible danger." The Chairman of the Council, however, looked at the situation quite differently. "It may be," he said, "that this decision will be interpreted in some quarters as ending hostilities. That is not so. Our dispute with the government still remains. . . . That is how I interpret the decision today, but in my view you have declared an armed truce."

That the Medical Association was in no mood to abandon its objectives was apparent in other resolutions adopted by the Representative Assemblies. It was decided that plans for withdrawal from the Service should go forward and that the defense fund should be strengthened by the maintenance of a special levy on all doctors, including consultants. It was further moved that an alternative health scheme be planned, so that in the event the practitioners should resign from the Health Service, they would not withdraw into a vacuum. Most important, perhaps, was the decision that the Council should "institute an inquiry into the whole field of publicly administered medical services in the light of the experience gained from the National Health Service since 1948." The investigation, it was stipulated, should be conducted independently of the government.[53]

There were some who desired to exploit the crisis so as to effect a permanent withdrawal, but their number seemed insignificant and they had no clear idea about what should be done once the doctors had resigned. *The Lancet* noted that there were those who "see this as the moment when a new Moses should unite his people to follow him out of bondage." "Before accepting such an invitation," admonished the journal, "general practitioners may well ask for detailed information of life in the wilderness."[54]

Whether the medical profession would ever have been able to muster enough unity to execute a successful withdrawal from the Health Service was doubtful. In spring, 1957, when feeling was at its peak, a secretary of the British Medical Association asked whether any plan for withdrawal was likely to succeed when no more than 60 per cent of the members were ever present at the peripheral meetings.[55] A French doctor who visited England during the remuneration crisis soon discovered that "most doctors expected others to resign for them. A doctor from Drypool-on-Sea callously remarked, 'I am quite in favour of the people in Manchester leaving the NHS,' but he had no intention of following suit. Another who lives at St. Ethelred-Super-Mare explained, over a cup of tea, that a man's first duty was toward himself and his family, and besides, he disapproved of the whole affair. Yet another respected member of the profession told me that England was a country of compromise and sweet reasonableness. Certainly doctors had asked for a 24 percent increase, but they might—indeed would—accept less."[56]

After more than a year's delay, the Association's Review Committee, comprising only doctors, was set up in fall, 1958, under the chairmanship of Sir Arthur Porritt. It was concerned with long-term policy and would conduct a co-operative inquiry into the Health Service under the aegis of the British Medical Association, the Royal

Colleges, the College of General Practitioners, and certain other medical organizations.[57]

While a subcommittee of the General Medical Services Committee was exploring the possibility of an alternative service, the Newsam Report was completed. Without equivocation, Sir Frank Newsam proclaimed that "it is unrealistic of doctors to think of withdrawing from the National Health Service." Should they do so "*en bloc* or in considerable numbers," he warned, "the almost inevitable result would be that the Government will be compelled to introduce a salaried medical service."[58] Unprepared to accept this and certain other conclusions, the Council quickly dissociated itself from the document. The British Medical Association remained committed to the strategy of withdrawal, and in spring, 1959, published a carefully prepared plan of action. In the event of a future dispute with the government that could not be resolved, complete separation from the Health Service and reliance on private practice were suggested as the "most effective and quickest way of securing a just solution." But the report emphasized that this plan would be possible only if there were complete solidarity and unity of action in the profession and a willingness "to take a stand on principles rather than on a matter of remuneration alone."[59]

Owing to the delay in the report of the Royal Commission, the British Medical Association pressed for another interim increase in remuneration. The Ministry of Health acceded to the extent of an additional 4 per cent boost in the basic pay of doctors and dentists, effective January 1, 1959. The capitation fee rose to 18s ($2.52) and the loading payment to 12s ($1.68). An upward adjustment was made in Initial Practice Allowances, Hardship Payments, Trainee Grants, and other fees. The average net income of medical practitioners now reached £2,426 ($6,792).[60] The two interim increases, totaling 9 per cent, fell far short of the 24 per cent originally demanded and the subsequently revised figure of 29 per cent, but the Association accepted the increments while awaiting the Commission's report on remuneration.

A rather accurate guide to medical thinking was the voluminous testimony presented to the Royal Commission on Doctors' and Dentists' Remuneration. Criticisms, suggestions, and recommendations were spread over many pages, but apart from the monetary problem, which was solvable, there were few, if any, issues that could be construed as a threat to the survival of the Health Service. The prevailing spirit seemed to be one of eagerness to improve and strengthen a program that had the loyal support of almost everybody.

Weary over remuneration crises that within a decade had twice disrupted an otherwise friendly relationship with the Ministry of Health, the British Medical Association proposed a plan for an annual review of doctors' salaries.   The scheme envisioned a permanent committee selected by the Prime Minister, with terms of reference that would be mutually acceptable to both sides.   An adjustment of remuneration would normally be made every three years, with the findings of the committee binding on all parties.[61]

Looking to the future, the medical profession hoped that a committee like the one now under the chairmanship of Sir Arthur Porritt might point the way to an improved National Health Service.   From various quarters came the suggestion that an objective review of the health program for the first decade would be helpful.   In urging that the faults of the Service be examined, *The Lancet,* however, seemed to feel that "certain weaknesses of the N.H.S. are inherent and must be accepted as the defects of its virtues."   For all the shortcomings the remuneration crisis had pointed up, the Service had abundantly justified itself in the eyes of that journal.   In seeking to improve it, the people were urged by this medical organ not to overlook what had been accomplished, the "unspectacular improvement of the hospitals; . . . the reforming ardour seen today in general practice, in the treatment of the mentally ill, and in the care of the old; and specially . . . this country's place in medical research and teaching."[62]

The long awaited Report of the Royal Commission on Doctors' and Dentists' Remuneration was published early in 1960.   The careful analysis of the testimony and statistical data and the balance and good judgment that characterized the recommendations resulted in a favorable response from almost all interested groups.   With alacrity the government welcomed the Report and offered it to the medical and dental professions as a "package-deal."   While some aspects of the Report were not completely to the liking of the medical profession, as a whole it was acceptable.   Certain points required clarification, and agreement had to be reached on the implementation of the recommendations.   To accomplish these ends, a Joint Working Party was set up.   In September of that year, the Report of the Working Party as well as the recommendations of the Royal Commission were formally ratified by a Special Representative Meeting of the British Medical Association.[63]   Immediately a new spirit of harmony replaced the former spirit of strife.

The Pilkington Commission found that the remuneration of doctors in 1957 was too low and that in the two subsequent years it did not increase as much as the incomes in industry, commerce, and the other professions.   To remove this inequity, the report proposed retroactive payments which would average about £478 ($1,340) per doctor. Effective January 1, 1960, the average net income from all official sources for practitioners under 70 years of age would be increased 22.8 per cent above the level which prevailed in the 1955-56 fiscal year. If distinction awards were taken into account, the over-all increase approached 24 per cent, which was not far short of the amount asked by the medical profession.

The Central Pool was to be continued "because of the practical advantages . . . and because the profession is accustomed to it and on the whole likes it," but group practice loans, private earnings, and Exchequer contributions to superannuation were no longer to be included in the calculation. Other minor modifications were to be made in computing the size of the Pool, but, as before, the size of the Pool was to be determined by reference to the number of doctors and not the number of patients. If the sources of additional income just mentioned were excluded, the average net income per doctor for 1955-56 was £1,975 ($5,530), instead of £2,222 ($6,221). The recommended average net income for 1960 from all official sources was to be £2,425 ($6,790), or £450 ($1,260) above the level five years before.[64] If private earnings and the other excluded sources were taken into account, then the practitioner would presumably receive an average net income of nearly £2,675 ($7,500).

The Joint Working Party fixed the capitation fee at 19/6d ($2.73). The loading fee was increased to 14s ($1.96) per patient, and the number of patients for whom the fee would be paid was extended by 200 in order "to distribute the greater benefit to those providing general medical services in all but the smallest practices." The new loading arrangement was made applicable to partnership lists of from 501 to 1,700 and to single-doctor lists of from 401 to 1,600. The practitioner with 2,000 patients would receive a gross remuneration of £2,790 ($7,812) from capitation fees and loadings; with 2,500, he would receive £3,277 10s ($9,177). Maternity fees, Initial Practice Allowances, Supplementary Annual Payments, Inducement Payments and Trainee Practitioner Grants were increased substantially, and some of the other fees for services were revised upward. A total of £1 million ($2,800,000) was reserved for finding "methods of making the best possible general medical service available to the public," and a second Working Party was to determine how this money could most effectively be used to accomplish that objective.[65] The Royal Commission felt that a merit award system should be created for general medical practitioners and suggested a special fund of £500,000 ($1,400,000) per year for this purpose. Still another Working Party would be set up to devise a scheme for rewarding distinguished service in general practice by additional remuneration.

In seeking to avoid the recurring remuneration crises, the Pilkington Commission proposed a standing Review Body of seven outstanding persons to be appointed by the government and to represent neither the medical and the dental profession nor any other interest. The deliberations of the Review Body would be conducted privately, and it would have the authority to initiate consideration of any change that should be made in the level of remuneration for doctors and dentists. The government, however, could seek the advice of this body and would transmit to it any representations that the professions might have. The Review Body would determine what factors were relevant at any particular time and would have access to all necessary data. Its function would be purely advisory, and the government would be free to accept or reject the recommendations, but in view of the eminence of the Review Body, its impartiality, and its thoroughness, the Royal Commission believed that the government would feel bound to accept the findings. Adjustments in remuneration would normally be proposed at infrequent intervals, the aim being to keep remuneration levels stable for periods of at least three years.[66]

The views of the medical profession and the Ministry of Health toward the Review Body were optimistic and hopeful. The abandonment of the Spens formula, which the British Medical Association had long defended, did not seem to involve any real regrets, because it obviously had become obsolete.[67] Since the government would not bind itself by a permanent arbitration arrangement, the most logical approach and the one that seemed to offer the most satisfactory possibilities of accurate adjustment in the income of doctors was the Review Body.

CHAPTER VII

Entry into General Medical Practice

ONE OF THE PRIMARY objectives of the National Health Service was to achieve a more equitable distribution of medical care. There were industrial districts in which the ratio was one physician to as many as 5,000 patients, and in them, of course, the maximum of 4,000 patients permitted on a Health Service doctor's list by the 1948 regulations was easily reached. Quite the opposite was true in certain rural and semi-urban districts, particularly in southern England, where the average was one doctor for every 1,100 to 1,500 persons. That number of patients prior to 1948 had furnished a fairly adequate income to many doctors whose patients were generally middle class, but these physicians under the capitation system of remuneration found their incomes drastically reduced. Most of their private practice disappeared. They had ample time for good doctoring but suffered a financial grievance, whereas the practitioners in under-doctored areas, although well paid, were burdened with too many patients and simply had too little time to maintain the highest standards of medicine.

It was this grossly unequal distribution of physicians that had brought the Medical Practices Committee into existence. Set up as a statutory body, it was granted authority to control the flow of practitioners into over-doctored areas. The British Medical Association, it will be recalled, had strongly opposed the idea on the grounds that it would constitute a threat to the general freedom of movement of doctors. Such fears were to prove groundless, since the Medical Practices Committee could not coerce and had no power to direct doctors into any area or to deny them the privilege to practice where they wished except in districts that already had too many physicians. Even in such areas, exceptions were made if circumstances required, and there as elsewhere partnerships could be freely organized. If a son or relative planned to join a practice or to become the successor in a single-doctor practice, no objection normally was raised, but the opening of new practices and the disposal of others vacated by death or resignation were subject to strict control in such districts by the new agency. It soon became apparent that such an arrangement was a definite benefit to doctors in these districts, who had little to gain from excessive competition.

Seven of the nine members of the Medical Practices Committee were general practitioners who, although appointed by the Minister of Health, were in reality the nominees of the medical profession. The Medical Practices Committee functioned as an independent agency, but it consulted freely with the General Medical Services Committee of the British Medical Association. The Executive Councils, with their large professional representation, played an important role in the functions of the Committee, as did the local medical committees. Periodically the Medical Practices Committee would make a survey to determine how each area should be classified, and it was the data and recommendations of these local bodies that largely influenced the decision of the central body.[1]

The classification of areas was determined by a flexible standard of measurement, subject to the changing needs of the Service. Regrouping of districts occurred from time to time and was duly publicized. Originally four, the number of categories of classification was reduced in 1952 to three—designated, intermediate, and restricted. The division between them could not always be sharply drawn, and so, for example, an area could be classified as wholly restricted or part restricted and part intermediate. A restricted district was one considered amply served by practitioners, and the admission of new doctors into it was allowed only in exceptional cases. An average of 1,500 persons or less per practitioner would normally place an area in this category. A ratio of between 1,500 to 2,500 people per doctor would usually result in an intermediate classification, which meant that each application for admission would be decided according to the specific circumstances.

In designated districts, the right to practice was automatically recognized, and a financial grant was made available to those desiring to set up a single practice. At first the grant was known as the Fixed Annual Payment. Following the Danckwerts award, a more liberal grant called the Initial Practice Allowance was made. Subject to a requirement of a minimum of two years of experience in general practice or a minimum of four years of registration as a medical practitioner, a doctor who took over a small list in a single practice or who endeavored to start a new single practice could claim a grant which in 1961 was £1,250 ($3,500) the first year, £900 ($2,520) the second year, £500 ($1,400) the third year, and £250 ($700) the fourth year, subject to an income limit for each year. The practitioner would normally be required to have 150 patients at the end of the first year, 500 at the end of the second year, and 750 at the end of the third year. In addition to the allowance, the doctor would be entitled to the usual capitation fees. Should a doctor's application for an Initial Practice Allowance be denied by the Executive Council, an appeal could be taken to the Minister of Health, who would be advised by a committee of six members selected by him and representing equally the Ministry of Health and the medical profession.[2]

In the over-doctored or restricted areas, the dispersal of small practices was another means used to improve the distribution of medical man power. If a member of a partnership died or resigned from the Health Service, the remaining partners, if they chose, could assimilate the patients of the former partner. Small single practices that became vacant frequently were not filled, and their patients were advised to select another doctor. The rate of dispersal of small practices in London, for example, was quite high, for at least 40 per cent of all single vacancies that occurred during the first ten years of the Service were not filled. In that city there was no shortage of practitioners. Even in 1949, when large lists plagued the northern industrial cities, the average list in London was 1,656, while a decade later it was only 1,534.[3]

The policy of the Medical Practices Committee was one of caution, and only the most impelling reasons would cause it to classify an area as restricted. It was the Executive Councils and the local medical committees that, favoring a stricter policy, urged that more districts be closed to new entrants. When in 1949 the Medical Practices Committee requested the Executive Councils to report areas which were "manifestly under-doctored," only a few were suggested.[4] Established practitioners tended to be resentful when a district which had been restricted was opened to more doctors. Complaints reached the floor of the Annual Representative Meeting of the British Medical Association about the opening of restricted districts, and a Welsh practitioner, for example, presented a motion in 1955 calling upon the Council "to keep a close watch on the activities of the Medical Practices Committee and to take action to safeguard the interests of the association members."[5] Contrary to expectations, the Committee seemed to be a more zealous guardian of the freedom of movement of doctors than the medical profession itself.

The proportion of areas classified as over-doctored remained small. Even London, with its high ratio of general practitioners, had only one borough, Chelsea, that was completely restricted in 1958.[6]

Taking England and Wales as a whole, only 7 per cent of the practitioners and 5 per cent of the people were in restricted areas in 1958, and these percentages had changed little during the six preceding years. The number of persons per physician in such districts averaged 1,594 in 1958, or 13 more than in 1952. The over-all picture had become so much better by 1958 that only 18 per cent of the population lived in under-doctored areas, as compared with 51 per cent in 1952. Intermediate districts in 1958 embraced three-quarters of the practitioners and about the same proportion of people. A greatly improved balance was being achieved in the urban and semi-urban communities. The advice of the Ministry of Health, "Go North, young man, go North," was being heeded, with the result that no longer was there such an acute shortage of doctors in that region.

In 1960, the average number of persons on general practitioners lists stood at 2,287, or 149 less than in 1952. The problem of uneven distribution of doctors and excessively large lists was slowly being solved, but with a substantial portion of the population (27 per cent in 1960) on lists of over 3,000, it was clear that more time would be required before anywhere near the ideal ratio could be established.[7] Ten years of the Health Service had nevertheless brought the patient not only "a bigger choice of doctors" but also "a better share of the doctor's time."

Keeping the classification of areas under review was only one phase of the work done by the Medical Practices Committee. The certification of partnerships and the admission of practitioners to the medical lists were likewise controlled by this agency. It was the policy of the Committee, however, to defer in most cases to the judgment of the Executive Councils in matters involving the assessment of man power needs and the filling of vacancies. But there were occasions when nominees were rejected or an Executive Council's recommendation to deny a doctor admission to its list was denied. If, for example, a practitioner in one Council area found it convenient to take patients in another, the Medical Practices Committee usually granted permission, even if the Executive Council in the second area opposed the idea. This, of course, led to some resentment, since the local Councils felt that they were in a much better position to appraise the situation.

A medical practice vacancy was one of the best known but least important of the avenues into general practice. As explained, remaining partners handled their own vacancies and as a rule selected whomever they wished without interference. Single vacancies resulting from death or resignation could be disposed of in various ways, depending on circumstances. The small single practices were usually dispersed. Otherwise, an assistant or deputy who had been associated in a practice for some time, or a relative, would almost invariably be awarded the vacancy without delay. If no such person existed, the practice was advertised in the *British Medical Journal*. The number of openings that were made competitive was never large, averaging perhaps not more than 15 per cent of all single vacancies. It was not strange, therefore, that these vacancies, so few in number, were to invite such a flood of applications.[8]

The procedure followed was pretty much standard. Once the decision to fill a vacancy was reached, the Executive Council would publicize the opening. In co-operation with the local medical committee, the Council would screen the applications, interview a small number of the more promising candidates, and then submit three or more names ranked in order of preference. The Medical Practices Committee, which met at least once a week, examined the qualifications of the nominees and held personal interviews with them before reaching its decision. An unsuccessful candidate had the right of appeal to the Minister of Health, who could reach a decision without an oral hearing or refer the appeal to a special appellate body consisting of a lawyer, a medical officer of the Ministry, and a doctor chosen from a panel nominated by the British Medical Association. The appellant could attend the hearing in person or could be represented by counsel if he wished. Only in a very few cases was the decision of the Medical Practices Committee reversed.[9]

The machinery worked smoothly enough for the most part, but it was the time element that most critics found objectionable. In the event of an appeal, it took a minimum of ten or eleven weeks to fill a vacancy; otherwise, seven or eight weeks were required.[10] Normally, this amount of time did not prove excessive, but in the case of a sudden death in a large practice, there sometimes were serious consequences, especially if there were unexpected delays in making the appointment. At the annual meeting of the Executive Councils' Association in 1957, reference was made to an important vacancy in Kent that, owing to a series of unfortunate mistakes, required five and one-half months to fill. Although exceptional, this case was used as evidence for a motion, which passed, favoring the adoption of the system of filling vacancies used in Scotland, where Executive Councils exercised the right of selection, with the Medical Practices Committee serving only as an appellant body and with no other authority having such jurisdiction.[11]

The British Medical Association urged adoption of this plan or a similar one, but the Ministry of Health denied the need for change. It was contended that such delays as had occurred were due not so much to defects in the selection procedure itself as to the time consumed in hearing appeals, and the right to appeal was also a part of the Scottish system.[12]   The Cohen Committee was of the opinion that the English system was more satisfactory, since it gave the practitioner, through the appointive power of the Medical Practices Committee and the right of appeal to the Minister of Health, double instead of single protection.   Since "local knowledge may also be local interest and prejudice," the English procedure, it was affirmed, was a better guarantee that the interests of all would be served.[13]

Some issues were to die hard, and one of these was the loss of the right to buy or sell the good will of a practice.   Prior to the inauguration of the Health Service, the leadership of the British Medical Association had strongly opposed the government in its determination to abolish the custom in the new Service.   The sale of good will, however, was incompatible with health centers and the controls entrusted to the Medical Practices Committee.   Quite obviously, if over-doctored areas were to be closed to new entrants and single vacancies were to be dispersed, advertised, or otherwise disposed of by a central committee, an open market for the sale of practices could not be tolerated.   On this issue the Ministry of Health was adamant and would not compromise beyond the pledge to reimburse all practitioners who entered the Health Service at the time of its inception.

In co-operation with the medical profession, the government fixed the total amount of this reimbursement at £66 million ($184 million), to be apportioned among practitioners in proportion to their average gross annual receipts for the two years prior to the so-called appointed day.   The sum would earn 2.75 per cent interest, and the principal would be payable at retirement or at death, whichever was earlier, although in case of hardship an advance payment would be made.   To insure fair treatment, the Practices Compensation Committee, a majority of whom were medical practitioners, was set up to assist the Minister in determining the value of each practice.   In case of disagreement, provision was made for arbitration.[14]

The few doctors who remained in private practice were as free as ever to sell the good will of their practices, but the loss of so many of their patients, with the resulting reduction in the value of their good will, left these doctors resentful.   Among some Health Service doctors, especially the older ones, there was strong feeling that the compensation offered by the government was inadequate or that the right to sell good will was essential to freedom of movement, economic security, and high professional standards.   In the Fellowship For Freedom in Medicine these doctors found a determined and militant advocate of the cause they favored.   This organization, however, represented only a minority of the medical profession, whereas the British Medical Association, with an all-embracing membership, chose to abandon the fight for the right to sell good will as the only realistic course.

It was in the Representative Assembly of the Medical Association that the issue was finally resolved. The test came in 1954. After some fiery speeches, the motion that "no further action be taken regarding the scheme for the restoration of the right to buy and sell goodwill" was carried, but only by a small margin of votes. It was evident that a strong minority was not prepared to relinquish this right. Yet the arguments, repeated so often before, that the loss of good will interfered with clinical freedom or that its restoration was a necessary defense against the establishment of a full-time salaried service left many of the delegates unimpressed. They were unable to see how the abolition of this right had actually infringed upon their liberty.

To the majority of the delegates it was clear, as the chairman of the Council explained, that the restoration of the selling and buying of good will was neither feasible nor advisable. Serious practical difficulties would be encountered in trying to implement the proposed restoration. The heavy capital outlay that would once again be required of young doctors, the division of sentiment in the medical profession over the issue, and the absence of support in Parliament for the policy were reasons enough for opposing the proposal.[15] In reporting the debate, the *Manchester Guardian* observed that "among the welter of speeches there was a touch of unreality as no one really attacked the present system. Rather they were putting the pros and cons of a hypothetical 'good thing.' The days have gone when the association made headline news, by metaphorically speaking, burning Mr. Aneurin Bevan in effigy."[16]

In 1956 one last attempt was made to get the British Medical Association to reverse its position on the issue of good will. After a spirited exchange of remarks on the subject at the Annual Representative Meeting, it was moved that the convention proceed to the next item in the order of business "before any further damage is done." The convention so agreed.[17] The matter was now dead beyond all hope of revival. Some years before, the editor of *The Lancet* had struck at the heart of the whole issue when he said, "What happened when general practitioners entering the service surrendered the good-will of their private practices was that they exchanged their private security for a promise of public security."[18]

On some issues there was a large measure of unanimity in the profession—the immediate payment of compensation for the loss of good will, for instance. The doctors were impatient to have this money. The amount had been computed in terms of 1948 money values, which, in subsequent years, suffered from the inroads of inflation. What once had been considered a fair interest rate no longer seemed adequate. Obligations that had been assumed by the government as the result of other nationalization had been paid in full. Under the circumstances, death or resignation seemed times too far removed for the payment of good will compensation, and the Representative Assembly in 1951 and again in 1955 voted that the entire obligation be discharged without delay. But the government refused to modify the original agreement on the grounds that it was "a once-for-all settlement which could stand irrespective of any changes in the level of values." Through the ordinary methods of payment, however, the total sum owed was gradually being reduced. By 1958, possibly half of it had been paid out or mortgaged.[19]

The abolition of the sale of practices did not mean a debt-free era for young doctors, as one wryly observed in a letter to *The Times* (London) in 1957. He had just purchased a home with office accommodations at a cost of £7,860 ($22,000). Financing this purchase involved a loan with interest charges of between 6 and 6.5 per cent. Any young man entering practice was indeed lucky, this young doctor asserted, to escape with obligations of less than £5,000 ($14,000).[20]

Such indebtedness, however, would have been much larger if good will had still been a factor. There was some danger that a sales contract might be used by a practitioner to recover a part of the good will value, and this subterfuge the government assiduously tried to prevent. A doctor wishing to sell his premises (home that included office facilities) to a successor could do so only if the price asked did not exceed the real market value for such property. Before completing the transaction and as a protection to himself, the selling practitioner could obtain a certificate from the Medical Practices Committee showing that the sale of good will was not involved. Since the certificate was optional, the lack of it did not imply illegality or dishonest intent. In the case of *Brown v. King* (1956), a doctor's premises were purchased without a certificate being issued. When the buyer later contested the legality of the transaction on the grounds that the price was excessive and included a charge for the good will of the practice, the court, in examining the evidence, held otherwise and ruled the contract valid.[21]

Partnership agreements offered to assistants were occasionally so unfair that there was a question whether or not indirect payments were involved in exchange for an element of good will. Here also a doctor could seek a certificate from the Medical Practices Committee to the effect that the sale of good will was not a part of the transaction. The Cohen Committee felt that if the certificates were made mandatory, such abuses and misunderstandings as had occurred could largely be avoided. This policy was recommended, but the formal statutory amendment required to implement it seemed to evoke little support.[22]

The sale and purchase of good will were not without at least one advantage—the facilitation of the movement of practitioners when they desired to make a change. Under the old system, an aging doctor who preferred fewer patients or a more pleasant environment could sell his own practice and purchase another which promised the conditions he desired. As a Health Service doctor, he could do neither of these things; he could only resign from his own practice. Getting another of preferred size or in a preferred area was almost impossible. About the only avenue open was to apply for an advertised vacancy, but so few and so competitive were these that an older doctor stood little chance of obtaining one. The Minister of Health was not indifferent to the problem, but there seemed to be little he could do about it.

The Medical Practices Committee did what it could to expedite the exchange of practices, but because of location, size, or other special characteristics, they could seldom be accurately equated. During the first nine years of the Health Service, only twenty-three exchanges occurred in England and Wales.[23] The British Medical Association set up a Practices Advisory Bureau in 1948 to assist doctors to find employment. While enjoying moderate success with helping substitutes, part-time assistants, and younger doctors to get appointments, this bureau accomplished little in improving the mobility of older doctors.[24]

Although younger doctors were generally more mobile than older ones, few doctors of any age found it easy to get precisely the type of practice they wanted. For the inexperienced doctor, moreover, entry into general practice often constituted a major problem, in spite of the Danckwerts award and the Working Party Agreement. Corrective measures stimulated the growth of partnerships and obtained certain other very definite gains, but they did not achieve a balance between the number of applicants and the number of openings of the sort desired. The abolition of the sale of good will caused some doctors to remain in practice longer than they otherwise would have—a situation that apparently was reversed in 1958, when the superannuation system came into operation. The rapid growth in the size of the medical register for the United Kingdom, which increased by some 11,500 doctors during the ten-year period ending in 1957, would of itself and regardless of other considerations have intensified competition for all types of medical jobs.[25]

Considering, however, the over-all picture of partnership, assistantship, and single-practice vacancies, it is clear that the opportunities under the National Health Service were not fewer but more numerous—and more attractive to young practitioners—than during any other period in English medicine. The steady increase in the number of principals, 2,400 between 1949 and 1958, was proof of an expanding service. The Medical Practices Advisory Bureau alone was able in 1957 to effect "606 successful introductions to general practice appointments" in Great Britain. Inquiries conducted by the chairman of this bureau in 1955, 1956, and 1958 revealed that "the amount of enforced unemployment in the [medical] profession as a whole is small indeed."[26] The number of doctors that became principals in 1951 and 1952 averaged 1,100 for each of those two years. In 1953 the total exceeded 1,500, subsequently declining to fewer than 950 in 1957 and then rising above 1,050 the following year. In 1960 the number was 929.[27]

It would appear that a very large proportion of young medical practitioners found, if not precisely what they desired, at least work that proved satisfying and rewarding, though for many of them simple good fortune was the cause. There were those, of course, whom the vicissitudes of a competitive situation left disillusioned, and some of these did not hesitate to give vent to their frustration in the *British Medical Journal.*

If entrance into practice was beset with obstacles, they were easily identified. Competing for an advertised vacancy offered little hope. Starting a new practice was hazardous and laborious, with all the uncertainties about the ultimate size of the list. The Initial Practice Allowances did much to offset the limited income during the initial years, but thereafter the earnings could be very discouraging. In view of the risks involved, a doctor hesitated to assume the heavy financial obligation necessary to acquire an automobile, premises, and medical equipment. It was thus not surprising that only 10 per cent of the entrants into general practice in 1956 started new practices—a proportion only a trifle larger than that which was able to fill advertised vacancies. In 1960 the percentages for these two types of entrants were 6 and 10, respectively.[28]

Financial aid from the government had its limitations, but without it fewer practices would have been created and many doctors already established would have been exposed to real hardship. In addition to the Initial Practice Allowances, there were other grants of assistance, among them the Supplementary Annual Payments, which were intended primarily for single-practice physicians over 60 years of age who had lists of more than 300 and less than 1,078 patients. The Supplementary Annual Payments were given in addition to the normal capitation and loading fees. They included a basic sum in 1960 of £335 ($938), plus 14s ($1.96) for each person on the list between 301 and 450, with a deduction thereafter of the same amount of money per patient. The entire grant was thus recovered if the list reached 1,078. There were 208 practitioners at the end of 1959 who depended upon the Supplementary Annual Payments for a part of their income.

For doctors in thinly populated areas or areas presenting similar obstacles to good medical service, there were Inducement Payments. Ranging from £200 ($560) to £675 ($1,890) in 1960, these were given to keep doctors in practices that had a small earning potential. Comparatively few physicians, however, were beneficiaries from such grants. Of even less significance from the standpoint of cost to the government were the Hardship Payments, which, similar in some respects to Supplementary Annual Payments and about the same in amount, were available in single practices to doctors aged sixty-five or over.[29]

An assistantship with a view toward partnership was the best and most certain course open to a young doctor interested in becoming a principal in general practice. There were, of course, many varieties of assistantships. Some offered partnership status after a few years, while others were designed as permanent assistantships without hope of such promotion. The terms were not always clearly set forth or fully understood, and sometimes misunderstandings were the result. Personal differences occasionally occurred. Some assistantships thus proved little more than blind alleys. Good openings usually required experience, and experience could best be obtained by serving in part-time appointments or contracting for a year of apprenticeship in what was known as the trainee scheme.

Part-time assistants were needed to fill temporary vacancies or to substitute for doctors who had to attend meetings or were ill or on vacation. In 1958, only 40 per cent of the demand for part-time assistants was met. The supply was inadequate partly because of the disappearance of the "professional" substitute. Booking a doctor for part-time work well in advance became increasingly difficult, for practitioners who were not permanently employed preferred to keep themselves available on short notice to consider full-time assistantship appointments.[30]

The trainee general practitioner scheme was designed to give inexperienced doctors a more thorough and systematic training in general practice than could normally be obtained in an assistantship for a comparable period of time. Initiated in 1948, this program did much to facilitate the transition from medical school and internship into general practice. The scheme was modified in the light of experience, with the British Medical Association playing a major role in shaping it. Since the program operated on a local basis, its success depended upon the vigilance of the local medical committee, whose senior members, together with representatives of the local University, composed the selection committee. Appointments as trainers were subject to annual review, and during the period of his appointment the selection committee was expected to interview the trainer in order to ascertain how well he was performing his duties. The medical profession, which had much to gain from the scheme, kept a sharp eye on its operation and did everything possible to insure its success.

To qualify as a trainer, a doctor was normally required to have ten years of experience in general practice and to be under 65 years of age. Attention was paid to his reputation, to the condition of his equipment and office, and to the nature of his practice, which should offer the trainee a varied experience, including, if possible, obstetrics. The trainer's list could not be more than 3,500, and he could have only one trainee at a time under tutelage. A formal agreement between the general practitioner and his trainee was required at the outset, and it was understood that the latter was not to be employed with a view toward partnership. The number of physicians approved as trainers was over twice the actual number of trainees, which usually averaged between 275 and 350. In 1960, the trainer was paid £150 ($420) per year for his services, while the trainee received £1,150 ($3,220), with an additional allowance of £200 ($560) for car expenses. The program was financed entirely by the Exchequer.[31]

The Walker Report, while recognizing that the trainee program was fundamentally sound, noted that trainers did not always carry out their obligations and that there was "a tendency to regard the trainee as a cheap form of help rather than as one who should be helped."[32] The Cohen Report pronounced the program a success and recommended that it be encouraged. The remedy for abuse, it was emphasized, "lies with Local Medical Committees who have the necessary powers and local knowledge to prevent this."[33] The strong support accorded the program by the medical profession was demonstrated when one member of the Annual Representative Assembly of the British Medical Association moved that the trainee practitioner scheme was unnecessary and expensive and should be abolished. The opposition to the motion was vigorous, with Dr. Talbot Rogers pointing out that there was no cause for apprehension, since the scheme was subject to careful observation by the General Medical Services Committee. The motion was defeated by a large majority.[34]

The right to employ an assistant was granted by the Executive Council, which shared with the local medical committee the authority to review at intervals that right. Otherwise, complete freedom was left to the principal, who selected the assistant and determined the terms and conditions of his employment. Usually the agreement was verbal, which left the assistant with little recourse in the event of a violation. In most cases the arrangement worked out satisfactorily, but there were some assistants who were employed with a view toward partnership and who discovered at the end of the trial period that "circumstances" had altered in the interim so that partnership was no longer open to them. To what extent bad faith was involved could not very easily be determined. In 1955, the chairman of the Council assured the Annual Representative Assembly that cases of actual abuse were rare. He stressed, however, the advisability of legal, written agreements for assistants, and the assembly went on record as favoring such a policy. It was further recommended that Executive Councils keep under more rigid review the right of a doctor to employ an assistant.[35]

When an assistant was hired with the expectation of being admitted to partnership, the assumption usually was that enough new patients would be attracted to make the arrangement profitable. The additional loading was not always enough to offset a fall in income from the division of earnings. Many physicians in single practice, especially the older ones, found it financially advisable to retain the services of an assistant but not to form partnerships.[36] The patient list was very high for such practices, the average in 1957 being 3,600.

Assistants were often in no position to bargain, and in expectation of better days to come they were willing to accept low incomes and other unfavorable terms. The average salary, including car allowance, offered to assistants in 1956-57, as determined from some 200 advertisements in the *British Medical Journal,* was less than £1,070 ($3,000). Two years later, however, the average gross annual remuneration for assistants was reported to have risen to £1,360 ($3,800).[37]

Prior to 1952, the number of assistants was more or less stabilized at about 1,700. In some respects, making the transition from assistant to principal was more difficult during the first four years of the Health Service than it had been before 1948. An assistant admitted to partnership no longer paid for a share of the practice. What is more, the formation of a partnership meant a reduction in the gross earnings for the senior member. There was little, if any, financial incentive to convert a single practice into a partnership. The Danckwerts award and the Working Party Agreement changed all this, and within a year 550 assistants became partners in practices in which they had served as assistants. By 1954, the number of assistants had declined about 12 per cent. During the next two years, the trend was reversed, but again in 1957, 1958, and 1959 there was a substantial drop in the total number of assistantships, even though the number leading toward partnership was the highest since 1953.

An assistantship had become indisputably the quickest and most advantageous way to achieve the status of principal and partner. Nearly 70 per cent of those entering practice did so as partners in 1958, and a good majority of these previously had been assistants in the same practices in which they attained partnership status. Although assistants were the major source of new partners, as a group they represented less than 7 per cent of the total of all general medical practitioners. Most assistants were relatively young. In 1958, for example, 37 per cent were under thirty and only 10 per cent were fifty or older.[38]

The Working Party Agreement of 1952 produced an immediate growth in the number of partnerships. In that year, 57 per cent of all principals were partners, by 1958 the total had reached 68 per cent, and in 1960 it touched 70 per cent. In rural areas, three-fourths of all principals had become partners, but in the urban communities the proportion was little more than one-half. About 80 per cent of the partnerships comprised two or three doctors; 7 per cent had five or more members. Fifty-five per cent of the doctors in partnership were under forty-five years of age in 1958, whereas only 36 per cent of the single practitioners were in that age group.[39]

The trend of a rise in the number of partnerships was welcomed by the medical profession, as well as the Ministry of Health. The government, being aware of the benefits that would accrue to patient and physician thereby, did everything it could to encourage partnerships and the type of organization known as group practice, which was even more effective. The advantages of a partnership were known to most doctors before the days of the National Health Service. An aging practitioner would often take on a junior partner who not only contributed a capital sum but did the larger share of the work, knowing that eventually he would acquire all of the practice. The abolition of the sale of good will, although its immediate effects were mitigated by compensation and pension benefits, did largely destroy the financial motive for forming partnerships, but this was restored to some degree by the loading arrangement. There were other incentives, however, besides the pecuniary ones, and these help to explain why the creation of partnerships did not stop during the first years of the Health Service.

In a partnership, expenses were shared, which meant a lower expense ratio than usually could be achieved in a single practice. Costs of ancillary help, such as a secretary-receptionist or a nurse, could more easily be met. Such assistance relieved the doctor of many routine tasks, giving him time to carry a larger patient load or to pursue special interests in the medical field. The heavy responsibility of caring for patients twenty-four hours a day, seven days a week, was considerably lightened in a partnership, in which the load could be distributed among the partners, although this advantage could be obtained by a simple rota arrangement with other doctors. A partnership was a very convenient way to provide for vacations and off-duty hours, one partner at such times doing the work of another. A greater willingness to co-operate was thus fostered by the partnership concept, and this could be viewed as a real gain, since the competitive spirit, strongest among single practitioners, was not an unmixed blessing. Most important of all was the professional stimulation which came from an exchange of views, a sharing of experiences, and a collaboration on cases.

There were, however, abuses and irritants that occasionally impaired partnership arrangements. Some of these can be put down to the frailties of human nature. More serious, perhaps, was the unfair division of money and work which often left a junior partner at great disadvantage. Since the entrant to a partnership brought no capital and often very little experience, he was seldom in a position to demand favorable terms. The junior partner received a disproportionately small share of the earnings and often had to work harder and accept more unpleasant assignments than was in any way equitable.[40] The *Medical World Newsletter* referred to partnerships of two doctors in which the senior partner received one-half or two-thirds of the income without ever seeing a patient.[41] While these were extreme examples and were relatively few in number, it was a common practice to give the entrant a share amounting to one-third of the earnings of the senior partner and not to accord him parity until ten or more years had passed.

Under a 1953 regulation, if less than one-third of the earnings of the senior partner was granted to the junior partner, there could not occur that division of patients among the partners necessary to obtain the maximum loading fees. Otherwise, the government refrained from any attempt to control the terms of a contract, except, of course, to prohibit the sale of good will. To what extent junior partners were exploited was a matter on which there was no general agreement.

The Medical Practitioners' Union was of the opinion that inequitable distribution of work and income had generated a certain amount of frustration and friction and that the remedy was for partnership agreements "to conform to criteria laid down centrally." Parity, it was felt, should be reached within seven years, and income should bear some relation to the amount of work rendered.[42] The Cohen Committee did not feel that the exploitation of junior partners was widespread, but recognized the existence of abuses. It urged certification by the Medical Practices Committee, parity after a maximum of seven or eight years, and expert legal advice in drawing up partnership agreements.[43]

In the appraisal of partnerships, reference to abuses should not be permitted to overshadow the fact that the great majority operated with comparative smoothness. Most of the partnerships examined by Stephen Taylor in his survey were found to be exceptionally good.[44] The Cohen Report, in illustrating conditions under which general practitioners worked, gave some interesting data concerning a partnership of six doctors and one trainee assistant that served 12,400 patients, of whom less than 100 were private patients. Five of the doctors shared the same building, which was modern in every way and included a laboratory equipped for simple pathology examinations. The ancillary staff consisted of a telephone operator, a receptionist-secretary, a manager, and a filing clerk. Eight automobiles served the partnership. The doctors had access to the local hospital and to the X-ray, physiotherapy, pathology, and outpatient departments. Each partner had one-half day off per week and a four- or five-week holiday every year. Duty at night, on Sundays, and on official holidays was rotated. General and clinical problems were discussed at meetings held twice monthly. Each partner was paid a fixed sum per month, and periodically any large balance was shared.[45]

This partnership was better than most and probably representative of the best. It approximated group practice, which presumably had replaced the health center as the more realistic approach to an improved practitioner service. The emphasis in group practice was on co-operation, which could be attained to a much greater degree than was possible in an ordinary partnership, in which doctors' offices were frequently in separate houses. Although it did not necessarily have the formal legal status of partnership, in effect group practice was usually that and more, having evolved into a much more integrated kind of organization. The members of a group practice, usually between three and six practitioners, shared premises, expenses, and earnings, employed secretarial, nursing, and other ancillary help, and worked as a team clinically and otherwise. Each practitioner had his own list of patients and made every effort to maintain a satisfactory doctor-patient relationship. But through consultation and collaboration with other members of the group, he sought to practice a more effective type of medicine. In a group practice, more time was normally available for professional improvement or sessional work in the local-authority clinic or a general-practitioner hospital.

Both the medical profession and the Ministry of Health strongly favored this approach as having the most to offer to patient and physician. "Group practice," declared the Minister of Health on one occasion, "besides lightening the burden of a doctor's life and enormously facilitating co-operation with his colleagues, also opens the door to increased co-operation in other spheres."[46]

A strong stimulus for establishing group practices was the Group Practice Loans Fund, which became operative at the beginning of 1954. Doctors desiring to organize a group practice could seek an interest-free loan for the erection of a new building or the conversion of existing premises. A committee representing the medical profession and the Ministry of Health took final action upon the applications to which the Executive Council, in consultation with the local medical committee, had previously given approval. The loans were recovered by systematic deductions from the remuneration paid by the Executive Councils. During the period in which the loan was in effect, the premises could not be sold, but as far as designing the building, arranging office accommodations, and operating the group practice were concerned, the doctors were permitted a large measure of freedom. The sum of £88,000 ($246,000) that was annually provided from the Central Pool for the Group Practice Loans Fund was enlarged as repayments were made, but each year the amount available fell short of the demand. By the end of 1960, £872,000 ($2,440,000) had been allocated as loans.[47]

Group practice could not accomplish all that was expected of it by those who viewed it as a practical substitute for the health center. The assumption that co-operation with the local health authority and other branches of the Health Service would be fostered through the group practice approach seems to have been borne out rather poorly. The members of a group practice owned or rented their office accommodations and otherwise retained full control over the management of their practice, subject, of course, to certain regulations administered by the Executive Council with whom the practitioners were under contract. The local health authorities thus were in no position to exercise jurisdiction over a group practice, and if co-operation were to occur, it would have to be voluntary. Co-operation of this kind was, in fact, manifested here and there, and there were prospects for much more of it, but group practice was on the whole disappointing in this respect.

When the Health Service took shape, it was the health center that aroused the liveliest expectations of doctors and laymen. The Interim Report of the British Medical Association in 1942 attached great significance to this type of practice and gave it a prominent place in the blueprint proposed for the future Health Service. The White Paper of 1944 and the great majority of doctors were no less enthusiastic about health centers, which, having such wide support, came to occupy a key position in the new law.

The enactment did not go so far as to spell out any of the details of health centers. It simply provided in Section 21 that such centers were to be provided and maintained by the local health authority, with facilities for any or all of the following: pharmaceutical, general medical, and dental services, specialist or other services for out-patients, and the statutory services required of the local health authority. In view of the growing specialization and interdependence of the various branches of medicine, the necessity for co-ordination was recognized, and so the proposed union of the practitioner, consultant, and preventive phases was warmly applauded. The need of the family doctor for diagnostic help from the pathologist and radiologist, for advice from the specialist, and for assistance from nurses familiar with therapeutic techniques was well understood. By bringing many of these skills together, the health center would, it was anticipated, do much to improve the quality of medicine.

Few could quarrel with the principle, but implementing it was another matter. How should the centers be built and managed? There were no clear conceptions about size, cost, design, or administrative policy. The only logical approach seemed simply to be to learn by experiment, but that would take time, and many in the government and the profession were impatient of delay. The most serious handicap was the lack of money.

The Council of the British Medical Association in 1948 made some concrete proposals. In a well-equipped building staffed with nurses, midwives, doctors, dentists, and pharmacists, the health center should unite curative medicine, the concern of the general practitioner, with preventive medicine, primarily the responsibility of the local health officer. It should offer a co-ordinated program embracing "general medical service, care of mothers and young children, care of school children, vaccination and immunization, antenatal and postnatal examinations, health visiting, home nursing and health education." Compensation for the practitioners should come from the Executive Council, the local health authority, and the regional hospital board, each paying for services rendered within its particular sphere. It was further suggested that the general administration of each center should be entrusted to a joint committee representing all of the professional personnel. A health center with eight doctors could serve an estimated population of 25,000. Before launching an all-out program of construction, the government was urged to experiment with different types of centers and during the period of experimentation to establish a central committee for co-ordination guidance.[48]

The most enthusiastic advocates of the health center concept were the Socialist Medical Association and the Medical Practitioners' Union. The latter in 1949 demanded the immediate erection of 100 centers and the completion of the entire program of health center construction within ten years.[49] While this organization was later to lose its crusading zeal for the centers, the Socialist Medical Association was to remain their staunch and unswerving ally. Although the Fellowship For Freedom in Medicine was at no time in favor of the idea, the medical profession as a whole accepted it at first as something very good, being impressed, it may be suspected, more with the theoretical aspects than the practical ones.

The program got under way very slowly. The Ministry of Health moved cautiously, uncertain about precisely what form the health center should take. A number of dispensaries and general clinics at the outset were approved as health centers and operated as such by the local health authorities, but comparatively few of the new centers provided for by law ever got beyond the drawing board. After ten years they were still in the experimental stage, and the authorities still had no clear conception what the prototype should be. As early as 1951, Dr. A. Talbot Rogers, an influential medico-politician who had been one of the most vigorous champions of the health center, acknowledged that "there now seems little likelihood that the national finance will permit of any widespread trial of the health center experiment perhaps for ten or twenty years" and that this would be "too long to wait." Like many others, he was beginning to feel that perhaps group practice would have to be accepted as the alternative.[50]

It was not merely a question of finance or a shortage of building material, as the Ministry of Health was to observe, but also a problem of personnel management. Staffing a health center on terms necessary for the creation of a smoothly working team was often impossible. Getting such divergent groups as the hospital, local authority, and Executive Council to co-operate was difficult, owing to the traditionally competitive character of British medicine. The doctors, in taking a second look at the health center concept, decided that what was good as an idea might not be to their interest in practice.

There were risks involved that discouraged participation. If a doctor joined a health center, would he not lose patients in the transfer, and if later he should wish to return to his old quarters, would he not sustain a further loss? The fact that another doctor might move into the vicinity where he had once maintained his office and build up a successful practice at his expense had its effect. The latent hostility with which general practitioners viewed the local health authorities was an obstacle. The control of health centers was considered a threat to the independence of the practitioner. There were the usual misgivings about what might happen to the doctor-patient relationship. Some shared the fear that in a health center general practice would evolve into "some sort of a glorified hospital outpatient department where intimate knowledge of the patient, continuity of treatment and the idea of the doctor as guide, philosopher and friend are sacrificed to a hurried, impersonal machine."

Because of its superior facilities and other special advantages, there was a certain amount of jealousy of those who joined a health center. An old dread was revived for those who saw the health center as a back door to a salaried service. The concern over competition from new health center doctors was also important. If none of the practitioners within a district would accept service in a new center, how should it be staffed? On this point the British Medical Association was emphatic—that if the local doctors would not serve, the Executive Council should have no right to advertise the vacancies elsewhere. With this policy the Ministry of Health disagreed, although it recognized the inadvisability of advertising elsewhere under such circumstances. To avoid the danger of a health center's becoming a white elephant, it was deemed prudent to negotiate in advance the contractual arrangements for staffing the building. But doctors hesitated to commit themselves in that fashion, since it was impossible to anticipate all conditions that might later arise.[51]

The fact that many of the foregoing fears were demonstrated to be groundless in practice did not seem to make doctors any more sympathetic toward health centers. The Postal Survey of the British Medical Association in 1951 disclosed that only 38 per cent of the practitioners approved of them. The Hadfield Survey of the same year showed a somewhat higher percentage, but still less than half. By 1956, the sentiment, if anything, was less favorable. The Social Surveys revealed that little more than a third of the practitioners supported the idea of a health center in their neighborhood.[52]

The health centers that came into existence were of three types:

those that were taken over on the appointed day, those that were established as new centers under Section 21 of the Act, and those that were planned and provided by bodies other than local health authorities. At the end of the first five years, there were in England and Wales twenty-five health centers in operation. Four of these were established under Section 21, and one was provided by a non-govermental agency. All the others had existed in one form or other prior to 1948. The Woodberry Down Health Center, Stoke Newington, cost more than £180,000 ($500,000), but considerably less was spent upon the other centers, and upon two of these only a few thousand pounds were spent for the renovation of some old buildings. At the end of 1958, there were ten Section 21 health centers in operation and a few others were under construction. The establishment of several more centers had already been approved, but it was apparent that the government preferred to follow a very limited program of health center construction.[53]

The type of center visualized by the founders of the Health Service was never fully realized. It was intended to be an institution where doctors and others would join in a common effort to cure illness and promote positive health. Too often it became a place where competition and an absence of unity seemed to be predominant characteristics. In many cases, the doctor retained his old quarters, using the health center only as a branch office. Many health center practitioners were not in partnership, each competing with the others for patients. Few of the health centers offered all of the services, some having only general medical, pharmaceutical, and dental services and others having general medical and pharmaceutical services, no dental service, but maternity and child welfare services. The centers were expensive to maintain, with income from office space often being far below the amount required to meet the initial and operating costs of the building. The Executive Council usually contracted for the office space from the local health authority and then leased it at a big discount. Even with this reduction, office space charges were considered burdensome by doctors who had their regular offices elsewhere.[54]

The Woodberry Down Health Center, one of the earliest constructed and the most elaborate of all, was opened in 1952 by the London County Council. Designed, as were most of the others, to meet the medical needs of a new housing development, it offered the full range of curative and preventive services. The center was equipped with six suites of rooms for general practitioners, a garage for each doctor, a small flat for the night physician, a common room for the medical staff, a room for minor operations, a medical storeroom, two dental offices and a dental workshop, a lecture hall, an ultraviolet and an X-ray room, laboratory facilities, space for child welfare, school health, and maternity units, a day nursery, and accommodations for health visitors and other nurses. The ancillary help in 1956 included an administrative officer, two clerk-receptionists and two nurses. None of the six doctors in that year was in partnership with any of the others, and all had offices elsewhere. The annual running cost of each suite of offices was about £964 ($2,700), of which slightly more than one-third was recovered in rent from the doctors. Designed to create the best possible working conditions for general practice and to permit the closest co-operation with the other health services, the Woodberry Down Center stood out as a model, albeit one that, because of its cost, would not soon be duplicated.[55]

More representative than Woodberry Down was the William Budd Health Center, Knowle West, at Bristol. Although it cost much less than the one in London, it had suites of offices for as many doctors and served several thousand more patients. With emphasis upon utility, office space was designed for use by the practitioners in the morning and evening and by the local health personnel in the afternoon. The ancillary staff in 1955 comprised a nursing superintendent and deputy, two secretary-typist-receptionists, one clerk, and three health center nurses. The nine doctors at the center in that year were members of five partnership firms. The services rendered —general medical, child welfare, school health, and maternity—were somewhat more restricted than those offered at Woodberry Down. Office rental per doctor was about one-seventh of the running cost of each suite of offices. The responsibility of each doctor for the treatment of school children and the prenatal care of mothers on his list tended to bridge the gap between the practitioner and the public health services. The William Budd center, for what it sought to accomplish, enjoyed a large measure of success.[56]

The operation of economical and flexible health centers designed to meet the special needs of a locality was considered by the Nuffield Provincial Hospitals Trust as the only way to surmount the difficulties that had so far retarded the health center program. Proceeding gingerly, this non-governmental agency established several modest centers which, as experimental ventures, won wide acclaim. The new and rapidly expanding housing area of Harlow New Town in Essex was selected as the most appropriate place for the new centers. They were small and strictly utilitarian. Doctors were willing to pay a rent that accurately reflected the cost of their quarters, since their practices were conducted almost exclusively from the centers. By putting all space to the most advantageous use, the investment in these center projects became self-liquidating. One of them, the first, evoked this evaluation from a doctor associated with the Nuffield Trust: "From Haygarth House we learned the virtue of smallness. There were many complaints about lack of space; but compulsory close living of doctors, dentists, local authority officers, health visitors, midwives, and secretaries, in the service of about 8,000 patients, helped to teach the value of co-operation and mutual help. Doctors and dentists became colleagues in diagnosis and treatment; doctors and health visitors colleagues in social medicine. The local-authority clinics were soon an everyday part of the life of the general practitioners; the county and area medical officers of health familiar friends."[57]

One other experimental venture must be mentioned, since its uniqueness brought it medical visitors from various parts of the world. Darbishire House, which served 8,000 or more patients, was a health center with a very special additional purpose—training of medical students. Associated with Manchester University and financed largely by the Nuffield Provincial Hospitals Trust, this center was opened in 1954. It took most of four years, with a two-year rent moratorium as a special inducement, to persuade four doctors to accept service in the center, but once they were established they became enthusiastic about it. Abandoning their old offices, they did all their practicing from the new center. Ancillary assistance, including X-ray and laboratory facilities, helped to simplify and expedite their work. In combination with child welfare, maternity, and social clinics, these practitioners were able to offer service free of the usual "over-lapping and duplication." To each doctor was assigned a final-year medical student for a period of two weeks, during which the student had the opportunity to observe some of the practical aspects of general practice. The success of this venture was beyond question, judging by the annual reports of the center and by editorial comment.[58]

The noteworthy achievements of this experiment and some of the others did not alter the general health center picture or offer much hope that health centers would become the pattern of the future. The Ministry of Health more and more adjusted its program in favor of group practice, without, however, abandoning its support of the idea of health centers. The Guillebaud Report could see a valid need for health centers in new housing areas or in densely populated industrial regions where the existing facilities were inadequate, but otherwise felt that the approach should remain experimental.[59]

The success of the National Health Service depended in large measure upon a sufficient number of adequately trained doctors. The medical schools did not lack students. Whereas before World War II the number of applicants did not greatly exceed the number of places, afterwards, and especially with the inception of the new health scheme, competition among students became very keen, and medical schools had ten times more applications than places. The London Medical College may not have been representative, but when the author visited it in 1954 he was told that 3,000 applications were received yearly, of which 600 resulted in interviews and 100 in actual admission. Students were drawn from all walks of life, but manual workers, who comprised close to three-quarters of the population, accounted for a disproportionately small part of the student body in medical colleges. In 1955, it was less than 20 per cent. Doctors' sons alone made up 17 per cent. The allegation that medicine was no longer a popular choice of career for the children of doctors was not confirmed by the data, which in that year showed that, among the sons of doctors admitted to colleges and universities, over half entered the medical course.[60]

Obtaining a medical education or any other type of university training was no longer beyond the reach of any properly qualified applicants. Local authority grants and grants to state scholars were available for those who otherwise could not afford to attend institutions of higher learning. In 1919, the University Grants Committee was established to investigate the financial needs of higher education and to advise Parliament in the matter. For some years the amount of money available to subsidize higher education was limited, treasury grants constituting not more than one-third of university income. But by 1950 the universities were receiving more than two-thirds of their income from Parliamentary grants. In 1938, only a fourth of the medical students were assisted by a scholarship or some other form of financial help, whereas the proportion in the 1950's reached three-quarters.[61]

When Harold S. Diehl and two other deans of American medical schools, at the behest of the American Medical Association, made their study of British medical education in 1949-50, they found academic freedom in no way threatened by state aid. The achievements of the University Grants Committee, declared the report of these deans, "had been so satisfactory that . . . medical education and medical research are not now and seem unlikely to become functions of the state, even though the state provides the greater part of their financial support." The American committee further observed that the greater influx of medical students led to a more careful policy of screening, and that each university enjoyed complete control over its admissions policy. Whether a student received financial aid was contingent upon his being admitted to a recognized university. The committee seemed impressed with the fact that economic barriers no longer meant the loss of gifted young minds to the medical profession.[62]

But there was a growing feeling in England that too many doctors were being trained. The medical schools, filled to capacity, were turning out practitioners at a much faster rate than population growth seemed to justify. The increase in the number of medical personnel was sharpest after 1948. More doctors were added to the hospital rosters, and each year saw a larger number of practitioners getting on the Health Service lists. An article published in 1954 by the dean of postgraduate medical studies at Manchester University was particularly disturbing. He observed that during the ten years preceding, the average annual increase in the medical register had been over 2,000. More than half of the general practitioners were under 45 years of age. For every advertised job, there was a flood of applications. If the medical schools continued to admit the present number of students, there would be a surplus, he predicted, of between 5,000 and 6,000 doctors by 1959.[63]

The Medical Practices Committee in 1954 raised the question of whether the saturation point in general practice was not in sight. In the same year, the Annual Meeting of the Medical Association resolved that "in view of the saturation of certain branches of the medical profession the Minister should be impressed with the extreme urgency of the situation." The Cohen Committee was not disturbed about the influx into general practice, which to it seemed reasonable, but felt that the British economy might not be able to sustain the expansion indefinitely. The Committee suggested that an inquiry should be made to determine what future needs were likely to be and whether there should be some limit imposed upon the number of medical students.[64] A committee of ten members under the chairmanship of Sir Henry Willink, Vice-Chancellor of Cambridge University, was accordingly appointed by the Minister of Health early in 1955 to explore the question of supply and demand in medical practice.

It soon became evident that the Medical Association did not favor any restriction on the number of entrants to the medical profession. In a memorandum to the Willink Committee, the Association acknowledged that the increase in doctors had been phenomenal but denied there was any substantial unemployment or that future man-power requirements could be accurately gauged. There were too many imponderables, among them the effects of an aging population, which by 1979 would number an estimated 9.5 million people in the old age group. In view of all the changes and the possible expansion that might occur in the Health Service, how could the future number of doctors, it was asked, be calculated with any accuracy? The rise of new specialities, advances in therapy, new concepts of social medicine, developments in occupational health, greater emphasis on preventive medicine, and new approaches to the problems of mental health were among the factors set forth that could render ineffectual any ceiling upon entry into medicine.[65]

The Willink Report, published in the fall of 1957, was cautious in its approach and restrained in its recommendations. The Committee frankly admitted that its findings, although based upon the most accurate data, might require modification in the light of subsequent developments. The evidence pointed to very little current unemployment among doctors. The difficulty of entry into practice combined with an intense competition for hospital posts to create the erroneous impression that there were too many doctors. The Committee noted a shortage of practitioners in some of the less attractive areas. If the average patient-doctor ratio were reduced everywhere to what many considered a more ideal proportion—one doctor for every 2,500 patients in the urban areas and every 2,000 in the rural areas—there would have been a noticeable dearth of practitioners in 1955. Exclusive of overseas students, the annual number of medical graduates in Great Britain approximated 1,825. This total, declared the report, was not too large for the current demand.

In seeking to determine the future needs of the practitioner service, the Committee examined such factors as the retirement trend, the emigration and immigration rates of doctors, the growth of population, and the need for physicians in the factory medical service, the pharmaceutical industry, and the clinics and other services of the local health authority and in the specialist and hospital services. It was none of these factors that seemed to warrant any ceiling on student enrollment, but rather the scheduled reduction in the size of armed services, which by 1962 would require 1,000 fewer doctors. The Committee accordingly proposed a 10 per cent decrease in the acceptance of medical students at the earliest possible date. Inasmuch as several years were required to train doctors, the effects of this decrease would not be felt before 1965. Looking further into the future, the Committee felt that beginning in 1971 the reduction would have to be removed and that by 1980 the output of medical schools would have to be increased by 200 above the current level. These alterations were considered necessary to offset changes in the age and size of the population, and the retirement and death of doctors. It was estimated that between 1955 and 1971 the number of active civilian doctors in Great Britain would rise 13 per cent, as compared with a 4.5 per cent increase in the population.[66]

The Willink Report shed light on several other areas, including the pattern of retirement and emigration for general practitioners. Sixty-nine per cent of those practitioners between sixty-five and sixty-nine years of age and 37 per cent of those seventy years and over were still in active practice.   These percentages were much higher than those for teachers and persons engaged in insurance and finance, but were not greatly out of line with those for most of the other professional groups.   Although the superannuation scheme for doctors would become operative in 1958, the amount of the pension for several years would be relatively small, so that early retirement would hardly be encouraged by the scheme.   But not even the maximum pension would cause many to retire at 65, since the average doctor, asserted the Report, "is sufficiently attached to his profession to wish to continue to practice as long as his health will allow."

Twelve per cent of the doctors practicing in Great Britain at the time had obtained all or the largest part of their training elsewhere. Most of these were from Northern Ireland, the Republic of Ireland, and the Commonwealth countries.   About 100 of the undergraduate medical students had come from the colonies and Commonwealth nations, and if there had been more room in the medical colleges the number would have been much larger.   In recent years, about 400 doctors of British origin had been emigrating each year, mostly to other parts of the Commonwealth.   Owing, however, to the desire on the part of those countries to draw their medical personnel from their own people and to develop their own training facilities, it was predicted by the Willink Report that the rate of emigration would diminish substantially within the next twenty years.   Conversely, as opportunities in Great Britain dwindled for outside doctors, their number would likewise decrease.   If the number of those who sought careers overseas in the recent past was balanced against the number of those from abroad who entered Great Britain to practice, an estimated net export per year of approximately 200 doctors was indicated, but this number, it was predicted, would shrink to one-fourth of its present size by 1970.[67]

The allegation that the National Health Service had caused an increasing proportion of medical men to leave Great Britain was questioned by the Board of Trade, which in 1958 disclosed that the number of doctors and dentists emigrating by sea from the United Kingdom declined between 1952 and 1957.   The net loss was actually greater in the earlier years (1951-52) than in subsequent years. In 1958, the British Medical Association prepared a memorandum based on returns from all but a few of the Executive Councils that showed that the emigration rate of doctors from 1948 to 1957 averaged annually 3.13 per thousand. The figures, however, revealed considerable fluctuation, ranging from 2.13 at the outset to 5 in 1951, then declining to 1.87 in 1954 and rising to 5.07 per thousand in 1957.[68] The crises over remuneration in 1951 and 1957 may have influenced the rates of emigration, but the over-all average for the ten years was comparatively low. The Pilkington Commission in its report of 1960 observed that the "available statistics give no grounds for supposing that the level of net emigration among doctors and dentists is higher than among the population as a whole."[69]

There was a net inward movement of doctors from South Africa, Pakistan, and India and a net outward movement to the United States, Canada, and a few other Commonwealth nations. Over 1,000 doctors from abroad were employed in British hospitals in 1957.[70] The interchange of experience and thought represented by this movement of medical personnel contributed much to the development of British medicine.

CHAPTER VIII

The Family Physician in His New Professional Role

MANY SURVEYS AND INQUIRIES have been made, some by doctors and others by laymen, concerning the type, volume, and effectiveness of the work done by the practitioner, his attitude toward various aspects of the health scheme, and the popular reaction to the general medical service. Together, they give a composite picture of the Health Service, although one not as sharply etched as could be wished. But a program so complicated and controversial might be expected to have various shades and colors. The evidence, in any case, does point to some very definite conclusions. Many of the more important surveys have already been the subject of comment, but there are others that should be mentioned.

Perhaps the best estimate of the practitioner's work can be obtained from the study by the Government Social Survey, which included information from a special inquiry in 1952 and from the Sickness Survey figures for 1950. An analysis by the Registrar General of the clinical records of thirteen practitioners, 1952-1954, is no less revealing. The report on a year of general practice by John Fry, a five-year study of a general practice by Alistair Mair and George B. Mair, and the studies of a general practice by Maurice Backett and two associates give a factual description of three large practices at work. By way of comparison with the prewar era, A. Bradford Hill's inquiries into the status of the practitioner have a special value. Nor should John Pemberton's consideration of eight general practitioners in 1947 be overlooked in any comparative treatment.

Dr. Stevenson's inquiry in 1952 analyzed the attitudes of some 60 practitioners. The poll conducted by the Social Surveys in 1956 covered an impressive list of questions addressed to a large number of doctors and patients. Less comprehensive but more recent was the canvass of public sentiment made in London and Edinburgh by J. F.

Brotherston and two associates. Few reports could have been more objective than the one prepared by Sir Frank Newsam, who had been selected by the British Medical Association to make an investigation of the family doctor's services. The conclusions embodied in this document, published in 1959, are most important.

Two noteworthy inquiries were conducted by Americans. The first one, in 1953, was done by D. Reid Ross, a graduate of the University of Chicago. In a 5 per cent random sample poll, he endeavored to appraise the sentiment of the people about the practitioner service in a typical industrial community. The second survey was made in 1956 by Professor Paul F. Gemmill of the Wharton School of Finance and Commerce, University of Pennsylvania. Through questionnaires and interviews, he covered 139 general medical practices in 48 widely distributed cities, seeking to determine what the medical profession and the patients thought of various phases of the Health Service.

The surveys were generally agreed that with the National Health Service came an improvement in professional co-operation that, however, had been achieved as much through the evolution of rota systems as through the growth of partnerships and group practices. Although the capitation system of remuneration was basically competitive in character, it did not prevent the stabilization of doctors' lists. Suspicion between practitioners thereupon tended to abate, and there emerged a greater willingness to form local practitioner associations. Such co-operative ventures existed before the war, but not until after the advent of the Health Service did they become general. A survey by the Medical Practitioners' Union in 1952 revealed that in the rural areas at least 50 per cent of the general practitioners belonged to a rota scheme, while in the industrial areas the percentage rose to 65. Rural rotas were usually too small to reach maximum effectiveness, but in the urban communities, where doctors were concentrated, rotas of five or more doctors were very common. More than one-half of all single practitioners in England and Wales belonged to rotas.[1]

Sometimes spontaneously and sometimes with encouragement from the Executive Council or the local medical committee, the practitioners within a locality would organize a rota for the purpose of assuring themselves more off-duty time. The arrangement made provision for week ends, mid-week half days, sickness, holidays, and nights. For a rota of five members, for instance, each practitioner had one duty-night per week and one duty-week-end every five weeks. The problem of obtaining substitutes was thus solved and provision made for an uninterrupted service for all patients. The duty-doctor was not normally overworked, since his services as a rule were required only in emergency. To prevent misunderstanding, no practitioner would accept on his list any patient from another physician in the rota. The scheme not only promoted a spirit of good will but tended to foster clinical co-operation. Cases were discussed and medical viewpoints exchanged in the rota meetings and between the duty-physician and individual members. To what extent rotas stimulated group practice could not easily be determined, but many of them "turned the sourness of professional rivalry into the sweetness of co-operation."[2]

One of the largest and most successful rota arrangements was that in Ilford, a community of 185,000 contiguous with East London. Organized in 1948 and comprising 65 practitioners, this rota was divided geographically into seven groups, each with its own secretary. All the groups, however, were served by a single clerk, who, during the period when the rota functioned, took the incoming telephone messages and relayed them to the appropriate duty-doctor, or, in the case of a serious accident, called an ambulance. Week-end calls averaged about 100 for the entire rota or 14 per duty-doctor. Night calls did not constitute much of a problem, averaging only one every other week end for each duty-practitioner. The scheme provided an exceptionally broad coverage, with provision for the care of a doctor's patients during any length of illness he might have. The plan operated smoothly and encountered criticism from only a small minority of the people.[3]

Not all practitioners were in a position to form a partnership or join a rota. To meet the need of such physicians for off-duty and leisure time, an Emergency Call Service was established in London in 1956. Organized along commercial lines, it was a standing deputizing arrangement which permitted any doctor who paid for the service to turn over all night and week-end calls to the agency. The British Medical Association was not enthusiastic about the plan, since it was open to abuse. It offered the physician an easy way to avoid work normally expected of him under his terms of service. For this reason, some doctors were critical of the scheme, and the General Medical Services Committee seemed to have misgivings about the future of such deputizing arrangements. The Emergency Call Service, however, did not appear to violate the regulations of the Health Service. If properly supervised and judiciously used, in full co-operation with the Executive Council, the scheme might, in the opinion of the Council of the Medical Association, "constitute a suitable supplement to the more usual methods of practice."[4]

If co-operation among the practitioners was good, it was even better between the medical profession and the Ministry of Health. The failure to adjust differences over remuneration amicably and speedily did not mean that government and doctors were unable to work together effectively on most other matters. Such co-operation through the years was attested to by various medical and lay officials. In 1956 the Minister of Health, in a not at all unusual statement, said:

I would like to record my thanks for the solid consistent help which I and my department receive from general practitioners as a body. At the national level we have the General Medical Services Committee, who are unwearied in conference and fertile in suggestions on all subjects affecting general practice. Next I would thank the individual doctors who have so willingly added to their other burdens by serving on departmental committees and working parties. I am not forgetting all the work undertaken (and to be undertaken in the future) throughout the country by local medical committees and their members, by which, with every month that passes, general practitioners in their own sphere are shaping the future of the National Health Service.[5]

The need for doctors to keep abreast of the most recent medical developments and otherwise to maintain and extend their professional knowledge was recognized as much by the Ministry of Health as by the British Medical Association. The National Health Service Act empowered the Minister to arrange postgraduate and refresher courses at the universities and to help finance the expenses incurred in taking them. Three main types of refresher courses were set up: intensive two-week courses, extended courses in which the sessions were spread over many weeks or months, and short, week-end courses. Some were general and others were more specialized, covering such subjects as dermatology, pathology, pediatrics, cardiology, infant feeding, obstetrics, and gynecology. For enrollment in a short course, the prior approval of the Ministry of Health was not necessary. The allowance, which in 1958 was £18 ($50) per week with which to pay a substitute and £2 5s ($6.30) daily for subsistence, was not considered adequate by the practitioners, but that did not seem to discourage enrollment, which grew steadily from 650 in 1950 to four times that number in 1960.[6]

In 1957, 700 British-trained doctors were engaged in research or postgraduate study. Not all, but a substantial number, of these were general practitioners. A Research Register showed that not less than 600 practitioners had a serious interest in research.[7] According to the Walker Report, about one-half of all family doctors had a special interest in a particular phase of general practice. The Hadfield Survey disclosed that almost two-thirds of the general practitioners were sufficiently alert professionally or had the opportunity or time to take refresher courses or attend clinical meetings and lectures, and almost three-fourths read at least one medical periodical.[8]

In the early 1950's, the College of General Practitioners was organized for the purpose of maintaining high standards in the field of general medicine. By 1960, it had more than 6,000 members and associates. To acquire associate status, a practitioner had to be in good standing in the profession, he had to have been qualified for seven years, and he had to agree to do postgraduate study from time to time. The primary purpose of the College was to supplement the scientific and educational work of the universities and the British Medical Association. One of its most useful functions was to arrange courses, symposia, and lecture-demonstrations for family doctors in their districts.[9]

In appraising the general practitioner, it must be kept in mind that there was no single pattern or norm to which all physicians could be reduced. Dr. Taylor, in his analysis, listed eight types of practices, including industrial, urban-residential, small-country-town, and rural. In many cases, the lines between the types were not sharply drawn. Included among the eight, but outside the Health Service, was private practice, but here also there was overlapping. A very small minority of physicians were in private practice exclusively, but many Health Service doctors had a few private patients and some practitioners who served only private patients accepted part-time hospital appointments or other sessional work in the Health Service. That the same physician could have an urban-residential practice, a sprinkling of private patients, and a "lock-up surgery" in a nearby industrial area served to emphasize the complexity of medical practice. To some degree at least, the quality and general character of a practice tended to reflect the environment.

Industrial practice, which primarily served factory workers, was in many respects the least desirable of all types. Here were to be found many doctors who resided elsewhere and were therefore inclined to neglect the appearance of their offices. Taylor observed that, although most of the industrial doctors were "good at their work and conscientious in its performance," there was a substantial minority who failed to "give their patients the service they have a right to expect." He ascribed the queues, so often observed in the industrial areas, to bad doctoring. Relations between the physician and his patients were nevertheless "friendly and uncritical." The industrial doctors had fewer links with the hospitals and less access to the pathology and radiology departments than almost any other group of practitioners. But Taylor noted that open-access service was becoming more common, especially in the smaller industrial towns. As for relations with the local health authority, they were "frail and tenuous." It was in this type of practice that the potentially good physician complained most often of frustration and that the need to improve the standards of medical practice was most apparent. Through slum clearance and new housing projects, many of the most objectionable features of this type of practice could be and were being removed.

Conditions were better in urban-residential practice, in which patients were mostly of the middle class and the upper industrial working class. Because they were "on the whole very healthy," it was easier for the practitioner to carry a large list. Partnerships were more numerous than in industrial practices, but one-half of the physicians were still engaged in single practice. Dr. Taylor noted two groups of doctors in the urban-residential area. The one, whose patients were clerical and skilled workers, had full lists and was contented. The other group comprised those who, prior to 1948, had a smaller but more select clientele of upper-middle-class private patients. To the great chagrin of these physicians, most of their fee-paying patients joined the Health Service. The additional patients and work which the Service brought them did not restore their incomes to the old level. Such doctors were often loud in their criticism of the new scheme.

Best of all was the country-town type, in which general practice seemed "to reach its finest flowering." Located in towns ranging between 5,000 and 50,000 people, this type was characterized by a relatively large number of partnerships and benefited greatly from ancillary help. More co-operation among doctors, a greater range of work, a keener interest in hospital assignments, and generally higher standards characterized the country-town type of practice. Less fortunate were the rural doctors, whose isolation usually left them at a great social and professional disadvantage. Work in the consulting room was frequently subordinated to visits in patients' homes. When ill or on vacation, these doctors had to employ substitutes, since rota schemes were often not feasible in rural areas.[10]

The majority of doctors' offices were a part of their homes. In some cases, the reception and consulting rooms represented an adaptation of space not originally designed for use as such. Some of the premises had been occupied by a succession of practitioners for more than a hundred years. In partnerships, each doctor often conducted his part of the practice from his own home, although joint-offices were not uncommon. In the poorer, heavily congested parts of large cities, the physician frequently maintained what was called a "lock-up surgery," which he used only during office hours. His residence usually was miles away. Such offices were often dreary, squalid, poorly heated, and badly furnished. It was in such industrialized areas that the larger percentage of substandard doctors' premises was found.

The extremes between the worst and the best accommodations ranged all the way from "ill-lit and ill-ventilated basement surgeries" to an "oak-panelled consulting room with furniture to correspond, and a waiting-room of luxury hotel standard." Such contrasts were observed by Dr. Stephen Taylor in his survey of 1951-52, but his general findings[11] differed little from those of Dr. Stephen Hadfield, who at the same time investigated a much larger number of practices. Hadfield found that two-thirds of the doctors' premises were adequate for the maintenance of a high clinical standard. One-fourth were fairly adequate, but lacked something essential. In the remaining 10 per cent, the rooms were "dismal and bare, dirty and inhospitable." Dr. Hadfield further discovered that 91 per cent of the practitioners had "the full range of essential equipment," including "the diagnostic instruments, auriscope, ophthalmoscope, stethoscope, sphygmomanometer, and urine-testing apparatus."[12] Patients polled by the Social Surveys in 1956 judged 12 per cent of the doctors' waiting rooms to be unsatisfactory.

The government reimbursed the doctors collectively for all practice expenses, but the method of repayment, as noted previously, was determined by the size of each physician's list and not by what he actually spent. The effect was to encourage minimum expenditures. But there were other reasons for substandard premises—uncertainty of tenure, refusal of landlords to redecorate, and the lack of suitable accommodations. Some of the poorer offices replaced better ones that had been bombed out during the war. Licensing restrictions, scarcity of materials and labor, and high costs were factors which had militated against the improvement of the reception and consulting rooms. The expectation of obtaining quarters in health centers served at first to discourage some physicians from renovating their offices. Many of these deterrents were only temporary, and as the years passed, there was a greater disposition on the part of practitioners to improve their premises. The Cohen Committee laid down certain minimum requirements, which included a lavatory for patients, a separate room for examination or a screened-off couch, a waiting room sufficiently large to seat the patients comfortably, and premises that were "bright and pleasant, well lit, well warmed, well cleaned and well ventilated."[13]

The Executive Council, acting independently or through the local medical committee, had the right to inspect the premises of any doctor and enforce compliance with the requirement of "sufficient surgery and waiting room accommodation." Such inspection seldom occurred during the early years of the Service, probably owing to the special situation that postwar difficulties had created, but in 1954 the Ministry of Health arranged with the General Medical Services Committee to sponsor a comprehensive survey of all doctor's premises. The local medical committees were to do the inspecting, and if any physician refused to meet the minimum standards he could be fined or struck off the medical register. The British Medical Association seemed glad of the opportunity to refute the allegations and exaggerations that had so reflected on the integrity of the medical profession. Twelve thousand premises were visited by teams of doctors. Nearly all practitioners co-operated willingly, but some viewed the procedure as a "grave intrustion into their professional privacy." Dr. Talbot Rogers, however, was quick to point out that, in view of the sentiment in Parliament, the government would have conducted the inspection if the British Medical Association had chosen not to do it.[14]

The nationwide inspection was completed in 1956, and the results were gratifying. The overwhelming majority of accommodations were found to be satisfactory, and in many cases the accommodations met the highest standard. The small minority of doctors whose premises did not at first pass inspection soon met, or took steps to meet, the objections raised. In some areas, however, existing accommodations could not be enlarged and improvements would have to await rebuilding schemes. In view of credit restrictions, banks were not always willing to lend money. Nevertheless, the general situation was good.[15] The survey in London, which covered 1,500 doctors' offices, disclosed that less than 4 per cent of them finally failed to meet the minimum standards. A few physicians had to seek alternative accommodations, which were not easy to find. Only a handful of practitioners refused to co-operate, and such cases were referred to the London Executive Council for action.[16]

In the registration of people on doctors' lists, duplications, inaccuracies, and the omission of vital data proved a very troublesome problem. Lists became inflated and the number of people registered on local lists sometimes exceeded the local population. It was not a question of fraud, but rather of carelessness by the patients and doctors and of a certain unwieldiness and ineffectualness in the machinery for registration.

When the Health Service was established, the government decided to base Health Service registration upon the so-called National Register, which assigned a number to each citizen, and as long as the national registration program continued, the system worked fairly well. Each person's number was on his identity card and ration books. Local National Registration Officers maintained accurate alphabetical records, and from them the Executive Council could get information not available from the Central Register. In 1952, national registration was terminated, but the Central Register at Southport was retained as the agency of the Health Service and national registration numbers were thereafter known as National Health Service numbers. Everyone was urged to keep his identity card and make certain that his number was correctly listed on his personal medical card. All persons born after the date of national registration termination, immigrants entering Great Britain, and others without a number would receive one when they registered on a doctor's list.

But many people misplaced or lost their medical cards, and in changing doctors such individuals were required to fill out a new form. Whether it was the receptionist, the physician, or the patient who did the writing, names were misspelled, and such pertinent information as the National Health Service number, the former address of the person, and the previous practitioner's name was frequently omitted or erroneously recorded. When the Executive Council received the form, it endeavored to obtain missing data, but often this was not possible. A new number would then have to be supplied by the Central Register, even though the individual might still be registered on a doctor's list elsewhere under the old number. Deaths, marriages, emigration, and conscription into the armed services were also sources of inflation. There was little that Southport could do, since the index was in numerical order, and identification was by number.

Inflation of lists did not affect the Exchequer, but it did distort payments to doctors. Those with inflated lists received more than their share from the Central Pool, while other physicians were underpaid. Apart from the embarrassment to the medical profession and the Ministry of Health, the inability of the Central Register to maintain an effective system of identification hampered the efficient operation of other branches of the Health Service, such as the Dental Estimates Board, which could not always check on a patient's record of previous treatment. Various proposals to help correct the situation were made, including one by the Executive Councils for an index based on date of birth. The British Medical Association and the Guillebaud Report urged that an alphabetical index be compiled at Southport as an adjunct to the numerical register. This proposal was finally adopted. The establishment of an alphabetical list was a major undertaking, requiring all of 1958 and the early part of 1959.[17]

The fact that among those receiving Health Service care were foreigners was a matter of irritation to many Englishmen. Although the law as amended in 1949 gave the Minister of Health the authority to require aliens to pay for all medical care, he chose not to use it. How many foreigners came to England for the primary purpose of utilizing the free medical service could not be determined, but the number was probably very small. Yet thousands of visitors from abroad did use the Health Service. In London, for example, the total increased from year to year, reaching 5,200 during the third quarter of 1959. In that year, Americans ranked second among such beneficiaries, being outnumbered only by visitors from the Republic of Ireland. The actual cost of the use of the Health Service by nonresidents, however, was insignificant. In 1957, it was roughly estimated at less than one-twentieth of one per cent of the gross cost of the Service.[18] Perhaps for that reason as much as his desire to foster a policy of good will toward foreign visitors, the Minister of Health turned a deaf ear to the many pleas raised in and out of Parliament that non-residents should pay for their medical treatment.

With the exception of visitors from the Commonwealth countries, it was the policy to deny admission to those coming to England for the sole reason of using the Health Service. Immigration officials were instructed to take prompt action in the matter if there were proof. As one Minister of Health explained, "If they saw a lady pushing a pram, and it would appear the pram was empty and soon might be filled, they would refuse that particular lady permission to land." Whether it was possible in most cases to determine the motive was doubtful, judging by the fact that in 1955 only six aliens were denied permission to land because their purpose was to obtain free medical care.[19]

The hope that other countries would grant to British nationals comparable medical benefits was realized only in a very meager fashion. The great difficulty was that most nations based their health programs on insurance, and reciprocation with a free health service such as Great Britain had was therefore very hard to achieve. By the end of 1959, full reciprocity had been arranged with Norway, Sweden, Denmark, and Yugoslavia, and partial reciprocity with Belgium, France, Luxembourg, and the Netherlands. While other limited agreements were pending, the results were on the whole disappointing.[20]

Englishmen soon discovered that, without the protection of insurance, traveling abroad could have catastrophic effects. This was especially true in America, where medical costs were much higher than they were on the continent of Europe. In 1955, for example, an elderly lady used her life savings to visit a son in the United States. She became ill and was hospitalized for three weeks at a cost of £241 ($675). Her two sisters, both old-age pensioners, had to send their own life savings to help meet the emergency.[21]   Equally unfortunate was a nurse from Manchester who in 1957 suffered an automobile accident in Los Angeles.   To pay the medical bill of £536 ($1,500), she was forced to accept employment in a hospital in that city.   A grant from a benevolent and orphan fund in England, together with money raised through British newspaper appeals, helped her to pay the debt so she could return home.[22]

Such occurrences could only reinforce the feeling that Health Service benefits for foreigners should be allowed only when a reciprocal arrangement existed for Englishmen in the country of origin.   It was apparent that there could be no reciprocity with the United States. In Parliament, a member in 1957 no doubt reflected the sentiment of many when he said, "The majority of tourists who come here can well' afford to pay.   There are cases in the West End of well-to-do Americans staying at expensive hotels, calling in doctors and claiming that the cost of the service they receive should be shouldered by the N.H.S.—in other words that the British Taxpayer should pay for it."

The National Council of Women in 1956 called for action to end free medical treatment for foreign visitors except in cases of emergency or where reciprocity existed.   One member sardonically suggested that advertisements in foreign newspapers should read "Come to Torquay and have your tonsils out" or "Come to Southport with your appendicitis."   The annual meeting of the Central Council of the National Union of Conservatives and Union Associates took a somewhat similar stand in the same year.   Since this assembly represented the rank and file of the Conservative Party, it was obvious that the feeling on the matter was rather general.[23]   There was almost enough sentiment in the 1956 Annual Representative Assembly of the British Medical Association to put that organization in favor of such a policy. In successfully opposing the resolution, Dr. A. Talbot Rogers, Chairman of the General Medical Services Committee, said that the amount spent on non-residents was less than most people realized and that Health Service benefits for foreigners were "one of the best advertisements for this country and one of the best producers of good will we can possibly have."[24]

When the Health Service was being planned, Aneurin Bevan reminded Parliament that for centuries the Catholic Church had freely offered treatment in its monasteries to all persons, regardless of nationality, and that it might be well for Great Britain to reassert that principle.   If unrestricted service were an example that Great

Britain was setting for the rest of the world, it was one that could be justified, despite the embarrassingly slow manner in which other nations were willing to reciprocate.

Apart from the element of good will, there was recognition of the fact that England had a certain debt to other nationals for their contribution to British medical progress. This was particularly true, for instance, in such a hospital as that of Stoke Mandeville in Buckinghamshire—an institution that had acquired a great reputation in plastic surgery and spinal injuries. Pioneering in the latter field, this hospital had accomplished much in developing techniques to help paralyzed people recover at least partial use of their muscles and thus find a new life. It was a middle-aged German Jew—a refugee from Hitler—who had established the Spinal Injuries Department in this hospital, and among his assistants were another German and a Czech. Serving the hospital in 1956 were 122 foreigners, whose work as nurses, cooks, porters, and members of the maintenance staff was vital to its smooth operation. In referring to the sixteen foreign patients then in the hospital, a writer who had carefully scrutinized the institution said he could not "believe that British people will want to deny to foreigners a share in something which foreigners had helped to create."[25]

Much was written about the role of the consultant in medical care and the threat it posed to the status of the general practitioner. In the eyes of the patient, however, the importance of the practitioner did not seem to diminish any. A survey in 1957 disclosed that, as between the hospital outpatient department and the practitioner, the latter was preferred by an almost 4 to 1 vote.[26] What the family doctor thought about the growing importance of the specialist was another matter. Did the practitioner feel overshadowed? As early as 1951, Dr. A. Talbot Rogers expressed the fear that the family physician was in danger of being reduced to a "sorting office in which it was decided to which specialist at which hospital a particular patient should be passed for the next installment of his examination or treatment."[27] Lord Moran, who for years served as President of the Royal College of Physicians, declared at the tenth anniversary of the Health Service that "an insidious decline in the status of the general practitioner" had occurred and that it was traceable not to the Health Service but "mainly to the condition of his life before the service." "It began," he said, "when the public felt that in serious illness they were safer in the hospital. It was mortifying to the practitioner that his patient at such a juncture should prefer to put himself in the care of a stranger. His *amour propre* was hurt. . . . Moreover, when the service came in he was no longer able to engage in a little specializing, which had lent interest to his working life. . . . In a sense his life was drained of what had been to him most interesting."[28]

But neither the Guillebaud Report, the Cohen Report, nor the Hadfield Survey indicated that the basic role of the general practitioner was in any way threatened.[29]   The Ministry of Health never tired in its emphasis on the importance of the role the family physician would always have in the Health Service.   Perhaps some who in their earlier years had aspired to become consultants may have nurtured misgivings about the future status of the practitioner, but not the great majority of family doctors, whose medical lives were too busy and full to give much thought to any threat posed by specialization.   There was, however, a widespread feeling that the practitioner and hospital services were not sufficiently co-ordinated and did not co-operate in a manner calculated to serve the best interests of the Health Service.

It was the general practitioner who determined what persons should be admitted as outpatients and inpatients and who decided which of his domiciliary cases should make use of the consultant services.   Yet the practitioner to a large extent was excluded from hospital work.   The trend toward more and more specialization left the family physician with a diminishing part in the hospital service. The diagnosis and treatment of most hospital patients was outside the training or experience of a busy family doctor.   As one specialist explained, "If the general practitioner is admitted to the hospital he could not replace the psychiatrist, the specialist in diseases of the ear, nose and throat and still less the radiologist or the biochemist." While this was true, there was work that general practitioners could do—that ordinarily performed by clinical assistants, for instance. Some beds were occupied by normal maternity cases and by patients who were there not by virtue of any need for specialist treatment but because home conditions did not permit the necessary medical care. Such patients could very properly be looked after by family physicians.

Many hospitals, however, being well staffed with consultants and registrars, deemed it administratively inexpedient to permit general practitioners to hold appointments or have the use of beds.   While only a minority of family doctors did hospital work before the advent of the Health Service, the proportion grew considerably smaller in the years that followed.   The Hadfield survey noted that the percentage had fallen from 28 in 1948 to 20 in 1952.   Urban doctors were less eager for sessional work in hospitals than country practitioners, who found the hospitals in smaller towns more flexible in their employment policy, but even these institutions showed a distressing reluctance to appoint family physicians.[30]   The great majority of practitioners had no desire for hospital work, but for those who did, the Ministry of Health and the medical profession felt that the opportunity should be granted. Virtually all reports and surveys concurred, especially in view of the need for greater harmony and more fruitful co-operation between two of the most important branches of the Health Service.

The British Medical Association on several occasions reaffirmed its position that family physicians should have access not only to diagnostic facilities but also to hospital beds.[31] The Ministry of Health was in accord with this policy, especially as it affected the hospitals in smaller towns, where such arrangements could more easily be made. In 1958, nearly 10,500 beds were available to family doctors for maternity and other medical purposes. Although this number was too small to satisfy the medical profession, it was almost a third more than had existed when the Health Service began. To make use of these beds, however, the family physician had to hold a hospital appointment. In 1958, there were over 3,000 such appointments, or 56 per cent more than in 1951.[32]

Almost three-fourths of the consultants approached in 1951-52 denied that any change had occurred in their relationship with the general practitioners. Nevertheless, the Walker Committee believed that all was not well in this area. Prior to the Health Service, the specialist was largely dependent upon the family physician for much of his clientele and accordingly cultivated his good will. After 1948, consultants, now salaried, were not dependent in this way and were free to develop a certain aloofness toward the general practitioner.[33] Whether this change in attitude actually occurred was a matter of opinion, but hospital policy was sometimes very frustrating to the family physician. The consultant's diagnoses of outpatient cases, for instance, were often slow in reaching the general practitioner. Family doctors were discouraged from visiting any of their regular patients under the care of specialists, and often the general practitioner got no medical reports from the hospital until several weeks after the patient had died or was discharged. The failure of some consultants to inform the family physicians promptly about the progress of their patients was viewed by many medical men as seriously interfering with the idea of "continuous treatment." When received, however, the reports were apparently considered adequate by all but a small minority of the general practitioners.[34]

The relationship between the family physician and the local health authority was complex. Long before the National Health Service began, the local authorities had developed health services of their own, largely in the field of preventive medicine. Such services were designed to meet a need which had not been adequately met by the practitioners themselves. Although welcomed by the people, who found maternity, school, and child welfare clinics extremely useful, these local services were not popular with the medical profession. The family physician, who resented any encroachment upon his sphere of responsibility, showed little disposition to co-operate with the clinics or the agents of the local health authority.

The effect of the Health Service was to narrow the gap between local authorities and practitioners. But co-operation came slowly. In most cases, a lack of knowledge about the complementary nature of the local health and practitioner services was to blame. No longer did family doctors stand to sustain financial losses because of free clinics, for practitioners were paid to look after all patients and received extra compensation for maternity cases, so that clinic services had no effect whatsoever upon their remuneration. The sessional work which many physicians did in the local clinics contributed to a better appreciation of their usefulness. Health employees such as the district nurse and midwife proved extremely helpful to many practitioners in their care of domiciliary patients. The Ministry of Health and the British Medical Association did what they could to create the proper climate for teamwork. Closer ties were effected through health committees, interlocking boards, and various conferences. Both the Cohen Report and the Taylor survey noted increasing co-operation and understanding,[35] and from government officials and medical leaders came recognition of the improved situation.

Where the general practitioner and the Medical Officer of Health got to know each other, the relationship was usually friendly, but in a large county with several hundred family physicians, all very busy, it was not easy to establish this personal basis for understanding. The paths of district nurses and practitioners frequently crossed, however, and here a working arrangement was established that proved highly beneficial. Attending principally the chronic sick, the district nurses became in a sense the main ancillary assistants of the practitioner in his domiciliary work. No less important in the life of the family doctor was the midwife. Much of the rivalry that at first tended to hamper good relations was cleared away when doctor and midwife discovered that their work was complementary. The physician received his obstetrical fee from the Executive Council without displacing the midwife, whose assistance in prenatal and postnatal work was significant.

Relations with the health visitor were often less cordial, owing to the fact that she was a field representative of the Medical Officer of Health and worked independently of the practitioner. But a high degree of co-operation was achieved in many cases. Her work covered a broad range of duties, including health education, school inspections, and home visits. There was also the domestic help service which, as far as it was available, proved a boon to the chronic sick and was therefore of indirect benefit to the family physician.

In order to maintain high standards, the Health Service endeavored to restrict obstetrical practice to doctors whose experience and training especially qualified them for that work. This policy was adopted largely under the influence of the consultants. Although the Ministry of Health laid down certain guiding principles, it was left to a local committee in each Executive Council area to determine what the qualifications should be. There was little uniformity. In some areas, virtually any general practitioner who made application was accepted, whereas in others a more selective policy was followed. In London, for instance, those who qualified as practitioners after 1950 had to have held a resident house post in obstetrics for six months in order to be certified for obstetrical practice. All other applicants were considered on the basis of their obstetrical experience. Only a minority of doctors qualified, the proportion in London being about one-fourth.[36]

The Hadfield survey showed that, though only a third of the family doctors had any real interest in midwifery, another third felt it was properly a part of general medical practice.[37] In view of these proportions, it is possible that some family doctors who desired to engage in maternity work were denied the right. Yet it was perhaps more for the sake of principle than for any other reason that the British Medical Association favored the automatic admission to the obstetric list of any qualified registered practitioner.[38] There was, however, much sentiment in the Association for carefully prepared lists, based upon the proper obstetrical qualifications. The Medical Practitioners' Union supported that policy, and so did the Cohen Committee.[39]

Practice of midwifery by those who did not qualify as obstetricians was restricted to the patients on their Health Service lists, but most of these doctors preferred to let others do the work. Over 97 per cent of the maternity cases handled by general practitioners in 1960 were handled by general practitioner obstetricians. Those who did qualify could concentrate exclusively on maternity cases, taking as few or as many as they wished, or they could combine such work with general medical practice. The terms of service required that all necessary care should be rendered to the patient, including not less than two prenatal examinations and one postnatal examination. Attendance at the confinement depended upon the condition of the expectant mother. Most of the doctors saw their patients far more than the minimum, but only in a minority of the domiciliary cases (19 per cent in 1960) were they present at the delivery.[40] It was generally recognized that a normal birth could be handled as well or better by a midwife than by a general practitioner, who often had less experience and not as much training. Midwives could not, however, use instruments, and if complications arose the doctor was called. When circumstance required, he could summon a specialist or rush the patient to a hospital.

The domiciliary consultant service was designed for persons whose condition did not permit removal to a hospital and for patients who could just as conveniently be accommodated at home. The resulting saving to the Exchequer was not overlooked by a thrift-conscious government. Consultants were frequently used in domiciliary cases to great advantage, but hospitals were preferred by most expectant mothers. Prior to 1940, less than 40 per cent of the births were institutional; by 1954, the proportion reached almost two-thirds.[41] In some of the urban areas, it even approached four-fifths. The trend, which had been accelerated by war conditions, continued afterwards because of a housing shortage and for financial and medical reasons. Confinement in the hospital cost the patient nothing and, in the opinion of many, involved less risk. With the need for economy in mind, the Ministry of Health endeavored without much success to reverse the trend by seeking to show that a domiciliary confinement had its own advantages and was perfectly safe.[42] To encourage home delivery, a special grant was given in addition to the regular maternity payment. Unable to find beds for all the expectant mothers, the hospitals gave priority to those who needed medical attention and to those whose home life made institutional confinement preferable.

When the expectant mother was accepted by a hospital, the practitioner generally lost jurisdiction over her, including the responsibility for all prenatal care. The paucity of maternity beds for use by the family physician rankled many doctors, whose protests reached the sympathetic ears of the Minister of Health. Hospital boards were urged to make more obstetric beds available to general practitioners, but the number grew slowly. In 1960, it was 3,685, or 18 per cent of the total of maternity beds for England and Wales.[43]

Although obstetrical standards were high and the obstetricians themselves were well trained, the maternity service was in need of reorganization. The weakness of the tripartite organization of the Health Service was nowhere more apparent than in the division of authority over maternity cases. The midwife was responsible to the local health authority; the general practitioner was subject to the jurisdiction of the Executive Council; and the consultant and the hospital were under the control of hospital boards. Administratively, each was independent of the others, and yet, practically, each was dependent upon the others for the successful operation of the maternity service. It was theoretically possible for a woman giving birth to triplets to use all three services. The midwife might deliver the first child and call upon the practitioner to deliver the second, and he might decide that the condition of the mother required the services of a domiciliary consultant or a hospital for the third birth. The Guillebaud Committee, which found so much that was sound in the Health Service, referred to the maternity services as being in a "state of some confusion, which must impair their usefulness and which must not be allowed to continue."[44] The Ministry of Health accordingly set up in 1956 a committee of twelve under the chairmanship of the Earl of Cranbrook to review the maternity service and to make recommendations for improvements.

Published in the early part of 1959, the Cranbrook Report covered a broad range of matters, only some of which affected the practitioner service. Under the terms of the Report, the obstetric list would be retained and made more selective. To qualify, a doctor would have to complete a six-month appointment in an obstetric unit of a hospital, and to remain on the roster, which would be reviewed every three years, he would have to average 20 cases a year and to attend one-half of the deliveries personally. Only the doctors who qualified as obstetricians would be paid for maternity work or have access to maternity beds. Clinical contacts would be encouraged between the obstetric specialist and the general practitioner obstetrician, and to promote greater co-ordination between the latter and the hospital, his fees for maternity work would be paid by the hospital service. The report accepted for the present the retention of the tripartite structure of the maternity service, but suggested that local liaison committees should be set up to insure more effective utilization of the facilities for maternity care and that local clinical meetings should be held for all those involved in maternity work.[45]

The *Medical World* applauded the Cranbrook Report, and *The Lancet* was well disposed toward most of its provisions. The *British Medical Journal* could see merit in many of the recommendations, but was critical of the proposed obstetric list and the exclusion of so many general practitioners from maternity work.[46] Impressed with the soundness of most of the recommendations, the Ministry of Health lost little time in commending them to the consideration of the local health authorities, the Executive Councils, and the hospital authorities.[47] It was apparent, however, that the implementation of the Report could be achieved only gradually.

There were other outlets besides obstetrics for general practitioners who desired more diversity or additional earnings. Some doctors served on hospital boards, Executive Councils, and medical committees. These appointments carried no remuneration, but sessional work in hospitals, local clinics, and the school health program was remunerative. Part-time factory medical work alone engaged several thousand physicians, but this assignment usually took only a few hours per week. Life insurance examinations and the administration of dental anesthetics were other examples of the minor commitments which took doctors outside the prescribed sphere of the practitioner service. Hadfield found that only one family physician in six engaged in no other professional duties beyond caring for his patients and that 13 per cent were engaged in considerable outside activity.[48] The Ministry of Health did nothing to discourage these extensions of responsibility, on the theory that they would enrich the life of the family doctor and add variety to the routine work of medical practice.

Some critics alleged that the practitioner was so burdened with paper work that it had superseded clinical work in importance. Doctors had long been accustomed to filling out medical certificates and other forms under the Health Insurance, but the volume of clerical work increased under wartime rationing and the statutory insurance plan of the mid-1940's, which embraced the entire population. Many of the benefits under this insurance plan were payable only after medical certification. The Health Service likewise increased the amount of paper work, much of which, however, had no relationship to the health scheme. Disgruntled doctors nevertheless were inclined to put the full blame for all the additional work on the Service. Recognition that there were too many clerical requirements led to an investigation by an Inter-departmental Committee that caused Parliament to modify the procedure in 1949. Under the new regulations, the number of certificates the practitioner had to fill out was reduced and those that were retained were simplified. With the curtailment and finally the abandonment of rationing and other controls which required certification, the burden of clerical work grew less onerous.

Paper work continued to be a source of annoyance to some doctors, but the great majority accepted it without protest as a necessary part of their medical duties. Taylor found "no serious complaints of excessive paper work." When they arose, they were due, he felt, to a "momentary irritation over an exceptional situation" or to the failure of the physician to appreciate the importance of the sickness or other benefits which the certificate would give the patient.[49] As a general practitioner, Dr. Talbot Rogers was not convinced that the abolition of certification for social benefits would appreciably diminish the amount of work he had to do. "Most of us," he affirmed, "consider that these burdens . . . are our responsibility."[50] While conceding that certification sometimes presented a problem, the Walker Report declared that if doctors who failed to take that aspect of their work seriously enough would "study the current regulations they would find them not so irksome after all."[51]

According to Stevenson's survey, only 25 per cent of the doctors were concerned about the administrative and clerical phase of their practice.[52] Gemmill's study disclosed that 61 per cent of the practitioners did not "find the volume of paper work very burdensome." A number of doctors informed Professor Gemmill that the increase in paper work had been largely, if not completely, "offset by the almost total disappearance of one especially unpleasant type—sending out bills for services rendered to private patients."[53] In a somewhat similar vein, a physician, in commenting upon ten years of the Health Service, asserted, "I think it is time we stopped this querulous nonsense about too much form-filling. We do less now than we did in the days of private practice; at least we don't have to keep accounts."[54]

Although there were about 40 forms available for use by doctors, only a few were regularly used. Among the more important were medical record cards, prescription pads, sickness certificates, request blanks for specialist, laboratory, and other hospital services, claim sheets for payment of services for emergency treatment, treatment of temporary patients, etc., and forms covering such matters as use of the ambulance, notification of infectious diseases, and immunization and vaccination. Most of the forms were very brief, requiring only a few moments of time to complete. Filling out a claim for payment for an emergency treatment or a request for an outpatient appointment or an authorization for a sight test required little more than the signature of the physician. But the form for the clinical information the practitioner sent to a hospital specialist might require up to twenty or more lines of explanation.

Most important perhaps was the certificate for sickness, which was required for insurance benefits. There were several kinds of sickness certificate—the first certificate of incapacity, the intermediate certificate (used if the incapacity continued for more than four weeks), and the final certificate of fitness to return to work. Sickness certificates were issued weekly during the first month of illness, after which the certificate issued every four weeks could be used. In 1959, provision was made for a long-term medical certificate for persons whose incapacitation had lasted six months and was likely to continue for some time. Under such circumstances, the doctor could issue a certificate covering thirteen weeks of sickness, even though he might have to see the patient more frequently than that. In case of permanent disability, no periodic medical certificate would be required.[55]

The amount of certification varied among doctors. Fry's study showed that 14 per cent of all consultations required the issuance of a certificate.[56] Other surveys disclosed a higher percentage, ranging from 20 to 25.[57] The evidence would indicate that the vast majority of doctors were careful in issuing sickness certificates. To what extent patients were able to inveigle certificates from doctors will never be known, but that some unjustified issuance of certificates occurred, especially in borderline cases, seems to be indisputable.

The law required records of the illness of all patients and authorized the Minister of Health, in consultation with the medical profession, to determine an appropriate form for this purpose, but it was never established. Medical record cards with envelopes were nevertheless supplied, although the type of notes made was left entirely to the discretion of the physician. The style and length of the medical observations thus varied greatly; yet the overwhelming majority of practitioners kept reasonably careful records. Even the patients were conscious of the diligence of their family doctors in making use of medical cards at the time of consultation.[58]

The prescription form was the simplest of all documents and one of the most widely used. The right of the physician to prescribe virtually any medicine he deemed necessary was recognized, and the prescription was honored by any Health Service pharmacist upon the payment by the patient of a nominal charge. If a drug store was not within a reasonable distance of his office, the practitioner himself was expected to dispense the medicine and collect the small fee. Some rural doctors were so situated, and although they were adequately reimbursed, they were able to dispense drugs at less cost than the average for the entire nation. But everywhere pharmaceutical costs were high, and since the mounting drug bill was largely determined by practitioners, who did most of the prescribing, their methods were subject to careful scrutiny. The purpose was to prevent over-prescribing and to encourage more prudence in the choice of drugs.

If a doctor prescribed an item not strictly a drug or prescribed extravagantly, the cost could be recovered. Once a year a physician's prescribing costs were reviewed by the Ministry of Health and a comparative analysis based on prescriptions issued several months previously was sent to him. Statistics were made available showing the average cost for an area and the nation as a whole, and if a doctor's prescribing costs seemed high by comparison, an investigation followed. Warning letters were used or, if the case appeared to be serious, a regional medical officer visited the physician. If circumstances warranted action, the abuse was referred to the local medical committee, but the final decision rested with the Minister of Health, who could seek the advice of three referees, one of whom had to be a general practitioner. Comparatively few cases reached the local medical committees, and even fewer resulted in a fine. In 1960, for example, only eleven cases were referred by those committees for formal consideration by the Ministry.[59]

It was easier for a doctor to prescribe a heavily advertised proprietary drug than to consult the British National Formulary for an alternative prescription that might be available at a much lower price. A standing committee endeavored to classify all new proprietary preparations according to their therapeutic value and to determine whether the equivalent could be had in a standard preparation. *Prescribers' Notes,* superseded in 1961 by *Prescribers' Journal,* was regularly issued to assist the physician in economical prescribing. The biggest difficulty seemed to be an absence of readily accessible information concerning the comparative costs of the more recent drugs. The advertising literature that flooded the doctors' offices was usually silent about prices. With 500 proprietary preparations on the market, a busy doctor had little time to check which drugs would represent the greatest savings to the Exchequer. To cope with this problem, the Hinchliffe Committee, which was appointed in 1957 to investigate the cost of prescriptions, proposed that the government prepare for quick reference a conveniently arranged loose-leaf prescribing handbook that would carry the latest data about comparative drug prices. Such a handbook was made available in 1960 to all doctors and final-year medical students.[60]

When the government imposed a shilling-per-item charge, the practitioners had a tendency to prescribe in larger quantities. Another cause of the rising cost of drugs was the tendency of the patients to take their minor ailments to the Health Service practitioner, who, they expected, would prescribe some medicine. It was hard to resist the assumption, and physicians undoubtedly had recourse to drugs whose value to the patient may have been largely psychological. Most important were the antibiotic drugs, whose therapeutic properties were little short of miraculous, but whose cost would have been prohibitive to many of the patients had they been forced to pay for them out of their own pockets. Such expensive drugs combined with inflation to shape the pharmaceutical budget. In surveying all aspects, the Hinchliffe Committee in its Interim Report could "find no evidence of serious irresponsibility on the part of doctors in prescribing. . . . We believe that, on the whole, the duty of prescribing drugs at the public expense has been discharged carefully and with due responsibility; nevertheless we think that some economy is possible without sacrifice of efficiency."[61]

Only the patients in the Health Service were entitled to free drugs and appliances, subject, of course, to the small fees which had been imposed by Parliament. The denial of free drugs and appliances to private patients rankled the private practitioners, who charged the government with a breach of faith. The Minister of Health in 1946 had promised that "all the Service, or any part of it, is to be available to everyone." Whether he had private patients in mind was not clear, but the law as interpreted gave them the same privileges enjoyed by Health Service patients except for free prescriptions. Private patients could obtain without cost maternity benefits, use of the hospital and consultant facilities, dental treatment, care of the eyes, and the domiciliary services available under the local health authority. In accepting such medical care, the private patient was treated the same as any other person. But should he desire to engage a particular surgeon for an operation, he would have to pay not only the specialist fees but also the full cost of hospital care.

In denying private patients the right to obtain drugs on the same terms as other persons, the government was not seeking to discourage private practice. In 1954, the Minister of Health gave emphasis to this point when he said: "Private practice, we believe, is and should remain a part of the N. H. S."[62] Government policy rested upon the position that the prescribing of medicine was an integral part of the general medical service and could not be used separately by doctors who were not under the statutory obligations applicable within the service. Permitting the use of the pharmaceutical service by private patients would involve additional cost to the Exchequer and also administrative difficulties that could be very troublesome. The Cohen Committee, which shared the government's view, refused to recommend that Health Service prescription forms be given to private patients.[63] Since so few people were not using the Health Service, there was little popular support for the necessary amendment that would be required to legalize free drugs for private patients. The Ministry of Health was cool to the idea, and in Parliament there seemed to be little enthusiastic support for it.[64]

The Fellowship For Freedom in Medicine was untiring in its fight on this issue, believing that the lack of free drugs for private patients was one of the biggest deterrents to private practice. The British Medical Association supported the same policy, but without the crusading spirit which characterized the activities of the Fellowship.

Yet in virtually every Annual Representative Assembly, a resolution was adopted advocating drugs for private patients, and the General Medical Services Committee continued to press for a change in the policy of the Ministry of Health.

Negotiations dragged on, without any clear evidence that the government would yield. In 1957, the Department of Health listed several points as a basis for further discussion. By 1959, however, the more serious obstacles apparently had been overcome as the British Medical Association revealed a greater disposition to concur in conditions that at first were viewed as objectionable. The registration of private doctors, the acceptance by them of legal contracts, and even the registration of private patients with the Executive Councils were among the terms agreed upon—all of which seemed to make the distribution of National Health Service drugs to private patients administratively possible. The way now seemed to be cleared for the government to ask Parliament for the necessary legislation.

Some doctors nevertheless had misgivings over the possible effect which the broadening of the pharmaceutical scheme might have in reducing the size of the Central Pool and the amount of remuneration Health Service doctors received. The excessively cautious policy of the Ministry left many observers uncertain whether the government was sincere or whether "it intended to postpone indefinitely something which was not desired, but which for political reasons the Minister did not wish publicly to refuse."[65]

The impact of the National Health Service upon private practice was tremendous. Often, private patients all but disappeared. Dr. Stevenson revealed that 50 per cent of the industrial and suburban practitioners whom he queried had abandoned private practice "as being more trouble than it was worth, for it had almost entirely disappeared in any case."[66] The Government Social Survey, based upon 7,000 interviews, showed that in 1952 only 1.5 per cent of the population were using private doctors exclusively and that another 2 per cent were on a Health Service list but were also attended by a private practitioner.[67] Free drugs for everybody might have boosted the percentage of private patients slightly, but it is doubtful that the number would have exceeded 3 per cent of the total population.

The Willink Report placed the number of general practitioners who were engaged wholly or mainly in private practice at 650, or less than 3 per cent of all general medical practitioners.[68] Most family physicians in the Health Service had only a few private patients, but some had none and did not want any. The Hadfield survey disclosed that 43 per cent of the doctors interviewed had no desire for private patients, while the postal survey reported 19 per cent in that category.

Two-thirds of the practitioners in the latter poll and one-third in the field survey wanted to include some private patients in their practice. In neither study was there more than a small minority of doctors who cared to have only private patients.

Some physicians did not want private patients because they were considered too much bother. Such doctors felt that much in private practice was "too far removed from real medicine." The desire for preferential treatment by private patients, the financial element in the doctor-patient relation, and difficulties in the collection of charges were other unfavorable factors. Other practitioners, however, believed that private practice was a challenge, that it provided the "correct relationship between doctor and patient," and that it "must be preserved or the standard of medicine would drop rapidly." The range of opinions varied greatly. One doctor, for instance, declared that it "doesn't make any difference to me whether it is a National Health or a panel patient or a private patient. I am always ready to attend to any ill person no matter who it is or whether he can pay or not. I think this is our duty." Another physician, in explaining his position, wrote, "I am quite happy about the present position—that is, the vast majority as Health Service patients, and just a few private patients (about 4% of my total number) as variety. I should dread a return to the old days of accounting, unpaid bills, self-dispensing, and the extra time and 'fussing' that private patients expect as their right. I am now able to concentrate on the patients' ills alone, without the frills!"[69]

Taylor noted a tendency for the children of private patients to join the Health Service. He further observed that many private patients were among those who could least afford private fees. One physician revealed that half of his private patients were gypsies who rejected "with horror the idea of registering." Some people remained private patients out of a deep feeling of loyalty to their family doctor who had served them for so many years. And there were those, even in the lowest income group, who would have none of the new Service because of the mistaken notion that it was charity. Private patients were in a better position to demand a home visit whether it was necessary or not and could claim more of the doctor's time. One practitioner put it this way: "Patients must realize that with the National Health Service, they cannot have it all their own way. If the service is to work, they have got to co-operate with the doctor. If they want unnecessary visits, then I tell them straight out they have got to become private patients."

No difference in the standards of medical treatment between Health Service and private patients was observed by Dr. Taylor.[70]

If private patients received preferential treatment, it was not apparent to the vast majority of Health Service patients. The Social Surveys disclosed in 1956 that 59 per cent of the Health Service patients whose doctors also served private patients were not even aware of the fact. Only 4 per cent were of the opinion that their physicians gave better treatment or showed more consideration to private patients.

The Fellowship For Freedom in Medicine did everything possible to sustain and advance the cause of private practice, printing in its bulletin data, testimonials, and even biographical sketches of private physicians who seemed to be doing well. Occasionally, a private practice was advertised for sale. Although the odds seemed against the survival of private practice, it somehow was able to maintain a small but tenacious hold. It was believed by some that free drugs and private medical insurance of the kind that had come into existence in the hospital field might offer a stimulus. There was also the hope that changes could be effected in the Health Service structure that might create a more favorable climate for private practice. The existence in the British Medical Association of a Private Practice Committee with a Private Practitioners Subcommittee attested to the fact that private doctors, although a small minority, were not without influence.

CHAPTER IX

The Medical Practitioner and the Patient

THOUGH HE WAS becoming more dependent upon the specialist and the laboratory technician, the general medical practitioner was in a position to offer a wider and more effective service than ever. Many diseases that once required hospitalization could now be treated in the home with new drugs. Improved therapeutic methods, better diagnostic procedures, and more knowledge about disease enhanced the efficacy of the family physician. The prolongation of life, with the rise in the incidence of chronic illness, was an important cause of the greater dependence of the people upon the practitioner. The growing interest in the problem of mental illness and the increased awareness of the effect of psychoneurosis upon physical health were equally significant. Separating patients who were in some degree mentally ill from those with organic ailments was a time-consuming process in itself. Being more conscious of the necessity of safeguarding their health, the people were less willing to nurse minor ailments without the benefit of a practitioner's advice. There was little question that society had greater use for the services of the family doctor than ever before.

Medical care, especially the hospital, specialist, and pharmaceutical aspects of it, had grown so expensive that it would have been beyond the reach of an estimated 80 per cent of the population if individual patients had had to pay for the services they received. It was this factor, more than any other, that had brought the National Health Service to Great Britain. With the financial barrier removed, the family physician was now in a position to administer freely to the needs of all people. Drugs, hospital facilities, and the consultant services were his readily available allies in the interminable fight against disease. If the doctor lost something by this arrangement, he also gained much. No one, asserted one medical authority, should "overlook the satisfaction the good doctor feels in being free, as never before, to practice his art without considering what patients can afford. In thus concentrating on needs and ignoring income, the Act realizes the best tradition in medicine; and in relieving the doctor of the necessity to profit by other people's troubles it goes a long way to rescue the profession from the commercialism by which it has latterly been permeated."[1]

In the years before 1948, many practitioners, although they were overworked, were grossly underpaid, and their plight was reflected in the inability of most people to obtain adequate medical care. The lot of most doctors improved materially under the Health Service. The number of general medical practitioners became more plentiful and their distribution more equitable which, of course, meant a better doctor-patient ratio, with a little more time for each patient. By 1958, the average list stood at less than 2,270, which, in the opinion of most physicians, was not too large for effective treatment, since a substantial minority of persons would have no need to see their doctor during the course of a year. How many patients a practitioner could expeditiously handle depended upon geography and personal ability and temperament. Only a third of the physicians had more than 2,500 patients on their lists, and another third had 1,500 or less. A substantial portion of the profession was thus not overburdened with an excessive number of patients.

In the opinion of some medical leaders, the maximum of 3,500 was not too many for able doctors.[2] The trend in sentiment was nevertheless toward smaller and more evenly distributed lists. If the British Medical Association seemed rather cool to the idea of a lower ceiling for the lists, there was nevertheless much support among the individual practitioners for such a policy. This was revealed in letters to the medical press and in the testimony before the Royal Commission on Doctors' and Dentists' Remuneration. The *Medical World Newsletter* was certainly not alone in the spring of 1959 when it looked with favor upon a reduction of the maximum list to 3,000 within three years, and later to 2,750.[3] Nor was lay support lacking in the matter. The Labor Party, in its 1959 statement of principles, accepted the 2,500 maximum as the ideal goal, to be achieved by stages, depending on the availability of doctors.[4] And the Newsam Report also specified such a figure as the maximum for first-class doctoring.[5]

Under the National Health Service, the doctor was in a better position to serve as a family physician, since all members of the family could avail themselves of early diagnosis and continuing treatment. In fulfilling this role, his freedom as a clinician was not threatened by the terms of service to which he had to subscribe. He was free to choose his patients, but once he signed any person's medical card he was under obligation to serve that person. The removal of a patient from his list could be effected within a week, however, simply by notifying the Executive Council. In seeking medical treatment, the individual was expected to produce his medical card if there was doubt about his identity; otherwise, he might have to pay a fee, which could be recovered upon application to the Executive Council. This was virtually the only charge which a practitioner was permitted to make to Health Service patients, except for the prescription fee that some rural doctors had to collect.

The general practitioner was required to render all the care normally expected from a family doctor. If the patient needed specialist or hospital treatment, the practitioner would make the necessary arrangements, furnishing whatever information was required. In prescribing medicines, he would do his own dispensing if a drug store was not accessible to the patients. He was required to issue the necessary medical certificates and to keep records of all illnesses he treated and the treatment given.

The location of his office and the schedule of his office hours were theoretically subject to the approval of the Executive Council, but in practice the doctor was free to handle these matters without interference. Likewise, the requirement that patients were to be attended in their homes, when necessary, was left to the discretion of the practitioner. For those who came to him with serious medical problems but who were not on his list, emergency treatment had to be rendered. In case of his absence or incapacitation, the physician had to make adequate provision for the care of his patients and was held responsible for any errors his assistant or deputy made unless the deputy was a practitioner on the medical list. The doctor could not be absent from his practice more than one week without notifying the Executive Council, and if he employed an assistant for more than three months he could do so only with the consent of that body or, on appeal, the Medical Practices Committee.

Although the Health Service requirements appeared to impose limits upon the freedom of the practitioner, they did not seem to hamper the effectiveness of the conscientious doctor as an agent of the Health Service. The medical profession as a whole did not find them objectionable. The rules merely sought to insure standards of medical practice that normally would be expected under any system. The policy was to leave the doctor as free as possible. Subject to the law of supply and demand, he was free to practice almost anywhere he wished. He enjoyed a large measure of freedom in practicing the medical arts. He could have private patients and engage in other types of work outside of his practice, and he could leave the Service whenever he chose by giving three months' advance notice.

The scope of the freedom enjoyed by the Health Service doctor was well understood by the medical profession. The polls and surveys almost without exception did not impugn it. Influential leaders in the British Medical Association gave recognition to it. Dr. Guy Dain did so on the occasion of the tenth anniversary of the Health Service,[6] while Dr. Talbot Rogers made a point, in 1955, of expressing his belief that "after seven years' experience of the new service . . . [the general practitioners] had achieved a remarkable degree of clinical and administrative freedom."[7] Sir Frank Newsam, in his survey, could find no evidence of undue interference by government officials with medical practice. Had there been "any instance of clinical interference by the government," he reasoned, it was difficult to believe that the British Medical Association would have let it pass unnoticed.[8]

The people also were allowed a large measure of freedom. Any individual was free to remain a private patient, though doctor fees and the cost of drugs discouraged this course. He could select his Health Service physician from a medical list available at the post office or Executive Council. If an individual had no preference or experienced difficulty finding a doctor, the Executive Council would assign the person to a physician. Comparatively few people required such assistance, although at first they were more numerous than in later years. For children, the mother selected the physician, or, if she could not do so, then the father or guardian selected him. Every person was entitled to medical care, either as a regular, emergency, or temporary patient. Students in boarding schools were usually treated as regular patients there and as temporary patients at home. Temporary residents registered only when they needed medical treatment and were then expected to provide their National Health Service numbers, whereas foreigners had only to give their home addresses.

If a patient wished to change doctors, he could do so without delay, providing he was moving to another address or had obtained the consent of the physician. Otherwise, there was a delay of fourteen days following notification of the Executive Council of his intention. During the initial years of the Health Service, the patient had the right to effect the change immediately, but in 1950 the policy of deferment was adopted because the medical profession demanded it. It was designed to grant as much freedom of choice as was "consistent with the need to discourage frivolous changes based, for example, on the wish of the patient to obtain easier certification or an unnecessary favourite proprietary medicine."[9]

The Social Surveys in 1956 disclosed that, excepting the instances when doctor or patient moved away, only 8 per cent of the people had changed practitioners since the beginning of the National Health Service. The Social Survey conducted in 1952 revealed that the annual rate of change of physician was about 7 per cent and that three-fourths of these changes were due to the movement of either the patient or the physician. Only one-tenth of all changes could be ascribed to dissatisfaction with the doctor.

The Social Survey further indicated that only 5 per cent of all adults had a woman physician,[10] which appeared to be a rather low proportion, considering that almost one-fifth of all active doctors were women. But since the number of women principals in general practice was only about 6 per cent, they had their share of patients. In filling a vacancy, the Medical Practices Committee seemed to have no strong views either for or against woman doctors.[11]

A study of a factory town in 1953 showed that almost three-fourths of the families had what might be considered a family doctor.[12] The Cohen Report placed the proportion of patients having a family physician at two-thirds and interpreted that proportion as further evidence that the advent of the Health Service had not "disturbed the relationship between doctors and their patients."[13]

Both Dr. Hadfield and Dr. Taylor undertook to evaluate practitioners according to the quality of their work. Taylor rated one-fourth of them as very good and another half as good. According to his survey, then, three-fourths of the doctors possessed adequate equipment and promptly examined their patients whenever the need arose. The remaining practitioners were not necessarily bad, but either their equipment was deficient, they were careless in their examination technique, or they were faulty in keeping records. In this group were the 5 per cent of physicians who were at serious fault in caring for their patients.[14]

Dr. Hadfield found that 69 per cent of the practitioners who came under his observation adequately examined their patients. Some of the physicians who did little in the way of examination seemed to have "an instinct or a sixth sense" for diagnosis, arising out of long experience. Yet Hadfield recognized that the line was pretty thin between such practitioners and those who "through over-confidence, tended too often to put their trust in spot diagnosis." Seven per cent of the doctors needed to revise their methods of diagnosis. The remaining 24 per cent were found to take chances and were not always sufficiently careful or thorough as clinicians, owing perhaps to the pressure of work. Critical though he was of the minority, Dr. Hadfield was proud of the standards maintained by the great majority of doctors. "Over 90 per cent of the practitioners that I saw," he asserted, "are undoubtedly interested and careful in the treatment of their patients. They give the necessary advice, supervise rehabilitation, prescribe carefully, and do dressings and emergency treatment. Not for them the mere hurried writing of prescriptions that I witnessed among a few."

In depicting the average practice, the Hadfield survey noted that the number of private patients did not exceed a handful. Where rota schemes existed, the doctor was able to have some leisure; otherwise, he was more or less on duty permanently. He was fond of his patients but indicated he would be happier if he could "purge his list of [a] hard core of inconsiderate trouble-makers." During his morning office hours he would see up to 25 patients, the great majority of whom would have a minor ailment or merely want a prescription or medical certificate. Possibly five would, from a clinical point of view, require more attention. While one patient might take 15 minutes, the next five or six combined could be dealt with in the same amount of time. Having treated most of his patients year after year, the practitioner usually knew how far he need go in his examination. Aside from an accident or a midwifery case, the day's work was fairly routine, with 15 to 30 visits daily during the winter and possibly half that many in the summer. The country doctor needed more time for his visits than the town practitioner, but spent less time on office calls. With only 10 to 15 minutes available for each visit, the physician had no time to socialize. An evening office session completed the day's work, except for emergency calls.[15]

The foregoing description, accurate though it may have been in a rough way, did not reveal the great variations between doctors. Among the practices observed by Taylor, the daily services per physician ranged from 27 to 87. In one urban practice—a partnership with a combined list of 7,900—each doctor averaged 70 services per day (40 office consultations and 30 visits to the home). Despite the heavy load, these practitioners were giving first-class clinical service, but without any frills. Since they were in their thirties, they were able to cope with all the work.[16]

Most of the surveys left little doubt that the British practitioner was a very busy man. Overworked doctors at the outset were commonplace, and crowded waiting rooms were almost the rule, but ten years of the Health Service had eased the pressure considerably. Patients still had to wait, and physicians still seemed to perform amazing feats in treating so many persons, but the picture was not what some critics painted it to be. Moreover, the pattern of British medical practice as a whole had to be considered in any appraisal of the family doctor.

A small fraction of general practitioners adopted the appointment system as a general policy, but only for special examinations and private patients was it used very widely. The consensus was that it would not work for ordinary consultations.[17] Yet the few doctors who adopted it found it reasonably effective in solving the problem of an overcrowded waiting room. The services of a secretary-receptionist were usually required, the patients had to be educated to the advantages of the system, and it had to be applied flexibly, with provision for those who neglected to get an appointment.[18] The need for an appointment system lost some of its urgency, perhaps, as the distribution of patients became more equitable. The practitioners with whom I discussed the problem did not feel that it was serious, and in some cases I was informed that the waiting period was seldom more than 30 minutes. Gemmill's survey disclosed that about four-fifths of the patients almost never had to wait as much as one and a half hours in the doctor's office.[19]

At least one-half of the practitioners had secretarial assistance, and another 25 per cent would have liked to have it. Secretarial assistance was one of the advantages of a partnership or group practice. By having the receptionist-typist attend to such tasks as filing cards, receiving messages, handling routine correspondence, and taking care of the paper work, the physician was free to do more for his patients. Ancillary help often made the difference between a practice that was well-ordered and efficiently managed and one that was not.

Between 60 and 75 per cent of all persons on a doctor's list made use of his services at least once during the year, but a small minority of patients were responsible for most of his work. Women and children made the heaviest demands upon the doctor's time, and among age groups, children under one year of age and adults over 65 required the most attention. The latter group, afflicted with chronic disorders, had one of the highest consultation rates of all. The study by Backett *et al.* revealed that, in a practice of more than 3,000 patients, one-sixth of all persons accounted for one-half the work and that chronic diseases accounted for one-third of all the work done.[20]

Contrary to expectations, the Health Service increased little, if any, the amount of work per person on the doctor's list. The prewar survey of Dr. Bradford Hill disclosed an annual average of between 4.81 and 5.39 consultations and visits per individual on the panel lists.[21] The Social Survey indicated that for 1950 the figures pointed to 4.8 items of service per person on the physician's list.[22] For Dr. Fry, whose practice numbered over 4,000 individuals, the proportions were 3.7 for 1949, 3.8 for 1950, and 3.28 for 1951.[23] The Department of the Registrar General, in its survey of 1952-54 covering 10 practices, found only 3.7 visits and consultations per year for each person on those lists.[24] Dr. Alistair Mair and his partner reported for their practice of 4,200 patients the highest rate of all, 5.45 services as the yearly average for the period, 1954-58.[25] The data thus made it fairly clear that the greater volume of work experienced by many physicians was due not to an increase in the amount of work per patient but rather to the new availability of medical treatment to the entire population.

The evidence further indicates that the patients were very cooperative in the matter of night calls. The Social Surveys of 1956, based on replies from 500 general practitioners, disclosed that almost three-fourths of them had fewer or no more night calls under the National Health Service than previously. Taylor found that night visits had become "a comparative rarity for most doctors," although he noted an increase in late-evening visits.[26]

Dr. J. H. Brotherston *et al.* made a survey of calls between 11 P.M. and 8 A.M. in a semi-rural, four-doctor practice of 9,000 patients. In so far as night calls were concerned, there was no reason to believe that conditions in this practice differed much from those elsewhere. Covering 19 months (1955-57), the study revealed an annual rate of 17 night calls per 1,000 patients. For two-thirds of the nights, the duty-physician was left undisturbed. Only 6 per cent of the calls were considered unnecessary. It was estimated on the basis of this survey that, in a practice of 2,000 persons with a similar rate of calls, a practitioner could expect to be called out 34 nights in a year and that on any one night his chances of having to visit a patient would be fewer than one in ten.[27]

In the matter of home visiting, the doctors seemed to be as conscientious as ever, but the rate of visits increased little, if any, under the Health Service. In the Social Surveys, only 30 per cent of the practitioners indicated that home visiting had increased appreciably. The Ross and the Mair and Mair surveys each showed that only one-fourth of the patients were visited in their homes.[28] The Registrar General put the figure at 28 per cent, and Backett *et al.* at 36 per cent.[29] The prewar ratio between office calls and visits in the home for panel patients was estimated at 3.3 to 1, a proportion that deviated little from the average under the Health Service.[30] It was thus apparent that the effect of the National Health Service on the frequency of home visits was negligible. Nor was the cause that doctors discouraged home visits, if the Social Surveys had any meaning. Only 9 per cent of the people interviewed seemed to feel that the practitioners minded visits to their homes.

It was in the doctor's office that the Health Service greatly increased the volume of work. Processing a score or more of patients in a single consulting session of about two hours required short cuts and a most careful utilization of time. In most practices, the average amount of time for a consultation was 10 minutes.[31] The great majority of the patients were "quickies" who, desiring repeat medicines or a certificate, required very little time. Progress cases, in which the diagnosis had been made and treatment begun, took between 5 and 10 minutes (examples were arthritis, pernicious anemia, and peptic ulcers). Uncomplicated new cases, such as abscesses, infectious diseases, and minor injuries took about the same amount of time. New cases that required careful diagnosis and treatment might necessitate 15 to 25 minutes. Some of the more baffling cases could not always be dealt with in an ordinary session, and an appointment for another time was therefore required.[32]

Although it was sometimes believed that the general practitioners in the Health Service had insufficient time for their patients, it is significant that Professor Richard Titmuss, a methodical scholar, was convinced from the available data that many of the doctors on an average had more time for each patient, if they chose to use it, than they did before 1948.[33]

The policy of referring minor surgery to the hospitals was a trend which the Health Service unwittingly fostered. Hospitals were better equipped for the work, especially for the treatment of casualty cases in which the danger of infection was very great. By letting the resident staff handle such cases, the practitioners escaped the risk of a liability suit if anything went wrong. The pressure of work and the absence of extra pay for minor surgery were also strong inducements to send such cases to the hospital. Exclusion from hospital facilities where some family doctors had once done minor surgery was another factor. Hadfield observed that a majority of practitioners did very little minor surgery, although the proportion of rural doctors who still did an appreciable amount was rather large.[34] Since antibiotics rendered unnecessary much of the surgery that had once been required, the indirect role of the family physician in this area was still significant. Taylor noticed that superficial abscesses and boils were opened and circumcision of infants was still performed by many practitioners,[35] but the transfer to the hospitals of an increasing amount of minor surgery was an undeniable fact. Many doctors did not view the trend as objectionable; others deplored it.

Vaccination, immunization, and the administration of injections were a part of the daily work of a family physician, but he seldom performed a blood count and did very little other pathological work. The great majority of practitioners had direct access to some pathological facility, although it was not always the laboratory of the local hospital.   Direct access to the radiological department was somewhat more restricted, but a majority of practitioners had this privilege, as well, and under the prodding of the Ministry of Health more hospitals were granting it.   The medical profession urged that such access be made even more widely available, and sentiment almost everywhere favored such a course.   Even though many pathological and radiological facilities were already available to general practitioners, however, not more than one-tenth of the X-ray, and an even smaller proportion of the pathological, work of the hospitals was done on their behalf. Where open access was denied, it was often because the facilities of the hospital were strained to the limit by work from its own outpatient and inpatient departments. In such cases, all patients requiring laboratory tests had to be referred by the family physician to a consultant.[36]   In commenting upon the improved lot of the medical profession under the Health Service, Sir Frank Newsam recognized that the general practitioner "now has better access to diagnostic facilities and is less isolated from the local health authorities than he used to be."[37]

The reference of so many persons to the outpatient departments of the hospitals was open to abuse.   Crowded reception rooms, it was alleged, encouraged physicians to refer to specialists cases that could have been handled satisfactorily in the doctor's office.   To what extent this was true could not easily be determined, since any reasonable doubt about a diagnosis was considered sufficient justification for getting the opinion of a consultant.   Patients often insisted upon it, since what first appeared to be a minor condition might later be discovered by the specialist to be a more serious one, requiring prompt treatment.   The Cohen Report perceived that the trend toward the "use of instrumental methods of investigation and treatment" and, as well, the "legal aspects of the doctor's responsibilities" were important factors in the greater utilization of the outpatient departments.   The Committee could find no conclusive evidence of abuse, though it was aware that, if abuse did exist, it was not likely to be easily discovered.[38]

A third of the general practitioners interviewed by Dr. Hadfield felt that the outpatient departments were crowded with minor cases that should not have been there.[39]   But if that service was misused, the patients did not think so, judging by the Social Surveys questionnaire of 1956.   Sixty per cent of the people interviewed had never been outpatients, and of those who had, only 1 per cent believed that the treatment should have been given by the family physician and not by the consultant. Fry's study revealed that somewhat fewer than 7 per cent of all his patients were referred for a specialist opinion. A survey by the Registrar General's Department disclosed an average referral rate of about 12 per cent.[40] Such percentages did not seem excessive in view of the increasingly important part the consultant was playing in modern medicine. The concern in Parliament, in the Ministry of Health, and in most medical circles was not so much with any abuse of outpatient facilities as it was with the amount of time that elapsed before outpatients could see a specialist. During the early years of the Service, that delay in some departments was as long as two and three weeks.[41]

A much-discussed aspect of general practice was the demands made by patients. To what extent were they unnecessary or unreasonable? Did the new health program foster irresponsible use of the medical services? In the opinion of the Fellowship For Freedom in Medicine, the provision of a free medical service gave the people "no incentive to economize or to take responsibility," and many patients visited their "doctor for every trivial complaint, even when surgeries were overcrowded."[42] Other voices were raised in apprehension about a scheme that gave people "the right to consult their doctors and consultants on the slightest provocation." Dr. P. T. O'Farrell, in his presidential address before the British Medical Association's Annual Assembly in 1952, expressed the fear that under a "so-called free service some patients may become too introspective about minor ailments and that the trammels of imaginary ills and anxieties may become self-nurtured to an unreasonable degree."[43]

The National Health Service had certainly brought a heavier patient load and no diminution in the number of minor ailments. According to the Postal Inquiry, 53 per cent of the doctors felt that "excessive numbers of unnecessary demands" were being made by patients, but Dr. Hadfield reported only 30 per cent. Significantly, neither these surveys nor the Walker Report expressed serious concern about the problem. On the contrary, there was a strong tendency to recognize it as a rather normal phase of medical practice. "I found few complaints," observed Hadfield, "that could fairly be labelled frivolous. It was exceptional for even the trivial case not to have something wrong."[44] "Who shall say without examining the patient," asked the Walker Committee, "whether a condition is 'trivial'?" "If patients," continued the Report, "are encouraged by the profession itself to seek medical advice in the early stages of illness they cannot wholly be blamed if some of them approach the doctor unnecessarily. What seems trivial to the doctor may not be so to the patient, who may have no one else to turn to for help in his problem. Some doctors, especially the younger ones without long experience, may not be aware how helpless the patient may feel in his small troubles and what relief a sympathetic hearing can give him."[45]

In Gemmill's survey, approximately one-half of the practitioners indicated that patients often took up their time with minor ailments. About what constituted a minor ailment, however, there was no agreement. The work expended on the so-called trivial cases was by no means unproductive, since any of them might prove serious if neglected. Pursuing this approach, Professor Gemmill asked his respondents, "Do you think that requests for medical attention for very minor ailments lead . . . to the prevention of serious ailments or to their detection while still in the early stages?" Eleven per cent said "often," and 60 per cent, "occasionally." Only 29 per cent replied "almost never."[46]

There was, of course, much sickness of a psychoneurotic origin. Overindulgence in alcohol, domestic unhappiness, financial worry, overwork, sub-standard housing, and the terrific pressure of modern living were among the causes. How many people were psychologically ill could not easily be determined, but the percentage was large. A surgical and psychiatric survey in 1953 and 1954 of outpatient gynecology disclosed that, of the 60 random subjects, only a small minority had any significant gynecological abnormality. The conclusion was that "emotional tension outweighs physical malfunction and disease as a cause in women who attend a gynaecology clinic."[47] The symptoms of almost a thousand new patients in the casualty department of a London Hospital in 1954 and 1955 showed that, of those who complained of pain, no organic cause was believed to exist in 26 per cent of the cases.[48] One practitioner found that over a third of 500 consecutive patients suffered from neurosis. Other doctors put the percentage at one-fourth, but few would place it at much less.[49]

The "bottle-of-medicine" habit, so strongly ingrained in the British people, was a major factor before the days of the Health Service. Not only in panel but in private practice as well, the " 'doctor's bottle' was encouraged as a part of the doctor-patient transaction." "However lengthy the examination, however sound the general advice," wrote one physician, "the patient who did not get 'a bottle' from the doctor's hands felt defrauded." High-pressure advertisements by drug companies reinforced even more the faith which people had in the healing power of drugs. All this carried over into the Health

Service. Neurotic and organically sick people continued to expect their prescriptions, whether the need existed or not, and busy doctors, who often knew little about psychoneurosis, found a prescription a convenient way to get rid of hypochondriacs and other patients considered a nuisance. The fear of losing patients may have made a few practitioners more accommodating in issuing certificates and prescriptions, but as a factor in medical practice as a whole it was negligible. Few patients changed doctors because of dissatisfaction over certificates and prescriptions, nor did the vast majority threaten to transfer or otherwise exert any undue pressure.[50]

The better family physicians recognized that if more time at the outset could be spent with emotionally disturbed patients, the result would be fewer chronic psychoneurotics later. Commenting upon this idea, one doctor explained that "the over-worked, over-anxious, under-paid or unhappily married patient who is brought to understand the nature of his troubles will not attend repeatedly for useless bottles of medicine, and neither in many cases [will] the frank psychoneurotic, who can often be given some insight into his condition." The extent to which patients were bothersome depended in many cases upon the efficiency of the doctor. Taylor observed that it was usually to the least efficient practitioners that thoughtless patients gave the most trouble. In a well-disciplined practice, there was a feeling of mutual respect and understanding between the doctor and his patients.[51]

Just as doctors were subject to regulations and could be disciplined, so it was felt by many practitioners that patients should be brought under a code of conduct. Any person had the right to register a complaint against a physician for failure to comply with the terms of service and an investigation would follow, but the doctor had no such recourse against a patient who misused the medical service. Under the Health Insurance scheme, disciplinary action could be taken against a panel patient, and such a policy, many doctors contended, would be good for the Health Service. Neither the Ministry of Health nor Parliament favored the idea, however. Unlike the doctor, the patient had no contractual relationship with the local Executive Council and therefore could not be made subject to sanctions unless new legislation were adopted. It was the judgment of the Cohen Committee that rules and penalties for patients were undesirable, since they would constitute a serious threat to the doctor-patient relationship.[52]

In 1951, the Council of the British Medical Association proposed that stringent rules and penalties for their infraction be drawn up by the Ministry of Health in consultation with the medical profession to prevent frivolous calls by patients. In 1956, however, the Council was convinced that an enforceable code of conduct for patients would be difficult to achieve. It even felt that a set of rules persuasive in character was unnecessary, since the great majority of patients were co-operative, since the problem was not a large one, and since the kind of rules proposed would serve no practical purpose.[53]

The Newsam Report recognized what most practitioners had come to accept—that the disciplining of patients was the duty of the family physician and could be accomplished most effectively through the process of oral education, although government propaganda would also play an important role in making "the public fully conscious of their obligations as citizens of a welfare state." Giving doctors the authority to fine patients was dismissed as being "repugnant to the underlying principle of the National Health Service."[54]

The disciplinary machinery of the Health Service was complicated and somewhat unwieldy. The delay in processing some cases was a source of irritation, and there were examples of practitioners' being summoned before the local medical service committee to answer charges that rested on flimsy evidence, but such doctors as a rule were quickly exonerated. Fines were sometimes considered excessive. There was little agitation in medical circles to revamp the disciplinary machinery, however. The British Medical Association found that it furnished adequate protection to a physician accused of violating the terms of service.

Cases were handled *in camera,* in order to protect the reputation of the doctor. Press releases on disciplinary cases seldom carried the name of the physician, and only when dismissal from the Service occurred were all particulars usually divulged. The respondent was given every chance to defend himself. Only if the complaint seemed to have substance was there a hearing, which was conducted before the medical service committee. Three of the seven members of the committee were doctors appointed by the local medical committee. Acting upon the report of the medical service committee, the Executive Council made its recommendation. If it involved expulsion, the case went immediately before the Health Service Tribunal; otherwise the Minister of Health, in consultation with a Medical Advisory Committee, decided what final action should be taken. If there was an appeal, the Minister could hold a hearing before a small *ad hoc* committee, but the final decision rested with him. Exoneration, a reprimand, or a fine were the usual alternatives. Disciplinary action was taken in any number of offences, including fraudulent certification, faulty treatment or neglect of the patient, irregular issue of prescriptions, professional misconduct, and unsatisfactory conditions of practice.

The Health Service Tribunal comprised three members—a doctor and a layman appointed by the Minister of Health and an experienced barrister or solicitor who, as the chairman, was selected by the Lord Chancellor. Although not a court, the Tribunal endeavored to equal the objectivity and thoroughness of a court of law. The Tribunal had the right to call witnesses, obtain evidence on oath, and impose costs. Any individual could be the complainant, but it was the Executive Council that invariably fulfilled this role, making representations and furnishing the evidence. If the complaint came originally from a patient, however, that person had to appear in the witness box and could be cross-examined. The practitioner could be represented in any manner he chose, including representation by legal counsel, and he could have a public hearing, if he desired, though none of the respondents on record preferred that alternative. If the Tribunal decided in favor of the respondent, the case was immediately closed, and the name of the doctor remained on the Health Service list. But if dismissal was recommended, the case could be appealed to the Minister, who had the power to affirm or reverse the judgment of the Tribunal.[55]

The Committee on Administrative Tribunals and Enquiries, known as the Franks Committee, proposed in 1957 that the decisions of the Health Service Tribunal should be final and that its jurisdiction should be extended to include less serious cases that had been appealed from the Executive Councils. The reason this Committee recommended that the Minister should be deprived of his appellate jurisdiction in disciplinary cases was apparently that the scales seemed to be weighted in favor of the doctor. Public hearings by the Tribunal were also urged in the more serious cases and in all others except those in which the appeals were initiated by the complainant.[56] Such proposals were vigorously opposed by the British Medical Association, which took the position that, since the present tribunal machinery worked satisfactorily, the appellate jurisdiction of the Minister should not be disturbed. To protect the doctor from reckless allegations, private hearings, it was contended, were best for everybody concerned. The Medical Association thus became the ardent defendant of the very machinery which it had once viewed with such fear.

To ensure that the administrative tribunals in Great Britain functioned justly and impartially, the government in 1958 set up a Council on Tribunals. As an independent organization, responsible only to the Lord Chancellor, this new body served in a supervisory and advisory capacity.   Among the large number of agencies that it kept under review were the National Health Service Tribunal, the Service Committees, and certain functions of the Executive Councils.   The Medical, Dental, and Pharmaceutical Associations were not pleased with the implications of the new arrangement.   They were afraid that the Council on Tribunals might use its influence to effect changes such as those recommended by the Franks Committee in the rules of procedure governing the disciplinary machinery of the Health Service.[57]

In disciplining medical practitioners, the Executive Councils seldom recommended removal from the list, and even more rarely did the Tribunal or Minister of Health sustain such recommendations.   An average of less than one medical practitioner a year was struck from the roster, and some years no such action at all was taken.   A few hundred cases involving violation in the terms of service were investigated by the medical service committees and reported to the Minister every year.   Appeals made against the decision of the Executive Councils seldom exceeded 50 and in some years dropped to less than 30.   In between two-thirds and three-fourths of the cases reported to the Minister, no action was taken, and with the remainder the discipline usually took the form of a warning letter or a reduction in the remuneration of the offender.   With few exceptions, the recommendations of the Executive Councils were upheld by the Minister of Health.[58]

Some cases seemed trifling, but they involved a question of professional dignity.   A certain Lancashire doctor, for instance, exasperated by the complaints of a patient, told him to "go to hell" and to get some other physician.   The Executive Council recommended a fine of £10 ($28).   Other cases were of major significance, such as the one involving a Kent practitioner who issued Health Service prescriptions to some of his private patients.   The gravity of this offense caused the Executive Council to propose a fine of £1,500 ($4,200), which was reduced by the Minister to £1,100 ($3,080).   For charging a fee for an emergency treatment, a Health Service practitioner in Derbyshire was fined £27 ($75), as recommended by the local Council.   The failure of a physician to visit promptly an aged woman before she died led to a severe reprimand.   A Gateshead doctor who was not punctual in holding office hours and who failed to make adequate provision for his patients during an illness was censured and fined £100 ($280).

Disciplinary action sometimes led to resignation, as it did in the case of a Lancashire physician who was faced by a fine of £500 ($1,400) for gross negligence.   The doctor failed to respond to a call shortly after midnight, and the patient died from "toxemia, peritonitis and a perforated duodenal ulcer accelerated by delay of medical aid." The physician claimed failing health, but the Executive Council refused to permit extenuating circumstances to soften the proposed disciplinary action. When the doctor offered his resignation, it was promptly accepted. An honest error in judgment, however, was not considered as prima-facie grounds for complaint. A doctor was exonerated who diagnosed the condition of a sick woman as rheumatism and later as a slipped disc and rheumatism, when within a few hours the patient had to be rushed to the hospital with a brain hemorrhage.[59]

During my six-month sojourn in England, I had the opportunity of interviewing a number of medical practitioners. Whether these doctors were typical of the majority I, of course, could not determine, but what they disclosed may not have been so very different from what many other physicians would have said had they been approached. One of the doctors was a junior member of a three-doctor partnership in Peterborough, a city of more than 50,000 people. He originally was a registrar in the hospital service, but an excess of registrars forced him and other senior registrars to leave the service. Entering general medical practice, he acquired a list of 2,000 persons, of whom 50 were private patients. Concerning the latter, he asserted that they often got inferior treatment because they could not afford the more expensive drugs. These patients, he said, were inclined to view the Health Service as charity and in their "stupid pride" refused to accept it. Most doctors, he asserted, would be better off without such patients, but the number of these persons was declining, and not a great many were left. Only one doctor in Peterborough was then exclusively engaged in private practice.

That junior partner believed that in the cities there was such competition for patients that doctors tended to coddle hypochondriacs. Refusal to administer to them would result in an unfavorable reputation that might impede the enlargement of the doctor's list. About 20 per cent of the patients of this particular practitioner he identified as hypochondriacs. The problem, he explained, was not an indictment of the Health Service, which had simply given to those people who otherwise could not afford it the opportunity to display their neurotic tendencies. Much more significant was the simple fact that under the present system nobody was neglected medically. Many doctors worked harder for less money, but the Health Service had not made medicine less interesting. Regulations on the whole were fair, although there was much paper work to be done. In winter, this practitioner treated 50 to 60 patients per day, as compared with

18 or 20 under the old system. Each week he got a half-day off, and every three weeks a day and one-half. In summer he had a four-week vacation. He said that doctors largely controlled the Health Service through their membership in the Executive Council and other boards and committees and that the scheme was efficiently administered, being above partisan currents. The Health Service, he claimed, certainly deserved some of the credit for the improved health of the nation.

The best part of one afternoon was spent in conference with two partners in Huntingdonshire, who together had a rural practice of 5,000 persons. They had no private patients and did not want any. The senior member disclosed that from 1948 to 1954 his income increased 50 per cent and was now in the neighborhood of £3,000 ($8,400). Some doctors, he conceded, were making less than they did prior to the inception of the Health Service, but the majority were doing better. Earning more, most physicians had greater security. They had, of course, no need to be concerned about unpaid charges. The senior member had two cars and a nice home with modern conveniences. He commented favorably upon the pension system, which would yield him superannuation benefits of £900 ($2,500) per year. Younger doctors, he said, would retire at as much as £1,180 ($3,300). He displayed great pride in his practice, indicating that he was at present involved in making extensive alterations in his office accommodations. Both practitioners agreed that the people overwhelmingly accepted the Health Service and that opposition in the medical profession was diminishing sharply and would disappear within twenty years. They pointed out that in the Huntingdon area only two doctors were positively antagonistic toward the Health Service.

The two partners in winter had alternate Sundays and one afternoon each week off; in summer, they got one full day every week, plus a month's vacation. There was no queuing in the reception room, and it was a rare person who waited more than 30 minutes. During an office session, a few patients might take 10 to 20 minutes of their time, but many required only a very few minutes. The amount of paper work, now cut to the minimum, was smaller than before the war. Doctors were free to do as they pleased, being subject to no bureaucratic controls. I was assured that the health scheme was bi-partisan, that doctors largely ran the program, and that individual initiative and freedom of expression were in no way hampered.

The tendency was to send patients to the hospital for minor operations and certain types of medical treatment—a trend which these doctors felt was good. Hospitals were much better than before the war, with better specialists, better facilities, and better service. For emergency cases, there was no delay in admission; for non-emergency cases, the period of waiting was never more than a year. Practical preventive medicine was being pushed hard, especially among children, who were periodically given thorough medical examinations. Prenatal and postnatal care was better than ever. It was not the policy of these partners, however, to give medical examinations to healthy adults. They, like so many other doctors, were too busy to practice this kind of preventive medicine. It goes without saying, of course, that if a man entered their office with a cough, he was examined thoroughly to determine the source of the trouble. In no other branch of the medical profession in the world, I was informed, was there so much honesty as the English. These doctors were aware of no fee splitting, but they reminded me that detection in this abuse resulted in expulsion from the Service.

In the same shire, but many miles away, I had a lengthy discussion with a physician who was not in partnership and who had qualified as a doctor in 1936. He lived in a very attractive home, and his office was located there. He had three children, one of whom, a boy, was in a private school costing £350 ($980) a year. Among his 2,100 patients there were a few private patients, but he discouraged any more from coming to him because of the difficulty of sending out and collecting bills. He said he favored the Health Service primarily because under the old system he hesitated to keep calling on a patient in need of his services out of the fear that the patient might believe that his visits were motivated by a desire for more fees. Now he could see such patients as often as he wanted, secure that they knew that what he did for them was governed solely by their needs. It was his observation that hypochondriacs were no more numerous than before 1948, and he, in fact, believed they were probably fewer, since, no longer paying fees, they were less likely to feel that they had purchased his time, for whatever purpose. Prior to the Health Service they were a main source of the doctor's income, but no more was that true.

Huntingdon was a closed area in which no more practitioners were allowed to enter because of the relatively great concentration of doctors there. The doctor with whom I was speaking said he would like to have more patients, and if he had 3,500 he would obtain an assistant. Competition among doctors was described as friendly. His patients received as good or even better service than before 1948. There was no queuing in his office, and no patient ever waited more than half an hour. His emergency cases were admitted immediately to the hospital, and for others there was a delay of from one to six months. Since the start of the Health Service, the local hospital had greatly improved. Primarily because of its superior facilities but partly because of the absence of a special fee for surgical work, the tendency was to send patients to the hospital even for minor surgery. Often, this doctor accompanied his patients and even performed some of the less difficult operations.

He denied that there was much bureaucracy in medical practice or an excessive amount of paper work. There were, he averred, no undue interference from Executive Councils and no obnoxious regulations. No political pressure hampered the physician, who was free to do as he pleased. Few if any doctors would now restore the old system, he believed, although at first 90 per cent opposed the Health Service. The pension system was good, he affirmed, and in general the Service brought security to the medical profession. The National Health Service, he emphasized, in no way had made medicine less appealing.

Doctors were by no means alike in their appraisal of the Health Service. The sharpest criticism came from the Fellowship For Freedom in Medicine, which took a dim view of what the new scheme had done to the prestige and standards of the medical profession. In discussing the matter, one spokesman for the Fellowship said that a patient used to be "looked after by" or "under the care of" a physician, whereas now the patient was someone on a "doctor's list" or someone for whom the doctor was "at risk." This change in terminology, it was claimed, symbolized the deterioration which had occurred in one of the most important phases of medical practice.[60]

An outspoken critic of the Health Service was Dr. Alexander Hall, an active member of the Fellowship For Freedom in Medicine. As president of the British Medical Association in 1956, he questioned the wisdom of the state's playing such a major role in the maintenance of health. "The people of the country should consider," he advised, "whether they are developing an attitude of mind to the N.H.S. which is more disease-conscious than health-conscious." He deplored so much "unreasoning faith" in the "bottle of medicine" and the "wonder drugs." The introduction of the state as a third party, he charged, had "interfered with the essential freedom of the patient and the doctor." The status of the practitioner, he declared, had suffered unduly from the enhanced prestige of the specialist, and much of the blame for this he attributed to the Health Service. Private practice, he felt, should be preserved and fostered, since it offered the most hope for an escape from "the cold blast of bureaucratic control."[61]

Those who believed that the doctor-patient relationship had suffered pointed to physicians who were denied direct access to hospital beds and to X-ray and pathological facilities. Some patients considered hospital treatment and diagnosis superior to anything the general medical practitioner had to offer. The patients' "irresponsible demands" and their tendency to view the doctor as a dispenser of prescriptions and certificates were likewise set forth as causes in the alleged loss of professional stature by family doctors. Also cited were the "breathless pace" of the physicians with large lists and the growing trend of transferring the minor surgery from the doctor's office to the hospitals.

To what extent these factors affected more than a minority of the doctors was not clear, and to what extent they were attributable to the Health Service was even more debatable. Many of the problems facing general practice had existed previously, a few were exaggerated, and others were perhaps a reflection upon the clinical and administrative efficiency of some of the family physicians. According to the Newsam Report, most of the difficulties "had been creeping on the profession for at least thirty years."[62] But there was reason to believe that at least some of them reflected new forces at work, to which some of the physicians had not made adjustment.

Whatever the cause or explanation for the problems, neither the medical profession nor the Ministry of Health was oblivious to their existence. In achieving a better distribution of doctors and patients, in encouraging hospitals to make beds and other facilities more directly accessible to practitioners, and in emphasizing the inviolability of the doctor-patient relationship, the government endeavored to improve the situation. Progress was made, but there were some problems that did not lend themselves to any easy solution and might well remain in existence for many years to come.

Functional illness, for example, did not always respond to the sort of clinical treatment that the average doctor was able to give. Unable to find a pathological cause for an illness which had its origin in psychosomatic disorders, the physician was frequently unable to arrive at the proper therapy, with the result that some patients tended to lose faith in their doctors. Even if the medical practitioner had been sufficiently trained in them, the application of psychiatric techniques would scarcely have been possible for the great majority of family doctors, owing to the volume of their work.[63] The problem obviously would have existed in the absence of the Health Service, although maybe not to the same degree. It was thus evident that the relationship between doctor and patient hinged upon many factors, some very complex, and that to ascribe to the Health Service any deterioration in the relationship, as some critics did, was a gross oversimplification.

Those who had formerly been panel patients were not so likely to observe any change in doctor-patient relationship as those who had been private patients and who joined the Health Service to escape the high cost of private medical care. As private patients, they paid fees based upon the service rendered and were therefore able to command more time and more courtesies from the doctor than they could reasonably demand as Health Service patients, for whom the practitioner received a flat capitation fee regardless of how many items of service were given. With a heavier patient load, the Health Service physician had to be governed by a more utilitarian approach, although he could be and usually was just as interested in his patients and as effective medically. A busy practitioner could hardly be expected to indulge a patient with a home visit when that person could just as well come to the doctor's office for treatment.

It came as a surprise to most family physicians that the bulk of the middle class entered the Health Service. Owing to high taxes, inflation, and a desire to educate their children in private schools, members of this economic group were caught in a financial squeeze which made it imperative that they accept the relief from direct medical costs offered by the Health Service. In spring, 1954, the *Manchester Guardian* published a number of representative middle-class budgets, and in the great majority medical expenses were conspicuously absent. Small token payments for dental treatment and prescriptions were occasionally listed, but only in a few isolated cases were medical costs an item of any consequence.[64] In joining the Health Service, a certain adjustment had to be made, but most middle-class patients were able to achieve it with good grace. There were a few, however, who wanted the same type of service as before and who became disgruntled when they could not get it. Such patients were usually told that if they wanted to be attended in their homes for trivial ailments they would have to become private patients or choose another doctor.[65]

The Postal Inquiry of the British Medical Association indicated that two-thirds of the doctors felt that the attitude of their Health Service patients who had formerly been private patients had changed, in some cases becoming more demanding and in others more considerate. The Walker Committee was of the opinion that middle-class patients who had formerly been served privately had not made excessive demands upon the Service. The Hadfield Survey found that the vast majority of practitioners discovered no adverse change among such patients. Some people, however, who formerly could not afford to call a physician very often now made greater use of the medical service. Most practitioners were impressed with the moderation shown by former private patients in using the Service, and only one-fourth of the doctors complained about increased demands from such individuals.[66]

In trying to determine whether there had been any impairment in the doctor-patient relationship, it should be remembered that there was, as the Walker Report pointed out, no standard by which the relationship could be measured in the first place. Nevertheless, the Report held that there had been some deterioration, but expressed surprise that "there have not been greater difficulties when the magnitude of the changes which took place in 1948 is taken into account." The Walker Committee believed that the evidence on the whole showed the doctor-patient relationship to be satisfactory. "The majority of practitioners," asserted the Report, "find that their relations with the majority of their patients are friendly. By most the general practitioner is regarded as a professional man and friend." The Committee seemed to feel that it was a small core of troublesome patients that had created "the general impression that the N. H. S. has brought about a deterioration of the doctor-patient relationship." The Committee was nevertheless concerned over the lack of time which prevented "a doctor from familiarizing himself with the 'totality' of his patient."[67] This, however, was a problem that could be solved by increasing the number of practitioners and decreasing the size of lists, and each year revealed improvements in these two areas.

The Cohen Committee was of the opinion that the available information sustained the "impression made by the evidence of individual doctors, that the [doctor-patient] relationship is good; in some respects indeed, it was found to be better than before, and this was attributed to the absence of the money bar and to increased co-operation between doctors." The Guillebaud Committee found that the great volume of evidence disclosed no decline in the quality of the practitioner service. In full agreement with the findings of the Cohen Report, the Guillebaud Committee observed that family doctors were seeing more patients and doing more work for each patient than before 1948. "As payment is no longer a factor to be considered," it was emphasized, "there is no reluctance on the part of the patients to seek the advice of a doctor on all matters connected with the family's health, and doctors generally welcome this freedom of approach, even if it occasionally be misused."[68]

On the tenth anniversary of the Health Service, Dr. H. Guy Dain could see considerable merit in the program. It will be recalled that, as chairman of the Council of the British Medical Association between 1943 and 1949, he had assumed a very critical attitude toward the proposed health scheme and had led the profession in its fight against certain features of the new law. It was thus significant that this man should recognize in 1958 that "to every inhabitant of the country, whether Britisher or visitor—[the Health Service] has been an enormous benefit and success." He willingly admitted that "the Service has been a boon" for the patients. "The absence of any financial barrier between the doctor and patient," he affirmed, "must make the doctor-patient relationship easier and more satisfactory." It was inevitable, he declared, that as the people took full advantage of the Health Service benefits and the practitioners attended their new patients, problems would arise, but "they have really been remarkably few." In no way, he declared, had clinical freedom been threatened. And the steady diminution of private practice seemed proof enough to him that the general practitioner had given an efficient service.[69]

In reviewing the first ten years of the Service, the chairman of the Executive Council for Cheshire, R. B. Howells, could observe no change in the traditional relationship between the patient and physician. In some cases, he felt, it had improved. "Experience points," he said, "to the existence of a relationship not only of a high order but of one increasingly so, and many defects in the service, or difficulties in the application of central policy to the local scene have been remedied or overcome by the initiative and good sense of the people most intimately concerned—doctor and patient."[70]

What did the doctors feel was the effect of the Health Service upon their practice? In seeking an answer, Professor Gemmill posed this question in his survey: "With your present list of patients, do you find it *reasonably easy,* or *difficult,* or *almost impossible* to give them what you regard as adequate medical care?" Less than 4 per cent said it was "almost impossible," slightly more than one-third found it *difficult,* and the remainder indicated that it was *reasonably easy.* Most of those in the first two categories had more than the average number of patients.[71] Only one-third of the practitioners queried in the Social Surveys of 1956 seemed to think that their relationship with their patients had become more impersonal, and about the same percentage as in the Stevenson inquiry thought that there had been any decline in the doctor-patient relationship.[72]

According to Dr. Hadfield, 90 per cent of the family doctors had friendly relations with their patients and felt the need "to fill the role of guide, philosopher and friend." A majority of the doctors, however, reported a tendency to be regarded by a minority of their patients as a "supplier of medicines rather than medical adviser," but, in the opinion of Hadfield, the irritation caused by this attitude tended to exaggerate its importance. Almost one-half of the practitioners applauded the fact that the Health Service had broadened the scope of their practice. "They speak with relief," declared Hadfield, "of being able to prescribe what the patient needs and to visit him as often as the condition requires, free from the inhibitive consideration of the patient's purse."

Dr. Hadfield reported that two-thirds of the general practitioners had adjusted themselves to things as they were. "Buoyed up as in some cases, by hope of improvements," he said, "they have not allowed themselves to suffer from a sense of frustration and loss of interest." Little more than one-fourth felt thwarted. Stevenson noted that 70 per cent of the doctors were reasonably content. The Postal and Hadfield surveys found a majority in that category,[73] evidence that is all the more significant when it is recalled that at the time these studies were made the Danckwerts award had not been announced and there was great unrest over the remuneration issue. Nor did the attitude of the practitioners toward the Health Service seem to undergo any fundamental change as a result of the second and more serious crisis over compensation, which occurred during the latter part of the 1950's. If such a change had occurred, it was not perceived by the Newsam Report. While recognizing that "the overall standard of general practice . . . falls short of what it might have been," this document noted that the "majority of family doctors are not frustrated. They work happily and have adjusted themselves to the idea of service to the public and general responsibility for the health of their patients."[74]

Even those who were critical of the general medical service could see merit in it. Such a critic was a young doctor, who summarized the advantages of the service in this way:

There is no doubt that the established young general practitioner in partnership practice to-day has a much easier time of it than had his predecessors. His nights are less frequently disturbed, mainly because there is now less domiciliary midwifery, and his off-duty time is much more regular with the inception of the rota system. Finally he has a secure, pensionable job. So far as his patients are concerned, there is greater continuity of care and incidentally of clinical records. . . . There is no longer a financial barrier between patient and doctor, who can prescribe freely without fear that the patient may not be able to afford his treatment. . . . Despite its many present-day failings, general practice remains a branch of medicine in which is to be found a great deal of satisfaction.[75]

And what did the people think of the role of the general medical practitioner in the Service? The Social Surveys in 1956 disclosed that approximately four-fifths of the people polled felt that their doctor was also a friend in whom they could confide, that he had done a good job, and that he gave enough time to patients. Only a very small fraction had noticed any change in the treatment or attitude of their physician since the start of the Service.   Ross's survey of a factory town revealed that 94 per cent of the families believed that the treatment they were receiving from their physicians under the Health Service was as good as it had been previously.[76]   The inquiry conducted by Brotherston *et al.* showed that only 17 per cent of those queried thought there had been any decline in the quality of medical care.   One-half observed no change, and the remainder noted an improvement.[77]

Patients were not all agreed about what they liked and disliked about the practitioner service, but Professor Gemmill undertook to record the consensus of those brought within the scope of his inquiry. In general, they disapproved of having to wait in the doctor's office, but were no longer troubled so much by this problem.   The small amount of time allowed for most consultations was more widely criticized, although "many patients state emphatically that their own doctors give all the time that is needed."   Some patients resented the prescription charge and even more the fact that foreigners received medical care free.   Among the patients' likes, all calculated to improve doctor-patient relationship, were that medical treatment was now "a matter of right and not charity"; that excellent medical care, once accessible only to the wealthy, was now available to the poorest; that the medical service was in no way limited in its coverage or comprehensiveness; and that the "cost of a catastrophic illness will not wreck a family's financial programme."[78]

CHAPTER X

Organization and Management of the Hospital Service

REFERENCE HAS ALREADY been made to the size and scope of the hospital and specialist services. The gross cost of this phase of the Health Program was almost six times greater than that of the general medical services. Absorbing all but 20 per cent of the personnel employed by the National Health Service, the hospital division stood as a towering giant in comparison with all other branches.

The hospitals that were taken over by the government in 1948 represented an extraordinary mixture of voluntary and local authority institutions. They were characterized by sharp differences in size, origin, internal organization, and standards. The voluntary hospitals, which represented slightly more than 40 per cent of the total number of institutions, had taken pride in their autonomy but for the most part were small and had suffered from financial difficulties. Some had distinguished themselves and were internationally famous, but the great majority had maintained a precarious existence and were inadequately staffed and deficient in most other respects. The local authority hospitals, which accounted for more than three-fourths of the beds, were of many types, including general, isolation, mental and mental deficiency, chronic, and tuberculosis. Some of the municipal hospitals were exemplary, but most of them were handicapped by overcrowding, inadequate staffs, and meager facilities. Many seemed unable to divest themselves of influence of their Poor Law origins. Perhaps the chief characteristic of the hospitals prior to 1948 was the lack of co-ordination among them and their reluctance to co-operate with each other. The rivalry between the voluntary and local authority hospitals was particularly unfortunate.

What was wrong with the hospital service was well known, thanks to the critical observations of experts and most particularly to the surveys published in 1945. There was little disagreement about the broad objectives that should be accomplished in a reorganization of the hospital structure. Larger planning areas were deemed necessary in order to create a balanced and well co-ordinated system with a better distribution of specialists and facilities to replace the highly competitive and chaotic one that had existed so long. But the specific methods by which this end should be achieved most effectively were not so apparent. There was a cleavage of opinion on how much control should be concentrated in the Ministry and what measure of authority should be left to the individual hospitals and on how sweeping should be the regrouping and reorganization. Local attachments were strong, especially in the voluntary hospitals, and any reduction in the autonomy of such institutions was sure to be resented. The local government officials, long accustomed to hospital management, were averse to the surrender of their prerogatives in that field.

The framework of hospital administration provided by the National Health Service Act of 1946 consisted of three tiers—the Ministry of Health, the regional hospital boards, and the hospital management committees, with the individual hospitals, of course, constituting still another level. Operating independently of this hierarchical arrangement, but directly responsible to the Ministry of Health, were the boards of governors of the teaching hospitals. Each level of authority was assigned a special role, but the jurisdiction of each was not rigidly delimited by law, with the result that there was a certain elasticity in the delegation and exercise of authority. The intent of Parliament was quite clear—in the simplest terms, to establish a national hospital service financed almost wholly from the national treasury and administered through a decentralized system, each element of which performed that function best calculated to insure a uniform quality of service.

The major responsibility for seeing that this intent was accomplished rested upon the Ministry of Health. The status this department occupied in the government and the control it was able to exercise over finance were primary factors in conditioning the development of the hospital service. When the Health Service was launched, the Minister of Health held a seat in the cabinet. Aneurin Bevan, who filled the post from 1945 to 1951, was able to exert a powerful influence in shaping the fortunes of the Health Service. Shortly after he left office, the Ministry of Health was reorganized, losing its jurisdiction over housing, which was transferred to another department. The removal of these extraneous functions seemed logical enough, but the effect was to reduce the staff of the Ministry of Health by almost one-half. In this truncated form, the Ministry of Health ceased to have cabinet status or to maintain headquarters in Whitehall. Its spokesman, now a junior minister, was at a disadvantage in defending the interests of the National Health Service. His loss of rank made the office less desirable, and this factor must have contributed to the short tenure of Health Ministers. Between 1951 and 1957, seven changes occurred in that office. In commenting on this situation in the House of Commons in 1958, Aneurin Bevan deplored the fact that the Minister of Health "did not acquire in that office sufficient stature to be able to stand up against the importunities of the Treasury."[1]

The story of hospital finance has many ramifications, with a number of agencies playing a part. Although the basic pattern remained unchanged, there was sufficient elasticity to permit some modification, particularly in the relationship between the Ministry of Health and the hospital boards and committees. In general, controls were more rigid during the early years of the Health Service, but after 1952 the Ministry of Health pursued a somewhat more liberal and less paternalistic policy toward the voluntary bodies that governed the hospitals. The Ministry, for instance, relinquished to the hospital boards the sole responsibility of approving the detailed estimates prepared by the management committees. In the matter of auditing, it gave to these boards the responsibility for any action necessary for the ordering of the accounts of management committees that had been examined by auditors from the Ministry of Health.[2] The greatest frustration, however, was not the controls—which in some degree were being reduced—but the paucity of funds, which seemed to force the hospitals into an ever tighter strait jacket.

The hospital budget was largely worked out in the fall and the early part of the winter. The hospital management committees were called upon to submit to their regional board an estimate of the amount required to maintain services at the current levels. If new wards were to be opened or other fresh expenditures were to be incurred, the additional funds that would be needed were specified. The regional boards verified and amended these forecasts, transmitting the total to the Ministry. The total figure for hospital expenditures was then negotiated with the Treasury, subject, of course, to final approval by Parliament. When notified what their shares would be, the management committees prepared a careful budgetary analysis, to be approved by their regional board. Price increases, wage raises, and other unexpected expenses that might later arise could be met by a supplementary budget, but the regional boards, themselves under pressure, made every effort to keep the management committees within the original budgets. Their efforts in this respect were surprisingly successful.[3]

The so-called hospital revenue expenditures embraced funds for development, including the enlargement of the staffs or plants. It was at the revenue expenditures, much more than at the so-called "static" or "inherited" estimates, that the Treasury took a careful look to see if any trimming should be done. How the development funds should be used was more or less discretionary with the Minister of Health, who, in distributing them, endeavored to correct in some degree the inequalities between the hospital regions.[4]

The regional boards enjoyed a large measure of freedom in allocating money within the total grant allotted to them. They determined how much should be given to each management committee and how much should be retained at regional level as a reserve. Most significant was the power of virement, or the right to shift funds from one division to another and to use savings realized in maintenance and administration to finance an additional development project. Use of this power was encouraged, since it stimulated thrift and resulted in the improvement of hospital facilities. Unspent funds always reverted to the Exchequer, and had it not been for virement, there might have been a tendency for hospital authorities to spend in a less beneficial manner the money allotted them. The power of virement, however, was subject to some criticism on the grounds that regional boards, in exercising it, might tend to make unwise reductions in the allocations to management committees. But there was little evidence of any serious abuses of the kind, and although irritations arose, the fiscal relations between hospital boards and their management committees for the most part seemed satisfactory.

The government was opposed to block grants and to carrying over unspent balances. During the early years of the Service, there was considerable sentiment in favor of grants covering expenditures for periods of three to five years. Financial strictures combined with an inflationary condition to render such a fiscal policy inadvisable.[5]

The Ministry of Health handled directly all large-scale development projects, such as the erection of major hospital buildings, but had to seek Treasury approval for the more costly ones. Although the regional boards were allocated substantial sums for most of the other types of capital expenditures, the Ministry of Health examined the major elements of expense and reserved the right to examine all elements if it wished.[6] Complaints were voiced over the delays caused by the way capital projects were scrutinized. It did not appear, however, that the Treasury was at fault, since the schemes submitted to it for approval were usually held for consideration no more than three weeks. Rarely would the Treasury turn down any scheme unless its cost threatened to upset the total fixed for all capital expenditures. It must be remembered, of course, that when the project reached the Exchequer for final approval, it had already been inspected by the surveyors, architects, engineers, and doctors of the Ministry of Health.

In the field of capital expenditures, the Ministry of Health endeavored to improve the hospital facilities in the less favored and poorer regions. This leveling process, in view of financial limitations, could be accomplished only gradually, but the policy was none the less apparent in the proportionately larger grants awarded hospital boards in Liverpool, Wales, Birmingham, Sheffield, Newcastle, and Manchester. The four metropolitan boards that administered the London hospitals received proportionately less, as did the teaching hospitals.

As the fiscal watchdog of the government, the Treasury was interested in whatever concerned government funds. The influence of this agency over the Whitley council that recommended Health Service levels of remuneration could be strong, even though the Treasury had no direct part in any of the negotiations between the management and staff sides. When Whitley Council awards of higher rates of pay were made, the Ministry of Health deemed it prudent to consult Treasury officials about what increases, if any, would be accepted by it. The Ministry might otherwise find its approval of a Whitley award being disavowed by the paymaster of the nation. Quite obviously, the fiscal department, if committed to an anti-inflationary policy, could not very well permit, for example, the salaries or wages of hospital employees to get out of line with those of civil servants because of the unsettling effect this imbalance might have upon the whole wage structure. Although the Ministry of Health frequently consulted the Treasury, formally and informally, the Ministry retained a large area of fiscal freedom. The Treasury never exercised any control over the size of the hospital service staff and in other respects left the Ministry of Health more room for action than most government departments seemed to enjoy.[7]

Other controlling agencies besides the Treasury were the Public Accounts Committee and the Select Committee on Estimates. They possessed a high degree of investigative authority, with the result that few phases of the hospital service seemed to escape the probes of one or the other of these powerful committees. Each served a specific purpose. The Public Accounts Committee exercised accounting control, while the Select Committee on Estimates was concerned with the broader problem of preventing waste and making sure that the people were getting the best medical value possible for the money spent. Appointed by the House of Commons and comprising some of its most experienced investigators, these committees produced, in their review of the fiscal and related aspects of the hospital service, some outstanding reports, with recommendations that the Ministry of Health could not ignore.

The Public Accounts Committee examined appropriation accounts for hidden subsidies and waste. Assisted by the Comptroller and the Auditor General, the Committee sought information principally from the Treasury's officers of accounts and the accounting office of the department being investigated. During the first ten years of the Health Service, the Public Accounts Committee examined hospital expenditures in five formal sessions, the first in 1950-51. In that session, a number of matters came under scrutiny, including the supplementary estimates of 1949, bulk purchasing, the financial management of farms and gardens, budgetary overestimates, and hospital cost accounting. The Committee became apprehensive when it discovered that some hospital employees were paid salaries above those established by the Whitley agreements—a revelation which caused the Ministry to put an end to the practice and to require that no exceptions to the officially approved pay schedules be permitted.

In the 1952-53 session, the Public Accounts Committee was disturbed to learn that a regional board authorized to purchase some property for a convalescent home had failed to use the property for that purpose. After leaving it vacant for a while, the board decided to utilize the property as a training school for nurses. The failure to inform the Treasury of the change in plans was disquieting to the Public Accounts Committee. Lack of funds had caused the board in question to modify its original plans, but the reason the Ministry did not systematically check the administrative decisions of this and other regional boards was in order to leave them with as much discretionary authority as possible. The critical attitude of this powerful Committee in such a minor matter is a good example of the pressure from above that helped to condition the conduct of the Ministry of Health. Yet the efforts of the Public Accounts Committee and the Select Committee on Estimates to foster greater centralization and more central financial control were, in the end, largely thwarted by the Ministry, which was eager to preserve the prerogatives of the regional boards.[8]

The Select Committee on Estimates, being much larger, was able to carry out much of its work through subcommittees. Its range of investigation could be extremely broad and thorough, as was demonstrated in the Sixth Report of 1956-57, which proved to be a mine of information about many phases of the hospital service. A large number of witnesses from the various levels of hospital administration were summoned for interrogation and much documentary material was submitted. Although much impressed with the improved efficiency and standards of the hospitals, the investigating subcommittee was none the less "depressed by the apparent lack of vigour with which some fundamental problems are being faced by the Ministry." Its recommendations, which need not be discussed at this point, touched on such matters as joint contracting, virement, departmental cost accounting, the domiciliary consultative service, administrative salaries, disparity in hospital standards, and the necessity of making medical students cost-conscious.[9]

As did the Public Accounts Committee, the Select Committee on Estimates made sure that the necessary follow-up action would be taken on its report. In the 1957-58 session, a subcommittee of the Select Committee received comments from the Ministry of Health on what policy was being followed in regard to the recommendations of the previous year. In the 1958-59 session, another subcommittee pursued the matter further, receiving oral and written testimony about what additional action had been taken. The evidence showed that the majority of the proposals had been or were being acted upon to the full or partial satisfaction of the subcommittee. Only in two or three cases did the subcommittee feel that the Ministry had been delinquent in implementing the recommendations or had failed satisfactorily to explain why more positive action had not occurred.[10]

Behind these committees stood Parliament. How far was this body able to affect hospital policy? One method of doing so was the Parliamentary questions, already referred to in an earlier chapter. Since time was strictly limited to one or two brief question periods each week and these periods were shared by several departments, only a few questions, with their supplementary queries, could be asked at any one time. If a member, however, was unwilling to take his place in the queue for an oral answer, he was always privileged to request a written one, which was forthcoming within a week. Possibly half the questions were of this type. An analysis disclosed an average of 300 oral questions on the hospital service for each of six Parliamentary sessions. Most of them seemed to touch on such matters as capital development plans, salaries, and staffing, and only a small minority were about the patient and his treatment. This perhaps can be explained by noting that members of Parliament often found it more convenient, when acting on behalf of a constituent, to request a written reply, which always received the Ministry's careful consideration.

Since a majority of the oral questions came from the opposition party, it can be assumed that they were not without at least some political implications. In the appointment of members to the regional boards and management committees, for instance, a sharp lookout was kept in Parliament on the role of party influence. The demand that ministerial circulars be used to execute certain policies or to standardize certain practices was usually resisted by the Ministry, on the grounds that such an encroachment upon the authority of the hospital boards and committees was ill-advised.[11]

Occasionally there was a major debate in Parliament on the hospital service or some other phase of the Health Service. In reading the Parliamentary Journals, one cannot avoid being impressed with the serious, constructive, and informative character of the discussions and their comparative freedom from partisanship. The high level of the debates in the House of Commons was well demonstrated when the Guillebaud Report came under review and in July, 1958, on the occasion of the tenth anniversary of the National Health Service. The latter discussion lasted more than six hours and touched on almost every element of the Health Program.[12] The debate in the House of Lords during the same month lasted almost four hours, but was devoted exclusively to the hospital service.[13] The friendly but critical analysis, especially on the part of the Lords, tends to dispel any illusion about the "corroding influence of politics" on the Health Service or the lack of awareness on the part of Parliament concerning the problems that faced the hospital service. In the give and take of Parliamentary discussion, the Minister of Health and the Permanent Undersecretary were both observers and participants. They could not very well remain indifferent to the logic, the evidence, and the weight of public opinion that found expression during the debates.

In creating the hospital service, Parliament made provision for a decentralized system of subordinate but semi-independent boards and committees. These bodies were made statutory, but their functions were defined in such broad terms[14] that only time and experience could determine the most effective relationship between them and Savile Row. Being charged with the full responsibility of maintaining an efficient hospital and specialist service, the Ministry of Health had largely to formulate the pattern of control itself, and in doing so used a somewhat variable procedure.

The staff at the Ministry's headquarters in 1958 numbered approximately 2,000, of whom about one-half served in a clerical capacity. The major part of the work was organized under some eight divisions—mental, Whitley, family practitioner and local authority, hospital and specialist, international health and food and nutrition, establishments (registry printing), public relations, and civil defense. In addition, there were specialist units, such as the Accountant-General's department, the supplies division, and the medical department.

So great was the responsibility of the hospital service that it required the assistance of several of the other divisions of the Ministry. Most important was the co-operation of the medical department. Its contribution to the hospital program was valuable in many ways, but of particular significance was the first-hand knowledge its officers gained through visits into the field to see how the hospitals operated. While fewer than 200 employees (clerical, secretarial, executive, and professional) were listed in the hospital and specialist division at headquarters, there were many times that number in other divisions that shared in the work of administering the hospital service.[15]

Aside from legislative enactments and the Parliamentary techniques of exerting influence, what were the influences upon policy at the Ministry of Health? Reference already has been made to the Central Health Services Council. It maintained nine standing committees—medical, dental, pharmaceutical, ophthalmic, nursing, maternity and midwifery, tuberculosis, mental health, and cancer and radiotherapy. Independent statutory agencies composed of experienced and even distinguished professional representatives, some from the field of hospital administration, these committees served in an important advisory capacity. Acting upon their recommendations, the Ministry issued a number of memoranda to hospital authorities. But whether the Central Health Services Council and its standing committees took as much initiative in their advisory role as was intended by Parliament was doubtful.[16]

Ministerial policy was further conditioned by a vast amount of practical information obtained from the hospitals themselves. Ministry officials regularly held conferences with the chairman and senior officers of the hospital boards. Regional officers of the Ministry of Health sat as observers at meetings of hospital authorities, and specialists from the Ministry (catering, medical, engineering, and nursing) visited the hospitals in the capacity of advisers and observers. The officials at headquarters regularly conferred with organizations like the Teaching Hospital Association, the Association of Hospital Management Committees, and the Association of Chief Financial Officers. Before issuing circulars, the Ministry, as noted elsewhere, often sought the opinion of the regional boards and management committees.

The Ministry of Health could draw upon a wealth of factual material and expert observations contained in inquiries, studies, and surveys. Some of the documents represented the work of individuals or committees from outside the Service, while other reports were made by officers in the Ministry or by mixed commissions of hospital authorities and Ministry officials. The Nuffield Provincial Hospitals

Trust and the King Edward's Hospital Fund financed special investigations. The Guillebaud Committee had much to say about the hospitals, but the more specialized reports covered such topics as hospital staffing, hospital supplies, bed occupancy, convalescence, welfare of children in hospitals, maternity services, outpatient waiting time, welfare of inpatients, the hospital pharmaceutical service, recruitment and training of nurses, care of the chronic sick and elderly, internal administration of hospitals, voluntary service in the hospitals, mental illness, midwives, and hospital cost accounting.

To what extent these documents influenced the Ministry of Health could not always be determined, but a sharp revision of policy, with the necessary Parliamentary action, sometimes followed the publication of a long-awaited report, as in the case of mental health. Often no action was taken or action was taken only after a considerable lapse of time. If a report seemed to meet an urgent need, the Ministry was not allowed to forget the fact, either by Parliament or by the medical or lay press. In general, it appeared that Savile Row was overly cautious in reacting to these documents, but it must be remembered that many factors were involved, including the brake of bureaucracy, from which few governmental departments are ever free. Conflicting interests could not easily be resolved. And, of course, the lack of funds, often a major factor, made the Ministry hesitant about any changes that involved additional expense.

Once a plan of action had been adopted by the Ministry of Health, how was it put into operation? What means were available for insuring compliance? Major regulations were usually issued as statutory instruments or extensions to the Health Service Act, and these had the force of law. Such rules, having lain on the table of the House of Commons, carried the full sanction of Parliament. The authority of the Ministry to audit the financial accounts of the management committees was an effective check on the degree of compliance with its fiscal policy. The general power of issuing administrative directives was a vital weapon of authority in the arsenal of the Ministry, since it commanded immediate obedience. But directives were used sparingly, in view of the desire of Savile Row to avoid dictation.

Should all other measures fail, the Minister could exercise his powers of default. If a regional board or a management committee refused to comply with a regulation or otherwise proved delinquent in performing its functions, the Minister could hold an inquiry and then dismiss the entire membership, replacing it with new appointees. As for removing an individual member of a board or committee, the Minister could do so only after a resolution had been adopted by the board or committee as a whole requesting such action on the grounds that the conduct of the member was detrimental to the effective performance of its duties.[17]   Since these bodies were voluntary and usually represented the most experienced and responsible citizens available, the Minister's use of his reserve powers would have signified a critical blow to the voluntary system of hospital management. Moral suasion was about all that the Ministry could use against the voluntary bodies if the spirit of co-operation and good will were to prevail.

Among the non-statutory methods of implementing policy were the circulars, which have been discussed in an earlier chapter.   There was little evidence that they were used to achieve more centralization in the hospital service.   The number of non-Whitley notices was not large, and the number of all circulars tended to diminish with time. Perhaps the circulars could have been briefer and could have been used in a more discriminating fashion, but it was apparent that they constituted the most appropriate channel for the transmission of policy statements and informative data from the nerve center of hospital administration to the periphery.

It was inevitable that complaints should arise.   It was the duty of the Ministry to hear them and see that justice was done.   All regional boards were urged to establish their own complaints machinery.   In most cases, the complainant sought satisfaction on the local or regional level, usually approaching the management committee if the matter concerned the detailed conduct of individual hospitals, or the regional board if broader issues were involved, such as admissions policy or over-all inadequacy in services.   The failure to adjust complaints on the lower levels would then necessitate action at the national level.   Many of the complaints reached Savile Row through members of Parliament.   Before taking action, the Ministry usually requested a report from the regional boards.[18]

In seeking a clear picture of the role of the Minister of Health, it should be kept in mind that the hospital service was the only public service financed almost entirely by Exchequer funds and managed by a government department in partnership with voluntary bodies.   Working out an effective relationship and a proper division of powers between the Ministry and these subordinate agencies could not be achieved at once.   There were certain functions which quite obviously only the Ministry could exercise, such as the formulation of basic policy, the co-ordination of all branches of the hospital service, the over-all allocation of funds, the planning of major capital developments, the establishment of the salary and wage structure, and the nationwide supervision of the service.   Since the Minister was held responsible to Parliament for the maintenance of an efficient hospital system, he had to proceed gingerly in determining precisely what part the regional boards and management committees should play.[19]

That the Ministry at first followed a somewhat contradictory course was not due entirely to errors in planning; the ambiguity in the law and the financial crisis that arose during the early years of the Service were also causes. Section 12 of the National Health Service Act provided that the hospital boards should administer their functions on behalf of the Minister and the management committees should do so on behalf of the boards. This principle of responsibility through a chain of command was in some measure contradicted by Section 13, which gave these subordinate bodies an independent legal status, with rights and liabilities "in all respects as if the Board or Committee were acting as a principal." The latter section thus provided for a decentralized hospital service, and the former seemed to endorse centralization.

When the law was in the formative stage, there were those who wanted to confer upon the regional boards only a planning and advisory function, but the government decided to yield to them in addition the power of supervision and administration. Once the hospital service began to function, however, the central organization tended more and more to bypass the regional boards by sending guidance memoranda directly to the management committees. The effect was greater centralization and a weakening of the supervisory and administrative authority of the regional boards. This trend was augmented during the budgetary crisis of 1949-50, when the Ministry of Health removed the power of virement from the regional boards and deprived them also of their control over the size of the staffs employed by the management committees. These steps were taken in the name of the most urgent economy, but they seriously impaired the prestige of the regional boards. To recoup the loss, some of them were guilty of interfering with activities that distinctly belonged to the management committees.

The Select Committee on Estimates was responsible for a reversal of this trend by its insistence that the regional boards either be reduced to advisory and planning agencies or be given greater administrative authority. The Ministry chose the latter course by restoring to the boards the right of virement and control over staff size. By 1952-53, the Ministry of Health had come to accept in practice as well as in theory the advisability of decentralization in hospital administration.[20]

Where the line should be drawn between central administration and decentralized voluntary control was not easy to decide in a system in which public responsibility was so great. The Minister of Health in 1956 explained to the House of Commons that anything "which can reasonably be decided and done at the level of the individual hospital should be done there, and, in the same way, anything which can reasonably be decided and done at the . . . hospital management level should be done there; and the regional board, and in his turn the Minister, should reserve to themselves only those functions which are inescapably theirs. . . ."[21]

In the practical application of this policy, the Ministry continued to move slowly—much too slowly for the Select Committee on Estimates, which in 1957 urged the abandonment of the controls that the Ministry and regional boards exercised over hospital non-medical staffs. After being importuned about the matter for two years, the Ministry in 1959 finally yielded and went even further by enlarging the delegated powers of the hospital authorities, particularly in the grading of their clerical and administrative staff. But in doing so, the Ministry took steps to keep in touch with man-power needs through the use of small teams of staff inspectors that would visit individual hospitals.[22] The elimination of Ministry controls over hospital staffs removed an important source of irritation, since management committees had always found it troublesome to obtain Ministry permission whenever they contemplated enlarging their staffs.

Relations between the regional boards and the Ministry seemed to be comparatively smooth. But in spite of periodic conferences and consultations between regional and Ministry officials, the feeling seemed to persist that the liaison between these two administrative levels could be strengthened.[23]

During the first decade of the hospital service, there were fourteen hospital regions; in 1959, the number of these administrative areas was increased to fifteen. In districting, the government gave some attention to geographical factors, but its primary consideration was the inclusion of at least one university with a medical school and a teaching hospital in each district. The existence of ten such universities in the provinces determined the number of provincial regions. London had an abundance of medical schools and teaching hospitals and was therefore sliced into four regions, each embracing a large area in the adjoining counties. Regional boundaries cut across local government areas, but within each region were many local authorities and Executive Councils. The size of the regions varied greatly, ranging from 4.5 million people and 65,000 hospital beds to 1.5 million people and only 14,000 beds. The largest region, which had more than 250 hospitals (South-West Metropolitan), and another region with almost 200 hospitals (Newcastle) each found it convenient to set up an area committee, with delegated authority, to assist in administration. All other boards were able to handle their duties by themselves.

The Welsh Regional Hospital Board, it should be noted, occupied a status somewhat different from that of the others, which were directly responsible to the Ministry of Health. In deference to Welsh sectionalism, the Welsh Board of Health, as it was called, was allowed to have jurisdiction over all health phases, including the general practitioner and local health authority as well as the hospital and specialist services. The work done by the Welsh Board of Health, however, was mostly routine, but even so the regional hospital board was subordinate to it. Welsh hospital accounts had the distinction of appearing separately in the budgetary statements presented to Parliament.

Only three other regions had fewer hospital beds than Wales, which was in area one of the largest regions. There was a difference of opinion whether some of the regions were too big for the efficient performance of their duties, but the consensus seemed to be that this was not so. The evidence which came before the Guillebaud Committee showed the larger regions to be as successful as the smaller ones in discharging their administrative functions.[24]

The regional boards varied in size from 20 to 30 persons. Members were appointed by the Minister not as representatives of any organization or group but as individuals, and they came from all walks of life, with business and the professions usually supplying the majority of the members. Doctors could not constitute more than one-fourth of the total membership. This ruling, when first imposed in 1957, invited a sharp protest from the British Medical Association, which endeavored unsuccessfully to raise the ceiling to one-third. There was also dissatisfaction over the fact that very few and sometimes no general medical practitioners served on the boards. When pressed about the matter, the Minister recognized that a general practitioner and a Medical Officer of Health should be included among the medical members, who, he felt, should nevertheless consist principally of doctors from the consultant staffs of the hospitals.[25] But the medical profession was not alone in having misgivings over its share of the membership on these voluntary agencies. In 1957, the Trade Union Congress expressed concern that trade unionists comprised only 7 per cent of the hospital boards and management committees.[26]

The regional boards usually met once a month, but committee meetings and other assignments made heavy demands upon the time of the members. Eight to ten hours per week were normally required of those who gave full service to the board, with most of the meetings occurring in the daytime. The chairman often contributed as many as three days per week. It would seem that only persons retired, self-employed, or financially independent, or persons whose work could be arranged to suit their entire convenience, could contribute such liberal service. An analysis of membership in 1951 revealed that about 60 per cent were less than sixty years of age, which indicates that a good majority were in the most productive period of their lives.[27] Dual membership was quite common. In 1956, for instance, 62 per cent of regional board members also served on hospital management committees and one-fifth of the chairmen of these subordinate bodies belonged to the regional boards.

The amount of work varied, depending upon the size of the region, the committee arrangements, and the general character of the board. There was no fixed pattern, each board working out its own procedures. A wide difference in the use of committees, for instance, prevailed between the Sheffield Board, with over 200 hospitals, and the East Anglia Board, with one-half as many. The Sheffield Regional Board was very elaborately organized, there being in 1956 seven standing committees, six standing subcommittees, many advisory committees, and about two dozen committees of consultants. The East Anglia Board, on the other hand, was virtually without a committee structure. The planning committee was defunct, while the finance committee maintained only a shadowy existence. All normal fiscal matters and most all other business were handled by the whole board.[28]

As a voluntary body, the regional board could not handle the routine administrative work. This was left to a permanent staff, usually organized in four divisions—secretarial, medical, treasury, and architectural and engineering. Most important among the officers were the regional secretary and the senior administrative medical officer. The latter, as his title implied, had jurisdiction over medical matters, and the regional secretary was largely the business manager, being responsible for supplies, capital works, and such other matters as did not come within the special province of experts. In a sense, his office was the clearing house for administrative work, especially that of a non-medical character. Unfortunately, it was not clearly understood which of the two officials was the senior executive officer, and a spirit of rivalry sometimes developed between the regional board secretary and the senior administrative medical officer, neither as a rule being willing to recognize the other as the ultimate authority.

Among other important officials were the treasurer, engineer, architect, and regional psychiatrist. While some boards had their own legal advisers, others availed themselves of the services of outside solicitors. Much of the architectural work likewise was farmed out. Including those employed in the X-ray and blood transfusion services, the staff at the headquarters of the regional boards totaled about 4,000 persons.

The law prescribed briefly the basic functions of the hospital boards, but regulations greatly amplified the list. In general, the primary purpose of the regional boards was to organize and administer the hospital and specialist services, excluding, of course, the teaching hospitals. More specifically, these boards, within their respective areas, planned capital works, allocated maintenance funds, approved estimates of expenditure, and determined for what purpose hospital buildings should be used. They appointed the chairmen and members of the hospital management committees, as well as all consultants and other members of the senior medical and dental staffs. Any increase, however, in the number of specialists required the prior approval of the Ministry of Health. The blood transfusion and mass radiography services were the responsibility of the boards. Many boards maintained specialist departments in the fields of nursing, psychiatry, engineering, architecture, and law, and they were therefore in a position to furnish a rather broad advisory service to hospital officials.

In addition to their role of current supervision, these boards were expected to plan for the future. The degree of planning varied, though much of it was short term. Few boards deemed it practicable to work out master plans involving detailed, long-range blueprints. The lack of sufficient data caused the majority of boards to keep such planning on a less precise but more flexible basis. Many, however, had fairly clear ideas of what their aims were.[29]

The day-to-day operation of the hospitals was the responsibility of the management committees. Their job was to maintain the equipment and premises, to purchase supplies, and to appoint all of the hospital personnel except members of the senior medical and dental staff. The management committees were also expected to maintain liaison with other health authorities and to deal with the public. The overriding purpose of these committees was to see that the patients received adequate care and treatment.

The number of management committees, originally 388, stood at 382 in 1961. In organizing the hospitals, the regional boards followed a flexible course, being influenced to a considerable degree by geography and local traditions and history. Without much concern for size, the boards grouped the hospitals either on a functional or area basis. In grouping hospitals in the latter way, the theory was to integrate all hospitals within a certain area so as to establish a more or less self-sufficient unit with a complete range of clinical facilities. Hospitals, however, which specialized exclusively in mental illness, infectious diseases, or orthopedics and tuberculosis were usually given a separate status. In some cities, for instance, all children's hospitals were brought together under one committee, but more often, as in the case of large mental hospitals, each specialty hospital was left as an independent institution with its own management committee.

The two methods of grouping hospitals fostered a great variation in the number of hospitals assigned to individual management committees. One-fifth of them controlled only one hospital each, usually mental, while, at the other extreme, a few committees had jurisdiction over as many as twenty hospitals each. In terms of hospital beds, the contrast was even more striking, ranging from fewer than 250 beds for some committees to over 2,500 for others. Where the number of beds was small, a highly specialized hospital was usually involved, and where the number was quite large, a mental or mental deficiency hospital was usually the institution administered. From region to region the number of management committees varied sharply. In the mid-1950's, for instance, one hospital region, the largest, had 53 management committee groups, while another, the smallest, had only one-fourth as many.[30]

In integrating the hospitals, the regional boards had to deal with facilities that were inadequate and unevenly distributed. The less fortunate areas were marked for special assistance, and they were among the first to feel the effects of the improvement. The disparity in facilities was a factor of some importance in the grouping of hospitals. It was recognized that between the hospital groups there should be no rigid barriers, and whenever it became necessary on medical grounds, patients were exchanged between groups and even regions. This was particularly true where there was a deficiency of certain medical specialties and where it was practicable to reduce waiting lists by patient exchange.

The hospital management committees were intended to represent the community served. In selecting members, the regional boards endeavored to maintain a balance between the various economic and social elements. A number of local organizations were consulted (this was a statutory requirement), but the names suggested by them were not always accepted.[31] While doctors in the hospitals were eligible to serve on the management committees or regional boards, all other staff officers were barred from such membership. In the interest of better liaison, it was deemed advisable to have in the management committees representation from the Executive Councils, the local health authorities, and the regional hospital boards.

The hospital management committees averaged between 15 and 20 members. The membership, as revealed in a 1951 analysis, was somewhat similar in composition to that of the regional boards, except for a smaller professional representation and a larger representation of housewives. Almost a fourth of the management committee members were women, as compared with only 15 per cent for the regional boards. Another difference was the somewhat younger age group which characterized these committees, only one-third of the members being in the sixty-and-older age brackets.[32]

Since membership on the management committees, as on the hospital boards and Executive Councils, involved considerable work and no remuneration, there was apprehension expressed from time to time about the problem of getting qualified people to serve. The Council of the British Medical Association was of the opinion that many members of the management committees were selected solely as representatives of various sections of the community, rather than as individuals qualified for the complex job of hospital administration. The Select Committee on Estimates in 1957 was confronted by conflicting testimony on the availability of suitable people,[33] but the study sponsored by The National Council of Social Services and King Edward's Hospital Fund for London and the reports made by the Guillebaud Committee and the Acton Society Trust[34] did not disclose any serious difficulties in finding competent people to serve on the hospital management committees. In certain areas, some difficulty was experienced in getting enough professional people and businessmen to serve, but there apparently was no lack of public-spirited persons willing to accept membership.

Relations between the management committees and hospital boards were for the most part good. The years brought about adjustments and better co-operation. The chief problem centered about the administrative controls, which, as applied, ran counter to the desire for autonomy at the management level. As agents of the Ministry, the boards had little choice in carrying out the stringent financial policies prescribed by the government. But in allocating maintenance funds, the boards perhaps could have pursued a more flexible policy and one better calculated to inspire confidence among management committees. Much of the resentment, however, was at root due to the paucity of funds—a matter which was almost entirely beyond the control of the hospital boards or even the Ministry of Health.

As the financial picture improved during the latter part of the

1950's, a somewhat easier fiscal policy seemed to characterize hospital administration. Although the right of virement was not and apparently could not be granted to management committees, some of the regional boards adopted a freer policy in permitting their management committees to shift funds from one division to another, providing that more than the total amount allocated was not spent. The so-called inherited pattern of budgetary planning, under which the first year of spending by a management committee became the basis for subsequent annual grants, did little to reward or encourage frugality and careful fiscal planning. This policy tended with time to become less rigid; and with the increased emphasis placed upon costing returns, the Ministry and boards were in a position to pursue a more realistic budgetary policy.

The question of man-power allocation and staff appointments more than anything else dramatized the issue of autonomy. The need to accept budgetary limits on spending seemed logical enough, but not the establishment of controls that denied to management committees the right to add the most menial workers to the payroll without permission from the regional board or the right, so far as remuneration was concerned, to promote any of the clerical staff. These restrictions, as already noted, were largely wiped out in 1959, and with them a major grievance. But other aspects of staffing remained troublesome. To many observers, for example, it seemed apparent that the management committees needed guidance in selecting their senior administrative officers. The Select Committee on Estimates in 1957 recommended that the regional boards always be invited to send representatives to the meetings of the management committees when group finance officers and secretaries were being appointed.[35] The mandatory character of this proposal was unacceptable to the management committees, which seemed afraid that it might constitute a threat to their prerogatives in making staff appointments. The need for advice and assistance in filling such key posts was nevertheless recognized by these committees, some of whom did invite board members to sit in at meetings involving such appointments.[36]

In the exercise of their controls, some hospital boards apparently permitted so few administrative duties to be performed by the management committees that these agencies felt their duties to be little more than custodial. Where the management committees were granted considerable scope in carrying out their administrative duties—and this was done in many cases—the relations between boards and committees were much friendlier.[37] The interlocking memberships between boards and committees and the conferences between their chairmen and the staff officers did much to foster understanding. In surveying this phase of the hospital service, the Guillebaud Committee declared that "we have been impressed by the improvement over the years in the relations between the Hospital Management Committees, the Regional Boards and the Ministry. . . . We have the feeling that all the levels of management now have a much deeper knowledge of each other's problems than they had perhaps four or five years ago, and they are learning to live together with due regard for each other's rights and responsibilities."[38]

The principal lay administrative officers who carried out the work of the hospital management committee were the group secretary, finance officer, and supplies officer. Assisted by deputies and a clerical staff, these officials were largely responsible for the operation of all the hospitals within the committee's jurisdiction. Among the smaller units, however, it was not uncommon for two or all three posts to be combined in one person, and in some cases one finance officer was shared by two or more groups of hospitals. But a substantial majority of the committees not administering mental hospitals appointed individual secretaries and finance officers. Of these, the group secretary was considered the chief administrative officer. He was broadly responsible for the co-ordination of the various departments and the over-all supervision of the daily functioning of the hospital service. He was expected to see that the policy of the governing body was carried out and to keep a watchful eye on the adequacy of the hospital personnel. He was often the secretary of the hospital which served as group headquarters, in addition to being secretary for the entire group of hospitals.

Unfortunately, the group secretary was burdened with so much committee and clerical work that he seldom had sufficient time for the immediate personal investigation and supervision that is essential to an administrative job. Moreover, his dealings with other group officers were not always direct enough to be conducive of the most effective co-operation. His relationship, for instance, with the finance officer was not clearly defined. Since the group secretary as a rule was not versed in financial matters and since the management committee and the regional treasurer required a direct report from the finance officer, that official sometimes had difficulty in viewing himself as subordinate to the group secretary. While co-operation between the two officers was ideal in some cases, generally speaking it was perfunctory.[39]

Neither the finance office nor the supplies office existed as such prior to the inception of the Health Service. The financial work, at least in the voluntary hospitals, was rarely performed by accountants, but instead by bookkeepers. The purchase of supplies was not concentrated in one office, but was done on a departmental basis without much regard to system. In integrating the hospitals on a group and regional basis, there were thus no well-established precedents about administrative responsibility in these fields, with the result that duties, relationships, and techniques had to be worked out by trial and error.

Successful hospital administration seemed to depend upon a proper delimitation of responsibilities and the acceptance of whatever adjustments were required—two conditions not easily arrived at by those whose administrative training and experience were obtained during the era of voluntary and local authority hospitals. The failure of such key administrators as the group secretary and the finance officer to become part of a smoothly working team was in the final analysis a personnel problem, which could be corrected through the establishment of a sound career service that would attract administrators with the proper training and the highest qualifications.

Prior to 1948, medical influence in hospital management was dominant, particularly in the municipal hospitals where a medical superintendent was in full charge. Under the National Health Service, that office was largely abandoned, except in tuberculosis, mental, and infectious diseases hospitals. Only a minority of the general hospitals continued to have medical superintendents, who no longer had authority over non-medical matters. It seemed obvious that the hospital service had become so complex that only specially trained administrators should be placed in general control. Finance, laundry, maintenance of buildings, catering and food supplies, clerical services, the supervision of non-medical personnel—all these elements of modern hospital management could be handled better by a qualified layman than by a consultant whose life's work had prepared him for clinical duties.[40] This was recognized by the medical profession, although the fear that lay administration would threaten clinical freedom caused many doctors to favor the medical superintendent system. The Council of the British Medical Association supported, as the best solution to the problem, a tripartite scheme such as the one advocated by the Bradbeer Committee.[41]

Under that arrangement, the lay authorities, while technically supreme, controlled only business matters, leaving to medical and nursing staffs absolute control over their own areas of activity. The tripartite scheme obtained the approval of the Ministry, which recognized that certain matters had to be left completely to the medical staffs, such as co-ordination of medical auxiliaries, management of outpatient clinics, supervision of medical supplies and equipment, notification of infectious diseases, and control over medical records, waiting lists, admissions, and discharges. Under the tripartite plan, a medical committee in each hospital administered such matters through its chairman. Each consultant, of course, retained full charge of the beds placed at his disposal and complete freedom in dealing with his inpatients and outpatients.

A strong medical committee was the best guarantee that the tripartite system would work satisfactorily.[42] Only where the committee was weak did the British Medical Association favor the appointment of a medical superintendent.[43] Where such weakness existed, the Bradbeer and Guillebaud Committees urged the selection of a clinical medical administrator by the hospital management committee and the representatives of the medical staff, acting jointly.[44]

The success of the tripartite scheme depended also upon the good will and the friendly relations between the professional and lay staffs. The system seemed to work quite well, and was viewed by many as a big improvement over the old authoritarianism of the medical superintendent system, which both the doctors and the lay administrators found unsatisfactory. Only in the mental and mental deficiency institutions was the necessity of medical superintendents recognized by most people. The character of these hospitals, it was felt, required the concentration of a high degree of authority in the hands of a psychiatrist of consultant status.[45]

The tripartite system was applied only to individual hospitals and not to administration at group level, where lay officials were in complete control. The choice, however, of whether their chief administrative officer should be medical or lay was left to the regional boards, which decided almost without exception in favor of lay control for all but the mental and special hospital groups. This decision met with some opposition in medical circles, but elsewhere was widely approved. The absence of a medical officer at group level did not have any serious effects, since the medical advisory committee representing the medical staffs of the various hospitals could exert considerable influence over the management committee as well as the group secretary.[46]

As for the third group in the tripartite arrangement, the nursing staff, it seemed to have lost influence under the Health Service. In the voluntary hospitals even more than in the municipal ones, the matron, as head of the nursing service, had enjoyed great professional prestige. Her supervisory control over certain non-nursing departments had virtually made her mistress of the hospital household. She had direct access to the governing body, being consulted on all matters within the broad area of her responsibility. The growing complexity of hospital administration, however, had encouraged the use of lay specialists in the management of catering, the laundry service, and the domestic staff. Even before 1948, it had become the policy of some hospitals to deprive the matron of jurisdiction over these departments; but the National Health Service, by accentuating the trend, seemed to attract to itself most of the resentment felt by those who had suffered a reduction in their prerogatives. In some cases, the matrons were even relieved of control over the nurses' homes on the theory that lay supervision was preferable to the old type of nursing discipline. This reduction in authority, combined with the fact that the matron's advice was not always sought by the governing body, tended to foster in her a strong sense of frustration.

Although nursing committees did exist and matrons were more or less responsible to the management committees, there was need to place the advisory and administrative role of the nursing staff on a uniformly stable basis. The Bradbeer Report accordingly urged the nurses to organize regular committees on the hospital and group level. Either the chairman of the group committee or a matron chosen for the purpose should advise the management committee on all policy affecting the nursing service of the area. In each hospital, the matron would function as nursing administrator, and in matters pertaining to nursing administration she would also be directly responsible to the governing body.[47]

The hospital group was officially viewed as a unit, with each individual hospital constituting a sub-unit or a part of the whole. The Ministry of Health did what it could to reinforce this idea, to the end that each hospital would function as an integral segment of a unified organism. Every hospital, however, had its traditions and local ties that could not easily be replaced by stronger loyalties to a managing body created by statute and usually located elsewhere. In practice, the individual hospital remained a "corporate body with a morale of its own" and sought to preserve its own individuality.

The management committee obviously could not effectively coordinate and supervise from day to day the detailed functions of each of the several hospitals that might be a part of the group. While the law made no provision for them, the necessity for a secretary and a lay committee in most hospitals was generally recognized. There was, of course, no need for such a secretary in the hospital in which the group secretary functioned in that capacity, and there was no need for a house committee when the governing body had responsibility over only one hospital. Whether house committees should be used at all was discretionary with the management committee, which in most cases chose to have them. Appointed by the management committee, the house committee more or less functioned as one of its subcommittees. The house committee usually included one or more members of the management committee, but otherwise was representative of the local community.

The Minister of Health made it clear that, in order to avoid fragmentation, house committees should not be delegated executive functions. They could not, for example, be permitted to appoint any part of the hospital staff or incur expenditures involving Exchequer funds. They might spend money from the endowment fund, but could not hold in their name any legacy or gift. Only the management committee had this right. The primary function of the house committee was to oversee the daily performance of the hospital, with special regard to the welfare of the patients and members of the staff. In some cases, the house committee was given considerable advisory control over expenditures and other executive matters, but in most cases it had little real power.[48]

The King Edward's Hospital Fund for London and the Acton Society Trust concluded that house committees had too little autonomy,[49] but the Bradbeer and Guillebaud reports took a cautious view toward the granting of any executive authority to these bodies, lest such a policy might contribute to the weakening of group unity.[50] All of these reports, however, agreed that house committees did excellent work, especially in promoting patient welfare and better public relations. Since the committees were close to the people, they stimulated a lively local interest in the hospital and strengthened the voluntary spirit which was the very basis of hospital administration. The interlocking membership with the management committee and the attendance of the group secretary and other officials at house committee meetings forged closer ties between the individual hospitals and the group administration. The house committees also served as the recruiting grounds for membership in the higher governing bodies.

The chief lay administrator of the individual hospital was the secretary. As a subordinate of the group secretary, he relayed orders and otherwise implemented policy. He was responsible for the supervision of the non-medical aspects of the hospital, and to him all departmental officers were responsible in general administrative matters. His knowledge of the inner workings of the institution gave him a key position as an advisor to the group secretary. His importance, however, depended upon the size of the hospital, the freedom of action permitted to him, and his relationship to group administration. The salary and responsibilities of the secretary's office did not always attract persons of the highest qualifications. If the secretary's status was that of a junior administrator who performed routine clerical work, there was a tendency for departmental heads to bypass him and go directly to the group secretary or one of the other group officials. Since his office was the potential recruiting ground for group secretaries and other higher hospital executives, many felt that it should be given more authority and made more attractive. The Noel Hall Report even recommended that the secretary should have a voice in the selection of his senior subordinates and entire responsibility for choosing the remainder of the subordinate staff.[51]

Hospital administration under the Health Service involved a revolutionary departure from the past. In most cases the same officials, though with new titles, with different responsibilities, and often with reduced authority, remained at the helm. Having served for long years under the old regime, these individuals did not find acceptance of the new order easy. The remarkable thing was that the change occurred with so little outward manifestation of disturbance. That there were inner conflicts and deep frustrations, however, was disclosed in a very revealing study made by the Acton Society Trust in the early 1950's. Three institutions were involved—a mental, a former local authority, and a former voluntary hospital. The last two, with four other hospitals, were under the same management committee, but the mental institution had its own governing body. All of the hospitals had greatly benefited from an improvement in facilities and medical staff.

The voluntary hospital had the most difficult adjustment of all to make, since the self-contained and democratic pattern of existence which had characterized it in the past was quite different from the administrative hierarchy of the new hospital service, with its triple tier of controls. Prior to 1948, this hospital was operated by a board of governors (several hundred subscribers to the hospital) and an elected board of management, assisted by several committees. The house governor and the matron were very influential with the governing body. Business was usually expedited quickly. Faced by a recurring financial problem, the hospital was relieved on this score by the new service, but the old way of life was swept away. All authority passed to a new governing body—the management committee—that was no longer accessible to the house governor, who, as the hospital secretary, was left little freedom of action. Although the house committee included several members of the old board of management, its role was mostly advisory, with no legal capacity to reach vital decisions. The power of the matron was curtailed. The loss of the endowment fund, the introduction of a new and more complicated staff records system, the greater rigidity of finances, and the making of policy by authorities removed from the scene of action, proved galling to those who had a loyal attachment to the hospital they had supported and directed for so many years.[52]

Already tax-supported and controlled by a government agency, the municipal hospital was in a better position to bridge the gap than the voluntary institution. But problems arose that could not easily be resolved. During the years that the county-borough council had jurisdiction, the hospital officials grew accustomed to having the seat of authority located elsewhere, and when the new group headquarters was established at this hospital, the old staff members viewed the arrangement suspiciously, fearing unwarranted interference by the group administrators. Contrary to the usual practice, the group secretary did not assume the secretarial post of the hospital, which was awarded to the former steward. The medical superintendent retained his title, but was required to surrender all control over lay administration to a man who had been his subordinate. The division of authority between the two was not clearly defined. Although responsible to the group secretary, the matron and the secretary continued to show deference to the judgment of the medical superintendent even on administrative matters.

The house committee, which included three members from the management committee, held monthly meetings, which were attended by the group secretary and the senior officers of the hospital. Periodic tours of the institution by the members of the house committee promoted a better climate of understanding, but the lack of authority for executive action caused some to view the committee meetings as a waste of time.

In this former municipal hospital, as elsewhere, there was a Joint Consultative Committee—an element of the Whitley Council machinery. By choice, the doctors were excluded. The representatives of all other trades and professions in the hospital met their management opposites for the settlement of grievances and to discuss matters of common interest. Questions of general interest or disputes that otherwise could not be settled were submitted to the Joint Consultative Committee, which brought the management and staff sides together in a hospital-wide conference. Only a minority of the hospital personnel, however, either voted in the elections or seemed to have much interest in the Whitley proceedings.

At the mental hospital, conditions were very much as before, except for an improved service and, in the opinion of some, a larger measure of autonomy. The transfer of this institution from local government control to the jurisdiction of the Ministry of Health did not seem to result in any objectionable bureaucratic interference. The policy of decentralized management left this hospital with its own group administration. The medical superintendent retained most of his authority while becoming less authoritarian. Between the office of the group secretary, who also became secretary of the hospital, and that of the medical superintendent there was some overlapping of functions, but the relationship between these two officials was harmonious. The medical staff, which functioned democratically, dealt largely with staff problems, while the medical superintendent handled matters of a more general nature. There was no apparent tension among the hospital personnel. Reactions to the Service were mostly favorable, the only apparent difficulty being some confusion as to the proper division of the duties between the administrator and clinician.[53]

In evaluating these three case studies, the Acton Society Trust recognized that they were not necessarily typical, although a wide range of evidence supported many of the findings of the studies. The picture painted was of the earlier period of the change, and the reactions and attitudes very likely were subsequently modified by the continuing process of change. As the older staff members were replaced by younger ones, as the hospitals became better oriented to to the new system, and as refinements were made in the administrative techniques, it was inevitable that a different spirit would permeate hospital thought.

The revolution in administration, which drastically altered the basic pattern of so many hospitals, was milder in its effects upon the teaching hospitals. Having occupied a somewhat privileged position before the establishment of the Health Service, they were permitted to continue as the aristocrats of the hospital world. They were given their own boards of governors, who were appointed by the Minister of Health. The purpose of these hospitals was to supply the universities with such facilities as were required for clinical research and teaching. Thirty-six boards of governors administered the teaching hospitals. Ten of the boards and roughly one-half of the beds were in the provinces.[54]

In size and composition, the boards of governors of the teaching hospitals were similar to the regional boards, except that the boards of governors had a larger proportion of doctors and a smaller percentage of members in the sixty-and-over age group, as revealed in one of the early studies.[55] The 25 per cent limit on the number of doctors serving as members of each regional board was not applied to the boards of governors, because of the nominations, mostly medical, which the university and the hospital medical staffs had the statutory right to make. There was also some difference in the type of work done. The boards of governors, having no management committees, performed all phases of supervision themselves, including the appointment of all staff members.

The great majority of teaching hospitals were former voluntary institutions. Some of them were very large, quite old, and internationally famous. The London Hospital, for instance, was founded in 1740. In spite of severe damages sustained in World War II, it could boast in the mid-1950's of over 1,000 beds, a medical staff of 250, and a nursing staff of more than 800.[56] Heavily supplied with doctors and nurses and always seeking to use the most modern equipment and the latest technique and to furnish the best in amenities, the teaching hospitals spent per bed what seemed to be a disproportionately large amount of money in comparison with the share allotted to the nonteaching institutions. The higher standards and greater costs created resentment and jealousy among the less fortunate hospitals, which demanded that the teaching hospitals be divested of their privileges. Voices were raised to insist that such hospitals be brought under the control of regional boards and that the funds be more fairly distributed among all hospitals.

To some extent there was a redistribution of available resources, the share allocated to teaching hospitals falling from 14.5 per cent of total hospital expenditures in the first full year of the service to 13.4 per cent in 1958. During the first four years, the cost of teaching hospitals increased only 4 per cent, as compared with 20 per cent for the general hospitals. But these percentages did not include the cost of consultants and merit awards. If these additional expenses were taken into consideration, the trend appeared somewhat less favorable for the nonteaching hospitals.[57]

On the subject of whether the teaching hospitals should be placed under the administrative control of the regional boards, opinion differed. Although the Labor Party in its statement of policy in 1959 supported the idea, the lay and medical consensus opposed it. In view of the special role performed by teaching hospitals, it seemed to many that independent administration was vital, just as it was necessary that medical schools, to preserve their academic standards, should be free of external controls. The selection of patients that was necessary for teaching hospitals might be curtailed if the separate status of these institutions were terminated. It seemed very doubtful to the Guillebaud Committee that costs could be reduced and a better distribution of nursing and medical man power achieved through a union of the two hospital systems. The integration of these hospitals, it was averred, would involve the threat of "over-standardization and uniformity"—"one of the dangers of a national hospital system."[58]

The Acton Society Trust was also unwilling to support a merger, but it drew a distinction between the London and the provincial teaching hospitals. The fact that postgraduate hospitals in that city served the entire nation, it was argued, precluded their subordination to regional boards. As for the undergraduate teaching hospitals, their beds were not required by the London regional boards, which already had enough for their own needs. Toward the London teaching hospitals, the staffs and graduates responded with the strongest sentiments of loyalty, and any attempt to submerge the identity of these institutions would have been strongly resisted.

The provincial teaching hospitals, it was explained, were different, in that they did not command such strong emotional attachment as the more famous ones in London. Moreover, in such places as Oxford, Bristol, and Cambridge, the teaching hospitals offered about the only general hospital services in those cities. Furthermore, and this was to some degree true of London, the evidence did not conclusively show that the teaching hospitals, as claimed, always functioned as centers from which medical knowledge and clinical progress were diffused throughout the entire area. The Acton Society was nevertheless convinced that the retention of the boards of governors in London was absolutely necessary, but it did not feel that the need for such a policy in the provinces had been so clearly demonstrated.[59]

Most authorities were in agreement that the solution lay not in the direction of merger but rather of closer collaboration between the teaching and non-teaching hospitals. Such collaboration did exist to a varying degree in all regions, but the effectiveness of it depended upon the willingness of the hospital staffs to co-operate. The interlocking of the boards of governors and regional boards was rendered possible, if not assured, by the statutory provision that one-fifth of the nominees for the boards of governors could be made by the regional boards. There was ample evidence presented to the Committee on Estimates and the Guillebaud Committee of effective co-operation between hospital boards.[60] The Acton Society Trust was particularly impressed with the Liverpool region, where interlocking membership of the board of governors and regional board, and of their medical advisory committees, had done much to foster unity of action and where there existed a common consultant staffing between them. A remarkable degree of informal integration was even achieved among the regional board, the board of governors, and the local health authorities through joint advisory committees.[61]

From what has been said, it should be clear that hospital administration was sustained by two important groups—those who were paid for their work and those who were not. The quality of the hospital service was no better than those who administered it. If the hospital staff did not measure up to expectation, the blame might well be laid to the absence of an attractive career system, and corrective action could be taken. But if the thousands of Englishmen who were needed as board and committee members or who otherwise voluntarily served the hospital in ways to be discussed later failed to come forward, then the whole theory of decentralized, popular control would have to be replaced by a new approach. But there was no apparent danger that such a new approach would ever be needed.

On the tenth anniversary of the Health Service, the Minister of Health in his remarks to the House of Commons observed that "one of the things which has turned out better than some people expected . . . has been that the strength of the voluntary spirit in our Health Service and hospital work has continued unabated, and we still have a very sound basis of voluntary work, freely given and highly regarded."[62] In the House of Lords, at about the same time, an authority in the hospital field declared, "In a long experience, I can certainly say—and it is curious, but very satisfactory to be able to say it; I should scarcely have expected it would be so—that the number of volunteers giving voluntary service in the hospital with which I am most familiar is greater than at any previous time in the 250 years' history of the Westminster Hospital."[63] None recognized more clearly the importance of the voluntary service or appreciated more fully the vigor it had demonstrated through the years than the Guillebaud Committee. "It seems to us," the Committee reported, "that the continuance and further expansion of voluntary service is one of the surest ways of maintaining the essential humanity and vitality of the hospital service and preventing the development of that enemy of human welfare—institutionalism."[64]

The voluntary phase of hospital administration could not in the long run be successful if the staffing program were defective. In seeking qualified replacements for aging hospital administrators, the authorities were faced with the need for a more attractive career service. Putting the administrative and clerical employees, more than 30,000 of them, on the civil service rolls was not possible in view of the decentralized character of the hospital service. Instead of one centralized employing agency with full control over the appointment and qualifications of the hospital personnel, there were several hundred employing boards and committees. Standards varied between hospital areas, but more serious was the lack of flexibility that seemed to characterize the training of junior administrators. Officers tended to become frozen in their jobs with little hope of promotion or recognition for meritorious service. Within departments and among hospitals, and between groups and regions, there was insufficient movement and at first virtually no systematic exchange of hospital staff. The need for a substantial improvement in career prospects was reflected in a decline in morale among some of the administrators.

Staffing controls, as noted elsewhere, only aggravated the problem. The reduction in the administrative personnel during the early 1950's and the prior approval necessary for any subsequent increase in the staff had proved frustrating to the hospital authorities. Such restrictions were finally lifted, and the management committees and boards were even granted considerable freedom to grade their administrative and clerical staffs. This more enlightened policy revealed a growing awareness on the part of the Ministry that a less rigid approach was needed to improve the staffing arrangement. In 1956, the Guillebaud Committee urged that a "proper career structure is a matter of the utmost importance."[65]

Even before the Guillebaud Report was published, the Ministry had advised the hospital boards and management committees to establish and expand programs designed to train selected staff members for senior posts. By being permitted to work in various departments and hospitals, junior administrators could get the broad perspective required for the more important appointments. Several of these regional schemes were established. Special training courses were instituted, and funds were provided to cover expenses incurred by administrators in taking them.[66] A significant contribution in this field was made by the King Edward's Hospital Fund. Beginning in 1951, this association set up a Hospital Administrative Staff College which offered a training program for senior administrative officials. A two-year training curriculum and many courses of three months and shorter duration, including refresher courses, were made available to group secretaries, hospital secretaries, finance officers, and others.[67]

Following the publication of the Guillebaud Report, the Ministry of Health inaugurated a three-year training scheme for hospital administrators, limited to sixteen carefully selected persons per year. That number represented about one-third of the annual loss of senior administrators. Adequate financial provision was made for the trainees, who were drawn from younger officers in the hospital service and from university graduates and other well-qualified applicants. Eight were to be trained by the Staff College of King Edward's Hospital Fund and the other half by Manchester University, each using a somewhat different approach. The training involved intensive courses in hospital management and related fields and broad practical experience in various phases of hospital work at different types of hospitals. In the third year, the trainee would be assigned to administrative posts, and upon the completion of the course he would be permitted to compete in the usual way for a suitable administrative appointment. From hundreds of qualified applicants, the selection committee chose its first batch of trainees, who began the course of study in fall, 1956. The only serious criticism of the program was the limited number of students involved, but it was experimental, and the Ministry had no desire to arouse among the older administrators the fear that their chance of promotion or their position itself was threatened by the program.[68]

All of these schemes were obviously limited in scope. A complete revision of the existing grading and salary structure was necessary. With this in mind, the Minister of Health in 1957 appointed Sir Noel Hall to investigate and suggest improvements in the administrative and clerical staffing program of the hospitals. The Report, published in the fall of that year, proposed a number of drastic changes. In place of the eight existing grades, he recommended five, two clerical and three administrative. The lowest or junior administrative grade was for training and probationary purposes—to qualify candidates for the basic grade from which appointments would be made to the higher grade in which the responsibilities were very weighty. To insure a fair and effective system of promotion and recruiting and to assist in the establishment of training schemes, Sir Noel proposed that a personnel advisory and information service be established, initially on the regional level, for all employing authorities of the Health Service.

The so-called "pointing" system that based the remuneration of an administrator upon the number of beds in his hospital was condemned. Should he decrease the total through efficient management and the careful application of medical science, the administrator would be rewarded by a reduction of salary. But the Noel Hall Report opposed any change in compensation that penalized meritorious achievement. The much-criticized pointing system should eventually be discarded, the Report recommended, but only after all hospitals had been carefully graded.

A sound staffing program required good career prospects, a careful selection of recruits, adequate post-entry training methods, and an effective system of promotion. The Report did not consider that the hospital service was in a critical position, since a sample of age distribution showed that the present concentration of hospital administrators was in the forty to fifty age group.[69]

Some of the proposals, such as the five grades, were readily adopted, but others required modification. The hospital management committees, for instance, objected to the recommendation that personnel records of all administrators be kept by an officer of the regional board, who, in an advisory capacity, would attend the meetings of these committees when they considered staff appointments. Less likely to offend the sensibilities of the management committees was the compromise scheme put forward by the Ministry. Under this plan, the staff register would be supervised by a committee representing the management committees, the regional board, and the board of governors. This committee would prepare a list of persons who could function as assessors, and from this panel one would be selected by the management committee to render assistance when administrative vacancies were being filled.[70]

In his investigation, Sir Noel Hall was confronted with an anachronistic grading structure that contained 130 different scales of pay for clerks and administrators. With the five new grades established, the next order of business was a revision in the pay schedules. The failure of the staff and management sides of the Whitley Council to reach an agreement on all phases caused the matter to be referred to the industrial court. The decision was rendered during the summer of 1958. All but the top administrators were affected by the new pay structure. Adjusted to the five clerical and administrative grades, the revised pay scales provided substantial increments. In seeking a fair basis for the remuneration of senior administrators, not included in this portion of the pay structure, the Whitley Council decided to set up a small fact-finding commission to determine the rates of pay for comparable work in other fields of activity. The Whitley Council would be guided by the commission's report in negotiating a salary schedule that would prove attractive in recruiting the ablest administrators.[71]

Owing to the rapidly changing pattern of medical science, no area of human activity would require more planning, more flexibility, or more inspired leadership than the hospital service. Whether the hospital system in its existing framework would continue to meet that challenge only the future could tell. But among the hospital authorities and the rank and file, the general opinion overwhelmingly rejected the idea of failure. This spirit was abundantly demonstrated to Sir Noel Hall in his probe of hospital staffing. He wrote that it was a "profoundly impressive experience to have seen at first hand the very great achievements in social engineering, the results of the co-operative efforts of thousands of men and women regardless of political views and, in many cases, of personal interests. I know of no case in the democratic world where a service which needs small-scale contacts with its public at all its points of action, and yet has to maintain a reasonable degree of uniformity throughout the nation, has been so successfully brought into being."[72]

There was little sentiment in favor of changing the basic features of the machinery that administered the hospital service. The whole idea of control being shared between the Ministry and the subordinate boards and committees was strongly endorsed by virtually every report that touched on the subject. There were occasional voices raised in favor of jurisdiction by a public corporation or by the local health authorities, but such proposals, because they were impracticable, found little acceptance in medical, hospital, or Parliamentary circles. Only an agency directly responsible to Parliament, such as the Ministry of Health, could be entrusted with sums of money as large as those expended by the hospitals—never a semi-independent corporation. The local authorities objected no less on these financial grounds, but additionally, the areas controlled by the county and county-borough councils were deemed much too small for effective hospital planning and administration.

The gloomy forecasts about inefficiency and waste that greeted the new hospital service proved ill founded. The various inquiries demonstrated that the people had got a good return on their investment in the hospitals. The Select Committee on Estimates, for example, observed that the costs per inpatient had risen little in real terms; and since the standard of service had improved, the Committee assumed that this increase "must have mainly been financed by economies resulting from increased efficiency, skill and individual effort."[73] The Acton Society Trust, the Guillebaud Committee, and Abel-Smith and Titmuss were similarly impressed with what had been achieved in the hospital service. Despite the limited funds available, much was accomplished in reconditioning old buildings, putting hospital beds to more effective use, reducing the waiting lists, making more adequate provision for the mentally ill and the aged sick, and improving everywhere the facilities and services of the medical and nursing staffs. These improvements will be discussed in detail in the next three chapters, but such gains should be noted here in order to keep in perspective the whole picture of hospital administration.

Whether the hospital resources could have been put to better advantage and whether greater efficiency might have been achieved were subjects fully explored by the Committee on Estimates. The feeling was that room for improvement existed and greater economy was possible. The Guillebaud Committee likewise recognized that certain innovations would lead to still better performance. The implementation of these Reports was proof that the Ministry was not the prisoner of the system within which it was operating. The Committee on Estimates within two years got action on most of its thirteen suggestions. Such recommendations of the Guillebaud Committee as an improved career service for hospital administrators, a new hospital cost accounting system, and a separate research and statistical department in the Ministry were eventually acted upon in a manner that must have gratified the authors of the Report.

The Acton Society Trust, in its survey of the hospital service, was of the opinion that the resources at the disposal of the hospital authorities had been wisely deployed and that the administrative tasks had been competently performed. But there were shortcomings that would have to be remedied if the service were to attain maximum efficiency. The inadequacy of money for hospital buildings was deplored. The slow response to some suggested reforms was noted. Hospital service leadership was not sufficiently dynamic, and there were too few top-flight administrators with the proper sort of background for their work. The Central Health Services Council was too large and met too infrequently to furnish the sort of guidance needed by the Ministry of Health in formulating policy.

Although the Ministry had established a statistical department, it was considered to be too small and not precisely what was required for the adequate evaluation and utilization of the vast flood of factual material that poured into headquarters. It was suggested that a Central Intelligence and Statistical Organization should be established which could keep under review all phases of the Health Service, as well as supervising research and interpreting statistical data. As an integral part of the Ministry, this agency could render notable service in planning for the future. It was in the area of long-term planning that the Ministry of Health seemed weakest. The Ministry was further handicapped by the junior rank which it held in the government and the lack of sufficiently trained liaison officers.[74]

Such were the friendly but critical observations of the Acton Society in its sixth and final publication on the hospital service. The Society had much to say in commendation of what had been accomplished—and in striking a balance it was of the opinion that what had been done was good, but the complexities of hospital administration required sharper tools, better trained administrative staffs, a new dynamism, and more streamlined techniques, all of which could be had without changing the basic framework of the administrative structure.

Sir George Schuster, chairman of the Trustees of the Acton Society Trust, experienced no trouble in outlining what might be done to give the hospital service "creative leadership." Among his suggestions were an intensive study by experts of the hospital cost structure, the use of various efficiency techniques, and the application of scientific principles to the practical problems of the hospital service.

He was very much impressed with the quantity and quality of work accomplished during the first decade. He seemed confident that the hospital service had the capacity to solve its problems and cope with all exigencies. As chairman of the Oxford Regional Board, he had found hospital work "as interesting and rewarding as is possible in any walk of life." Looking into the future he believed that there were ways that a "state directed service [could] be an instrument of dynamic progress and provide scope for individual enterprise and initiative." It was important, he emphasized, that these ways be found, and then "it will be possible to make our British national hospital service truly the finest in the world."[75]

CHAPTER XI

The Hospital Service in Operation

THERE APPARENTLY were no wholly reliable measures of the efficiency of a hospital. Such factors as the age, character, location, and condition of an institution had much to do in determining performance and operating costs. A new building had a lower maintenance cost than an old one, and a London hospital had a higher overhead than a provincial one. The cost of a bed per week for a chronic or mentally ill patient was considerably less than for a maternity patient or one suffering from an acute illness. Between hospitals of the same type, however, there were criteria for roughly gauging efficiency or inefficiency—the staff to patient ratio, the length of patient stay and rate of patient turnover, and the levels of bed occupancy. More convincing, perhaps, were statistics on the net inpatient cost per week, but they also had to be used cautiously because there were so many variable factors.

The steadily growing cost of the hospital service created a strong urge on the part of the Ministry of Health to strive for more efficiency. There was little or no evidence of obvious waste, but the feeling persisted that more economy was possible if the proper techniques were employed. Under the comparatively simple interim system of accounting established in 1950, it was difficult to make any accurate comparison in patient costs between departments or even hospitals. The system used was subjective, the expenditures being classified for the entire hospital under such headings as provisions, fuel, and wages and salaries. What private beds, outpatients, or any specific service or department cost could be computed only in a notional or very arbitrary manner. Without accurate information, it was impossible to measure performance in terms of cost to detect extravagance.

Recognizing the need for an accounting system that would determine the costs of individual departments and services, the Ministry set up a working party to create one. Its report in 1955 became the basis for a new and comprehensive system of departmental costing.[1] Known as the "main scheme," the plan provided that expenditures would be calculated not only for each service but for individual departments in which they were incurred. Costs for all wards would be combined for most of the hospitals that used the main scheme, but in a few selected ones, ward costs would be broken down by specialities, such as general medical, private patient, general surgical, tuberculosis, geriatric, pediatric, and maternity. The cost of nurses' homes and operating theatres would likewise be analyzed. Because of the expense involved in introducing this accounting arrangement, it was recommended that the main scheme be instituted on an evolutionary basis. Only the largest hospitals were eligible at first to adopt it. For all others a modified system of subjective costing was used, but it was expected that gradually the system of departmental and unit costing would replace the older system. The proposed scheme became effective in the 1957-58 fiscal year.

For the first time, there were accurate figures on the average cost per week of an inpatient. The charge for private beds could now be correctly calculated. Among the 135 non-teaching hospitals that used the new scheme during the first year, the disparity in figures was most revealing. The inpatient net cost per week ranged from £15 10/10d ($43.51) to £35 9/7d ($99.34), the average being £22 6/2d ($62.47). The higher costs did not necessarily imply waste or inefficient management, as the working party had pointed out, but the comparison was valuable to show where inquiries should be made. By investigating costs that were greatly out of line, appreciable savings might be effected. The first published results from the new scheme were used by the Ministry as a lever to achieve greater economies in hospital management. Regional boards and boards of governors were requested to submit reports by the middle of 1959 indicating what action had been taken on the basis of the analysis of comparative costs and, where practicable, the amount of savings that could be expected from the introduction of economy measures.[2]

In seeking to make the hospital authorities cost conscious, the Ministry in 1955, for example, sponsored a fact-finding inquiry to establish the reason for such apparently wide differences in the cost of provisions, fuel, light and power, and drugs and dressings. Eight teaching hospitals were selected, four in London and four in the provinces, each group of four comprising the two institutions with the highest costs and the two with the lowest. The catering adviser of the Ministry investigated such matters as the dietary standards in these hospitals, the type of individuals fed, and the methods of buying and controlling the stores. The causes for the higher costs were appraised and brought to the attention of the four high-cost hospitals, which were then encouraged to conduct inquiries of their own.

In regard to drugs and dressing, it was established that the variation in cost among the eight hospitals was due primarily to the differences in the type of patients being treated. The investigation, however, could not be carried much further at this time, owing to the absence of a costing system that would reveal the separate costs for inpatients and outpatients. The inquiry into the inpatient costs per week for fuel, light, and power was more successful. It was observed that much of the disparity in costs could be explained by the use of different bases for measuring cost. Some of the hospitals, for example, had their own laundries, and the inclusion of the fuel and power costs of this service had a disproportionate effect on the cost structure as a whole. When the accountable differences were eliminated, the gap was reduced appreciably. The inquiry suggested that the hospitals with the highest costs might be able to reduce them by using a lower grade of fuel, by making the staff more economical in the consumption of utilities, and by determining whether purchasing electric power was not more economical than generating their own, as some did.[3]

The Ministry set up an advisory service in the mid-1950's to promote greater efficiency in domestic management, catering and dietetics, and the hospital laundry. Experts were made available on demand to hospital authorities who wished to reorganize these services. Two laundry engineers were appointed to assist hospitals in the more efficient use of machinery, materials, and labor and to give advice on reconstruction schemes and the renovation of old plants. Personnel administration and the techniques of processing soiled linen were among other subjects investigated. In the conservation of fabrics and the reduction of operating costs, substantial savings were effected. Comparable achievements were realized in the other two fields. Advisers on catering and dietetics assisted hospitals in rearranging and remodeling their kitchens and in selecting equipment that would best serve their special needs. In the field of domestic management, Ministry experts were prepared to advise hospital boards and management committees on the training, organization, and effective utilization of domestic and ancillary employees.[4]

Among the measures taken to reduce waste, none received more acclaim than the Hospital Organization and Methods Service, which was instituted experimentally in 1954. By 1959, it had become firmly established as an integral part of the Ministry, with an assistant secretary in charge. Hospital boards were then urged to appoint full-time senior officers to assist in the development of this work. The

Organization and Methods Service sent teams of efficiency experts to any hospital, upon request of the regional board or management committee concerned, for the purpose of studying some specific operation and advising how the work could be more expeditiously carried out. Studies were conducted in such areas of hospital activity as stores and supplies, finance and accounts, kitchen work, medical records, the blood transfusion service, general administration, laundry and linen arrangements, X-ray clinical procedure, nursing administration, and domestic services. Hundreds of recommendations were made. The information gathered in the course of each study was made available to other hospitals.

The special assistance in the field of outpatient arrangements and clinic organization took the form of a very helpful publication on outpatient waiting time. This report was the first of a series, and others on chest clinics, medical records, and domestic service followed. So successful was the Organization and Methods Service that the Ministry of Health decided to broaden its activities to include large-scale investigations requested by hospital boards. In 1959, an Advisory Council for Management Efficiency was appointed, its first assignment being to concentrate on the improvement of administrative efficiency in the hospitals, including the introduction of efficiency techniques recommended by the Organization and Methods Service.[5]

To supplement the work of the Organization and Methods Service, trained industrial consultants were brought under contract to make highly technical surveys. The hospitals also made use of work-study projects. Such ventures often originated at the grass roots of the hospital service and had the full support of all grades of employees. These research schemes, although applied to some small phase of hospital work, yielded surprising benefits. A work study project at the Westminster hospital, for instance, showed how more than £1,430 ($4,000) a year could be saved in the cleaning of syringes. So encouraged was the hospital over this achievement that it decided to employ three work-study engineers for a period of three years to explore other possibilities for economizing in money and man power.[6]

In the search for economy, the Minister did not overlook hospital supplies as an area in which substantial savings could be effected. There was some question as to the level of administration at which such goods should most appropriately be purchased. The policy of the Ministry was that the greater part of the purchases should be made at group level or on a joint-group basis. Individual institutions might find it advantageous to buy such items as perishable foodstuffs and, if their needs justified, a somewhat wider range of commodities;

but all hospitals were urged to depend in large part on bulk contracting by their management committee.

The Ministry of Health felt that certain standardized items used by all hospitals could be more profitably purchased at the national level. The sentiment at first favored a gradual broadening of central buying, but in taking a more careful look at inter-group purchasing, the Ministry decided instead to encourage expansion in that area. Central procurement of hospital supplies came to represent about 10 per cent of the total amount spent for such supplies by the hospital service. Some of the goods were purchased for delivery to government stores, from which they were redistributed to the hospitals. In this category were blood transfusion equipment, hearing aids and batteries, stationery and office equipment, X-ray equipment (much of which was shipped directly to hospitals by contractors), laboratory apparatus and glassware, and special drugs when these were first put on the market or were in short supply. Among the items centrally contracted for but ordered by the hospitals direct from the contractors were spectacles, mattresses, antibiotics, hormones, X-ray films and paper, rubber goods, hardware, cleaning materials, and, in the case of Wales, drugs as well.

The supplies division of the Ministry of Health had access to a tremendous amount of information concerning prices, trade conditions, and sources of supply. The tradition in England seemed to be that where a public service was subject to national financial control, there should be a large degree of central contracting or purchasing. In permitting 90 per cent of the hospital supplies to be procured by decentralized units, the Ministry seemed to be flying in the face of what was considered sound practice. The policy of Savile Row was nevertheless sustained on the basis of the investigation made by the Committee on Hospital Supplies.

Appointed by the Central Health Services Council, this Committee devoted three years to a study of the problem, issuing an interim report in the spring of 1956 and the final report two years later. The Committee felt that joint-group contracting offered the most economical approach in the procurement of hospital supplies, although foods and certain other items, depending upon geography and transportation, should be obtained either on a group or individual hospital basis. There was no need to expand the central supply system, which, if anything, should be reviewed to see whether some of the contracting could not be done just as well by inter-group committees.

The Committee on Hospital Supplies did not favor the application of any rigid or uniform pattern, but instead advocated a flexible course adapted to the needs and interests of each area. The argument that standardization would result in "drab institutional uniformity" was, in the opinion of the Committee, no more valid in the hospital world than in the hotel or catering industry, where large-scale buying was a normal practice. A single contracting committee for the joint-group could handle all its buying responsibilities, or they could be divided among a number of area committees. The estimates from the various hospitals would be combined, bids advertised, and contracts placed by the joint-group or area committees, but delivery would be made to each hospital in such quantities as were specified by it. In this way, hospital groups could obtain all the benefits of central contracting without abandoning any part of their autonomy. The entire undertaking would remain purely voluntary. A high degree of co-operation, it was explained, would be required from the engineers, catering officers, pharmacists, and others concerned, with the supplies officer playing an especially important role, but the final responsibility for the supply arrangements of the group would be that of its chief administrative officer.[7]

Group contracting schemes were very common from the earliest years of the National Health program, but joint-group arrangements made slow progress at first. The type of supplies organization that evolved in a particular area seemed to be governed largely by the location and background of the hospitals involved. Former local authority institutions were more amenable to group buying than former voluntary hospitals, which preferred the course to which they had been accustomed—contracting on an individual basis with local firms. Through circulars and moral suasion, the Ministry endeavored to stress the advantages of group and inter-group supply schemes, but some hospitals were slow to respond. When it became apparent that competitive bidding was not always adhered to by some of the institutions, the Ministry in 1956 circulated model standing orders designed to insure the acceptance of the lowest bid unless there were good reasons for not doing so.[8]

Following the publication of the interim report on hospital supplies, the Ministry circulated a questionnaire that disclosed surprising progress in the field of co-operative buying. Over 100 joint-contracting schemes had come into existence, including all or some of the management committees in every one of the hospital regions in England. Drugs and dressings were the most commonly listed item, but a wide variety of other goods were included, and in some cases provision was even made for joint-contracting for certain foodstuffs.[9]

A good example of bulk purchasing was that practiced in the Manchester Region, where all the management groups embarked upon a joint-contracting program in 1954. At first experimental, the scheme proved successful and soon acquired permanent status. Originally only textile products were involved, but soon drugs and other items were added. No central organization had to be established, and no additional expense was incurred. Several management committees were selected as contracting committees, each having jurisdiction over the negotiation for one or more items. There was no need for depots. Each management committee ordered items as it desired from the contractors whose bids had been approved, paying the stipulated price.[10]

While joint-group contracting was the most publicized of the inter-group co-operative ventures, there were other joint-service arrangements. By pooling the resources of hospitals in a single group and between groups, substantial savings were realized in bakeries and laundries. In the case of the latter, especially, did joint-service become common. Financial and advisory assistance from the Ministry rendered possible the renovation and enlargement of certain laundry plants so they could provide service of this character. To some degree, transportation facilities were also organized jointly. Hospital engineers likewise found it convenient to co-ordinate maintenance work on a joint-service basis.[11] In other areas of hospital administration there were inter-group conferences, consultations, and varying degrees of co-operation. The progress made by hospitals in group and joint-group endeavors during the first decade of the hospital service was impressive and a factor of real significance when measured against the competitive and individualistic pattern which so completely dominated hospitals prior to 1948.

In seeking to put hospitals on as sound a fiscal basis as possible, the Ministry was confronted with the problem of hospital farms and market gardens. When the Health Service was initiated, many of the hospitals, especially the mental and mental deficiency ones, operated farms for outdoor patient therapy and also as a source of vegetables and milk. Some institutions, however, had a tendency to acquire more land than was necessary to achieve these purposes. A survey in 1953 revealed that hospital farms represented a total of at least 40,000 acres, and the market gardens almost 4,000 acres. There were 14,000 head of cattle, 25,000 pigs, and a considerable number of sheep and poultry. A committee appointed to investigate the matter reported that with the increasing mechanization of agriculture only a small number of patients could benefit from occupational therapy on the farms and that full-scale farming was no longer desirable or necessary. Market gardening and poultry-raising, it was held, still served a useful purpose.

Acting upon this report, the Ministry issued a memorandum in spring, 1954, advising that it had no authority to operate farms unless they were essential to the hospital service. The only purposes for which land could be held were necessary seclusion, patient therapy, recreational space, and sites of future development. The hospital authorities were advised to determine whether the land held or the farming activities carried on were justifiable in this light. The fact that some of the farms incurred heavy losses could no more be overlooked by the Ministry than by the Public Accounts Committee. The surveys made by regional boards in some cases led to a complete abandonment of farming and the disposal of thousands of acres of land. But such liquidation of a long-established activity moved slowly.[12]

The cost of the hospital service, as noted elsewhere, was borne almost entirely by funds from the national treasury. Fees for private and amenity beds and for certain appliances in the outpatient department produced about the only revenue from patients in a service that was otherwise free. There were other minor sources of revenue—canteens, farms, the lodging and board of the hospital staff, auto accident insurance, and certain specific services accorded to local authorities. In addition, there was the revenue from the endowment fund.

When the hospitals were brought under national jurisdiction, endowments belonging to the non-teaching hospitals were put into a central fund, which totaled about £20 million ($56 million). The money was invested in government bonds and other securities, and the income was divided among the regional boards and management committees in proportion to the number of hospital beds which each controlled. The total annual distribution was £713,000 ($2 million), which averaged 30s ($4.20) per bed. The share allocated to the regional boards for the most part was transmitted by them to the management committees. The teaching hospitals did not have to surrender their endowments. Significantly, the law provided that no future legacies or gifts granted to the hospitals would be absorbed into the central endowment fund. The management committees would henceforth exercise jurisdiction over any benefactions that might be made to hospitals within their group.

The income from the endowment money could be spent on amenities for patients or staff, such as television sets or comfortable furniture, or it could be used for research or almost any other hospital purpose. A number of small capital schemes were financed out of the money—a practice with which the Ministry of Health was careful not to interfere.

The government had no desire to discourage new legacies. Although the endowment fund had been freed from all trust stipulations, the government gave assurance that the terms of all trusts made and accepted since the adoption of the Health Service Act would be honored. While legacies and gifts were welcomed and hospitals continued to receive them, the Ministry was opposed to charity appeals sponsored by any of the hospitals. At the beginning, some of them, wishing to increase their amenity funds, participated in fund-raising campaigns, but the Ministry of Health put a stop to such practices on the grounds that people would naturally resent being asked for voluntary subscriptions when the hospital service was financed out of tax money.[13]

Another source of income was private and amenity beds. The creation of such beds was not primarily motivated by a desire for revenue but was rather intended to satisfy the medical profession and those who felt that in a free hospital service some accommodations should be made available to persons willing to pay for the privilege of having privacy. Consultants, eager to have some fee-paying patients in National Health Service hospitals, demanded private beds as a part of the price the government would have to pay for their acceptance of the new law.

For the convenience of private patients, each hospital set aside a few "section 5" beds, as they were called, but the full cost of the rooms, including all services and overhead charges, had to be paid by the users. The rate varied among the hospital regions, but it was highest in the teaching hospitals of London. In three regions surveyed in the mid-1950's, the rates in maternity hospitals for pay beds ranged from £15 ($42) to £25 ($70) per week. Hospital costing figures revealed a substantial increase in fall, 1958. The *British Medical Journal* reported that in some institutions the cost of "section 5" beds rose to £36 ($100) or more per week.[14] The medical profession from almost the outset of the Health Service decried the "high" charges, demanding lower rates on a grant-in-aid basis. Such a proposal was contrary to the law and never appeared to elicit much sympathy from the officials at Savile Row. The Guillebaud Committee doubtless reflected the overwhelming sentiment of the nation when it held that the "user of the pay bed should pay the full cost of the accommodation and services provided."[15]

The charges must have discouraged the use of pay beds and may well explain why the number of such beds was only 5,628 in 1960, compared with over a thousand more when the service started. No less significant was the fact that during the first decade of the Health Service an average of not more than 50 per cent of these beds were occupied daily by paying patients. Not all of the remaining beds stayed vacant, since one-half or more of these were filled by Health Service patients who, on medical grounds, were permitted to utilize them without charge.[16]

Surgeons' fees were subject to maximum limits in all but a small percentage of the private beds. In 1958, for example, and for some years previous, the charge for a series of treatments for the same condition normally could not exceed 75 guineas ($220.50), though when the treatment was long and complicated, the fee could rise to a maximum of 125 guineas ($367.50). Under the schedule of charges that was published in the spring, 1953, and that remained in force for many years, a barium meal, complete tract radiodiagnosis was not to exceed 3 guineas ($8.82), while the provision and fitting of contact lenses carried a maximum fee of 10 guineas ($29.40). Operations for simple hernia, non-acute appendicitis, or an abscess of the prostate gland had a ceiling charge of 25 guineas ($73.50), whereas a double hernia, a perforated ulcer of the alimentary tract, an acute appendicitis, or a tumor of the brain could command a fee of no more than twice that amount. Only in special circumstances could the specified fees be exceeded.[17]

The surgeon's fee for possibly 15 per cent of the private beds was unrestricted. A case was cited in the *Spectator* of two private patients, known to each other, who underwent the same type of surgery in the same hospital. One had a restricted bed and was charged 75 guineas ($220.50) by the specialist, while the other patient, who managed to get into one of the few unrestricted rooms, had to pay a fee of 260 guineas ($764.40).[18]

Aneurin Bevan deplored the existence of private beds. In 1958, he disclosed to Parliament that every week letters reached his office about paying patients who were able to "jump the waiting list" because of their financial advantage and not their medical need. While acknowledging that the practice was not universal and did not "impair the service," he protested that it nevertheless "has caused great grief."[19] A campaign pledge in 1954 committed the Labor Party to the abolition of pay beds when it came to power. In the election of 1959, the party was just as opposed to pay beds but no longer categorically demanded their elimination. By replacing large wards with small ones and establishing more single and double rooms and day rooms, the hospitals, the Party believed, would make "the need and cause for private pay beds disappear."[20]

Since private beds constituted only slightly more than 1 per cent of the total number of staffed beds in the hospital service, the impact of queue-jumping, even if it were prevalent, could not have been very serious. Whether the existence of pay beds had created a two-standard service, as some alleged, was never demonstrated, though private patients did seem to be more quickly admitted than most non-emergency Health Service patients, could engage their own specialists, enjoyed a more liberal arrangement for visitors, and were able to obtain more but not necessarily better nursing. In the fall, 1954, the Conservative Minister of Health denied that the abolition of pay beds could be of any possible benefit to the Health Service. "If a man wants to pay his coppers and his shillings every week to a hospital contributory scheme," he averred, "rather than spend it on pools, so that he and his wife or children if they are ill may have some privacy—well, what on earth is wrong with that?"[21]

For those Health Service patients who preferred to avoid the wards with their twenty or more beds, there were amenity beds, otherwise known as "section 4" beds. Prior to 1961, the charge was 12s ($1.68) per day for accommodation in a single room, or half that amount for accommodation in a small ward with two or more beds.[22] If the patient required privacy for medical reasons, there was, of course, no assessment. In some years "section 4" beds totaled more and in other years less than the number of private beds, but the difference between them seldom exceeded a few hundred. There was little more demand for amenity beds than for pay beds. A considerable number of amenity beds stood vacant, and upwards to a third were occupied by non-paying patients who were assigned such beds for medical reasons. Impressed by the fact that only 46 per cent of "section 4" beds were occupied in 1955 by amenity patients, the Select Committee on Estimates recommended that the Minister of Health encourage the hospitals to publicize the availability of these beds and otherwise seek to induce paying patients to use them. The Minister did so, but without much success.[23] Apparently, the British public did not find the wards, with their curtained beds, unpleasant.

In spite of the fact that private patients in pay beds did not represent more than 1 per cent of all the inpatients in Health Service hospitals, it could not justifiably be assumed that the desire for private hospital care would completely disappear. Hospital provident societies in 1959 gave protection to not fewer than 950,000 persons. At least three such associations existed in the United Kingdom, but only one, the British United Provident Association, had attained any size. Its membership accounted for at least two-thirds of all who carried hospital insurance. Founded in 1947 from the amalgamation of several provident associations, this organization experienced a phenomenal growth. In 1959, it had an annual subscription income of £3 million ($8,400,000), of which 85 per cent was paid out in claims. While not antagonistic to the National Health Service, the

British United Provident Association was designed to render private treatment possible in private nursing homes, private hospitals, and in the pay beds of Health Service hospitals. To those who desired to make their own hospital arrangements and to have the medical attendants of their choice, this type of insurance was attractive.

All persons under sixty-five years of age were eligible for membership in the United Provident Association, but the premium rates were too high to attract many from the working classes. The scale of premiums determined the amount of the benefits. Five different schedules were available. The least expensive plan in 1960 for a subscriber aged 50 with two or more dependents cost £11 15s ($32.90) per year; the most expensive, £39 11s ($110.74). Each scale carried the same range of outpatient and inpatient benefits, covering such items as home nursing, surgeon's fee, X-ray therapy, ancillary specialist services, and hospital pay bed, but the amount payable for each varied greatly. The coverage for a hospital bed was limited to ten weeks each year at the maximum rate of £13 13s ($38.22) per week for the least expensive policy mentioned above and nearly three times as much for the most costly. The amount allowed for the other services was in the same ratio.[24]

The British United Provident Association in 1959 expanded its program to include a general practitioner scheme open to those who were insured under the standard hospital program. Two alternative scales of benefits were made available in that year. Exclusive of the first two, three, or four attendances, depending on whether the subscriber was single or had one or more dependents, the fee allowed for each consultation was either 12/6d ($1.75) or £1 ($2.80), with a proportionately larger sum for a minor operation. The yearly maxima in the two schedules were £50 ($140) and £80 ($224) for each insured person. The annual premiums were £2 10s ($7) and £4 15s ($13.30), respectively, for a single subscriber, plus less than half that amount for each dependent. The age limit upon eligibility for membership was fifty-five years, although during the first year of the scheme subscribers to the age of sixty-five were accepted. That this plan, launched as an experiment, would have the same appeal as hospitalization insurance was doubtful.[25] The absence of any provision for drugs was a handicap. The Fellowship For Freedom in Medicine was nevertheless pleased over the implications which this scheme held for the future of private practice. But for all the jubilation this association showed about the rapid growth of the provident societies,[26] the fact remained that after ten years of the Health Service, only 2 per cent of the population had any kind of private hospital protection.

In establishing the National Health Service, the government exempted some 250 nursing homes and hospitals from nationalization. They were considered to be unsuited for a role in the new scheme. The majority of them were run by religious orders. Such institutions were free to continue accepting patients on whatever terms they chose, but their facilities were usually meager and inadequate and the quality of service they offered was in no way comparable to that available in Health Service hospitals.

In surveying the hospital program at the tenth anniversary, Parliament took deep satisfaction in what had been achieved. In spite of outmoded plants, the hospitals had done surprisingly well in meeting the tremendous demand that a population of 45 million made upon a free service. The Minister of Health disclosed to the House of Commons that during the ten-year period the number of staffed beds had increased 6.5 per cent, 29.5 per cent more patients were being admitted to the wards, the ratio of treatment to beds had improved 22 per cent, the waiting list had fallen 11.5 per cent, and 12 per cent more outpatients were being treated. Aneurin Bevan, whose role in founding the Health Service was not forgotten on this occasion, commented upon the improved health of the British people. He said that the new Service deserved much of the credit for the rapid decline in tuberculosis and children's diseases and the sharp reduction in infant and maternal mortality. Under the old system, he reminded Parliament, the medical facilities and drugs would not have been available to all people in need of them.[27] Reference was made in the House of Lords to the comparatively high bed occupancy rate and the 30 per cent increase in the medical and dental staffs.[28] Inspiring as were these and other observations, neither house failed to ignore the limitations that remained to be overcome.

The waiting list was perhaps the most widely questioned aspect of the hospital service. In 1949, there were 500,000 persons waiting to enter the wards, but by 1956 the total had dropped to 431,000. During the next three years, the downward trend was reversed. In 1960, the waiting list again registered a decline, but even so it stood at 465,000 in December of that year. Whether these figures denoted the actual count of persons requiring hospital treatment was quite doubtful. In the opinion of some observers, the number was inflated by possibly 25 per cent. A few hospitals accepted the names of only those who could be accommodated within two or three months, and in some cases a booking arrangement was used. The majority of institutions, however, preferred to compile their lists without reference to their size or the time factor. The names of patients might remain on a list for 12 or more months before they received a call from the hospital. Since 48-hour notices were often given, refusals were rather frequent. While some hospitals endeavored to check every three months or so in order to keep their lists up-to-date, others failed to do so, with the result that there were many names that should have been deleted.[29]

The waiting lists tended to be longer in the northern part of England than elsewhere. In proportion to the number of beds, teaching hospitals had the largest group of patients seeking admittance. The movement of people into suburban areas or the rapid growth of some new industrial community greatly affected the volume of hospital work. Some of the larger hospitals, with a greater variety of consultants, drew proportionately larger waiting lists than those whose facilities were not as well suited to handle the more complicated cases.[30]

Emergency patients were promptly admitted to every hospital. It was only among the non-emergency cases that a waiting period existed. The delay varied between departments within a hospital even more than between hospitals. General surgery drew the longest lists, which, combined with the ear, nose, and eye department, accounted for more than half of the national total. Statistics for 1960 revealed that such specialties as gynecology and traumatic and orthopedic surgery also had sizable waiting lists. In such areas as infectious diseases and diseases of the chest, the waiting time had become negligible.[31] With the development of so many highly specialized fields of surgery, it was necessary to sectionalize beds, each specialty getting a certain number. Adjusting beds to meet the fluctuation in surgery trends, which also varied on a seasonal basis, was difficult, for the demand could not always be anticipated or provision made for the prompt transfer of beds from one department to another.

The longest delay in admission was to be found in the ear, nose, and eye specialty. In non-teaching hospitals, the average period of waiting in this department was reduced to 4.5 months by 1956. In the same hospitals that year, the waiting period averaged 5 days for general medicine, 4 for diseases of the chest, 32 for the chronic sick, 53 for general surgery, and 73 for gynecology. In most of these categories, the teaching hospitals had somewhat longer waiting periods.[32]

The experience of individual doctors in getting their patients hospitalized seemed to show considerable variation. The Hadfield Report (1951-52) revealed that 70 per cent of the general practitioners interviewed had to wait six months or more to get their non-urgent cases into the hospital, the greatest difficulty involving the aged and infirm.[33] But four years later the Social Surveys reported that only 42 per cent of the doctors that answered the questionnaire had any trouble in having their patients accepted without delay. In appraising the Health Service in 1958, two medical writers were of the opinion that at least 60 per cent of the patients awaiting surgery in the provincial hospitals were admitted within three months.[34]

From the foregoing evidence, it is apparent that a definite reduction in the waiting time had occurred. But immediate surgery for most patients had never been a part of the Health Service pattern. The existence of waiting lists could not be regarded as an abnormal phenomenon when all the people were suddenly given free access to the hospitals. In fact, waiting lists were common even before 1948. The need to reduce the waiting period was never lost sight of by the officials at Savile Row, who recognized that this could be done only through the more effective utilization of the hospital resources.

What London could not effectively accomplish in the elimination of its waiting lists, it was able to achieve in the accommodation of emergency cases. Necessity left that great metropolis little choice in the matter, but whatever the motivation, it got an Emergency Bed Service that functioned with extraordinary success from the inception of the Health Service onward. Founded in 1938 and operated by the King Edward's Hospital Fund, the Emergency Bed Service was designed to co-ordinate information on vacant beds in the hospitals of the Greater London area and to assist practitioners in finding space for patients requiring immediate hospitalization. If a physician had difficulty in placing a patient, he referred the matter to the Emergency Bed Service, which moved quickly into action. It operated day and night and kept constant check on bed vacancies. In the event that, because of overcrowded conditions or for some other reason, no hospital volunteered to accept the patient, the matter was immediately brought to the attention of a medical referee, who had the authority to force admission. From the initial call of the practitioner to the acceptance of the patient by a hospital, less than 30 minutes was normally required. A sensitive graph in the operations room of the agency recorded the weekly rise and fall of the sickness rate, and through a warning system, the Emergency Bed Service kept the hospitals informed if a critical situation arose.

During the first decade of the Health Service, the Emergency Bed Service averaged more than 60,000 cases a year. The success of this agency was attested to by the fact that in the 1956-57 year approximately 95 per cent of all general acute cases in the London area were admitted to hospitals. Some of the applications were withdrawn by the doctors, but in that year no person was denied admission if need was established. The record of other years was almost as good, but the use of pressure on hospitals, unavoidable on certain occasions, was an unpleasant element of a scheme that otherwise functioned in a spirit of amity.[35]

When the hospital service began, there were over 50,000 unstaffed beds. By the end of 1960, the number had fallen to 21,000, which was 4 per cent of the total bed complement in the hospital service. This achievement was largely accomplished by overcoming an acute shortage of nurses. By 1960, the number of whole-time nurses stood at 162,000, or 29 per cent more than in 1949, while the number of part-time nurses had reached 44,000, an increase of 91 per cent. With 54,000 student nurses enrolled, 17 per cent more than were enrolled 11 years earlier, the general nursing picture promised to grow even better.[36]

The number of beds per thousand persons was 11.6 in England, compared with 9.7 in the United States. Perhaps because of the out-patient and the domiciliary consultant services and the greater range of home care available under the National Health Service, the number of admissions per thousand persons in England and Wales was only 80, whereas in the United States it was 124. In America, the turnover of beds was thus much greater, and proportionately more people became inpatients than in England.[37]

By shortening the length of stay for patients and by reducing the number of unstaffed beds, the British hospitals were able at the end of ten years to accommodate almost 30 per cent more patients than when the Service began. Comparatively few new beds were added and not one new general hospital was opened during that period. But more effective use was made of the old beds. While it was commonly believed that the maximum rate of bed occupation was between 80 and 85 per cent, some hospitals had demonstrated that a 90 per cent level was practicable. Taking all beds into consideration, that percentage was reached in 1953 and more or less maintained in subsequent years, but if mental and mental deficiency beds were excluded, the occupation rate did not rise above 83 per cent, which, in the opinion of many hospital officials, was very good.[38]

Substantial progress was made in the bed turnover rate, and it was therefore possible to treat more people. Between 1953 and 1958, the average length of stay for patients in most departments was reduced by from one to three or four days, but in a few specialties, such as chest diseases and chronic illness, the reduction was much greater. In 1960, the average hospital stay for ear, nose, and throat was 5.3 days; general surgery, 12.1 days; gynecology, 9.5 days; and chronic illness, 142.1 days.[39]

When the hospital service was in the planning stage, the feeling was that the number of beds would have to be substantially increased to take care of the expected patient load. The hospital surveys during the latter part of World War II indicated the need of 8 or more non-mental beds per thousand persons, and a later memorandum on the development of the consultant service proposed a goal of 14 beds per thousand persons. Exploratory studies made by the Nuffield Provincial Hospitals Trust and the Oxford Regional Hospital Board, however, suggested that the earlier predictions were excessive and that the existing number of beds might even be sufficient.[40]

It was apparent that more adequate outpatient diagnosis and treatment, further development of the domiciliary service, and improved co-ordination of all branches of the Health Service would lessen pressure on hospital wards. Since social conditions accounted for the hospitalization of some individuals who otherwise might be treated at home, the continued improvement of the housing situation also promised to be of help. In comparison with some of the other Western countries, the average duration of stay in English hospitals still seemed too long and could be further reduced. And the replacement of obsolete hospital buildings with new ones, it was held, would permit a vastly more efficient use of beds and diminish the need for so many.

The wards were not the only part of the hospital service that had to cope with an expanding volume of work. Before the inception of the Health Service, many hospitals were either poorly equipped or completely unable to handle X-ray or pathological examinations. In improving the hospitals, the Ministry of Health devoted careful attention to these two fields. As noted elsewhere, a majority of the institutions made these facilities directly accessible to the general medical practitioners, while others were pledged to do so as soon as it became feasible, but the overwhelming bulk of work came from the hospital inpatient and outpatient services themselves. During the four-year period ending in 1957, the number of pathological examinations increased 33 per cent, while the amount of work in the X-ray division expanded 14 per cent.[41]

In the Manchester hospital region, to cite one example, every hospital center was furnished with a comprehensive laboratory service accessible to all practitioners. In removing the deficiencies which prevailed there in 1948, 20 new laboratories were provided and the others renovated at a cost of £300,000 ($840,000). During the first three years of the Health Service, the number of pathological examinations increased by more than a third, and during the next two years by another third. All hospital centers were likewise supplied with up-to-date X-ray facilities, to which family doctors were also given direct access. At a cost of £500,000 ($1,400,000), nineteen new radiological departments were established and the old ones modernized. Each year witnessed an impressive increase in the amount of X-ray work performed by the hospitals of this region.[42]

Every available weapon was pressed into the fight to reduce the ravages of tuberculosis. Most spectacular was the miniature X-ray camera, installations of which in mobile units the Ministry expanded from 36 in 1948 to more than twice that number within six years. Originally under central jurisdiction, this mobile X-ray service was later transferred to the regional hospital boards, which were able to X-ray 3.3 million people in 1958, compared with less than one million in 1948. Some 27 million examinations were made during the first ten years of the health program. By concentrating on the more congested and poorer areas, where the incidence of tuberculosis was likely to be the highest, the mobile units detected thousands of cases annually. Other respiratory diseases, as well as lung cancer and heart abnormalities, were brought to light by mass radiography. Chest clinics and outpatient departments were provided with the miniature cameras, and they contributed to the successful campaign against tuberculosis. Under the auspices of the local health authorities, many adults and an even larger number of school children were vaccinated against this disease. Although most tubercular patients were treated in British hospitals, more than one thousand persons were sent to two sanatoria in Switzerland under an agreement that was in force between 1951 and 1955.

As a result of the general progress of medicine and a determined effort by the health authorities, the number of deaths from tuberculosis fell from 22,000 in 1948 to one-fifth of that figure a decade later. The heavy demand for space in the sanatoria gradually moderated, and a substantial proportion of the beds in them were freed for other purposes. The waiting list, once very large, became negligible. By 1958, the number of cases detected by mass radiography had fallen to 1.9 per thousand, or one-half the rate of ten years previous.[43]

The improvement of the radiological and pathological departments was paralleled by the betterment of surgery facilities. During the early years of the service, the Manchester Regional Board, for example, erected 4 twin operating suites and 9 single operating theaters, in addition to making major alterations in existing facilities. The record of the South-East Metropolitan Region, which built 14 new single and twin operating suites, was as good.[44] The interest of the Ministry of Health in this area of hospital work was reflected in a comprehensive study on *Operating Theatre Suites* published by it in 1957.

Among the services rendered by the hospitals, none was more necessary than blood transfusion. Established as a wartime necessity, the Blood Transfusion Service continued to function after the war, at first under the Ministry of Health and in 1948 under the supervision of the regional hospital boards. There was need for more blood in the casualty departments, in cardiac surgery, and in many other phases of hospital treatment. To increase the number of donors, the Blood Transfusion Service resorted to films, television programs, press advertisements, pamphlets, and posters and other display material. The demand was more than met each year, with a good safety margin, by a steadily increasing supply of blood. In 1960, 853,000 persons gave over 1,000,000 donations to the blood bank, which represented well over twice the amount contributed in 1949. To insure the greater safety of transfusion, extensive research on human blood groups was carried out in the laboratories.[45]

The fitting and dispensing of medical appliances to patients with physical handicaps was another function of the hospital service. The hearing-aid service was one of the most highly regarded by elderly people. Hundreds of hospitals provided specialists for testing and prescribing, but the fitting and repair work was done by a much smaller number of institutions. By 1957, the waiting list was no longer a major problem, with most of the distributing centers being able to supply a hearing-aid within a month. The service was entirely free, including repair work and the supply of batteries. Seeking to improve the original model, the Electro-Acoustics Committee of the Medical Research Council carried out extensive testing and experimenting. In 1958, a new transistor type, weighing 3 ounces with battery, was introduced in limited quantities, with the expectation that it would eventually replace the older and heavier model.[46]

To Aneurin Bevan, this service to the deaf was worthy of special comment on the tenth anniversary of the Health Service.

Deafness is a most disabling disability. It is worse than blindness; it is stupefying. Large numbers of people could not attend their work, could not take part in normal social intercourse, because of this terrible misfortune. How many there were we did not know. . . . The number of Madresco hearing aids issued between 1948 and 1957 amounted to 580,000. . . . When people are talking about the cost of the National Health Service, I hope they will keep such facts as that in mind; because not only does the Service rescue people from a kind of twilight life, but their rehabilitation is of an enormous economic advantage. People are able to go about their normal avocations and to lead happy and contented lives, rescued from what was a near death.[47]

Among other free appliances were artificial legs and arms, artificial eyes, invalid chairs, hand-propelled tricycles, and motor and electric tricycles. They were purchased centrally but distributed by certain hospitals that specialized in prescribing and fitting the artificial limbs and eyes and determining how the need for vehicles could best be met. Storage sheds with repair parts were maintained at numerous locations to ensure that the vehicles were kept in operating condition. Continuous research endeavored to improve the design, convenience, and effectiveness of the appliances. In 1960, 23,000 motor and electric tricycles, hand-propelled tricycles, and invalid chairs were issued to Health Service patients, many of whom were veterans. In that year about 11,000 artificial legs, 2,000 artificial arms, and 9,000 plastic and glass eyes were supplied to handicapped persons, for whom the hospital service sought speedy rehabilitation.[48]

One aspect of the health program not easily expressed in terms of facts and figures was medical research, which had broad ramifications involving hospital doctors and technicians, the universities, private foundations, the Public Health Laboratory Service, and the Medical Research Council. Among these, the last was perhaps the most important, since it not only sponsored a vast range of investigations touching almost every field of medical science but also served as the co-ordinating agency for much of the research done by the other groups.

Founded in 1920, the Medical Research Council was charged with the responsibility of promoting all types of research in the cause, prevention, and cure of disease. No phase of its work was more vital than clinical research, which required access to patients and close collaboration with the hospitals. The Council used most of its resources to maintain research teams in major hospitals and universities as well as in remote places throughout the world. A small part of its funds came from benefactions, but most of the money was derived from the national treasury. In the 1959-60 fiscal year, the Council was awarded by Parliament a grant-in-aid of £3,500,000 ($9,800,000), or four times more than in 1948. The permanent staff employed by the Council had grown to 2,250, most of whom were scientists and laboratory technicians.[49]

The National Health Service Act authorized the Ministry of Health to engage in research and to encourage other agencies to do so. Direct power was also granted to the hospital boards and management committees to undertake research. To insure that the clinical research facilities of the nation were utilized to the best advantage, a permanent Clinical Research Board was set up by the Medical Research Council, in consultation with the Ministry of Health. This Board gave advice to the Council on matters affecting clinical research and took a special interest in encouraging and supervising the major, long-term clinical research schemes in the hospitals. Such projects were financed by the Medical Research Council.

Short-range investigations of the hospital service were left to the regional boards and were administered and financed by them. Each regional board and board of governors was instructed by the Ministry to appoint, in consultation with the regional university, a research committee for the purpose of advising how the money available for decentralized research should be spent. The projects financed by Exchequer money were restricted in scope and cost, but where non-Exchequer funds were involved, no such limits were imposed.[50]

The role of the Public Health Laboratory Service was of special significance. Administered for years by the Medical Research Council, this agency was transferred to the jurisdiction of the Ministry of Health in 1960. The Public Health Laboratory Service functioned in many parts of the country and, with a highly trained staff, maintained constant vigilance in the prevention and control of infectious diseases. In searching for new and dangerous micro-organisms and the means to combat them, this Service carried out nationwide surveys of foods and large-scale vaccine trials.[51]

The Nuffield Foundation, the Wellcome Trust,[52] the British Empire Cancer Campaign, and above all, the universities, played major roles in medical research, which during the era of the Health Service seemed to command more support than at any previous time. When Harold S. Diehl and his two associates, all deans of American medical schools, completed their survey of British medical education in 1950, they had formed a very high opinion of British medical research.[53] Sir Harold P. Himsworth, head of the British Medical Research Council, visited the United States in the fall of 1958 and spoke glowingly there of the vigor of British medical research and the growing strength which it had demonstrated since 1948. Highly selective in their choice of personnel, government-financed research programs, he explained, were attracting able medical scientists for lifetime careers.[54]

A formidable list of research projects was set forth in the reports of the Council. Three fields in particular promised to command a greater part of the research effort—heart diseases, cancer, and mental illness. Growing concern in Parliament over research on mental illness may have been what prompted the Medical Research Council to make a full-scale inquiry into the subject. In spring, 1959, the Council decided to establish two new committees, one on clinical psychiatry and the other on the epidemiology of mental disorders.

The purpose of the latter committee was to provide a more realistic appraisal of the methods of treatment.[55]

The work done by the Social Medicine Research Unit of the Medical Research Council was of significant potential. Located in the new research building of the London Hospital, this agency was concerned with the relationship between health and disease on the one hand and social conditions on the other. By studying, for instance, the housing, working, and other social conditions of patients afflicted with a heart disease or some other chronic ailment, this research group hoped to gain important further knowledge of preventive medicine. Such research began at the point at which the care of patients by the clinical departments tended to stop. The growing importance of degenerative diseases, it was believed, increased the need for greater knowledge about the effect of social conditions on preventive treatment.[56]

In caring for patients, the hospital service had to cope with the long convalescent period some of them required and had to provide rehabilitation facilities for others. The regional boards shared with the local health authorities the responsibility for making provision for those whose condition required some nursing care but no longer the elaborate and expensive services of a hospital. The lack of effective co-ordination between the hospital and convalescent services left some patients under hospital care longer than circumstances really warranted.

Placing patients whose recuperation would be gradual in convalescent homes was considered advisable medically and was certainly less expensive for the Health Service, but this policy could not always be followed because of the shortage of convalescent beds. Such homes were a part of the hospital pattern long before the National Health Service began. Some were private and were operated for profit, but the majority were non-profit institutions founded by Friendly Societies, churches, trade associations, and other local groups and voluntary societies. When the Ministry of Health nationalized the hospitals, only the nursing homes that had facilities for medical treatment were acquired; all others, representing the greater portion of such institutions, were not nationalized. The number taken over had a total complement of less than 6,000 beds, and these were unevenly distributed.[57]

The need for additional convalescent beds caused regional boards to make special arrangements with private convalescent institutions. In some areas, sufficient accommodations were obtained in this way, but in other regions waiting lists developed. The southern part of England had the larger proportion of these homes. The demand for convalescent beds seemed to be greater in the summer than at any other season. Although a majority of the voluntary homes, especially in the London area, provided competent service, there were many whose standards needed to be raised.

The changing pattern of medical care created a serious financial problem for some of the voluntary convalescent homes. At the outset of the Health Service, there was great need for pediatric convalescent beds. The more effective control of children's diseases joined with full employment, better housing, and free or inexpensive school lunches to improve the health of children greatly. Beginning in 1951, there was a sharp decline in the need for children's convalescent beds. By 1958, at least one-third of these beds were closed. Some of the homes accepted elderly patients for the first time, but the required alterations, including the installation of elevators and the creation of more ground floor space, were expensive and discouraged many from making the transition. There was also the new hospital policy of placing patients in convalescent homes at an earlier stage of recovery. This involved a somewhat different standard of service, with more nursing and other added expenses. But financial assistance was available from some quarters. In the London area, for example, the King Edward's Hospital Fund was generous in aiding some of the voluntary homes to meet the changing convalescent needs of the hospital service by financial grants and by giving technical and other advisory assistance.[58]

Local health authorities also made use of convalescent beds, but unlike the National Hospital Service, which charged nothing, they required their patients, if financially able, to pay some of the cost. Although in theory a distinction was supposed to exist between the regional hospital patient who had to have "nursing or medical care" and the local authority patient who stood in need of a "recuperative holiday," both types of persons were seeking rest and in many cases received very much the same type of care. Whether called a nursing or a holiday home, the same institution could and sometimes did accommodate patients from both groups. A somewhat anomalous situation resulted, since it was the sponsoring authority rather than the condition of the individual that determined whether he should have to pay a charge of £3 ($8.40) or more a week or no charge at all.

The great majority of patients discharged from the hospitals were soon able to return to their jobs, but the disabilities of a small minority prevented them from doing so. The hospital service, with the cooperation of other agencies, undertook to rehabilitate such patients. What the hospitals did was only part of an over-all attack upon a problem about which the British people had grown increasingly conscious. Various laws in the interest of the disabled were adopted in the mid-1940's, some being merely improvements of earlier legislation and others going much further than any preceding legislation. Provision was made for the education and training of disabled children, for special assistance to handicapped persons in securing employment, for more adequate benefits to persons physically unfit for work, for larger pensions to those who suffered occupational injuries or diseases, and for general improvements in the welfare of persons "permanently handicapped by illness, injury or congenital deformity." Under the National Health Service Act, such persons could claim medical treatment and whatever surgical appliances were needed, but in addition they were the beneficiaries of a special rehabilitation program designed to assist in their restoration to a useful life.

The rehabilitation services which the hospitals offered depended upon their type and size, but a very high percentage of acute hospitals had physiotherapy departments. Designed to restore a specific bodily function and to improve general physical well-being, physiotherapy utilized electron therapy, massage, and group and individual remedial exercises. There were over 3,900 physiotherapists in 1960, or roughly one-fifth more than during the first year of the Service. Exclusive of group exercises, individual treatments were given in 1960 to 764,000 inpatients and a larger number of outpatients.

Occupational therapy was not as widespread. There were less than 40 per cent as many practitioners in this specialty as in physiotherapy, but the number of occupational therapists was expanding at a faster rate. This type of therapy seemed to have greater value in the mental and mental deficiency hospitals than in the others. Like physiotherapy, occupational therapy undertook to restore the mental and physical capabilities of the individual, but the emphasis was on creative activity. An attempt was made to relate the remedial work to everyday tasks. For men, then, carpentry, metal work, and machine tools might be employed, and for women, model kitchens and living rooms. With the aid of simple gadgets, these people were taught to recover confidence in themselves and to learn to live with their disabilities.

Among others active in the rehabilitation service were the remedial gymnasts, whose entrance into the hospital field was a recent development. There were fewer than 225 of these in the hospital service in 1960. Where a hospital lacked the services of a remedial gymnast, group exercises were frequently provided by the physiotherapist.

Almoners and psychiatric social workers played a significant role, but they also were in short supply. Less than 1,000 of the former and not more than 430 of the latter served the hospitals in 1960. While the almoners were associated more with the general hospitals and the psychiatric social workers with the mental institutions, both performed somewhat the same type of work. Both supplied the doctors with relevant data concerning the social and industrial background of the patient. They also assisted the patient in the adjustment to his home life and job and brought to his attention the services that were available for his welfare.[59]

In a minority of the hospitals, resettlement clinics were established to assist the most difficult cases. These special clinics were served by the psychiatric social worker, the almoner, the occupational therapist, the physiotherapist, the disablement resettlement officer, the consultant in charge of the case, and a doctor familiar with the status of local industry. The patient would be interviewed and his papers carefully examined. The clinic would then assess the patient's capabilities and determine what further training or treatment, if any, he should have, and what other agencies could be of help.

While the hospital service could diagnose and treat the patient, the assistance of others was required in the rehabilitation and resettlement phase. The local health authorities and the general medical practitioners were helpful, but more important were the industrial rehabilitation units distributed at strategic points throughout the nation. Although these retraining centers were not a part of the hospital service, a substantial number of persons were referred to them by hospital specialists. Only individuals who could return to gainful employment were accepted, and all expenses were paid by the government. Each unit was provided with a schoolroom, a gymnasium, and a garden and with workshops where the patient for 8 to 12 weeks was taught some job under conditions that closely simulated those which existed in industry. Members of the staff, including a social worker, a remedial gymnast, an industrial psychologist, and several occupational supervisors, assisted the patients in their efforts to regain self-confidence and master a new skill. Upon the completion of the course, a full assessment was made of each rehabilitee, who was then advised what steps he should take to find his rightful place in society. The local office of the Ministry of Labor helped to place the patient in a job. Among the 10,000 persons who annually attended these rehabilitation units, the overwhelming majority completed the course of study and found employment.

In 1953, a committee was appointed by the Minister of Labor to appraise the rehabilitation program and to make recommendations. Reporting in the fall of 1956, the Piercey Committee seemed pleased with the general character of the hospital program and had little criticism to offer. It advised, however, that resettlement clinics should be established in all major hospitals and that more physiotherapy facilities should be made available in rural areas. Local authorities were urged to build more hostels and more social and occupational centers for disabled persons. The Piercey Committee was convinced that the existing approach was sound but that it should be carried forward on a broader front.[60]

One of the busiest services was obstetrics. Its importance was enhanced by the growing preference among women for institutional confinement. During the early years of the Health Service, the proportion of births in hospitals increased substantially, reaching a ceiling of 65 per cent in the mid 1950's. Only the shortage of beds kept the national average from climbing higher. Some hospitals accepted maternity cases without discrimination, but the majority gave priority to those women who had to be admitted for medical and social reasons. The policy of the Ministry of Health was to encourage normal births at home, but for many expectant mothers, having their babies in the hospital had become the accepted pattern.

The availability of maternity beds varied greatly throughout the nation. In some areas—London, the Isles of Scilly, Bath, and Southport, for instance—more than 80 per cent of the births were institutional in 1957, but in such places as Middlesbrough, Norfolk, and Great Yarmouth the proportion was less than 40 per cent. The occupancy rate also varied sharply between regions. Emergency admissions, staff shortages, and the necessity of closing wards because of epidemics were among the factors that explained why some hospitals were able to keep no more than 60 per cent of their maternity beds full, while other institutions averaged 95 per cent.[61]

The number of maternity beds in 1960 was nearly 20,000, or 4 per cent of all staffed beds. There had been little change in the total since the earliest years of the Health Service.[62] In a careful survey of the maternity service, the Cranbrook Committee recommended that the number of these beds be increased by 5 per cent, so as to permit 70 per cent of all births to occur in the hospitals. This proportion, it was believed, would insure institutional care for all who required it. The Committee was satisfied that the domiciliary service, involving the practitioner obstetrician, the specialist obstetrician, the local clinics, and the midwives and home nurses could provide adequate service for the remaining confinements. The Committee was convinced that for many, childbirth at home had certain advantages.

Some hospitals assumed full responsibility for the maternity patient from the beginning while others permitted a part of the care to be rendered by the family physician or the local health authority. In some cases, the hospital staff held special examination sessions in a local clinic or participated with the local health authorities in joint examination sessions. Cases that were first handled by local pre-natal clinics or by midwives and general practitioners and that sub-sequently were taken over by the hospital service sometimes lacked proper continuity in care. To promote greater co-ordination among all parties, the Cranbrook Committee recommended the establishment of local liaison committees and local clinical meetings, as well as the use of a standard "co-operation card" on a national basis. The co-operation card would be issued at the outset to every expectant mother. Appropriate entries would be made on it by all who rendered any obstetric service. Co-operation cards would do much, the Committee claimed, to prevent the duplication or the omission of care. In stressing the importance of better co-ordination in the maternity service, the Committee did not see any necessity for the establishment of unitary control over the three branches of the maternity service.[63]

In 1960, the average length of stay in the hospital for maternity cases was 10.3 days. While recognizing that in America a shorter stay was the practice, the Cranbrook Committee felt that this abbreviation could be attributed largely to the high cost of hospitalization and the near absence of breast feeding. To avoid the complications that sometimes developed during the first week or so of breast feeding and otherwise to safeguard the health of the mother and child, the committee accepted the ten-day period as the normal hospital confinement.

The most serious problem that faced the maternity service was the shortage of midwives. When the Health Service began there were too few, and ten years later the situation had failed to show adequate improvement. The role of midwives in obstetrics was so important that they usually delivered the child even when a doctor was present. In 1956, for example, 80 per cent of all babies were delivered by midwives. The total of those qualified and willing to perform this skill remained more or less stationary in the domiciliary service and did not increase sufficiently in the hospital service to keep pace with the expanding birth rate and the larger number of institutional confinements. The result was understaffed maternity wards and an excessive work load for many midwives. The Working Party on Midwives in 1949 believed that, in view of the rising obstetrical standards that often necessitated a dozen or more visits to the patient's home, the midwife should be responsible for no more than

55 births each year. Yet the pressure was so great in the domiciliary field that some of them had to handle 100 or more cases.[64]

The difficulty was not due to any lack of students of midwifery or midwives but to the fact that the majority of those who qualified did not remain in the profession. They preferred to become health visitors or to accept other posts in the field of nursing that required training in midwifery. More than 3,500 students enrolled annually as midwives during the first decade of the Health Service, but only a minority of them chose to make a career of midwifery. That a large proportion of the domiciliary midwives served also as health visitors and district nurses made it difficult for any system of interchange to be worked out with the hospital service, where the shortage of midwives was even more acute.[65]

The larger hospitals were better staffed with pediatricians, obstetricians, anesthetists and pathologists than the others, but the government's attention to the deficiencies of the hospital service had immeasurably improved the standards of all. Concerning the care received by patients, there was conflicting evidence presented to the Cranbook Committee. Some witnesses complained about the lack of personal attention, the rigid routine, the noise, and the rather casual treatment, but the majority of women were contented with the service.[66] The Social Surveys of 1956 reported that virtually all those contacted in the poll who had been confined in a hospital were satisfied with the way their confinements had been handled. In the letters on the subject to the editor of the *Manchester Guardian,* there were some adverse comments, but most correspondents paid tribute to the kindness, thoughtfulness, and consideration shown by the hospital staff. One individual, writing about her second Caesarean baby, declared that "when I returned . . . after nearly four years had passed, I found almost all the same faces there—doctors, sisters, receptionists, and many orderlies. One need not feel alone, or cut adrift from sympathy and understanding if one's baby is not born at home."[67]

Staff shortages, the inconvenience of some of the older buildings, the patients' lack of familiarity with hospital routine, and the confusion of the overcrowded wards were factors that the Cranbrook Committee believed had conditioned the thinking of the critical minority. Recognizing that many of these were directly related to hospital planning, the Committee proposed that "maternity hospitals should be organized in self-contained units of such size that one sister can be in charge of both lying-in and labour wards and if possible in charge of the antenatal beds as well."[68]

An inquiry into maternal deaths during the period from 1952 to 1954 disclosed that 40 per cent of all deaths associated with pregnancy and childbirth could have been prevented. Among the causes were very few cases of bad midwifery. Possibly a quarter of the avoidable deaths were due to the lack of co-operation on the part of the patient—failure to obtain medical advice or refusal to carry out the advice when it was given. Even more important were the errors of omission found chiefly in domiciliary practice—inadequate prenatal care, the failure to request specialist assistance when it was needed, and the failure to send risky cases to the hospital. This report was sent by the Minister of Health to the local health authorities, the local medical committees, and the hospital authorities with the plea that discussions be held about what should be done in order further to reduce the number of toxemia cases.[69]

Excluding abortions, the maternal mortality rate per 1,000 live births was 0.95 at the outset of the Health Service and 0.39 in 1957. During the same period, the neonatal death rate (under four weeks) declined from 21.1 per 1,000 to 16.5, but the stillbirth rate fell less slowly—from 24.0 to 22.5. Comparative figures for 1956 revealed that only in the last of these categories was the record in the United States appreciably better. The maternal mortality rate was about the same in both countries, but the neo-natal rate was lower in England and Wales, as was the infant mortality rate (under one year).[70]

In seeking to cope with chronic sickness, the hospital service was faced by a complex problem. The growing proportion of aged people meant a higher ratio of cardiac diseases, senility, arthritis, cancer, arteriosclerosis, and muscular, bronchial, and nervous disorders. Loneliness, inadequate care at home, and other social factors added to the mental problems and physical disability of those for whom some provision had to be made. Precisely who should assume responsibility for these cases and what should be done about them was not always easy to decide. The hospital service was willing to admit for treatment and care the acute sick, the chronic bedfast who required prolonged nursing care, and the senile patients whose mental condition made it impossible for them to live with others in the community. The Ministry of Health, however, took the position that the local health and welfare authorities should retain jurisdiction over those who had minor illnesses, infirm persons who had to have some assistance in taking care of their personal needs, and those in welfare homes who, with only a few weeks to live, had become bedridden and could not benefit from any nursing or treatment beyond that which could be rendered by the attendants. Since many in need of care were borderline cases, mistakes in judgment occurred, and patients were mistakenly assigned to welfare homes instead of the hospitals and vice versa.

To meet the growing demand, the hospital service by 1959 was able to increase the number of staffed beds for the chronically ill 14 per cent above the total in 1948. Even more significant was the fact that 46 per cent more chronically ill patients were accommodated in 1959 than eight years earlier. No less gratifying was the phenomenal increase in geriatric outpatients, who within the same period of time increased more than fourfold. While they numbered 10,000 in 1960 and there were many times that many geriatric inpatients, the outpatient geriatric service signified a new and important trend in the treatment of the chronic sick.

Despite the greater capacity for treatment in the hospitals, the waiting list for beds for the chronic sick during the first nine years of the Service showed a small annual increment and reached a total of 10,500 in 1957. The next three years, however, disclosed a substantial drop in the total, which by the end of 1960 stood at less than 5,700.[71] But the waiting list was not a very accurate criterion by which to judge the inpatient service. A survey of the chronic sick and elderly in 1954-55 revealed that in many hospitals the names of those who had died or recovered were not eliminated from the list for long periods of time. The inquiry further showed that urgent cases were usually accepted immediately or at worst within 36 hours.[72] The King Edward's Hospital Fund disclosed that a canvass which it had conducted annually in the London area suggested that half of the names on the waiting list for chronic sick beds should have been removed. Its investigation in 1958 indicated that 71 per cent of the chronically ill patients were admitted within a week.[73]

It seemed apparent to many that the need was not for more chronic sick beds but for a better distribution of the existing ones. Whereas the South-Western, Oxford, and East Anglia Regions had 1.7 chronic sick beds per 1,000 population, which was somewhat better than the national average, the North-West Metropolitan Region had less than half that number. With a more realistic utilization of the available resources, it was believed that adequate provision could be made for the chronically ill without additional beds. This belief was based upon the new and encouraging developments in geriatrics and the expectation that all branches of the Health Service could co-operate more effectively.

The need for better co-ordination was evident from the fact that in 1955 there were 4,500 patients, occupying 8 per cent of the chronic sick beds, who no longer needed hospital care and could have been discharged if the necessary care had been provided by their relatives or by the local health authorities. The proper care was, of course, vital, since many of the patients were in frail health and ran the risk of relapse. During the same year, an estimated 2,000 persons in welfare homes were in need of hospital treatment. Although patients were frequently transferred between the welfare homes and the hospitals, the exchange arrangement stood in need of improvement.[74]

What may have been an encouraging aspect was the bed occupancy rate of the chronic sick, which approached an average of 90 per cent and in some regions was even higher. Even more important, perhaps, was the improvement in the bed turnover rate, which came about in part because more patients were being rehabilitated and were leaving the hospital. In 1958, the number of discharged patients from the chronic sick wards in the London area for the first time exceeded the deaths.[75] Earlier admission of patients and better remedial treatment offered more hope to the chronic sick. With more geriatric units for inpatients and geriatric departments for outpatients and more ancillary services, the hospital service was in a stronger position to deal with the problem of chronic sickness.

It was recognized that at least 40 per cent of the persons described as chronically ill could be rehabilitated and made physically able for discharge. The Ministry of Health urged that such patients should be given treatment in a geriatric unit under the supervision of a geriatrician consultant or physician, assisted by the proper ancillary staff. By the end of 1959, 95 geriatric units had been established, with 17,000 beds. Patients that did not respond to treatment were placed in the long-stay units under the jurisdiction of the same doctor in charge of the geriatric services, so that transfer back to the acute wards could be quickly effected if the situation justified it.

As a part of the program, the Ministry also advised the hospital authorities to establish geriatric outpatient departments. Staffed by occupational therapists, physiotherapists, almoners, and chiropodists, that service was useful in determining priority of admission to the wards. It also assisted the patient who was waiting to enter the hospital and provided after-care for those who had been released. A geriatric outpatient department, the Ministry contended, not only facilitated the discharge of patients but prevented many of the chronically ill from ever becoming inpatients. A considerable number of these departments were established.[76]

The success of the geriatric outpatient department at the St. James Hospital in Leeds gave proof, if proof was needed, that that kind of service performed important functions. This department treated 407 patients in 1957, two-thirds of whom were seventy years or older. Sessions were held twice weekly for a full day. The service had access to a remedial gymnasium and the X-ray and laboratory facilities and enjoyed the assistance of the hospital staff. Local authority ambulances furnished the transportation. About 40 per cent of the patients responded to treatment. The condition of over one-third remained stationary, while that of one-fifth continued to deteriorate. Thirteen per cent were finally admitted to the geriatric unit of the hospital, and 3 per cent either died or remained at home. In seeking to provide help, the staff carefully assessed each patient socially as well as medically, exploring such matters as housing, social difficulties, financial support, and the type of therapy that offered the most hope.[77]

The day hospital performed somewhat the same role as the geriatric outpatient department. Designed to treat psychiatric illness as well as chronic sickness, this type of service was based upon the assumption that some patients needing hospital treatment could get it without having to occupy a bed. More individuals could be cared for in this way, and respite could be given to relatives by taking the elderly sick off their hands during the day. The patients themselves benefited from the change of environment and the therapy. Comparatively few hospitals offered day facilities at the end of the first decade of the health program, owing to the experimental character of this service. But where established, the day hospital seemed successful and enjoyed the full commendation of the Ministry of Health.

Some hospitals shared the care of the chronic sick with their relatives. By arranging a short stay at the hospital for the patient in the Social Rehabilitation Unit and returning him to his home for an equal period of time, the relatives found that they could cope with a responsibility that otherwise might have become intolerable and might have led to permanent assignment of the individual to the chronic sick wards. Where it was available, this arrangement was rarely abused.[78]

The first Social Rehabilitation Unit was established at the Langthorne Hospital in London and met with a warm response from both the patients and their relatives. Within a period of 18 months, two special wards had accommodated a total of 100 patients on an alternating basis of six weeks in the hospital and six weeks at home. The patients were furnished with attractive quarters and given the benefit of physiotherapy, occupational therapy, and chiropody. The social life fostered among the patients did much to dispel loneliness. Thirty per cent of them had been the responsibility of their daughters, one of whom in commenting upon the program said that the "temporary stay procedure has made a difference to me between existing and living."[79]

For the chronic sick who no longer needed active treatment and required only a short period for recovery, there were short-stay convalescent wards or annexes. A number of convalescent homes for this purpose were made available to some of the London hospitals by the King Edward's Hospital Fund, with the understanding that the regional boards would provide the maintenance funds for these institutions. By 1956 more than 6,000 elderly patients had been beneficiaries of these homes, where they were free from much of the routine of hospital life.[80]

What could be accomplished in the more efficient treatment of the chronic sick was demonstrated by a doctor in Sunderland, who established an active geriatric department along the most modern lines. In a hospital of 570 beds for the chronic sick, he was able within six years to increase admissions from 500 to more than 6 times that number by reducing the average stay from 2½ years to 28 days. The waiting list was abolished and some of the beds were no longer needed.[81]

The lack of sufficient staff seemed to plague the chronic sick service more than any other department. Reference has already been made to the shortage of almoners, physiotherapists, and occupational therapists. Owing to the shortage of geriatricians, physicians and consulting physicians who had no special training in geriatrics often had to be appointed to supervise chronic sick departments. Although the nursing force for the hospital service as a whole experienced a healthy growth, its number remained almost stationary in the chronic sick wards. Recruitment of nurses for this department was apparently discouraged by the poor working conditions, the slow turnover of beds, and a feeling that this type of nursing resulted in a loss of status.[82]

Nowhere else in the Health Service was the need for new buildings more pressing than in the hospitals for the chronic sick. The heating and lighting left much to be desired, and in most cases the general layout of the rooms and facilities had become dreadfully obsolete. Protests about such conditions were frequently made in the lay and medical press, and some individuals went further to dramatize the great need for new wards. The geriatrics specialist at St. Luke's Hospital in Bradford, for instance, tendered his resignation in fall, 1957, partly because of the "appalling" situation which prevailed in that institution. But in spite of the handicap, the hospital, under his direction, had done amazingly well. A unit of 700 beds was established, the waiting list had disappeared, and an average of 100 patients were being rehabilitated every month.[83]

Although little had been done by the end of the 1950's to replace the obsolete buildings, a considerable amount of money had been spent in renovating them and a few had been transformed into comfortable institutions with completely redecorated rooms and modern facilities. Some of the buildings were structurally unsuitable for modernization, but until they could be replaced, they had to be used on a makeshift basis, principally as long-stay annexes. Amenities were nevertheless introduced in all of the hospitals to a varying degree, and the aged sick were incalculably better off than they had ever been before.

The average cost per week of maintaining a chronic inpatient was £10 18/7d ($30.60) in 1960. The only patients costing less were the mentally ill and the mentally deficient, their weekly average per person being, respectively, £7 12/8d ($21.37) and £7 ($19.60). The maternity and acute departments were among the most expensive, averaging £27 3/5d ($76.08) and £25 16/7d ($72.32), respectively, for each patient per week in the general hospitals. The cost varied between institutions and regions, but was higher in London than elsewhere. Teaching hospitals avoided accepting chronic sick and mental patients, preferring instead a variety of acute cases for instructional purposes. For such institutions in 1960, the weekly average cost per inpatient was £36 9/7d ($102.14) in London, compared with £30 4/11d ($84.69) in the provinces.[84]

When the government took over the hospitals, the need for a large capital outlay was apparent. A critical housing shortage and an urgent demand for new schools, however, took priority in the allocation of the limited funds and building materials. The unexpected cost of the Health Service further restricted the amount of money that was available for capital projects. As a result, an average of only £10 million ($28 million) was spent annually during the first ten years of the hospital service for this purpose. Approximately one-half of the amount went to general hospitals, one-fifth to mental and mental deficiency hospitals, and only 5 per cent to chronic sick hospitals. Engineering services, ward accommodations, and special medical departments, including operating theatres, absorbed more than half of the money; and when provision was made for the other projects—laundries, kitchens, accommodations for the staff, and out-patient and casualty departments—only 16 per cent of the money remained for new hospitals and major additions to the existing ones.[85]

Not until 1955 was the government prepared to sponsor a major program of hospital construction. Although of modest proportions at first, larger sums were soon granted. Within four years capital expenditures doubled. Scores of schemes were launched involving plant modernizations, new ward blocks, new surgical blocks, and new maternity, outpatient, and casualty departments. In November, 1959, the Minister of Health disclosed in Parliament that since the inception of the Health Service three new mental deficiency and three new general hospitals had been opened and that nine others, mostly of the latter type, were under construction. The hospital boards, he explained, had been asked to complete their planning for several other major projects. Looking into the future, the Minister gave assurance that the building program would continue to expand, with £31 million ($86,800,000) scheduled for capital expenditures in 1961-62, compared with £25,500,000 ($71,400,000) for 1960-61.[86]

The medical profession nevertheless remained unimpressed with what the government had done about obsolescent buildings. In spring, 1958, the Central Consultants and Specialist Committee of the British Medical Association invited two experts, A. Lawrence Abel and Walpole Lewin, to investigate hospital construction. Reporting one year later, these men were convinced that capital expenditures were much too small to permit replacement of the outmoded structures that consumed disproportionate amounts of maintenance funds and handicapped the efficient operation of the hospital service. According to these experts, the situation was not only discouraging but dangerous, because of the growing threat of sepsis from overcrowded and inadequate facilities. Many of the operating theatres were not air-conditioned; few wards had dressing rooms; in many of the hospitals there were an insufficient number of bathrooms and lavatories and not enough privacy; and the general layout of the wards in relationship to the ancillary departments was very inconvenient. Most of the mental and mental deficiency hospitals were judged unsatisfactory in design and structure. In some of the new areas of population concentration, there was a pressing need for more hospital accommodations. To accomplish what should be done in Great Britain, the report recommended an annual expenditure of £75 million ($210 million) for ten years.[87]

The Annual Representative Meeting of the British Medical Association in 1959 accepted the sum proposed by Abel and Lewin as the minimum that should be spent on the new hospital building program.[88] The growing demand for more action was reflected in the campaign manifestos issued by the political parties in 1959. The Conservative Party promised to double the existing capital outlay during the next five years, while the Labor Party specifically recommended a total expenditure of £50 million ($140 million) per year.[89] With the political leadership pledged to an accelerated program, the prospects for an eventual solution of the problem no longer seemed remote.

During the first decade of the Health Service, much had been learned about hospital planning. It was apparent that, in view of the changing pattern of medicine, hospital structures should be made more flexible. When the Health Service was launched, for example, there was need for many additional sanatoria, but the subsequent decline of tuberculosis would have rendered many of them superfluous had they been erected.

Other factors had to be considered in hospital planning. The future role of the outpatient departments, short-stay units, day and night hospitals, the general practitioner service, and the domiciliary program held the prospect of a greatly modified use of and diminishing need for inpatient beds. It was thought by some that special diagnostic centers erected for the convenience of family physicians might further ease the pressure on the hospital service. There was also a possible trend toward integrated hospitals in which full provision was made for the care of all types of patients, including the chronic sick and the mentally ill. With a common nursing staff trained to handle all such cases, greater mobility and a better equalization of professional skills could be achieved. A hospital that comprised many well-planned buildings and was designed for all persons requiring institutional treatment could perhaps serve the needs of the sick much better than specialized hospitals, which varied so much in their standards of care and treatment. But whatever the future pattern might be, it seemed obvious enough to the hospital authorities that the common denominator of all planning was flexibility in design, size, and organization.[90]

CHAPTER XII

Mental Health

NO PHASE OF THE hospital service aroused greater interest than mental health. Even before the inception of the National Health Service, there was a growing consciousness that the old approach should yield to new concepts of treatment. The prevailing prejudice against those afflicted with mental disorders began to change slowly as more and more persons recognized that mental illness can be cured or ameliorated by proper care and therapy and that many patients can be restored to a productive role in society. Even mentally defective persons respond to the right sort of treatment and training, and for many of them there is also hope for a more useful life.

The need to cope effectively with the problem was emphasized by what appeared to be the growing incidence of mental illness. Between 1920 and 1957, admissions to mental hospitals quadrupled, with 44 per cent of all hospital beds in the latter year being occupied by mental and mentally deficient patients. In 1920, however, only the more severe cases were admitted as certified patients, and so comparative figures tend to be misleading. Quite possibly, the proportion of persons afflicted in that year with some form of psychosis or psychological disorder was as large as in later years, but there was then little room in the hospitals for the less extreme cases and the facilities to help such individuals otherwise were very meager.[1] Mental illness carried a stigma, and that must have encouraged many to bear their condition in silence. But with the new and more effective methods of therapy, a greater knowledge concerning mental disorders, and a more tolerant attitude on the part of the public, there was less reluctance to seek psychiatric treatment.

The incidence of mental illness could not easily be measured, since there were so many different types, ranging from mild forms of neurosis to extreme cases of mental disability. The number of persons in institutions was known, but to calculate the total afflicted with some form of mental disturbance was quite a different matter. General practitioners, using their own criteria, variously estimated the number of their neurotic patients to be as low as 2 per cent and as high as 70 per cent. More meaningful was a study of 171 medical practitioners made in 1955-56. That study suggested that 1 in every 15 patients who visited the doctor suffered from psychoneurosis. This represents a national total of over two million such persons under the care of family physicians during any year. A survey in World War II revealed that, in a period of six months, one-tenth of the employees in engineering factories suffered from "definite and disabling neurotic illness" and an additional 20 per cent from "minor forms of neurosis." Between one-fourth and one-third of all absences for sickness were caused by neurotic illness.

It was almost as difficult to ascertain the amount of mental deficiency, since there were many gradations of subnormality or arrested mental development. The picture was further complicated by the fact that mental defectives were, of course, not immune from psychosomatic and psychoneurotic disorders. The Report of the Mental Deficiency Commission in the mid-1920's suggested that, for every 10,000 persons in the general population, there were 80 mentally defective persons who would require at some time or other the type of care furnished under the Mental Deficiency Acts. This number, however, did not include the milder cases of subnormality that were not treated by the special mental health services but that nevertheless required some care and could even profit from some form of occupational training.[2]

Prior to 1948, the care of mental and mentally deficient patients was almost solely the responsibility of the local authorities. By virtue of the Lunacy and Mental Treatment Acts and the Mental Deficiency Acts, the counties and county-boroughs were required to provide institutional care and some measure of domiciliary care for such persons. It was left to the Board of Control, a centrally appointed body, to supervise the local officials in the performance of their duties under these laws. Visiting committees or joint-committees, usually selected by the local authority, were given wide supervisory jurisdiction over the mental and mental deficiency hospitals. Among the powers of these committees were the dismissal of hospital officers, the formulation of general rules regulating the staff, and the appointment of the superintendent, who exercised paramount authority in the hospital.[3]

Overcrowded and cheerless, the buildings usually were situated where the patients could easily be isolated from other people. Owing to the traditional attitude of the general public, it was felt that mental patients should have as little contact with the community as possible, and these institutions therefore tended to serve as places of confinement where a great many of the patients were detained under the compulsory powers of certification. The emphasis was placed on the custodial function, although the mental deficiency hospitals, more than the mental institutions, recognized the importance of active treatment and training. There were many patients, however, especially among the elderly, who no longer required further treatment but simply had no place to go. For them, the hospital had become a "permanent asylum."

Errors of judgment and poor planning sent some mentally defective and mentally ill patients to public assistance institutions, while some senile persons who had merely become a little confused were committed to mental hospitals. As a result, many who could not benefit from psychiatric treatment or special nursing care occupied mental hospital beds that were needed by mentally sick patients who were assigned to homes for the aged, long-stay annexes, and chronic hospitals in which little or no psychiatric treatment or training was then available. Other persons in need of psychiatric care remained in the community, owing to the general shortage of institutional beds. A shortage of nurses, psychiatrists, and other trained staff members contributed to this discouraging situation.

In the field of preventive mental care and social care—duties which devolved upon the local authorities—the situation left much to be desired. Since these functions were more optional than obligatory, many local authorities were negligent in fulfilling the role intended for them. In so far as general social care was provided for mentally ill persons, it was available only for hospital patients and those discharged from the hospital and was furnished by voluntary organizations or by local authority personnel working from the hospitals.[4]

In general, such was the picture during the era before the inauguration of the Health Service. In 1948, mental health and physical health were brought together in one comprehensive service for the first time. A mental health advisory committee was appointed to serve the Ministry of Health, which had the responsibility of coordinating and supervising all phases of the mental health program. Nearly 200 hospitals for mental patients and 150 institutions for mental defectives were removed from local control and placed under the jurisdiction of regional boards. In most cases, each institution was administered by its own management committee. As "designated" hospitals, these nationalized institutions continued to receive certified cases. Provision was also made for the treatment of mental illness in such institutions as neurosis hospitals, long-stay annexes, and day hospitals, where patients entered on their own free will. Subject to certain conditions, voluntary patients were also accepted by the mental hospitals.

The community health service for mentally disordered persons no longer remained an isolated branch of the local health service. The prevention of all types of illness, mental as well as physical, and the care and after-care of patients suffering from mental defects and mental illness as well as physical sickness now emerged as a unified service. The power to make whatever arrangements were necessary for the care of the mentally ill and defective did not involve, however, a mandatory obligation on the part of the local authorities to achieve specific standards of service, and performance therefore varied greatly throughout England and Wales. A health committee usually administered the single service on behalf of the local health authority, although in many areas a special subcommittee had jurisdiction over the mental health phase.

The supervisory functions of the Board of Control were transferred to the Ministry, but the Board retained its quasi-judicial functions. It continued to be responsible for the admission and discharge of all certified patients and for the periodic review of their status and to have authority over all matters affecting their liberty. In addition, the Board of Control was given the responsibility of managing such specialized hospitals as Rampton and Moss Side, which had custody over mental defectives considered dangerous, and Broadmoor, which housed mental patients with a criminal record. To the Ministry of Health was entrusted the general administration of these institutions.[5]

The new approach to mental health tended to reduce the barriers between the mental hospitals and society. People became more inclined to view mental disorders as they would other illnesses that required early treatment.[6] Information programs on television and in other media helped to give the public a better understanding of the nature of mental disturbances and what modern therapy could achieve. The Report of the Royal Commission on Mental Illness and Mental Deficiency in 1957 shed further light on the subject. In Parliament, the prevention and treatment of mental illness were fully explored. The adoption of the Mental Health Law in 1959, which embodied a thoroughly enlightened approach, did more than anything else to underscore the change that had occurred in the climate of public feeling.

In hospital admissions is found the most striking proof that the old fear of mental institutions was becoming less of a barrier to treatment. More people were seeking psychiatric help and hospital care than ever before. During the first ten years of the Health Service, the number of admissions to designated mental hospitals increased by two-thirds, but more significant was the fact that, while voluntary admissions multiplied 130 per cent, the number of certified admissions declined 60 per cent. In 1959, only 10 per cent of all admissions to these hospitals were certified.

Equally remarkable was the brevity of the stay of most patients. More than half of those admitted in 1954 were discharged within three months, and 69 per cent were discharged within six months. An even better record was established during the following years. Only 20 per cent of the admissions in 1956 remained in hospitals at the end of 12 months. It should be noted, however, that at least 40 per cent of all admissions were readmissions, which may be explained in part by the inadequacy of the local authority after-care service but which was much more the result of the belief that for many patients several short-term admissions might be better than a long, continuous period of confinement.

Owing to the rapid turnover of the great majority of admissions, the bulk of the residents at any one time in designated mental hospitals were long-term patients, most of whom were certified. The growing influx of voluntary patients, however, had the effect of reducing the proportion of certified residents from 85 per cent in 1949 to a little over 50 per cent in 1958. No less important was the fact that, in spite of the tremendous increase of admissions, the total number of patients residing in designated mental hospitals was smaller in 1958 than when the Health Service began. Until 1954, there was a steady increase in the number of such patients, the total then standing at 152,000. Because of improved methods of treatment and other factors to be presently examined, the number of resident patients began to fall, reaching 133,000 in 1959. Chronic patients once deemed hopeless were now being rehabilitated and discharged.[7]

From a statistical point of view, the progress achieved in the mental deficiency hospitals was much less spectacular than in the mental institutions. The rehabilitation of mental defectives posed greater difficulties, required more time, and yielded less apparent results than the rehabilitation of mental patients. Working with minds that were subnormal presented different problems and often seemed to offer less hope than dealing with patients who, although afflicted with a neurotic disorder, were once normal and could become so again. The discharge rate from mental deficiency hospitals nevertheless almost doubled between 1951 and 1958, which suggests that the improved methods of treatment were bearing fruit. With only 38 per cent as many beds as the mental hospitals had, the mental deficiency institutions were faced with a chronic shortage of accommodations. Although the number of staffed beds by 1959 was nearly 12 per cent more than at the beginning of the decade, the waiting list stubbornly remained in the neighborhood of 8,000. In comparison, the list for the designated mental hospitals was negligible.

It was evident from the larger and more evenly distributed medical and nursing staffs that both the mental and mental deficiency hospitals were better able to cope with the patient load as a result of the improvements wrought by the Health Service. At the end of the first twelve years of the Service, the number of mental health consultants reached 679—an increase of 67 per cent, compared with a 39 per cent increase in all types of hospital specialists in the same period of time. By 1960, the number of mental deficiency nurses had grown by two-thirds and the number of mental nurses by one-third. Initially, there was a grand total of 32,000 student, whole-time, and part-time nurses serving the mental and mental deficiency hospitals; twelve years later the number stood at 42,000. There were more psychologists, psychiatric social workers, and physiotherapists, but still too few to meet the demand.[8]

In addition to the so-called "statutory beds" established under the Lunacy and Mental Treatment Acts, there were other beds available for persons with mental disorders. Within a period of five years the number of such beds almost tripled, reaching more than 8,000 in 1958. They were located in neurosis hospitals, short and long-stay annexes for the aged, "dedesignated" units of mental institutions, and acute general hospitals. While constituting in that year only 5 per cent of all Health Service beds for mental patients,[9] they represented a new trend that the Royal Commission in 1957 viewed with an approving eye. Patients were admitted to such beds as they were to regular hospital beds, without formality. It was recognized that this course should do much to dispel fear and to encourage people with mental illness to seek treatment early, when it would be most effective.

The problem of mental illness was attacked on many fronts, with day hospitals, outpatient departments, and domiciliary visits by psychiatrists all playing a part in the campaign. In seeking to treat neurotics and other mentally disturbed individuals and to keep them from becoming inpatients, the hospitals expanded their outpatient psychiatric services. By 1958, there were over 500 of these adult clinics, only one-fifth of them being in mental hospitals. The work done at first was chiefly diagnostic, but gradually the clinics were enlarged, staffed, and equipped so they could offer treatment. Each year saw a steady growth in the demand for this service. By 1958, the number of attendances at these clinics had increased to over one million, or 134 per cent more than in 1949. Many patients who previously would have been hospitalized were now enabled through outpatient treatment to remain in the community as breadwinners or housewives. Inpatients were discharged earlier, and under the care of the psychiatric outpatient department were less likely to be re-admitted to the hospital.

As part of the mental health service, psychiatrists attended patients in their homes if the need arose. In 1959, there were 28,000 of these domiciliary visits, or five times more than during the first full year of the Health Service.

The day hospitals, as experimental ventures, held forth considerable promise for the future. From one or two such hospitals at the outset, the number reached 35 by the tenth anniversary of the Health Service.[10] One of the most widely publicized of these ventures was the so-called Worthing Experiment. With financial assistance from the Nuffield Provincial Hospitals Trust, the Graylingwell Hospital in 1956 set up a day hospital at Worthing. Fully manned by a team of nurses, occupational therapists, social workers, and psychiatrists, Worthing offered a comprehensive psychiatric outpatient service which undertook to screen all patients referred to it by the general practitioners. The home environment of each patient was investigated and all other factors were evaluated to determine whether effective treatment could be given at Worthing. Dangerous patients had to be sent elsewhere.

There were 20 beds for the treatment of those who had to be kept there during most of the day. Thirty or forty other patients were treated by appointment, some in the evening after their day's work. Using psychotherapy and modified insulin and electro-convulsant treatments, the staff was able to treat a much larger proportion of the patients in the community than hitherto had been possible. During 1957, nearly 1,300 patients were received at Worthing. Only 284 required highly specialized care and treatment such as pre-frontal lobotomy or deep insulin-therapy, and they were admitted to the Graylingwell Hospital. In the area covered by the Worthing service, admissions to Graylingwell in that year were 56 per cent less than in 1956, while in the rest of the hospital district they increased 6.9 per cent. The record in 1958 was even more impressive. Worthing thus proved what other day hospitals and outpatient departments had demonstrated in a less dramatic fashion—that treatment in the community could be effective, even more effective for many patients than treatment in a hospital ward.[11]

In seeking to improve the mental hospital facilities, the government was faced by a difficult task. Enlarging staffs, improving the outpatient services, and introducing modern techniques of therapy proved more practicable than transforming into suitable quarters the barracks-like, Victorian buildings that housed most patients. The modernization of many of the old Poor Law structures was not feasible, and until new hospitals could be erected, many of the patients were forced to live under conditions that were deplored in Parliament and the press. But some hospitals were reconditioned, the wide corridors and the single rooms being converted into lounges, dormitories, and dining rooms with modern conveniences. Others were made more cheerful by simply plastering the interior brick walls, redecorating and refurbishing the rooms, and making minor alterations in the floor plans. Pictures were hung on the walls, new furnishings were acquired, and other amenities such as radio and television sets were made available. Much was done, yet in some institutions conditions remained shockingly bad at the end of ten years of the Health Service. But during the latter part of the fifties, the capital outlay for mental and mental deficiency hospitals was substantially greater. New hospitals were brought to completion. One very encouraging sign was the reduction in the amount of overcrowding in mental deficiency hospitals, which during the six-year period ending in 1959 declined from 12.4 to 9 per cent.[12]

Some corrective measures could more easily be applied than others. An example was the diet. The traditional view was that mental patients required only one substantial meal per day and very simple, monotonous fare. In kitchens with few modern conveniences, as many as 2,500 meals were prepared at midday by a poorly trained staff. Breakfast and the evening meal often lacked protein and were too small. The amount of milk, fresh fruit, meat, and vegetables was inadequate, resulting in a diet low in nutritive value. The average weekly cost in 1955 of feeding a patient in the mental institutions of the metropolitan area was only 16/6d ($2.31), compared with £1 6/9d ($3.74) in the general hospitals. To remedy this situation, the Ministry of Health, beginning in 1956, allocated a special grant to the mental and mental deficiency hospitals to improve the variety, quality, and nutritive value of the patients' diet. The Ministry also suggested measures that should be taken to raise the standards of catering and thus more nearly to approximate the pattern that prevailed in the general hospitals. The situation thereafter grew better.[13]

In almost every way the care and treatment of mental patients showed improvement. Revolutionary in scope, the new approach seemed to offer such great possibilities that visitors from America, the Commonwealth countries, and elsewhere came to see how the new methods were applied. The pattern varied between hospitals. Some were much more progressive than others, but none could remain indifferent to the techniques that were being used with such success.

The newer forms of therapy, such as the insulin or electrical courses or the tranquilizing drugs, were employed where the need existed, but many patients, it was discovered, responded more readily to social treatments. It was upon these that the hospital authorities were inclined to concentrate their thinking and planning. They had learned from experience that, if patients were treated as individuals, with more understanding and a larger measure of freedom, better results were obtained. As much as possible, the hospital should simulate the outside community, but without its tensions and anxieties. The patients should be given a feeling of responsibility and through ward committees permitted a voice in various matters affecting their lives. The strait jacket, the padded room, the locked doors, and the constant surveillance of the patients by unsympathetic attendants should be replaced by freedom of movement and a new spirit of co-operation and mutual trust. The concept of the mental hospital as a custodial institution should yield to the concept of it as a "therapeutic community." Through group and occupational therapy, the lonely, isolated, uncommunicative patient should be given every chance to become a self-confident and useful citizen.

The abandonment of the traditional restraints actually led to fewer disturbances, fewer escapes, and less need for sedatives. The establishment of industrial units, which re-created more closely the economic activities of the outside world, proved to have a greater therapeutic value for many patients than the old fashioned handicraft departments. Assembling umbrellas, making ball-point pens, or manufacturing other useful products seemed to offer the patient new hope for an early release. In addition to occupational therapy, there were clubs, dances, and other social activities, with less segregation of the sexes. The primary purpose was to foster a more normal atmosphere, in which the dignity of the individual became a part of the institutional pattern. The results were measured in a more rapid turnover of patients and the restoration to society even of long-term residents for whom there had been little hope. Whether recovery was something more than just temporary depended upon many other factors—home environment, the attitude of the community, and the effectiveness of the after-care which the outpatient department and the local health authorities could offer.[14]

In the Parliamentary debates on the occasion of the tenth anniversary of the Health Service, the new spirit and achievements of the mental hospitals were the subject of comment. A very prominent member paid this tribute:

We have heard about the colossal mental hospitals, many of them 100 and 150 years old, but the astonishing thing is that the atmosphere in these hospitals has completely changed. The old padded cell . . . has practically disappeared. Eighty per cent of the patients are voluntary boarders. That is a remarkable achievement. It means that the stigma which is attached to mental disease is disappearing. An individual who, perhaps, feels himself to be a little unstable is prepared to go to a mental hospital for treatment. That is remarkable. The shock treatment and tranquillisers . . . have given infinitely more freedom to these patients. There has been a dramatic change.[15]

What could be done by fully utilizing the new techniques was amply demonstrated by the Glengall Mental Hospital, Ayr. When its experiment began, there was only one unlocked ward. Only a small proportion of the patients had regular work. There were domestic duties and a few odd jobs for some, but the great majority of patients spent most of their time sitting on benches in the wards. Serving a population of 300,000, this hospital with its 710 beds had a comparatively low admission and discharge rate. Many cases were rejected because of the lack of accommodations.

Beginning in January, 1956, the Glengall Hospital underwent a complete transformation. The wards were redecorated, the diet was improved, and each patient was furnished new clothing. A carefully planned program provided a full schedule of work and social activity for all. Games, parties, and dances were held and clubs and discussion groups formed. Week-end leaves, visits from the community, and other outside contacts were encouraged. More patients were employed on indoor assembly and outside farm work, and as an inducement to accept such work they were given incentive pay. Where occupational and group therapy proved inadequate, tranquilizers and convulsion therapy were used. All doors were unlocked except those on one male ward. Reporting at the end of eighteen months, the deputy-physician-superintendent revealed a rapid rise in the admissions rate. Patients were no longer turned away. The yearly discharge rate climbed to more than 90 per cent, while the resident population declined 7 per cent. During this period, 56 chronic patients who had been in the hospital more than two years were able to leave. A much better feeling toward the institution had developed in the community. All this was accomplished without a substantial increase in the staff or in the cost per patient.[16]

The transformation in the approach to mental deficiency was no less noteworthy. As therapeutic centers, the mental deficiency hospitals increasingly recognized that treatment and not detention should receive the emphasis. The admission of a patient was usually determined not so much by the degree of the defect as the absence of intelligent and sympathetic care at home. According to the most advanced views on the subject, mental deficiency should not be considered so much a disease as a "state of social incompetence" that responded in some degree to treatment if it was begun early enough. Some authorities even held that there was no fundamental difference between mental deficiency and mental illness. The same causes, it was argued, operated in both cases, but with the mental defective they began earlier and thus led to a more catastrophic result— arrested mental development. It was estimated that a careful application of the present techniques of therapy to mental defectives could result in the ultimate discharge of at least half the patients, of whom not less than 30 per cent would be able to live at home and not less than 20 per cent to do some type of productive work.

Improvement in the condition of mental defectives was often painstakingly slow. Habit training was followed by the teaching of simple activities. Elementary handicrafts were taught and then more complicated ones. Each stage had to be reached gradually. The use of coercion was scrupulously avoided. Instruction was given in cleanliness, correct speech, proper dress, and leisure-time pursuits. Occupational, social, and group therapy were utilized. When the individual had progressed sufficiently, he was granted more freedom. He could visit his home and do simple shopping in the stores. Those who could were allowed to obtain work near the hospital and eventually to move to a hostel. Seeking always to discover and develop every facet of intelligence in the patient, the hospital continued to supervise his activities until he was decertified and returned to the community.[17]

The transition from the sheltered existence of the mental deficiency hospital to independence in the outside world could not be made too abruptly, and for that reason hostels were maintained as a part of the hospital service. A patient well on his way toward recovery might spend several weeks or months in a hostel, where he would no longer be under the influence of the hospital ward and where living conditions more closely approximated those in the community. Here by stages he would acquire self-reliance, so that, upon being discharged to his home or to suitable lodgings provided by the local health authority, he could more easily make the adjustment.[18]

An important group of mental patients and one that promised to grow even larger consisted of those sixty-five and older. During the first nine years of the Health Service, the admission of such persons rose 84 per cent. Attracting the closest attention of the hospital authorities, this group came to represent one-fifth of all admissions and a third of the resident patients. It was apparent that many of those who had become residents of mental hospitals need not have been there. Surveys revealed that nearly one-fourth of these elderly patients were more suited for the chronic sick hospitals or old people's homes. Some could have been returned to the community if relatives or the local health authority had accepted the responsibility for their care.[19]

The shift of the mental hospital from its traditional role of asylum or place of detention to the role of institution for the treatment and rehabilitation of the mentally sick could not be achieved at once. The inertia of the past and large fiscal needs tended to slow down the transition. Other hospitals and units would have to relieve the mental institutions of custodial work and such phases of treatment and rehabilitation as could be performed more appropriately elsewhere. The Ministry of Health accordingly favored the establishment of short-stay psychiatric units and long-stay annexes. The former would serve in the diagnosis and short-term treatment of aged patients. Few of these were created. Long-stay annexes were designed for elderly patients who required psychiatric supervision and special nursing care but not the special treatment available in the mental hospitals. More than a score of long-stay annexes, with a total of nearly 2,500 beds, were in operation by 1957, and there were similar units attached to the mental hospitals that performed the same function. But it was apparent that much more would be necessary to cope with the rising rate of elderly admissions to mental hospitals. The problem would have to be attacked on a broader front.

Day hospitals and outpatient psychiatric departments had demonstrated their usefulness. Equally important was the need for more effective co-ordination between the chronic, general, geriatric, and mental hospitals so as to insure that these institutions received the type of patients for which each was designed. The role of the general practitioners, the voluntary associations, and the local health authorities could be of tremendous importance in easing the hospital patient load.

The mental hospitals proved that a great deal could be done for elderly patients. The old theory that all hope should be abandoned when an aged person entered such an institution was exploded by statistics. The death rate among the elderly in mental hospitals was reduced by one-fourth, and the annual discharge rate of elderly persons rose to 40 per cent. For some categories of mental illness, such as senile psychoses, which involved the progressive deterioration of the mind, the psychiatric services had the least to offer. This type of mental illness showed the highest incidence of death. But for affective psychoses which represented a "sustained depressive or manic symptom complex," the proportion of patients discharged was high. Nearly 50 per cent of all cases of mental illness among the aged belonged to this group.[20]

Mentally ill children who required treatment and care were admitted to special units, most of which were administered by a neurosis or mental hospital but were in buildings separate from those used by adults. In 1958, there were nearly a score of these units in England and Wales. Others were planned, but since the number of children requiring institutional treatment was comparatively small, there was little need for many units. The result was that it was often necessary to send a mentally ill child far from home. That arrangement had the unfortunate effect of reducing the number of visits from friends and relatives.[21]

Between existing facilities and those contemplated there were areas in which experiment was required to help charter the best course. The new approach to mental health implied further change and still better techniques. Many organizations and agencies, some public and others private, were active in helping to shape the future pattern of mental health. Among these were the Nuffield Provincial Hospitals Trust and the King Edward's Hospital Fund for London. Reflecting the growing interest in the new role of the mental and mental deficiency hospitals, these non-profit foundations allocated substantial sums to a carefully selected list of projects which often had a beneficial impact upon the hospital service out of all proportion to the actual financial outlay.

The Nuffield Provincial Hospitals Trust, in collaboration with a regional hospital board, opened a residential home for deaf children who were emotionally disturbed. Elsewhere, in co-operation with various authorities, statutory and voluntary, this organization established a number of special cerebral palsy units. In addition to the Worthing venture, which has already been mentioned, the Trust helped to finance an experimental Day Hospital Service for mental defectives. Other projects included an occupation center, a social psychotherapy center, a work therapy unit, and a special unit for the treatment of mental defectives who suffered from severe neurological conditions. The Trust also sponsored a study of the effects of incentives on long-stay psychotic patients at one of the leading mental hospitals.[22]

The King Edward's Hospital Fund for London was eager to initiate improvements in occupational therapy, catering, social and recreational facilities, and amenities for patients and staff. Club rooms, cafes, day hospitals, sport pavilions, residential annexes, gardens, and social centers were of special interest to this foundation. In 1958, the Fund made sixteen grants totaling £159,250 ($445,900) to help meet some of the current needs of the mental and mental deficiency hospitals. Most important of all the Fund projects was the establishment of a social therapy center and a pioneer psychiatric center.[23]

There was a difference of opinion about what the role of the general medical practitioner should be in the mental health program. Since most family physicians had little, if any, training in psychotherapy and had been tutored in the traditional concepts of medicine, they were not qualified to work in the field of mental health and had no desire to do so. The great majority were much too busy to apply the complex techniques of psychiatry, even if they had known how. Yet it was also evident that it was especially important for the practitioner to be able to distinguish accurately between psychological and physical disorders. If the physician were unable to help the patient, others would do so, and early treatment could be started.

In the lay and medical press there was a sharp interest in the subject of the family doctor and mental health. The Report of the College of General Practitioners in 1958 reflected this new attitude. The importance of psychiatry and the part it could play in general practice were stressed. In the medical schools, more time was given to mental health, and the students were able to observe psychiatric patients treated in the general and teaching hospitals. Postgraduate refresher courses were offered in this field, and the response was encouraging. In many areas, psychiatric clinics and case conferences were attended by family physicians. The Tavistock Clinic, the most widely known of all, gave practical training in psychiatry to many doctors.[24] Significant as was this trend, it should not be assumed that the average family physician was showing much interest or enthusiasm in psychotherapy as a technique useful in his practice. But the medical schools had it within their power to modify this attitude among future doctors, and there was some indication that this was happening.

One of the main changes accomplished by the National Health Service was to impose upon the local health authorities a greater responsibility in developing their domiciliary services. The entire trend in the Health Service, which the Royal Commission on Mental Health and the new law on mental health strongly supported, was to keep in the community all patients who did not actually require the type of institutional care and treatment that only the hospitals could give. An adequate program of care and after-care by the local health service would reduce the number of persons who otherwise might become hospital inpatients and would facilitate the early discharge of inpatients and reduce the readmission rate. Aside from the monetary savings such a policy might produce, it was deemed better for the patient to be treated in the community, amid familiar surroundings, if his condition permitted. To do this, the local health authorities had to provide clinics, home nursing, domestic help, hostels, residential homes, and training and occupational centers. Valuable allies were to be found in the general practitioner service, the outpatient psychiatric departments, and the domiciliary consultant service—all financed by Exchequer funds.

The best results could not be achieved without a close liaison between the community and hospital services. The effectiveness of this co-operation was largely a voluntary matter, depending upon the willingness of the local health and hospital authorities to work out a plan. In many areas the relationship was only perfunctory, but in others there was excellent collaboration. With full encouragement from the Ministry of Health and the Royal Commission on Mental Health, the trend was toward a closer working arrangement among the principal parties that were responsible for the care and treatment of mentally disordered patients. In 1956, the Report of the Mental Health Advisory Committee of the Central Health Services Council pointed out that such a policy "would enable co-ordinated arrangements to be made whereby new patients, according to need, could be sent to a mental or geriatric chronic sick hospital, to welfare accommodation, or left in their own homes, with possible attendance at a day hospital."[25]

One of the most successful examples of the co-operative approach in the treatment of mental illness was achieved at York. Begun as an experiment in 1953, the scheme won wide commendation. It was designed to integrate closely the work of the local mental health and welfare departments with that of the psychiatric hospital. A mental health center was created under a joint mental health subcommittee representing the York City Council and the hospital management committee. Both the Medical Officer of Health and the superintendent of the mental hospital kept in active touch with the center, and the health visitors, the psychiatric social worker, the assistant psychiatrist, and other staff workers met there for weekly case conferences. The status of patients to be discharged as well as those who had already left the hospital was carefully reviewed. Local problems affecting mental patients were likewise considered. The mental health center was also used for care and after-care services, for outpatient treatment, and as a club for ex-patients. Financed jointly by the local health and hospital authorities, this comprehensive service was believed to be less expensive than the haphazard arrangement that had formerly existed.[26]

A scheme started even earlier was the one at Oldham, in the Manchester area. The local health authority and the regional hospital board shared the services of a psychiatrist, who worked closely with the Medical Officer of Health. The outpatient clinics at the hospital as well as case conferences in the local health offices were attended by the staff of social workers. The local authority provided adult industrial and occupation centers, while the hospital authorities provided domiciliary consultation. Most significant was the day hospital, which drastically reduced the admission of patients to the wards.[27]

Any appraisal of what was achieved in mental health by the local health authorities would be difficult in view of the variety of the services they provided. In some phases of mental health, however, considerable progress was made. Most noticeable were the occupation and training centers for mental defectives. When the Health Service began, there were slightly over 100 of these centers. Within ten years, the number had more than tripled. Combined with similar part-time centers, they were able to accommodate over 15,000 individuals, or nearly four times more than at the outset. By 1958, only a few local health authorities were without such centers, but there was a need for more facilities. At first, only limited provision was made for mental defectives over 16 years of age, but more training centers were subsequently furnished for adults. Makeshift quarters were used during the early years, but later buildings specifically erected for the purpose were made available. Children and adults with subnormal intelligence who could not benefit from the regular educational system were admitted to the occupation and training centers where a special staff under general medical supervision endeavored to help each individual develop as much as possible. In 1960, 53 new training centers were opened and plans for 37 other centers were approved. By the end of that year, 84 per cent of the mentally subnormal children in the community who were deemed suitable for training were getting it.[28]

A substantial number of mental defectives remained in their homes, and over such persons the local health authorities exercised supervisory control. In addition to regular visits by appropriate staff workers, social centers or clubs provided a varying amount of guidance. Holiday excursions were occasionally arranged for the patients and their parents.

During the first decade of the Health Service, few occupation or social centers were provided for mental patients. Such activities remained principally the function of the hospitals. The after-care of mental patients was largely shared with the hospitals, great dependence being placed upon the outpatient service. Psychiatric clubs were established in many parts of England, but in general the contribution of the local authorities to the rehabilitation of mental patients was meager. The shortage of properly trained mental welfare officers was particularly unfortunate.[29] Meals on wheels, home help services, and other domiciliary aids were furnished in varying degree to aged mental patients who resided at home. A shortage of personnel and funds rendered these services less than adequate, but much was accomplished—a subject that will be explored in a subsequent chapter.

Providing residential facilities for the elderly, infirm, and handicapped persons was the responsibility of the local authority, and during the first ten years of the Health Service the number of persons thus accommodated increased more than 70 per cent. So great was the demand that often there were no beds for mentally ill patients who were ready to leave the hospital. Overcrowding and obsolescence characterized many of the welfare homes, but conditions steadily improved. The passage of time saw many of the dwellings modernized and new ones constructed. Reinforced by the day hospital, the outpatient department, the domiciliary consultant, and the local health and general practitioner services, the residential home and the hostel were viewed as playing a major part in the prevention and after-care of mental illness.[30]

It became the stated goal of the government, through substantially larger financial grants, to foster the expansion and improvement of residential accommodations, to encourage the building of more hostels as well as occupation and training centers, and to improve the general quality of the local mental services. In 1955-56, the expenditure of the local health authorities on mental health was less than £26,785,000 ($75 million). Nearly twice as much was spent in 1959-60, and a further increase was provided for the following year.[31]

A small proportion of mentally ill and mentally defective patients were furnished living quarters through agreements with voluntary organizations. Voluntary associations assisted at occupation centers, and they furnished short-term care and recreational facilities for patients. The National Association for Mental Health offered courses for the training of staff workers at occupation centers and, in addition, opened specialized homes for mental defectives. The Mental After-Care Association maintained more than a score of residential accommodations for the mentally ill. Such groups as the British Red Cross, the Order of St. John, the Women's Voluntary Services, and the National Leagues of Hospital Friends were helpful in many ways. Their services in the mental and mental deficiency hospitals and in the domiciliary field eased the work of nurses and other staff workers and proved of incalculable value in making institutional life more cheerful for the patients and in helping them to adjust to normal living in the community.[32]

If the mental health program had made substantial gains during the first decade, it promised to achieve much more during the next ten years. Two milestones pointed the way—the Report of the Royal Commission on Mental Health, published in May, 1957, and the Mental Health Act of July, 1959. With a few minor exceptions, the second document translated into law the recommendations of the first, and both reflected in a more explicit way the new and enlightened spirit that had shaped the British approach to mental health since the mid-1940's.

Under the chairmanship of Lord Percy of Newcastle, the Royal Commission labored for three years in the preparation of its report. The warm response which greeted the document showed that the nation was in agreement with the findings. Certain anachronisms had survived from the past and these, the Commission urged, should be removed so as to bring practice more into line with theory. The mental health service had not yet achieved full integration with the National Health Service. This could largely be accomplished, the Commission believed, by abolishing the designation of the mental and mental deficiency hospitals and permitting patients with mental illnesses or defects to be admitted for treatment with the same informality as all other patients.

The role which the hospital and the local authority should fulfill in the mental health program was sharply defined in the Report of the Royal Commission. The local health authority should accept full responsibility for the preventive services and should provide all types of community care for patients who did not require continued nursing attention or specialist inpatient treatment, or who, having been inpatients, no longer needed these specialized services. The Commission declared that it should be the duty of the local government to provide diagnostic clinics, hostels, and other residential accommodations, as well as occupational, training, and social centers for all mentally disordered persons who stood in need of such care. Regular case conferences between the local authority personnel and the hospital staff were advocated as the most appropriate way to decide what form of care and treatment was best suited to the needs of the individual patient.

The expansion of the medico-social services in the counties and county-boroughs was one of the few proposals of the Commission that required no new legislation, although the Mental Health Law was to make the Commission's intent unmistakable. Its Report centered upon the local health services, and around the recommendations in this area hung all the other recommendations. The local authorities had been negligent in providing preventive treatment and after-care for all mentally disordered patients. Responsibility for the care of mental defectives had been accepted as mandatory by the local governments, but mental patients were left largely to the jurisdiction of the hospital. This situation, it was emphasized, must be changed. All patients should be treated with the same measure of consideration. The Minister of Health, who already had the authority, should require the local health authorities to assume this obligation.[33]

The Minister of Health did not wait for the enactment of the new law, but in spring, 1959, issued a circular recommending expansion of the local health authority services in accordance with the suggestions of the Royal Commission. The county and county-borough councils were reminded that co-ordination of the hospital, general practitioner, local health, and welfare services could be effected through case conferences and the joint employment of medical staff and social workers. Reference was made to the pressing necessity for hostels and occupation centers that would meet a wide variation in individual needs. It was revealed that at the end of 1958 only one-half of the mentally defective adults who needed help in a training center were receiving it.[34]

More definite action was taken immediately after the passage of the Mental Health Law. In a directive, the Minister required the local authorities to provide services, including residential accommodations, for every category of mental patients. The local authorities were instructed to submit to the Minister by April, 1960, proposals as to how they planned to carry out their new duties.[35]

The certification of patients was another anachronism which the Royal Commission wanted abolished. Only when absolutely necessary should a mentally ill person be held against his will; and to insure the individual against wrongful detention a new system of safeguards was necessary. Admission and discharge for all other patients should be voluntary. The removal of the stigma of certification would encourage patients in need of psychiatric treatment and nursing care to seek it in the same spirit that other patients sought surgical treatment in a general hospital.[36]

It was believed that the voluntary policy would tend to eliminate the worst features of the old system, under which patients were sometimes kept in custody long after the need had passed. The press gave publicity to several tragic cases of individuals who had been unlawfully held for years in mental institutions because they were friendless and had no one to intervene in their behalf. In 1957, the matter of unlawful detention was aired in Parliament and in the annual meeting of the National Council for Civil Liberties in London. While recognizing that mistakes were made—in a widely cited case, a woman who was released after seventeen years of illegal detention—the government denied that the rights of any person had been willfully violated. There were, of course, hundreds of individuals who stayed on because they had no place to go and the local authorities would not assume responsibility for their care.

The alleged abuses under the mental deficiency laws doubtless gave the government all the more reason for welcoming the decertification of patients and the dedesignation of the hospitals. These policies were proclaimed as a big step forward in giving greater protection and freedom to patients and in finding a more wholesome way to deal with mental illness. The Ministry of Health could even view the new approach as "a great adventure."[37]

It had been the policy of the government to permit voluntary admission only for mental patients who were capable of signing an application form. Mentally deficient persons were all certified. Early in 1958, the Ministry of Health decided that it had the authority to permit the informal admission of mental defectives. Circulars were then sent to the mental deficiency hospitals recommending such a policy as standard procedure and requesting a review of the certification of all patients. By the end of 1958, one-half had been decertified and accorded the status of voluntary patients. Over 60 per cent of the new admissions in that year were voluntary, which meant an almost complete reversal of the old procedure for mental defectives. A similar policy for mental patients had to await the adoption of the new law. Mental hospitals were then enabled, as the normal method of admission, to receive patients without formal commitment, and steps were taken to decertify all patients who could be given voluntary status. Such persons were then privileged to leave the hospital when they wished.

Into the new mental health law went the most careful planning. Nearly five and one-half years elapsed from the appointment of the Royal Commission to the final adoption of the law. The enactment was evolutionary, in the sense that it gave legal sanction to the accepted trends, with increased emphasis upon the expanding role of the com-

munity mental health service.   The act was also revolutionary in
effecting drastic changes in some of the administrative and procedural
aspects of mental health.   Both compulsory segregation and designation were brought to an end.   The distinction between the mental and
mental deficiency hospitals and all others was abandoned, and mentally disordered patients could enter any hospital for treatment on a
voluntary basis.   No person could be coercively detained except in
his own interest or for the protection of society.

Elaborate safeguards protected the patient against wrongful detention.   Except in an emergency, two medical recommendations
were required to admit a patient to a hospital under compulsion.
One of the doctors had to have some knowledge in psychiatry, while
the other, if possible, had to have a previous acquaintance with the
patient.   In each hospital region, a voluntary Mental Health Review
Tribunal was set up.   Comprising a medical, a lay, and a legal member chosen from a panel, this agency had as its purpose the protection
of the liberty of the individual.   The patient could appeal periodically
to this tribunal, which had the authority to order the person released.
The power of discharge also could be exercised by the doctor who
treated the patient or by the managers of the hospital.   The nearest
relative likewise had the right to obtain the release of the patient if
he was not considered dangerous.   In the case of psychopaths and
subnormal patients under the age of twenty-one, obligatory detention
was permitted for purposes of treatment, but these persons could not
be held after the age of twenty-five unless they were deemed to be
a threat to society.   They would then have the right of appeal to the
tribunal.   As a further safeguard against abuse, the authority to de-
tain a patient, unless renewed, terminated at the end of fixed periods.

A new terminology was established, and such designations as
mental defective, idiot, moral defective, and imbecile were no longer
to be used.   Four categories of patients were recognized: mentally ill,
severely subnormal, subnormal, and psychopathic.   Defectives who
were not aggressive were classified either as subnormal or severely subnormal, depending on their condition.   The psychopathic category
included those with a persistent mental disability which resulted in
"abnormally aggressive or seriously irresponsible conduct."   In the
treatment of the mentally ill and the subnormal, a less rigid division
was recognized than had been applied previously.   The Lunacy and
Mental Treatment Acts and the Mental Deficiency Acts, which had
served England for so many years, were repealed.   Henceforth, the
same set of basic procedures would be applicable to all patients with
mental disorders.[38]

Among other important changes was the abolishment of the Board of Control, whose functions were divided between the Minister of Health, the local and hospital authorities, and the Mental Health Review Tribunals. Jurisdiction over registration and inspection of nursing homes and private and charitable hospitals was transferred from the Ministry of Health to the local authorities. Rampton, Broadmoor, and Moss Side were to be administered directly by the Minister of Health, but these institutions did not become a part of the Health Service. Under the old procedure, a judicial order was required for the detention of all mentally disordered persons. This practice was abolished, but the courts retained the power to send a patient to a hospital or put him under guardianship when ordinary penal measures seemed to be inappropriate or ineffectual.[39]

Such were the more pertinent provisions of the Mental Health Act. It represented a monumental achievement—the culmination of more than a half century of legislation and experimentation in the field of mental health. The measure was a bipartisan triumph. It enjoyed the solid backing of the medical profession and the public. It was recognized, however, that the success of the program would largely depend upon the co-operative efforts of many groups and agencies. Even with adequate financing of the community and hospital phases, a transitional period of some duration would be necessary to bring to full fruition the goals set forth so well in the Report of the Royal Commission on Mental Health. There were some observers who felt that the pendulum might swing too far in the direction of early discharge from the hospital to community care, but the prevailing spirit was one of genuine optimism about what the new policy could offer to those whose lives were blighted by mental illness.

CHAPTER XIII

Hospital Personnel and the Welfare of the Patient

BEFORE THE ADVENT of the Health Service, the uneven distribution of specialists and the relatively high fees they charged greatly restricted their usefulness. Many of the patients who were confined to their homes because of serious illness or disability could not afford the services of a consultant. Some gratuitous work was done by the specialists, but this approach was never adequate, nor did people want charity. General practitioners frequently had to do without the judgment of a medical expert in cases in which it was most needed.

The new health program provided a domiciliary consultation service free to all patients who for medical reasons could not go to the hospital. The service was recognized as a major step in facilitating closer relations between the hospital, the specialist, and the general practitioner services. The scheme, moreover, proved economically advantageous. Many of the patients that were attended in their homes did not have to seek admission to the hospital where the cost of their treatment and care was much higher. The interests of all were thus served, but the family physician seemed to gain most from the arrangement. He was now able to deal more effectively with difficult cases and to keep under his jurisdiction patients who otherwise would have become hospital inpatients. In exercising his right to call upon the aid of a specialist, the general practitioner was put under no obligation, as previously was sometimes the case when the consultant visited a patient unable to pay his fee. The general practitioner and the specialist now worked as equals, and through mutual co-operation they could offer more to the patient.

In 1949, there were 130,000 consultative visits in the homes and over 5,000 specialists available for such work. Ten years later, the total of such visits had more than doubled while the number of consultants under contract for domiciliary visits had increased 35 per cent. The great preponderance of the work was diagnostic and advisory, with the operative procedure being employed in only a small minority of cases.

Virtually every specialty was represented in the domiciliary consultation service. General medicine and general surgery together accounted for 60 per cent of the visits in the first year of the program, but this proportion declined to 47 per cent by 1958. Gynecology and obstetrics also lost some ground in relationship to the other specialties but remained among the four most important. Such specialties as psychiatry, traumatic and orthopedic surgery, pediatrics, radiology, geriatrics, and diseases of the chest showed surprising gains. They represented in 1958 nearly 30 per cent of all domiciliary visits, compared with less than 15 per cent during the initial year of the service. Although neurology, neuro-surgery, thoracic surgery, radiotherapy, physical medicine, and plastic surgery remained among the specialties less frequently employed in the domiciliary field, they also enjoyed increases during the ten-year period.[1]

The day-to-day administration of the domiciliary consultation service was at first entrusted to the hospital management committees. Lists of the available specialists were furnished to all general practitioners, who applied to the hospital bureau whenever there was need for a domiciliary consultation. Because this machinery proved cumbersome and ineffectual, it was largely abandoned in 1951. Thereafter, the general practitioner was authorized to address his request directly to the specialist of his choice. The consultant had to be under contract for such work, but approval was not required to arrange a visit by him. If no one of consultant status were available, then a qualified senior hospital medical officer could be summoned. The domiciliary consultation service now became the sole responsibility of the regional hospital board, to which the specialist submitted all claims for remuneration. If there were irregularities, the most practical control was to withhold payment of the fee.[2]

During the early period of the Health Service, domiciliary consultations were handled almost exclusively by part-time consultants, who were paid a fee for each visit. Although such work was considered a part of the duties of whole-time consultants, they usually preferred not to do it, since they were busy with a full schedule of regular hospital assignments and received no extra remuneration for domiciliary consultation. The Spens Committee made no distinction between whole-time and part-time consultants in recommending additional compensation for domiciliary visits. In 1955 the medical Whitley Council accepted a modified version of this approach by agreeing that fees should be paid to whole-time consultants after the first eight visits in any quarter. Many of these specialists were now willing to participate in the domiciliary program, although they objected to the policy of having to do a number of "free" consultations. The Pilkington Commission in 1960 could see little logic in the arrangement, but nevertheless refused to recommend any change in the basis of payment or the amount of the fees, which the medical profession contended should be increased substantially.[3]

A visit initiated by a hospital to supervise treatment or to investigate the urgency of a proposed admission to the wards was not considered a domiciliary consultation. To qualify for the fee, a specialist had to go to the home of the patient at the request of the general practitioner and normally in his company, the purpose being to give advice on diagnosis or treatment. The amount paid for a visit was 4 guineas ($11.76), with an additional payment if a portable X-ray or electro-cardiograph apparatus were used or there were an operative procedure. Where more than one consultation occurred in the same residence, the rate of payment was reduced for all but the first patient. Provision was made for travel expenses. The maximum which a specialist could earn in a year from domiciliary visits was 800 guineas ($2,352), but comparatively few ever received that much from this source and most of them fell far short of it.[4]

The success of this phase of the Health Service was recognized by most observers, and in the opinion of many it was comparatively free of abuse.[5] The Select Committee on Estimates, however, became concerned in 1957 about the rapid increase in the number of domiciliary consultations, which raised the question of excessive visits. The absence of an appreciable number of general practitioners from domiciliary consultations also aroused misgivings. Not all family physicians were convinced that it was always necessary for them to be with the patient during the visit of the specialist, whose advisory opinion could be communicated by telephone. But the terms of service more or less required that the family doctor be present, and general medical opinion seemed to endorse such a policy.[6]

There appeared to be little evidence of any serious irregularities. The Ministry was keenly aware of the difficulty of ascertaining abuse, since what was concerned was "essentially a question of clinical judgment in individual circumstances at a particular time." The officials at Savile Row took the view that the domiciliary consultation service was experiencing a healthy and necessary growth, the effect of which was to reduce the demand for hospital beds. Where examples of abuse were reported, medical officers from the Ministry were authorized to make a personal investigation and take appropriate action.[7]

Significant as were domiciliary consultations, they represented only a minor phase of the work done by specialists. The scope of the inpatient service has already been noted, but even more important was the outpatient service, if the criterion is the number of individuals examined and treated. In 1960, four million inpatients were discharged from the hospitals, compared with three times that many new outpatients who received courses of treatment. Including casualty cases, outpatient attendances in that year totaled nearly 42 million.[8]

To a large degree, the outpatient service was the cornerstone of the entire medical edifice. The advisory opinion and the special skills of the specialist were indispensable to good doctoring. The consultant was potentially an effective link between the major divisions of the Health Service. In helping to keep people from becoming inpatients or making it possible for inpatients to be discharged earlier, the consultant strengthened the role of the general medical practitioner and the local health authority by permitting more patients to remain in the community.

Although the experience of doctors varied, that of a general practitioner in Kent may not have differed greatly from many others'. In 1957, 13 per cent of his patients required radiological and pathological investigations. Another 7 per cent were referred to consultants, but less than half of these were admitted to the hospital.[9] Ross's survey of a factory town disclosed that about 6 per cent of the population annually made use of outpatient clinics.[10] During the first decade of the Service, the number of new outpatients increased 13 per cent. In some specialties the rate of growth was much larger. In gynecology it was 27 per cent; in the medical departments, 33 per cent; in mental health, 50 per cent; and in obstetrics, nearly 80 per cent.

In removing the deficiencies that initially characterized the outpatient departments of many hospitals, the Ministry of Health systematically enlarged this phase of the hospital service. In 1960, the number of specialists (whole-time and part-time) was 7,416, or 39 per cent more than twelve years earlier. The rate of increase in the number of specialists was much higher during the early years than later. The growth in the number of consultants in the five largest divisions during the twelve-year period was: general surgery, 10 per cent; general medicine, 37 per cent; anesthetics, 80 per cent; pathology, 60 per cent; and mental health, 67 per cent. Radiology experienced an increase of 61 per cent; orthopedic surgery, 53 per cent; and pediatrics, 42 per cent. The expansion in the ear, nose and throat specialty was 11 per cent, while in ophthalmology it was only 2 per cent. Two of the smallest departments showed the most phenomenal development of all: plastic surgery and thoracic surgery, each over 110 per cent. The size of the specialties in 1960 ranged from 37 consultants in infectious diseases to 883 in general medicine.[11]

Not all the hospitals maintained on their staffs consultants from every specialty, but there was a fairly equitable distribution of those whose services were normally required. A peripheral institution that was too small to support certain specialties had access to the larger hospital centers within the area. Wherever possible, the hospital group was made self-sufficient in all but the more rarely used specialties, which were available in key institutions.

Plastic surgery, for instance, was new and existed in comparatively few hospitals. Prior to World War II, it was a negligible element of British medicine, but war casualties increased its importance. Several new centers sprang up, and by 1960 there were 58 plastic consultants in the Health Service. The scope of the work was broadened to deal with burns and injuries, and facial blemishes that constituted a serious handicap.[12]

Two cases involving Americans came to the attention of the author when he was in England. A girl four years of age, the daughter of an officer in the United States Air Force, sustained terrible burns over most of her body when her gown caught fire from an electric heater. An eminent plastic specialist in London began the difficult task of grafting skin, and the work was done with consummate skill. Because of the recurrent growth of scar tissue, the girl was likely to have to submit to plastic surgery for many years. The officer told the author that he dreaded the prohibitive cost that would be entailed when he returned to the United States. In England there was no charge. The other case involved a Fulbright scholar who was touring England by car when he had a head-on collision near Stranraer. He, his wife, and an eight-year-old daughter were severely injured. The child required the services of a bone surgeon and a plastic surgeon, and all three of the victims were destined to spend considerable time in the hospital. Again, they bore none of the cost themselves.

Only the major hospitals were staffed with specialists in thoracic surgery, neurosurgery, neurology, and dermatology. A wide range of dental care was made available to hospital patients, but staff shortages made it impossible to put all patients in a state of dental fitness. Every effort, however, was made to achieve this goal for long-stay patients. In 1959 there were 260 dental consultants in England and Wales who took care of oral surgery and handled the major dental operative treatment in the Health Service hospitals. In that year, there were 440 fully equipped dental departments in the non-teaching hospitals. Within a six-year period (1953-59), the number of weekly dental sessions in all the hospitals increased over 50 per cent. In the field of orthodontics, remarkable progress was made in providing consultant advice and treatment in most of the hospital regions.[13]

Nearly one-third of all outpatient attendances were treated by the casualty department. Largely because of the antiquation of the buildings in which this department was housed, the casualty service was subject to unfavorable criticism. Owing to the distance between the reception halls, the X-ray departments, and the wards, there were dangerous delays. The same nurses and doctors frequently served a great variety of cases, and in turning to a newly arrived patient, the staff did not always function as a well-integrated team. Yet considerable progress was achieved during the first decade, with many new casualty departments being established. Some thoughtful observers felt the casualty work should be left to the better equipped hospitals in each group, where highly trained teams of specialists, radiologists, anesthetists, nurses, and blood transfusion experts, with the most modern facilities, could concentrate on this type of work. Such a policy, however, was not favored by the smaller hospitals.[14]

As noted in an earlier chapter, some of the work done in outpatient clinics seemed to belong by rights to the general practitioner. The Guillebaud Committee stressed that the outpatient department should be largely consultative and that all cases which the family physician was competent to handle should be returned to him for treatment. In the opinion of the Select Committee on Estimates, this policy was not always followed. But if the outpatient service were improperly used, there was little awareness of the fact among patients, who seemed well satisfied with the character of the treatment they received. In the Ross survey, for instance, only one-half of one per cent had any complaint about their experience in the outpatient clinics.[15] It can be assumed that the outpatient departments deserved a share of the credit for the low admission rate of inpatients. In the early 1950's, the rate was 78 per thousand of the population in England and Wales, compared with a much higher figure for the Scandinavian countries.[16]

Non-urgent outpatient cases often involved a delay of two weeks, depending on the specialty and the hospital, but some clinics were able to reduce the maximum waiting time to one week. While a waiting period of even a fortnight was not objectionable to most patients, an unduly long wait in the reception room was a source of irritation. As a result of a memorandum issued in 1954 by the Ministry of Health, the hospitals reviewed their procedures and the vast majority were able to reduce the average waiting time to 30 minutes. The so-called open clinic system and block method of appointments yielded in most institutions to a system of individual appointments or appointments for not more than two or three patients within a given period.[17] The appointments scheme worked smoothly enough for the most part, although the absence of some patients led to a policy of scheduling somewhat more appointments than could comfortably be accommodated. In 1958, a report by the Hospital Organization and Methods Service verified the fact that the practice of scheduling patients too early to offset possible absences was the major cause why some individuals had to wait so long. The report indicated that if more than one-fourth of the patients waited over 30 minutes or if more than 3 to 5 per cent waited over an hour, the appointments situation warranted a careful investigation.[18]

Chest clinics were in a special class, owing to the necessity of taking X-rays and processing the film before the consultation. The minimum time required on the premises for old patients was 30 minutes and for new patients an hour. Because of failures to coordinate the various stages in the clinic procedure, some patients were detained two to three hours. The need for more careful planning and timing so as to eliminate bottlenecks was urged in 1959 by a report on chest clinics.[19]

Many hospitals made considerable improvement in the reception and guidance of outpatients by using lay receptionists and voluntary workers. Putting patients at their ease was primarily the work of the receptionist, and where this was done there were fewer complaints over the appointments system. In some hospitals, the patients were also furnished with literature which explained hospital procedure and gave other helpful information.[20]

In reviewing the progress achieved in the hospital service during the first decade, Lord Moran, former President of the Royal College of Physicians, was much impressed with the new and improved status of the consultants. Especially noteworthy were their redistribution, the increase in their number, and their availability "without financial anxiety" to domiciliary patients. It was the decentralization of the specialists, he observed, that made possible the nationwide improvement of the hospitals. The remuneration and distinction awards meant that the specialist's "material prosperity now depended on his professional efficiency."[21]

Dr. Ffrangcon Roberts, in his evaluation of British medicine, spoke of the specialists, or a majority of them, as having achieved "affluence" in the Health Service. He referred to their earlier plight by way of contrast. Only by serving ten or more years in junior appointments at a pittance was it possible for the specialist to secure an honorary appointment in a hospital. When such an appointment was obtained, which was seldom before the age of thirty-five, it took several years to gain a reputation and through it a lucrative private practice. Even then, the position of the specialist remained precarious because of relentless competition, and unless he was able to distinguish himself, his income usually dwindled at the age of sixty. Under the Health Service the picture was much brighter. The junior hospital posts had become much more remunerative. Consultant status brought the payment of a good basic income at once and of an attractive pension upon retirement.[22]

But acquiring the coveted title of consultant was no easy achievement. At the outset of the Health Service, it was necessary in each hospital region to appoint small committees of eminent specialists, some of whom were retired, to assist in the difficult task of determining which doctors were qualified to be consultants. Many months were required to complete the assessment. Not all who did the work of a specialist were deemed worthy of the formal appointment as one. The title of senior hospital medical officer was used to designate those who could perform clinical duties but whose training was not considered sufficiently comprehensive or rigorous to merit consultant status.

Once the Service became stabilized, a fixed pattern took shape. Whoever aspired to become a consultant had to follow a long and arduous road. In the case of general and special surgery, three years of post-graduate study and a year or so of practical experience were required before the doctor was permitted to take the final F.R.C.S. (Fellow of the Royal College of Surgeons) examination. If successful, he underwent one or two more years of surgical training before becoming a senior registrar. Not less than four and sometimes six or more years in this post were necessary before the election to a hospital staff as a consultant came about. Since appointment was for an unlimited tenure, subject to retirement at sixty-five, or in some cases seventy, years of age, there were usually few openings. Each vacancy had to be advertised, and competition often was severe. Being qualified was no guarantee of an appointment. Very few consultants were elected before the age of 32, and many were 40 years or older when they received their appointments.[23]

A survey in the South-East Metropolitan Region during the period from 1952-56 disclosed that the length of training for consultant status, which included 2 or more years of military service, averaged between 12 and 16 years after qualification as a doctor. A senior registrar had one chance in three of becoming a consultant.[24]

Many who thus spent years in the hospital service were unable to realize their ambition. Some, having become senior hospital medical officers, could go no further, while others seemed to be frozen as senior registrars. The post of registrar was at first primarily regarded as a training grade, but the tremendous need for registrars in the hospital service soon caused the post to be regarded more as a staff grade. Although senior registrars remained potential consultants, this grade was overstaffed, especially during the early years of the Health Service when the demand for specialists was greatly overestimated. Having completed four or five years of training as senior registrars, many doctors were faced by the frustrating realization that there were no openings for them as consultants. Known as "time-expired" senior registrars, some stayed on in hospital work, while others emigrated or became general practitioners. The number of senior registrars was finally brought under central control, the normal period of service was increased from three to four years, and a better balance was achieved. But the problem did not disappear.[25]

Lord Moran on one occasion referred to the hospital posts as a ladder reaching toward consultant status. He said that "all people of outstanding merit, with few exceptions, aimed to get on the staff." But many fell off the ladder. While admitting that some family physicians were "men of extreme ability" and that economic conditions forced off the ladder doctors who were competent to climb, he left the impression that, generally speaking, those who failed to attain consultant status were somewhat inferior in ability and qualification. Since he was chairman of the Merit Awards Committee and a man with a distinguished reputation in medicine, the statement created a furor in medical circles. Quite obviously, it was too broad a generalization, since there were many, including foreigners, who held short-term junior hospital posts for training purposes and who had no aspiration to become consultants.[26]

What was the hierarchy of hospital grades? At the very bottom was the house officer post, which involved routine medical work and ran for six months. To qualify as general practitioner, a doctor had to hold two of these appointments, normally one in a medical post and the other in a surgical post, although a midwifery post could be substituted for either of them. Above the house officer grade were six others—senior house officer, junior hospital medical officer, registrar, senior registrar, senior hospital medical officer, and consultant. Their duties were never sharply defined.

The post of senior house officer was open to any doctor who had completed 12 months as house officer. The appointment carried some additional responsibility and was for one year only, although some general practitioners held more than one of these posts. The junior hospital medical officer grade was occupied during the early period of the Health Service by doctors who were not specialists or in training to be specialists. The tenure was often, but not always, of limited duration.

The other grades have already been the subject of comment, but a word more should be mentioned about the senior hospital medical officer, whose tenure, unlike that of the senior registrar, was unlimited. Although this grade presumably required less clinical skill than the consultant possessed, the work done was frequently indistinguishable from that of the highest grade. In view of the disparity in remuneration, the senior hospital medical officer was not happy about his status. But there was no evidence to bear out the allegation that this grade was a blind alley, since several hundred senior hospital medical officers were elected to consultant posts during the late fifties. The ratio was one such promotion for senior hospital medical officers to every two for senior registrars.

The grade of consultant accounted for well over one-third of the entire hospital medical staff. Next numerous were the registrars and house officers, who together totaled less than the number of consultants. By the end of the first decade, all grades except senior registrars and house officers became more numerous, some substantially so. The number of registrars had increased 85 per cent, while the number of senior house officers showed an even more spectacular growth.

In only two grades was there an apparent shortage. Most serious was the lack of sufficient registrars who, in spite of the phenomenal increase in their number, were unable to meet the demand in certain areas. Had it not been for a high proportion of doctors from overseas who wanted the experience in this grade, the situation would have been much more critical. Among consultants, the alleged shortage was not so obvious except in such specialties as pathology, anesthetics, radiology, and psychiatry.[27] The Willink Committee found no appreciable dearth of consultants. The Ministry endeavored to maintain a systematic and balanced expansion in the various specialties, but the need could not always be anticipated or the demand adequately met.

The shortage of junior hospital staff did not seem as serious to the Willink Committee as it did to some. The Committee predicted that the deficiency would be made good partly by younger doctors staying longer in the hospital service and partly by more general practitioners undertaking part-time hospital work.[28] Those who thought the problem grave noted that it seemed to show little improvement in the years that immediately followed the Willink Report. The non-teaching hospitals, especially the peripheral ones, were the most seriously affected by the shortage.[29]

It was apparent to many that the staffing arrangement could be improved and that the existing grade structure should be carefully reviewed. The shortage of registrars, the somewhat anomalous position of the senior hospital medical officers, and the problem of time-expired registrars were most in need of investigation. In summer, 1958, the Ministry of Health and the Joint Consultants' Committee set up a working party to study "the principles on which the medical staffing structure in the hospital service should be organized."

In the meantime, steps were taken to improve somewhat the plight of the two grades that gave cause for the greatest concern. Senior hospital medical officers who undertook work commensurate with that performed by consultants were paid a larger salary than those who did not. Senior registrars unable to secure a higher post were retained in their grade, pending the report on the staffing structure. A limited number of designated senior registrar posts with security of tenure and a higher rate of pay were created for senior registrars who had completed their training. These appointees were free to compete for higher appointments.

Under the chairmanship of Sir Robert Platt, the Joint Working Party on the Medical Staffing Structure in the Hospital Service completed its report in December, 1960. While recognizing the key role of the consultant, the report also noted his dependence upon the assistance of other doctors, some of whom needed hospital training in preparation for a different type of medical career and some of whom wished to make a permanent career of hospital work. For the latter, the Working Party proposed a new grade of unlimited tenure—medical assistant. It was proposed that the training arrangement for senior registrars should be improved and that the senior hospital medical officer and the junior hospital medical officer grades should be discontinued as part of the permanent staffing structure. The most striking fact that came out of the investigation was the large proportion (41 per cent in 1960) of hospital doctors among the registrars and other lower grades who were born outside Great Britain.[30]

At the very top of the hospital medical staff stood the consultant. The facilities of the hospital were at his disposal. He was assisted by a team of skilled workers, but the ultimate responsibility for the treatment and care of the sick rested on his shoulders. Appointed by the regional hospital board, he was not subject to local pressure. He had complete clinical freedom. Tenure was unlimited, subject to compliance with the terms of service, though a contract could be terminated for a post at a particular hospital if there were no longer need for the specialty. Prior to 1959, a person who thus lost his job had to compete openly with others for a new appointment, but regulations were amended in that year so as to permit any regional board to re-employ such a consultant on a non-competitive basis.[31]

This more flexible approach grew out of an important case involving a consultant who was wrongfully dismissed. The individual, a gynecologist employed by the Manchester Regional Hospital Board, was discharged in spring, 1952, for his alleged failure to comply with the terms of service. His professional technique in an operation was under question, and he was charged, as well, with having failed to give sufficient information in death certificates and to issue birth or death certificates in respect to certain premature births. In resisting what he considered to be a grave injustice, he waged a prolonged fight that lasted seven years. A panel of experts appointed by the regional board eventually exonerated the consultant of any culpability, and a high court of justice awarded him over £7,150 ($20,000) to cover unpaid salary and damages for breach of contract. Pressure exerted by the medical profession and others cleared the way for new employment rules and the reappointment of this consultant to another post.[32]

The consultant grade was unique in the sense that the overwhelming majority (approximately three-fourths) of the doctors in it were part-time employees. Only a few of the senior hospital medical officers were under part-time contract, and in the lower medical grades part-time employment was of negligible importance. Being in a position to bargain, the consultants at the outset demanded and obtained a statutory prohibition against the introduction in the hospitals of whole-time employment for all specialists. The Ministry of Health did nothing to discourage part-time employment, and even urged regional boards, subject to the needs of the hospital service, to let the successful appointees decide on what basis they preferred to work and to permit whole-time consultants to change to a part-time schedule if they wished. The trend at first favored full-time and later part-time employment, but at the end of the decade there had been relatively little change in the ratio. Nearly two-thirds of all the work done in 1959 by consultants in the hospitals was accomplished on a part-time basis.[33]

Part-time employment had its advantages. The right to engage in private practice was denied to those under full-time contract. Except for a few well-established specialists, however, the financial gain from this source was comparatively small, and for the younger men it was almost nonexistent. Yet the doctors, influenced by the traditional pattern of medical thinking, continued to equate private practice with professional freedom and a high standard of performance. There seemed to be a feeling that part-time service carried with it higher professional and social prestige.

The part-time consultant with a private practice could claim tax-exemption on automobile, equipment, and office expenses, whereas the whole-time consultant could not do so, since the facilities required for his work were supposed to be furnished by the hospital. Part-time consultants, it will be recalled, were paid for all domiciliary visits, whereas those who worked whole-time received no fee for the first eight visits each quarter. Consultants under part-time contract received travel expenses from their home or office to the hospital and back (up to ten miles each way) and were paid for travel time (up to one-half hour each way). Whole-time consultants were granted none of these benefits.

Even more important was the method of computing part-time remuneration. All hospital work was expressed in terms of notional half-days. A notional half-day was the equivalent of three and one-half hours of work, which need not be performed in a single session. The full-time consultant was required to spend eleven notional half-days in the hospital per week; the part-time consultant was allowed a maximum of nine. In computing the time of the part-time specialist, a special weighting was used that was based upon the recommendation of the Spens Committee. The consultant who did not work full-time, it was held, should be paid proportionately more of the whole-time rate, owing to the "continuous responsibility for the patients in his charge, which must extend beyond the limits of the time he contracts to serve."

The regional board accordingly estimated the number of hours per week, including travel time, needed by an average doctor to discharge the duties attached to the part-time post. The number of hours per week assigned to the consultant was then divided by three and one half to get the number of notional half-days, but any fraction left over was counted as a whole half-day. Thus any time over three and one-half and up to seven hours was recorded as two notional half-days. Each notional half-day was allowed one-eleventh of the whole-time basic rate of pay, plus a fraction varying from one-quarter to three-quarters. An estimated working time of three to eight notional half-days carried the maximum fraction, which meant that a specialist working not less or more than this period of time would receive over £215 ($600) per year more than the proportionate amount paid to the whole-time consultant.[34]

The disparity in the rate of pay was even greater prior to April, 1954. In one large hospital region, the evidence indicates that the part-time consultant was then paid 33 per cent more than the full-time specialist per notional unit of work. Where several part-time specialists were involved, each working only a few sessions per week, the differential between part-time and whole-time cost for the same amount of work was as much as 80 per cent. Even the maximum-part-time specialist could be very expensive, but when he performed the same duties as the full-time specialist there was little variation in the cost.[35]

There was a difference of opinion about the relative merits of part-time appointments. Critical voices were raised in Parliament and elsewhere. Although the Socialist Medical Association favored a full-time hospital service, the medical profession as a whole did not support such a view. The testimony presented before the Guillebaud Committee and the Royal Commission on Doctors' and Dentists' Remuneration was largely opposed to the abolition of part-time contracts.

Among the arguments against part-time service was the assertion that it fostered a divided loyalty between the consultant's private practice and his work for the hospital service. From the floor of the House of Commons came the statement that in the "opinion of well informed circles . . . the payment of a consultant by the session encourages him to keep his out-patients' department fully occupied and his beds full."[36] The cost factor seemed to be the most effective point cited, but there were other and less persuasive allegations—that part-time service contributed to the abuses associated with pay-bed facilities, for instance.

The advocates of part-time service noted that without such an arrangement, many eminent consultants would have refused service in the hospitals. The improvement of the hospital service, especially in the more remote regions, was achieved, they observed, through the co-operation of part-time as well as whole-time consultants. They claimed that emergency cases requiring surgery and skillful treatment were often dealt with more effectively and at less cost by two part-time specialists than by one full-time consultant. They called attention to the fact that a large proportion of the part-time specialists worked more hours than were required by their contracts—a practice, of course, just as common among whole-time consultants.[37]

The Guillebaud Committee recognized that part-time consultant appointments were in the best interest of the hospital service but held that the financial arrangement should be no more attractive for part-time than for whole-time employment. The Pilkington Report, appearing four years later, was in agreement with that point of view, but went further by specifically condemning such practices as weighting and the payment of travel expenses to and from work. It did not, however, advocate the immediate abolition of such benefits, in view of the hardship which such a course might inflict. The report recommended that they be withdrawn gradually, so that future appointees would mainly be affected.[38] The implementation of this proposal seemed reasonably certain after the government and the medical profession indicated acceptance of the Pilkington Report.

At least 60 per cent of the part-time consultants were under contract for nine notional half-days per week (the maximum permitted), while 85 per cent worked six or more. All but a small part of the income of such consultants came from hospital contracts, the remainder being derived from sundry sources such as domiciliary visits, private practice, instruction in the medical schools, and services for insurance companies, other agencies, and hospital boards with which the doctor had no contract. The greater flexibility of earning capacity enjoyed by part-time specialists may explain why their income was usually larger than that of full-time consultants. During the 1956 fiscal year, for instance, their income averaged £3,600 ($10,000), which was £600 ($1,680) above the level received by whole-timers.[39]

Just as the general medical practitioners found remuneration to be an issue, so did the hospital medical staff, and for the same reasons. The fifties as already noted, were a decade of inflation, straitened government finances, and economic adjustment. Twice during those ten years hospital doctors demanded higher pay, and like the general practitioners, they obtained a satisfactory revision both times, but only after a frustrating delay. The lessons learned from the two major conflicts were not lost on the government and the medical profession. The Pilkington Report cleared the way for new machinery which, as explained in an earlier chapter, promised a more rational and peaceful adjustment of compensation issues for dentists and medical doctors.

The two controversies over remuneration did not disrupt the hospital service or foster any real ill will between the personnel and the Ministry of Health. To the hospital medical staff and especially the consultants, the National Health Service had proved a great boon. A comparison of the status of the hospital doctor before and after the Health Service quickly dispels any doubts in the matter. The Spens Report on the Remuneration of Consultants and Specialists provides ample data on their earlier economic position. In order to determine the proper range of professional compensation for specialists and those who aspired to that grade, the Ministry of Health in 1947 set up the Consultant Spens Committee. Reporting in 1948, this group laid the basis for the salary scale in the various medical grades of the hospital service. The recommendations it submitted were the result of an examination of the status of the hospital doctors in the prewar era.

The Spens Committee observed that the prewar specialist, having waited years for an appointment, was willing to serve on the staff of a voluntary hospital with little or no pay. Whatever his age, he "had to face the risks, hardships and uncertainties involved in the effort to build up a private practice." The Committee also took cognizance of the trying and often hopeless financial struggle of the junior staff members, whose difficulties were "progressively accentuated throughout the training period." Those who lacked private funds had to turn to outside work. Many who would have preferred to become specialists, unable or unwilling to pay the high price in effort and privation, were forced to leave the hospital service and find a career in general medical practice.

The Spens Committee took the view that "in a public service intending specialists . . . should not be called upon to pass through a stage of comparative penury and hardship," nor "should they be tempted to spend too much time in supplementing their income from other sources when they could be more suitably occupied in their professional studies." The potential specialist, it was emphasized, should be paid a salary commensurate with the "growth in his skill and the increasing responsibility of his work." His remuneration should be "maintained at a consistent level until the age of retirement is reached," and he should "enjoy financial security in marked contrast with the uncertainties of private practice." To draw the "best possible recruits," the Spens Committee felt that for a "significant minority" there should be given "the opportunity to earn income comparable with the highest which can be earned in other professions."

The Spens Report proposed what was deemed an adequate salary scale for the various grades and, in addition, recommended merit grants for consultants who distinguished themselves. Three levels of merit wards were proposed: £2,500 ($7,000) for a total of 4 per cent of the specialists; £1,500 ($4,200) for 10 per cent; and £500 ($1,400) for 20 per cent. Under the provisions of the Report, the most outstanding specialists would command from salary and merit payments a maximum income of £5,000 ($14,000).[40]

The Report was promptly accepted by the medical profession and the Ministry, but the terms and conditions of service had to be worked out. It was also necessary to make adjustment in the proposed rate of remuneration, which was based upon the monetary values of 1939. By the middle of 1949, an agreement was reached providing for a 20 per cent increase in the pay scale. The interim contracts that were signed by the consultants in 1948 now yielded to permanent ones, and hospital staffing was placed on a more secure basis.

What had been judged sufficient remuneration in 1948 was considered inadequate a few years later, however. To offset the steady depreciation in money values, the consultants in June, 1952, asked for an adjustment in compensation. Four months previous, the pay controversy of the general medical practitioners had been happily adjudicated by Justice Danckwerts. A precedent had been set for the betterment of medical salaries, but the claim of the consultants was nevertheless rejected by the government, which was primarily concerned about the dangers of inflation. The government was unwilling to agree to arbitration, in view of the high cost to the Exchequer that had resulted from the Danckwerts award. Within the framework of the Whitley Council system, negotiations dragged on until spring, 1954, when an acceptable revision in remuneration was adopted.[41]

The inflationary spiral continued to erode the salaries of the consultants, who in 1956 made common cause with other members of the medical profession in seeking a further boost in income. The vicissitudes of the struggle as it affected the British Medical Association and more particularly the general practitioner have already been treated and need not be reviewed here. It should be mentioned, however, that the controversy, which spanned nearly four years, resulted in two interim increases for hospital doctors as well as general practitioners. In 1957, the hospital junior medical staff received a 10 per cent raise in pay, while the senior staff got 5 per cent. In the early part of 1959, both were granted an additional 4 per cent increase. Then in 1960 came the long awaited report of the Royal Commission, which in general recognized the validity of the claim of the British Medical Association for a substantial improvement in remuneration for all medical doctors.[42]

In gathering data, the Royal Commission took a careful look at comparative professional incomes in 1955-56. The total career earnings for consultants between the ages of thirty and sixty-five averaged £3,342 ($9,357) per year. Consultants, then, had the highest professional incomes. Second highest were actuaries, and then came the hospital doctors. Below them were barristers and solicitors. Next were the general medical practitioners and the general dental practitioners, both averaging £2,257 ($6,319). Architects, surveyors, engineers, and university teachers all ranked lower in total career earnings, but graduates in industry had a somewhat larger yearly average than general medical practitioners.

The median income for consultants at their peak earning capacity (age fifty-five to sixty-four) was the highest received in all professions in that or any other age group. The median income for general medical practitioners at their highest period of earnings (age forty-five to fifty-four) was exceeded in that age bracket only by consultants, hospital doctors, and actuaries. The median earnings for dentists at their best years (age forty to forty-four) were surpassed in that age category only by consultants and hospital doctors.

In surveying all factors, the Royal Commission was of the opinion that the earnings of dentists and doctors in 1957 had been too low. During the two subsequent years, the incomes of doctors, hospital dentists, and, to a smaller extent, general dental practitioners did not increase as much as incomes in commerce, industry, and the other professions. The young doctors had been underpaid to a greater extent than the older ones, but this was not true of the young dentists.[43]

The increase in remuneration (above the 1956 level) that the Royal Commission proposed for the hospital medical staff was between 40 and 58 per cent for the junior hospital grades, but only from 21 to 26 per cent for consultants. House officers would receive £675 ($1,890) the first year, and £750 ($2,100) the second, and a comparable increase would be provided in the third year. For senior house officers, the pay would be raised to £1,050 ($2,940) if they were under the age of twenty-eight or £1,100 ($3,080) if they were twenty-eight or older. Registrars, who were considered underpaid "both absolutely and in relation to senior staff," would receive under the new scale £1,250 ($3,500) the first year and £1,400 ($3,920) the second and any subsequent year. To ease the plight of the time-expired senior registrar, provision was made for eight annual increments, the new salary rising from £1,500 ($4,200) to £2,100 ($5,880). The remuneration of the senior hospital medical officer, who also was deemed inadequately paid in comparison with the other grades, would begin at £2,000 ($5,600) and rise to £2,700 ($7,560). If he were in a consultant's post, the additional £550 ($1,540) that had already been granted would give him a maximum income of £3,250 ($9,100).

The minimum pay for whole-time consultants was £2,550 ($7,140). Beginning at the age of thirty-four, there would be nine annual increments, boosting the maximum basic salary to £3,900 ($10,920). Distinction awards, which had undergone no change since originally proposed, would now be increased to £3,000 ($8,400) for "A" awards, £1,750 ($4,900) for "B" awards, and £750 ($2,100) for "C" awards. One hundred "A-Plus" awards of £4,000 ($11,200) each were proposed as an additional inducement for achievement. The consultant who had made an especially noteworthy record in the field of medicine could now look forward to a possible annual maximum of £7,900 ($22,120). Few persons elsewhere in professional life could ever hope to reach such a level of earnings in the British Isles.

The new salary schedule was to become effective on January 1, 1960. No provision was made for retroactive pay as such, but a lump sum of £9 million ($25,200,000) would be distributed to rectify the underpaid status of hospital doctors and dentists from March, 1957, to the beginning of 1960.[44]

The upward revision of compensation would affect the amount of the retirement pension. The superannuation arrangement for part-time specialists was the same as that for the general practitioners. For whole-time hospital medical doctors, the pension was calculated on a different basis. One-eightieth of the average annual remuneration for the last three years of employment was multiplied by the total years of service (up to a maximum of 45) to determine the annual pension. Since whole-time consultants and other hospital doctors usually reached the peak of their earnings just before retirement, such an arrangement worked to the interest of these individuals. But for part-time specialists and general dental and medical practitioners, whose peak income was more likely to be attained in the middle of their lives, the other basis for computing the pension was deemed more equitable. This, it will be remembered, was 1.5 per cent of the total compensation received during the entire period of employment in the Health Service. So satisfactory was the superannuation system that it invited no serious criticism from hospital doctors or others.[45]

Perhaps the most noteworthy aspect of remuneration in the hospital service was the distinction awards. They were available to a total of 34 per cent of the consultants and, once granted, were payable until the recipient retired or reached the age of seventy. They were, moreover, included in the calculation of the retirement pension. The probability of a consultant receiving one of the awards at some time during his career was as high as 43 per cent, if he entered the grade in his mid-thirties. Most of the "A" awards were won by those in the fifty and above age group, while the other two awards were extensively conferred in the forty to fifty age group. A surprising number of "C" awards were even given to consultants under forty years of age.

In order to insure a just distribution throughout England and Wales, the awards available each year were divided equally between London and the provinces and subdivided in proportion to the number of consultants in each region. Deaths, resignations, and the annual increase in the total body of consultants determined how many awards would be made in any one year. In 1960, for instance, 404 were conferred. The total held in England and Wales at the end of that year was 88 "A plus" awards, 265 "A" awards, 707 "B" awards, and 1,413 "C" awards.

The merit awards system was administered by a standing advisory committee of fifteen persons, virtually all medical men, who were nominated by such bodies as the Royal Colleges, the Medical Research Council, and the universities. Under the chairmanship of Lord Moran, the committee established the program on a sound and impartial basis. In order to determine which consultants were entitled to recognition, the chairman and members of the advisory committee annually visited all the hospital regions and conferred with hospital committees and various key figures. Consultants who seemed most deserving were carefully screened and interviewed. Other sources were tapped, such as the Royal Colleges, which appointed their own committees to canvass for eligible candidates. In each specialty the merit awards committee had assessors. Acting upon the decision of the advisory committee, the Minister of Health made the appointments. Actual payment of the awards, however, was left to the boards of governors and the regional hospital boards.

The distribution of merit awards left a variable pattern, however equitable it may have been. In the Liverpool Hospital Region only 27 per cent of the consultants held awards in 1958; in the London Metropolitan Regions, 39 per cent; and in most of the others, 30 per cent. Consultants in the teaching hospitals possessed 54 per cent of all the awards, and they also accounted for 85 per cent of the "A" awards and 67 per cent of the "B" awards. Only 14 per cent of the consultants in the field of mental health and anesthetics had awards in that year, compared with 63 per cent in the field of neurology and thoracic surgery. In plastic surgery, general surgery, and general medicine, more than 50 per cent of the consultants had been honored, but in radiology and dentistry only 21 per cent. As between part-time and whole-time consultants, awards seemed to have been conferred without discrimination. The amount of the distinction award under a part-time contract was in proportion to the number of notional half-days of hospital service.[46]

All awards were given in an absolute secrecy that caused resentment in some quarters. Some members of the profession—so it was reported in the House of Lords—referred to the condition as "diabolical secrecy."[47] The Annual Representative Assembly of the British Medical Association in 1957 moved that "in any revision . . . of the medical services there should be no secrecy about any special payments made for merit."[48] But those who understood the workings of the program were convinced that secrecy was essential. The Royal Commission shared this opinion in so far as the names of the award-holders were concerned, but held that the policy had been carried to extremes in withholding statistics which showed the distribution of awards by specialties and regions. By publishing facts hitherto unknown in these matters, the Royal Commission set a precedent. The refusal to divulge the names of the award winners was largely based on the feeling that such publicity would not serve the best interests of hospital harmony.[49]

Some favored replacing merit awards by responsibility payments, but this would have completely altered the entire basis of the program. Seniority, rather than outstanding achievement, would then have been rewarded. A motion favoring such a policy was adopted by the Representative Assembly of the Medical Association in 1956, but the Council chose to shelve the proposal. The Central Consultants' and Specialists' Committee rallied unanimously in support of the system as it existed. While it was recognized that "some of the criteria of merit are necessarily subjective" and that there was a possibility of favoritism, the consensus was that distinction awards furnished special encouragement for good work. Those in private practice could vary their fees according to their professional standing and most employees in other fields could anticipate promotion, but whole-time consultants did not have the benefit of either of these incentives. In appraising all factors, the Royal Commission came to the conclusion that "the awards system is a practical and imaginative way of securing a reasonable differentiation of income and providing relatively high earnings for the 'significant minority.' "[50]

The medical and dental staff represented only 4 per cent of the half-million employees that were part of the hospital service. The professional and technical staff other than nurses and doctors constituted another 4 per cent, the administrative and clerical staff 7 per cent, and the nursing and midwifery staff 43 per cent. The remaining 42 per cent embraced a heterogeneous group, which included maids, ward orderlies, porters, cooks and other members of the kitchen staff, laundry workers, carpenters and other artisans, members of the cafeteria and canteen staff, stokers, linen room employees, garden laborers, telephone operators, engineers, and operating theatre attendants.

The professional and technical staff represented over a score of grades, the most numerous being physiotherapist, radiographer, medical laboratory technician, occupational therapist, pharmacist, almoner, assistant in dispensing, and darkroom technician. Except for chiropodists, ophthalmic opticians, and speech therapists, only a negligible part of the work done by the professional and technical staff was on a part-time basis.[51] Some of the grades, such as radiographer, physiotherapist, and hospital pharmacist, suffered from a shortage of personnel during the latter part of the 1950's. In the case of pharmacists, the retail trade had been more remunerative for qualified pharmaceutical graduates, but in 1960 hospital work for such persons became more attractive owing to the higher rates of pay established by the Whitley Council. Other grades also were beneficiaries of better salaries.[52]

In 1960, Parliament established seven of the medical ancillary services on a professional statutory basis. This action involved the dietitians, occupational therapists, chiropodists, physiotherapists, X-ray technicians, remedial gymnasts, and medical laboratory technicians. Prior to the adoption of the law, these professions existed on a rather informal basis, but now general standards were prescribed. Each profession was to have its own registration board, and over all would be a supervisory council representing the seven professions, the medical doctors, and the government. The registration boards would determine such matters as the training courses and the qualifications for registration. A code of conduct would likewise be formulated, with disciplinary procedures.[53] As these professions were given a more responsible constitution, the hospitals stood to benefit, as did the entire Health Service.

All divisions of the hospital service experienced a healthy expansion in man power during the first decade. The professional and technical staff (non-medical and non-nursing) led all others, with an increase of slightly over 50 per cent. The medical staff (including consultants) was next highest, with a growth of approximately one-third. Close behind were the domestic and maintenance staff and the nursing and midwifery staff. The smallest increase in personnel, about 25 per cent, was registered by the administrative and clerical staff.[54]

The nursing staff was not only the largest numerically but the most expensive in the hospital service. In the 1958-59 fiscal year, it absorbed over 40 per cent of the salaries and wages, and one-fourth of all hospital maintenance expenditures.[55]

At the outset a big shortage of nurses existed, but as the years passed it grew less serious. Recruits for the nursing profession became more numerous, and the number of trained nurses during the first decade increased by 35 per cent. Yet not all the hospitals were fully staffed. The growing supply of nurses never overtook the demand, which expanded even more rapidly. The reasons were obvious enough—the larger number of inpatients, the reduction in nurses' hours, and the greater claims that the advances in medical practice and surgery made upon the nurses' time.

In seeking to enlarge the nursing force, the government was confronted by a high drop-out rate among student nurses. The hospital service not only needed more recruits but more students who would complete training and make a career of nursing. In the campaign to enlarge the supply of nurses, the responsibility for the publicity and central recruiting activities at first rested primarily with the Ministry of Labor and National Service. In 1957, however, this duty was transferred to the Ministry of Health, although the Ministry of Labor and National Service continued to operate a placement and advisory service for nurses. In carrying out its new assignment, the Ministry of Health was served by the National Advisory Council on the Recruitment of Nurses and Midwives.

Prior to 1957, the Ministry of Health restricted its publicity activities to the circulation of general information about nursing and midwifery, including remuneration and the conditions of service. Under the new arrangement, the Ministry broadened its activities. Regional hospital boards were urged to establish local recruitment plans, to provide career talks, to organize mental health exhibits, and to staff mobile nursing recruitment exhibits. Assisted by the Central Office of Information, the Department of Health distributed literature, slides, films, posters, and other display material. In seeking to combat the shortage of nurses in the mental and mental deficiency hospitals, the Ministry expanded its program of public enlightenment on mental health matters. Leaflets were issued describing mental nursing and the new approach to mental illness. So successful was this phase of the campaign that in 1958 the hospital authorities began to shift the recruiting emphasis to other categories of nurses that were in short supply. The three nursing exhibition vans that toured the country in that year were visited by organized groups from nearly 500 schools.[56]

The nursing service no longer lacked recruits, whose number was enhanced by the rise in the birth rate which began in the early 1940's. Popularly referred to as the "bulge," the higher birth rate had its first impact upon the employment market in 1958. With applicants becoming more plentiful, the Ministry now began to urge a more selective policy of recruitment. The fact that an estimated nine out of every ten girls aged 16 would marry before the age of 30 could only mean a heavy loss of student and trained nurses, irrespective of the most careful policy of recruitment.

The employment of young persons between fifteen and eighteen years of age in hospitals came under critical review. While actual nursing training did not commence until eighteen, the early introduction to hospital work, it was believed, would stimulate interest in a nursing career. The work assigned to such juveniles, however, was not always appropriate to their age. In 1954, the Ministry of Health issued a memorandum providing that the practice of using juveniles on nursing duties should stop and that more emphasis should be placed upon their taking educational courses. Young persons should remain in school.[57]

It was quite obvious that the improvement of working conditions would strengthen nursing as a career. The Report on the Work of Nurses in Hospital Wards by the Nuffield Provincial Hospitals Trust in 1954 disclosed that trained nurses had to do considerable work (some of it administrative and non-bedside) that could be done as well by less skilled personnel. Too much of the nurse's time was spent away from the patient. The situation was further aggravated by a lack of labor-saving devices in many of the hospitals and an insufficient supply of nursing equipment. The re-assignment or elimination of certain routine tasks and the revision of the working hours was urged by the Report, which recognized that the "whole nursing care of the patient" should remain the primary concern of the nursing profession.[58]

Corrective action was eventually taken in many of the matters stressed in the Report, but some of the proposals could be achieved only after being carefully tested. The recommendation that the total nursing care of a limited number of patients should be left to a definite group of trained nurses became the basis of a series of experiments in a selected group of hospitals. Known as group assignment, this plan was at variance with the traditional procedure (work assignment) under which the individual nurse was charged with one specific portion of the care of many patients in the ward. The subcommittee of the Standing Nursing Advisory Committee, which supervised the experiments, was so impressed with the results that it advised the introduction of group assignment into the hospitals as soon as feasible. This system, it was averred, "should have the effect of raising standards of training and nursing care, reducing wastage and improving the status and satisfaction of the nursing staff."[59]

Improved nurses' homes replaced many of the substandard ones, and in virtually all of them amenities were added. More important was the reduction in working hours and the increase in pay. By 1956, no day nurse worked more than 48 hours per week. A recommendation by the Nurses and Midwives Whitley Council in spring, 1958, caused a large proportion of hospitals to introduce the 44-hour week. In many institutions, nurses who took their turn at night duty were still required to work 12 hours, but a report by the Royal College of

Nursing in 1958 strongly urged a reduction of night duty to 8 hours, and it appeared only a question of time before this reform would also be adopted.[60]

The scale of remuneration varied according to the size and type of the hospital. A series of pay increases over the years carried the pay scale to a level that for matrons in 1961 ranged from a minimum of £805 ($2,254) per year in the smallest non-training hospital to a maximum of £1,565 ($4,382) in the largest nurse-training institution. The comparable figures in that year for a nurse in charge of a ward were £605 ($1,694) and £850 ($2,380), respectively; and for a staff nurse, £485 ($1,358) and £675 ($1,890). Student nurses in general hospitals received a minimum of £285 ($798) per year and a maximum of £320 ($896), but those in mental hospitals were paid an additional sum of approximately £150 ($420).[61]

Like other Health Service workers, the nurses were reasonably well protected in their jobs, and if discharged had the right of appeal. During the early part of 1960, a matron was dismissed after twenty years of service for refusing to apologize for a letter she had written criticizing the efficiency of the hospital management committee. She appealed her case to the regional board. After a three-hour hearing conducted by an appeals committee, the board decided that the nurse had been unjustly fired and instructed the management committee to reinstate her. If the regional board had ruled against the matron or had refused to hear her appeal, she could have carried the case to the Minister of Health.[62]

The nursing profession was in a position to protect its interests. Two organizations served the nurses—the General Nursing Council, a statutory body, and the Royal College of Nursing, a voluntary association. The former agency, some of whose members were elected by the nurses themselves, determined the conditions for admission to the nursing register. The inspection of hospitals that trained nurses and the supervision of syllabuses and examinations were also a part of the work done by the General Nursing Council. The Royal College of Nursing was the professional association of the trained nurses. As the bargaining agent of the nurses, it sought higher wages and improved working conditions. The Royal College was also interested in obtaining a uniform standard of training, a better selection of student nurses, and more specialized training and post-certificate study. In full support of these aims, the General Nursing Council advocated the reintroduction of an educational entrance test for student nurses and the provision of more clinical experience in their training.

Three years of training and two examinations (the preliminary and the final) were prerequisites that had successfully to be met before a student nurse could qualify as a state registered nurse. There were lower grades of nurses, of course—the nursing auxiliaries, the nursing assistants, and the enrolled assistant nurses. They did much of the practical and less specialized work in the wards and were toward the bottom of the salary scale for the nursing staff. Among these categories, the enrolled assistant nurse had to undergo the most training. She was useful in all hospitals, but the chronic sick institutions had the greatest need for her services. It was thus a source of disappointment to the hospital authorities that recruitment for this grade, unlike that for the others, had not met much success. A report in 1954 attributed the lack of interest in this type of nursing to the absence of incentives. Corrective action was proposed. In 1959 and 1960, the downward trend seemed to be reversed in view of a 6 per cent increase in the number of enrolled assistant nurses.[63]

In the training of nurses, extensive use was made of films covering such subjects as the prevention of cross infection, techniques of lifting patients, blood transfusion, antibiotics, neuro-psychiatry, and the importance of gaining an insight into the problems of the patient. In an effort to offer nurses more diversified training and to encourage closer relations between the general and special hospitals, the Ministry of Health resorted to an important innovation in the early 1950's. Student nurses in general hospitals were invited to take part of their training in tuberculosis sanatoria, and later the program was expanded to include mental and mental deficiency institutions. The scheme did not prove popular, and only a small minority of general nursing students were willing to go into the special hospitals. But those who went benefited greatly, and some became interested in taking supplementary training.

Other experimental training schemes emerged. A combined course of study was set up to prepare a student nurse for both general and mental nursing. Integrated training was also offered that qualified the individual nurse for health visiting and midwifery as well as general nursing. The Queen's Institute of District Nursing in 1957 announced a new plan which would enable a student in one comprehensive course lasting four years to train as a district nurse, health visitor, and general nurse. An additional six months of training would also qualify the student to become a state-certified midwife.[64]

Nurses, like doctors, were encouraged to take postgraduate courses. Hospital officials could grant nurses leave of absence with pay to do advance study. A substantial number of nurses benefited from instruction offered by the Royal College of Nursing.   Short courses were arranged by some of the regional hospital boards.   The King Edward's Hospital Fund, a pioneer in this field, annually scheduled refresher courses for staff nurses and ward sisters.   The courses, all well attended, varied from a few weeks to several months in length, while one of them, designed especially for administrators, took a year. The training of prospective matrons in the Residental Staff College stood out as one of the most noteworthy contributions of the Hospital Fund to the National Health Service.[65]

The foregoing discussion of nursing indicates a willingness to experiment where experimentation was necessary.   A sense of purpose and a feeling of pride were the mainsprings behind the drive of that profession to improve the quality of the hospital service.   It is a matter of some significance that what the nurses have done and are doing in the general and special hospitals throughout England and Wales has attracted as observers a steady stream of foreign visitors.[66]

Hospital personnel, especially the medical staff, were faced by the problem of legal liability for malpractice.   In the early 1950's, the courts began to put a new interpretation upon the law of negligence. Whereas the policy had been to make hospital doctors the sole defendants in liability suits, the courts now took the view that the hospital itself, as the employing agent, had to share responsibility and could also be sued.   The principle was clearly set forth in the case of *Cassidy v. Ministry of Health* (1951).   Following an operation on a patient's hand, the surgeon had failed to give the necessary medical attention, with the result that the hand was left useless.   The hospital involved in the unsuccessful operation was also made a defendant and held liable by the courts under the doctrine of vicarious liability or responsibility.

The Health Service itself was in no way implicated in this particular decision, since the negligence had occurred prior to 1948, but the defendant hospital was a local authority institution and the defendant doctor was employed by it on a full-time salaried basis.   Since the specialists and other staff members in the Health Service hospitals were also paid employees, the Cassidy Decision made their employers—the regional boards, the boards of governors, and the management committees—fully subject to the doctrine of vicarious responsibility.   In so far as the law of liability was concerned, the courts could see no difference in the relationship between the medical staff and these administrative bodies and that which existed between servants and employers anywhere.

The number of claims against hospitals and their staffs increased sharply during the first five years of the Health Service.   There was no evidence that this trend was due to any deterioration in medical treatment or to any decrease in the standards of care. The fact that hospitals as well as staff members could now be sued seemed to encourage more suits. Some people who would have hesitated to start legal proceedings against a voluntary hospital may have viewed the state-operated institutions as fair game in seeking damages. More important, certainly, was the Legal Aid and Advice Act of 1949, which furnished assistance to those who previously could not afford litigation.[67]

The medical profession viewed this situation with alarm. The specialists were afraid that the doctor-patient relationship would be jeopardized by the growing claims against the hospital authorities, who, to protect themselves, might impose bureaucratic controls and otherwise seek to interfere with clinical freedom. The doctors preferred to retain full responsibility for the treatment of their patients and to be the sole defendants in any liability suits for negligence. In this way, it was felt, their professional freedom could be effectively safeguarded. In 1956, the Representative Assembly of the British Medical Association went on record that it did not believe it was in the "best interests of British medicine and the British people that the hospital doctors in the country should have the legal status of technical servants of the hospital authority." The Central Consultants' and Specialists' Committee took a similar stand.[68]

Hospitals that had to pay liability claims endeavored to recover as much of the money as possible from the defendant doctor. If a settlement could not be reached out of court then the hospital authorities would resort to legal action—a procedure that was viewed in some quarters as undermining the mutual good will that prevailed between the regional boards and the senior staff members. To protect their interests, the doctors and dentists turned to defense societies for legal protection against liability claims. Two such organizations existed in England and Wales, the Medical Protection Society and the Medical Defence Union. The latter, which was the larger, had a membership in 1958 of over 45,000.

In spite of the forebodings of the medical profession, the doctrine of vicarious liability in practice did not appear to pose a very serious threat to the professional independence of the consultants, nor did it affect the general relationship between the medical staff and the hospital. As the years passed, the matter receded as an issue of importance. Several factors contributed to this decline. In 1954, Parliament imposed a three-year statutory limitation upon claims for damages arising from negligence in the hospital. Action not taken within that period presumably faced dismissal from the courts. In the same year, the medical profession, the defense societies, and the Ministry of Health arranged that any claim by a hospital against a doctor for the purpose of sharing damages would be settled out of court. If no agreement could be reached in determining the apportionment, then each automatically would pay 50 per cent of the amount. The dental profession accepted the same scheme, which seemed to work very well for all parties.

The belief that access to clinical records would be flagrantly misused was not sustained by the daily operation of the hospital service. While the medical history and other pertinent data concerning a patient was the property of the hospital, it was the view of the Ministry of Health that as a general policy such records should not be made available to any other agency without the knowledge of the specialist and permission of the patient. The Ministry assured the British Medical Association in 1949 that if a doctor were subject to a liability suit for defamation as a result of entries on a patient's clinical record that was later lent to the Ministry of National Insurance or the Ministry of Pensions, the doctor would be fully indemnified for the cost of such litigation. Family physicians who revealed confidential data to tribunals were also covered by this pledge.[69]

In rendering judgment in claims for damages, the courts exercised restraint and moderation. In the case of *Woolley and Roe v. Ministry of Health,* the judge proclaimed that "We should be doing a disservice to the community if we imposed liability on hospitals and doctors for everything that happens to go wrong. Doctors would be led to think more of their own safety than of the good of their patients. Initiative would be stifled and confidence shaken. . . . We must insist on due care of the patient, but we must not condemn as negligence that which is only misadventure."

Injections were a source of frequent litigation. In the case of anesthetics, if the harmful reaction was due entirely to the "personal idiosyncrasy" of the patient, no liability was involved. But negligence would probably be found, explained an authority on the subject, if the wrong drug were given, or possibly if the administration of a drug like insulin were delegated to the patient without clear and complete instructions as to how it should be used. While an error in diagnosis did not necessarily involve negligence, it frequently was the basis for litigation. Accidents by the surgeon, it was disclosed, were not necessarily the result of negligence; but using the wrong solution, or an excessive amount, or making the injection into an artery rather than a vein was construed as negligence in some of the decisions.[70]

Three cases in 1958 might be cited by way of illustration. The two that ended in damage awards involved the use of drugs. The amount of £12,500 ($35,000) was allowed in one case in which the patient, who was known to be sensitive to penicillin, died from an injection of it.   In the other case in which a damage award was allowed, a nurse failed to follow instructions and gave more injections of streptomycin than had been prescribed, which caused the patient to lose her sense of balance.   Her disability caused her to stagger as though she were drunk.   The damages awarded totaled £3,000 ($8,400).   In the third case, the court held that a mistake in diagnosis, even though it caused an injury, did not necessarily constitute negligence.   The patient had a small lump on her breast that was erroneously diagnosed as a malignant cancer.   As a result of X-ray therapy for which there was no need the individual suffered severe ill-effects.   While characterizing the diagnosis as unfortunate, the judge could find no evidence of negligence and disallowed the claim.[71]

The total compensation paid by hospital authorities and Executive Councils for all kinds of legal claims increased from slightly over £23,636 ($66,180) in 1950 to a record £159,047 ($445,231) in 1954.   The following year, there was a significant decline in the total paid, and in the ensuing years the amount remained at a level far below the 1954 peak.   In 1958, the total was £100,000 ($280,000).[72]   The fear of larger and larger claims, with more and more litigation, proved groundless, as did many of the other apprehensions about the doctrine of vicarious liability.

By and large, then, the evidence was that hospital personnel had gained substantially from the Health Service.   A careful student of the British Health Program, Professor Richard M. Titmuss, observed that doctors, nurses, and other members of the hospital staffs enjoyed better conditions than had ever existed before.   Nurses and other ancillary workers were more adequately paid and worked under improved arrangements.   Doctors could use their skill according to need and without reference to the financial status of the patient. Almoners no longer were compelled to give consideration to whether or not a patient was a Poor Law case.   "An analysis of changes in functions among different professional groups," he concluded, "would show the extent to which the National Health Service had led to an enlargement of professional freedom."

Such gains were impressive, but in solving some problems, others emerged that aroused certain fears among observers, myself included. One danger was that those who worked in the hospitals might tend to operate the service in their own interests rather than in the interests of the patients.   Something of the sort had occurred in the monasteries during the Middle Ages and might recur in the hospitals if the true objectives of the service became "dimmed by excessive preoccupation with the means." With the increasing development of specialism, there was a possibility that the growing number of medical experts might become more impersonal and lose touch with the patient as a human being. While recognizing that hospital personnel were not deliberately callous, Titmuss was nevertheless concerned about the forces at work that might tend to make it more difficult for the staffs to appreciate fully the fundamental needs of the patient and to show the warmth and the proper spirit of understanding so essential in medical care and treatment.[73]

If past achievements were any guide to future developments, there were grounds for hope. In spite of shortcomings, the record of the service had been good, and many of the dire predictions that were intoned at the inception of the program had been disproved. Long before the popular mind was prepared to support a nationalized hospital service, a Parliamentary committee under the chairmanship of Viscount Cave warned that state intervention in this field would prove disastrous. The committee warned "that the money loss to the state would be a small matter compared with the injury which would be done to the welfare of the sick, . . . the training of the medical profession, and the progress of medical research." Elaborating further on the dreadful consequences, the Cave Committee declared that the "personal relation between the patient and the doctor and nurse which is traditional in voluntary hospitals . . . would be difficult to reproduce under an official regime."

The King Edward's Hospital Fund carried this quotation in its report for 1957 to show how completely the national hospital service had revealed such fears to be groundless. No organization in England had the well-being of the hospitals more at heart than the Hospital Fund, and so it was with undisguised pleasure that this association noted what the Guillebaud Committee had to say about the hospital service. While "allowing for the manifold shortcomings and imperfections inherent in the working of any human institution, we have," declared the Committee, "reached the general conclusion that the Service's record of performance since the Appointed Day has been one of real achievement."[74]

But the Hospital Fund did not need the Guillebaud Report as proof that the hospital service had been undergoing steady improvement. The quadrennial inspection of the London hospitals by the visitors of this association in 1956 revealed that gratifying progress had been made since their previous round of visits four years earlier. Many of the criticisms made in 1952 could no longer be voiced.[75]

Was the betterment due to nationalization? At least one important hospital official did not think so. Lord Cottesloe, Chairman of the North-West Metropolitan Regional Hospital Board, did not believe that the extraordinary improvement in the hospital service came about because of any virtue inherent in nationalization. "It is due," he claimed, "to the fact that those concerned in the service, doctors and nurses and lay administrators alike, have made up their minds that they would make the nationalized system work, and work well for the benefit of the patients: and, in that they have splendidly succeeded in spite of the system's defects."[76]

It would indeed be difficult to fix responsibility for the success of the hospital service, since so many individuals and groups were involved. The evidence indicates that the Ministry of Health, the Central Health Services Council, Parliament and its watchdog committees, the hospital personnel, the hospital boards and committees, the voluntary associations, and the professional organizations have all made their contribution. It was the loyal support of such associations and agencies, backed by strong popular sentiment, that held the best hope for the future of the hospital service.

Of primary concern was the welfare of the patient. The Parliamentary discussions on the hospital service and the memorandums of the Ministry of Health seldom strayed far from the general theme of what would serve the best interests of the patient. The Central Health Services Council sponsored in 1953 the Report on the Reception and Welfare of In-Patients. It touched on such matters as better diet, use of heated trolleys, redecoration of the wards, acquisition of more suitable furnishings, provision of hairdressing and other personal services, availability of books and magazines, access to chaplains, and reduction of noise. The report recommended that bed curtains should replace screens in the wards so as to give the patients more privacy; that earphones or pillow phones for radio reception should take the place of loud-speakers; that visiting periods should be fairly short and frequent; and that patients should not be awakened before 6:00 A.M., and preferably later. More hospitals were urged to establish canteens for the benefit of visitors as well as patients. Television, while not so suitable for general hospital wards, was recognized as ideal for the wards in long-stay hospitals.

Special importance was attached to the personal interest that the staff at all times should take in the patient. It was recognized that, while increased specialization tended to make relationships more impersonal, many hospitals were "already making conscious efforts, which deserve the highest praise, to fill the gap in human relations which has been caused by these developments." The Health Service had given the public a "definite stake" in the hospitals, and people were now less willing to accept peremptory decisions and instructions without adequate explanations. The old attitude sometimes adopted toward charity patients was no longer tenable, since the right to use the hospital service with dignity now belonged to all people. Keeping in touch with the needs of the patient was considered indispensable.

In seeking to improve the service, many management committees annually held public meetings, but experience had demonstrated that detailed criticisms were not so easily obtained by this method. It was more effective for a lay officer to interview patients at the time of discharge and record their comments. Weekly meetings of the departmental heads proved successful in arousing the interest of the ancillary staff in the welfare of the patient.

The report on the welfare of inpatients offered suggestions covering the admission and discharge of patients. Many general hospitals provided brochures containing information on the subject, some entirely factual and others more informal. Such literature was viewed as helpful. Waiting lists should be kept current. When a bed became available, a letter giving the necessary instructions was considered more suitable than a postcard. The admission of the patient should be handled courteously and smoothly, preferably by a lay receptionist. All necessary information concerning hospital routine, rules, facilities, and other pertinent matters should be supplied freely, and the nursing staff should endeavor to inspire a feeling of confidence. Too often the patient remained in doubt about what course of action was contemplated in his case. Where practicable, the ward sister or a member of the medical staff was urged to volunteer such information. In most hospitals, an interview with the house officer or a consultant could be arranged by the patient on request, but it would be better, the report suggested, if there were recognized administrative machinery and regular times for such interviews. Inquiries by relatives should not be brushed aside or handled in an impersonal or general manner, as was sometimes done by telephone operators. A nurse who had accurate knowledge of the case should reply to such inquiries. When the patient was discharged, his own physician should be informed promptly; and in the case of personal difficulties, the patient should be assisted by the almoner or some other member of the hospital staff.[77]

Between such recommendations and their implementation there was a wide gulf which only time and a purposeful effort on the part of hospital officials could bridge. The Ministry requested and received from the hospital boards detailed reports on what had been accomplished in putting the recommendations into effect. It was found that "the general picture which emerges is one of genuine and continuing effort to diminish, as far as possible, the institutional aspects of hospital life and to make the patient's stay in hospital as congenial as possible." Financial restrictions delayed action on some of the proposals, but steady progress was nevertheless made on most of them. Virtually all hospitals had libraries, and practically none was without radio facilities, although earphones were not universally used. The Ministry was pleased to learn that television was becoming increasingly common and that for long-stay patients there were concerts, film shows, dances, outdoor and indoor games, occupational therapy, and courses of study. The Ministry noted with pride that more satisfactory arrangements were being made for hospital visits, the admission of patients, and the gathering of constructive criticism.[78]

The progress achieved in hospital catering was especially gratifying. Reference has already been made to the remodeling of kitchens and the acquisition of modern cooking equipment. Through the use of posters, leaflets, memorandums, and films, the Ministry endeavored to raise the dietary standards in all hospitals. Emphasis was placed upon personal hygiene of the kitchen staff and better techniques in the preparation and distribution of food. Dietary experts from the Ministry of Health advised the catering staffs on nutritive diets. King Edward's Hospital Fund provided sets of weekly menus for guidance and also operated a school in hospital catering where hundreds of students were trained.[79]

A particularly troublesome problem was noise. The human voice was the greatest single cause of it, but there were many other sources— buzzers, scraping screens, squeaking trolley wheels, clanking bedpans, banging doors, and the external sounds which came from street traffic. Little could be done about the last source but the others could be dealt with by corrective measures. Rubber trolley tires, rubber door stops, and silent elevator doors were among the more effective devices. Many hospitals did what they could to mitigate noise, but the Ministry of Health was dissatisfied with the progress achieved and decided toward the end of 1959 to set up a committee to examine anew the problem and advise what could be done about it.[80]

The welfare of children in the hospitals commanded so much interest that a committee was appointed by the Central Health Services Council to study the matter. Under the chairmanship of Sir Harry Platt, the committee in 1959 made its report, which established a more definite pattern for future hospital policy toward children. The feeling was that the child should be protected as much as possible from the effects of leaving the security of his home for the strange environment of the hospital. Children should be admitted to the hospital only when there was no other possible alternative and should be separated from adult patients and always shielded from alarming sights. Since it was not practicable to have children's hospitals for all children, the regular hospitals would have to be used. But children should be kept in a separate unit, preferably in company with their own age group. They should be carefully prepared for admission by suitable instructions, and it was sometimes advisable for the mother to be admitted also, especially if the child were under five years of age. A staff properly trained in child psychology should provide the treatment and care. Frequent visits of the parents should be permitted. Adequate educational and recreational facilities should be furnished. By 1960, there was ample evidence that many of these recommendations had gained wide acceptance among hospital authorities.[81]

The policy of continuing the education of children in the hospital had been well established many years before the Platt Report was published. In 1956, the Ministry of Education sent a communication to the local authorities asking them to review their educational program for children in the hospitals and to make more comprehensive arrangements. There were at that time no less than 120 hospital schools with 6,500 pupils, and another 1,400 children receiving individual tutoring. Keeping such children in active contact with their school work was considered of great psychological value.[82]

Closely identified with the welfare of patients was the voluntary work of a large number of organizations. Prior to 1948, their efforts were largely confined to the voluntary hospitals, and when the Health Service was inaugurated, it was predicted that this type of service would pass out of existence. At first there was reason to believe that that might indeed happen. The volume of voluntary service declined and some of the local groups disbanded. But the trend was soon reversed when it became apparent that the need for voluntary help was greater than ever. Soon it surpassed all previous records and became one of the most dynamic phases of the hospital service. So important was it that the Minister of Health in 1955 declared, "Without voluntary service the National Health Service would wither and die. Without voluntary effort I would not want to be head of the Health Service."[83]

The list of voluntary associations was impressive, but most important were the Women's Voluntary Services, the British Red Cross, the Order of St. John, and the Leagues of Hospital Friends. These have already been mentioned. There were others that specialized in helping cripples, invalid children, the mentally ill, tuberculous patients, the blind, and convalescents. The work done by these organizations included visiting patients, running the hospital library, assisting with the canteen and trolley services, arranging outings or concerts, providing occupational therapy, and rendering a great many personal services for inpatients. The Leagues of Friends was active in raising funds to provide additional amenities and comforts for the staff and patients. The tremendous significance of voluntary effort for the chronic sick, the mentally ill, and other types of patients could not be measured in monetary terms, but rather in the profound gratitude of the countless thousands of lonely and friendless souls who were helped.[84]

All social classes made extensive use of the hospital service. In their study of the cost of the Health Service, Abel-Smith and Titmuss discovered, however, that if the higher illness and mortality rates of the semiskilled and unskilled groups were considered, it would seem that the professional and middle classes made fuller use of the hospital service than did the lower class. The upper class appeared to be more willing to go to the hospital for treatment in the early stages of a disease. It was more concerned about minor symptoms and took greater advantage of the curative facilities offered by the general practitioner and consultant services than did the lower class.[85]

Although the hospital service was popular with all groups, the reaction of individuals varied widely, depending upon the variable conditions they experienced as inpatients. Efficiency and physical comfort, which left much to be desired in some institutions, were directly related to the problem of personnel shortages and the obsolescence of buildings and equipment. While the over-all improvement in the service had been impressive, it would take much time and large sums of money to eradicate all the blemishes.

Unfriendly critics had no difficulty finding flaws in the everyday performance of the hospitals. There were mistakes in judgment, but there were also the examples of medical science at its finest. An example of each might be cited, one occurring in 1959 and the other in 1960. A patient of sixty-five who was refused admission to a hospital died shortly afterwards. The hospital doctor who had examined her could find nothing seriously wrong and directed the ambulance to take her home. Upon reaching her bedroom she collapsed, and in a coma was admitted to the hospital, but it was then too late. Since she suffered from softening of the brain and hardening of the arteries, perhaps nothing could have saved her, but the hospital concerned received a blot upon an otherwise excellent record.

The other case involved a woman in a nursing home who had a bad hemorrhage one hour after her baby was born. A call to a London hospital brought an obstetrician quickly to her bedside. An anesthetic was administered in order to remove the placenta, but the heart of the patient stopped beating. Within four minutes, the obstetrician had opened the chest wall and, by massaging the heart, had restored it to beating. Once more it stopped, and an injection of adrenalin was given to restart it. When the woman stopped breathing, artificial respiration was used. Later her lungs were inflated with oxygen and the incision was closed. Transferred to a hospital, she recovered consciousness within eight days and eventually returned home in good condition.[86]

The following comments selected at random are revealing, although not necessarily representative. Seen through the eyes of inpatients, the picture in the wards was not always rosy, but usually there was a brighter side. In 1952, a patient in a communication to *The New Statesman and Nation* grumbled about the food which, although "eatable" and "nutritionally adequate," was "nasty" and "ill-cooked." He was able, however, to pay "tribute to the care and skill and kindness of the nurses." He declared that "nothing except a sense of vocation can explain the devotion, and indeed affection, with which they contrived to understand and anticipate the varying wants of a ward-full of patients, differing in age, ailment and temperament. . . . Here in microcosm is something approaching the classless society. Sick men are equal—and almost as naked—before their nurses as before their God."

In the same journal, another patient a few years later said, "Since I contracted polio in 1950 I have spent years in various hospitals. I cannot believe better treatment could have been than I received under the Health Service, but sometimes the lack of peace nearly drove me to the screaming point."[87] Mixed comment was made in 1958 by a father who visited his young son in an isolation ward. Shocked at the unsatisfactory accommodations, he wrote to the editor of the *Manchester Guardian,* "The care and attention of the nursing and auxiliary staff, and the skill and kindness of the doctors and surgeons is beyond all praise, but how long must their labours of mercy be conducted under such primitive conditions?" Another patient complained some months later in the same newspaper about the food, the noise, and the inadequacy of the lavatory facilities, but he was impressed with the care given to the patients in his ward. "Opposite me," he observed, "was a man in his eighties. He was like a skeleton. . . . He absorbed blood and then food through rubber tubes, and emptied his body of its poisons through another. The two tubes accentuated the impression that he was poised between life and death. The nurses cared for him every moment; the doctors or the surgeon came every few hours. The voices of the nurses speaking to him and his own whispered thanks were chastening to hear."[88]

Such were a few of the more candid comments on hospital life. The adverse remarks were directed principally at the outmoded facilities that obstructed the smooth running of the service. The hospital personnel were much less open to criticism. Indeed, a great deal was written in their praise. What the General Purposes Committee of the Manchester Regional Hospital Board stated in the mid-1950's was not exceptional: "It is invariable that former in-patients speak in enthusiastic praise of the kindness and care and the skilled treatment which they received whilst in hospital."[89] Carried away by her own enthusiasm, a matron in a hospital within that region said, "There is not anywhere in the world a finer service than in the hospitals of England today—from the humblest member of the staff to the highest. Loyalty, thoroughness, skill and devotion to duty are outstanding, and while, as in all services, the occasional 'dreg' gets through it is eventually removed."[90] However immoderate her opinion may be, it is the pride and the *esprit de corps* which it reflects that make it significant. This type of spirit was what was counted upon to make the hospital service the viable force envisioned by the founders.

CHAPTER XIV

Role of the Local Health Authorities

WHEREAS CURATIVE MEDICINE was the primary concern of the Executive Councils and the hospital service, preventive medicine was left largely to the local health authorities. The elective county and county-borough councils had the responsibility of administering the health functions which Parliament delegated to the localities. Most of these duties had been a part of the local governmental pattern for a considerable period of time, but the Health Service strengthened and expanded them. Some that had been optional became mandatory, and more funds were made available for their implementation. The loss of jurisdiction over the hospitals did not diminish the importance of the local health authority in the field of public health. Indeed, the role of this body became more significant.

The health of a community is determined by many factors—pure water, clean air, adequate sewerage, good housing, proper food, and vaccination and immunization. Health education is very necessary. Provision has to be made for the aged poor, the mentally deficient, the physically handicapped, and others in need of care and treatment. The local authorities bore the major responsibility in most of these areas, though they depended, of course, upon the aid of the general medical practitioner and hospital services. In the performance of their assigned role, the local governments made use of home nurses, health visitors, domestic help, the ambulance service, prenatal, postnatal, and child welfare clinics, day nurseries, and domiciliary midwives. They handled, as well, the distribution of welfare food, the provision of residential accommodations, and the inspection and coordination of the environmental health services.

Supervisory control over the above services was allocated to committees selected by and made responsible to the county or county-borough council. The health and welfare services were normally managed by separate committees, although some councils entrusted the two phases to one committee. The latter course was favored by the Guillebaud Committee, which recognized that the domiciliary services provided by the National Assistance Act of 1948 and the National Health Service Act of 1946 were complementary and could be integrated more effectively under a single committee or a joint subcommittee than under separate committees.[1]

The Health Service made the creation of a health committee mandatory. This committee, a majority of the members of which had to be members as well of the county or county-borough council, could exercise all the functions of the local health authority except to borrow money or to control the tax rates. The County of Essex, typical of many, established such a committee on a broad basis. The regional hospital board, the Executive Council, the local medical committee, the more important voluntary associations, and the area subcommittees were given a voice in deliberations through representation on the health committee. To oversee each of the eleven health areas into which the county was divided, a subcommittee was set up that also included representatives from the groups most directly concerned. Such decentralization had been recommended by the Ministry of Health. The health committee was served by other subcommittees which dealt with such matters as mental health, finance, policy-making and the ambulance service. Since the County of Essex was a more or less self-contained unit, it did not feel the need, as did some of the other counties, to make joint arrangements with neighboring counties, except for the more economical operation of the ambulance service.[2]

The chief public health official in the county was the Medical Officer of Health, whose office had existed for more than one hundred years. Not only did he have to be a medical doctor, but to qualify he had to take additional training and acquire a special diploma. His duties ranged over the broad area of public health and health education. He was assisted by a team which, in the larger counties, included dentists, specialist doctors, home nurses, health visitors, sanitary inspectors, midwives, health education officers, mental health workers, statisticians, occupational therapists, speech therapists, and ambulance drivers. Under his leadership, this corps of workers was responsible for combating such adverse conditions as impure food and water, air pollution, inadequate sewerage, substandard housing, unsanitary schools and work places, overcrowding, inadequate nutrition, and occupational hazards. The heaviest demands were made in the field of personal health, in which the team was active in providing the domiciliary services.[3]

Unlike the hospital doctor or the general medical practitioner, the Medical Health Officer had civil service status. Although employed by the local government, he could appeal to the central department if he were dismissed. His remuneration was determined by action of the Whitley Council. In spring, 1959, new salary scales were announced that overshadowed in size all previous adjustments. The increases represented roughly one-third more than the 1951 rate of pay for Medical Officers of Health and an even larger addition to the remuneration of Assistant Medical Officers. The salary schedule was determined by the degree of responsibility. It rose to a maximum of £3,575 ($10,000) if the office served between 400,000 and 600,000 people. Above that number, the compensation was left to the discretion of the county or county-borough council.[4]

In the era before the Health Service, the family physician did little to conceal his resentment toward the maternity and child welfare clinics and sometimes was alleged to go so far as to greet the Medical Officer of Health with the admonition, "Back to your drains!" No longer was that true. Once viewed as a competitor, the Medical Officer now appeared more of a friendly ally. The joint conference between the College of General Medical Practitioners and the Society of Medical Officers in 1959 attested to the improved spirit between these two medical groups, although the vestiges of distrust still lingered in the minds of some practitioners.[5]

The total net cost of the local health service in the 1959-60 fiscal year was £62.5 million ($175 million). How was this money allocated? The ambulance service absorbed 21 per cent, or £13 million ($37 million). The care of mothers and young children took 15 per cent, domestic help 14 per cent, and home nursing 12 per cent. Midwifery, health visiting, mental health, and the prevention of illness (care and after-care) followed in that order and together represented about 27 per cent of the local health expenditures for that year. Vaccination and immunization accounted for 3 per cent of the budget, while health centers, still in the experimental stage, took a fraction of 1 per cent. If the last two items appeared negligible as cost factors, they nevertheless showed a phenomenal increase in the annual amount spent during the first decade. Domestic help likewise experienced a rapid rise in cost which carried it from less than £2.5 million ($7 million) in 1949-50 to more than £8.5 million ($24 million) in 1959-60. The figures for mental health were £1.3 million ($3.5 million) and £4 million ($11 million), respectively, for those years. For none of the other elements of the local health service was the rise in cost during the eleven-year period much over 100 per cent; for midwifery it was 44 per cent and for the care of mothers and young children it was 24 per cent.[6]

During the pre-Health Service era, the ambulance service functioned haphazardly. The Health Service Act required that the local health authorities either maintain an adequate ambulance service or arrange for others to do so. When necessary, all persons suffering from mental disorders or physical illness and all expectant or nursing mothers were to have ambulance transportation to and from the hospital. In complying with the law, the local authorities had to submit the details of their ambulance program to the Minister of Health for approval. The use of voluntary effort was encouraged, with the result that the British Red Cross and the St. John Ambulance Brigade were utilized by many of the county and county-borough councils for the purpose of supplementing the official ambulance service. These organizations proved helpful in giving first-aid training to ambulance personnel.

The demand upon the ambulance service was heavy. The number of patients carried and the mileage run increased steadily until 1956, when they leveled off. In 1960, 16.5 million patients, or twice as many as in 1950, were transported by ambulance. The number of miles traveled in 1960 (106 million) was somewhat larger than in 1956 and 19 per cent more than in 1950. Yet the average number of miles per patient was reduced from 9 to 6.3 during that decade.[7]

How could more patients be carried without a comparable increase in mileage? Beginning in 1951, the Ministry published general data on the ambulance service costs, showing such statistics as the cost per patient, the cost per vehicle mile, and the number of miles per patient in each county and county-borough. The information was classified so that a valid comparison could be made between areas with the same degree of urbanization. In 1954 and 1955, local surveys were made by the Ministry that revealed how the most efficient service could be provided. It was found that effective liaison was necessary between the ambulance and hospital authorities and that this liaison could be achieved when the Medical Officer of Health assumed an active role in directing the ambulance service and the hospitals set up a transport officer to co-ordinate the calls for ambulances. While there were many reciprocal arrangements between neighboring county officials, some of the agreements stood in need of revision. It was also observed that, where radio-control existed, a far more effective deployment of the ambulance resources could be attained.[8]

Circulars were issued by the Department of Health to underscore the need for the adoption of these and other techniques that were proving successful. The response was heartening. Since rail transportation for patients was more economical for long trips, it was used increasingly. Where the occasion demanded, such as a deep snow, helicopters were employed to effect the speedy removal of patients to the hospital. One-stretcher dual-purpose automobiles, in many ways more suitable than the old-style ambulances, were put into service. Other types of modern vehicles were also acquired in a systematic replacement program rendered imperative by the large number of obsolete conveyances that were in operation when the Health Service began. By 1958, radio control had been adopted by two-thirds of the local authorities. The operational efficiency of ambulances was so much improved by this innovation that fewer vehicles could run fewer miles and yet haul a larger number of patients. More liaison committees, transport officers, and satisfactory reciprocal arrangements added strength to the service. In meeting the need for ambulance stations, a substantial number were erected during the latter half of the 1950's. Since hospital doctors and general practitioners largely determined when ambulances should be used, every effort was made to educate them in their proper use.

While volunteer effort was encouraged as much as ever, there was some decline in this type of service due to the extension of radio control and the resulting elimination of small sub-stations. There was also wider use by local authorities of their own multi-seat ambulances. In 1960, the number of ambulances and sitting-case cars operated by the local health authorities was in the neighborhood of 4,500, or 32 per cent more than when the service started. The total of full-time paid drivers and attendants had risen to over 10,000—an increase of 77 per cent. Owing largely to higher wages and salaries, which accounted for 60 per cent of the total ambulance expenditures, the gross cost per patient rose from 15/5d ($2.16) in 1950 to 16/9d ($2.34) ten years later. Since this represented only an 8 per cent increase per patient, compared with a much higher ratio for other health services, the ambulance authorities had reason to be proud of their achievement.[9]

In a service of this character some abuse was inevitable. Outpatients as well as inpatients were privileged to use the service whenever it was medically necessary and special transportation was required. A survey in the casualty department of a London hospital during the latter part of 1954 and the first month of 1955 showed that nearly one-half of 52 casualty patients brought by ambulance did not actually need this mode of conveyance.[10] The Guillebaud Committee found that some abuse existed during the early years but that the more flagrant types had been eliminated. The evidence further indicated that the local health authorities had been able to operate the ambulance service more efficiently each year, and that they were in a much better position than the hospitals to manage it. The Ministry of Health received comparatively few complaints, although there was some criticism from outpatients of delay in being picked up by the multi-seat vehicles.[11]

Since preventive medicine was the overriding preoccupation of the local health authorities, health visiting, with its educational and advisory work, was of special importance. The antecedents of this service went back almost to the middle of the nineteenth century, but it was the National Health Service that revitalized health visiting, making it a statutory obligation of the local governments. To insure high standards of performance, the Minister of Health laid down regulations requiring that health visitors should "possess a specialist qualification for the work." Circumstances, however, forced him to relax the standards, so that many of the posts were filled by those who were not fully qualified. While 1,400 were initially in the category of those not qualified, the number was reduced two-thirds by 1959. The qualified staff enjoyed a slow, steady growth, but the shortage of trained personnel continued to plague the service, particularly in industrial communities.

In 1960, there were 6,700 health visitors, the great majority of whom served part-time. Most of them combined health visiting with tuberculosis visiting, midwifery, or home nursing. Such an arrangement in some regions was necessitated by economic and geographical considerations. In many cases, the same person functioned as school nurse and health visitor—a practice that was endorsed by both health and education authorities.

The number of home visits by health visitors did not fluctuate sharply during the first twelve years of the Health Service. In 1949, there were slightly more than 10 million visits, and in 1960 the total was only 16 per cent higher. The trend, which at first moved upward, was reversed in the years that immediately followed 1954. The steady improvement in child and maternal health, together with a declining birth rate during much of that period, doubtlessly affected the pattern of domiciliary visits. With a larger number of health visitors, there was more time for each call, and this was all to the good in view of the greater emphasis upon social work in the visits.[12]

The health of mothers and children continued to absorb much of the energy of the health visitor, and most of the families with children were visited one or more times. Usually the health visitor was allotted a small region in which she attended clinics, went to the schools, and called at the homes. She was particularly interested in advising mothers on the care of their babies, and among the things which she emphasized was the desirability of vaccination and immunization. The study on health visiting conducted under the chairmanship of Sir William Jameson and published in 1956 considered that the dramatic drop in the maternal and child mortality rates was in part due to the influence of the health visitor.[13]

School health, tuberculosis, communicable diseases, the prevention of illness, the care of the aged sick, mental hygiene, and the rehabilitation of the handicapped were of concern to the health visitor and promised to command more of her time in the future. In these areas also her work was largely advisory. It served to bring her into contact with the welfare of the entire family, and it was in this broader range of duties that she had the opportunity "to act as a common point of reference, a common source of information, . . . a common adviser on health teaching—in a real sense, a 'common factor' in family welfare." Because of her strategic position in promoting family health, she could contribute to a better understanding of the social aspects of illness by the general practitioner. Moreover, her potential role as a co-ordinating agent between the general practitioner, hospital, and public health services was not overlooked by students of the National Health Service.[14]

To qualify for health visiting, four and one-third years of training were required—three years as a student nurse with state registration, six months in midwifery, and nine months in public health. The Jameson Committee, which viewed such a program as being too disjointed and compartmentalized, proposed a course of training in which all of these aspects, together with social work, would be integrated so as to provide "a clear picture of family health and welfare services." It was contended that all training should be practical, involving a knowledge of home management, social service, family welfare, and mental hygiene. The length of training would remain the same, but it was suggested that refresher courses should be available to all, and for some, advanced training in the universities. By 1959, three institutions that trained health visitors had inaugurated an integrated course of study.[15]

The Jameson Report proposed that within ten years the total of whole-time health visitors or their equivalent should be increased 44 per cent. To accomplish this end, the number of students being annually trained would have to be boosted from the current level of 640 to 1,100—a feat which, it was recognized, would not be easy to achieve. Improvement of the conditions of work and the financial incentives for health visitors was deemed essential in attracting more recruits.[16]

In a joint circular, the Ministers of Health and Education indicated general agreement with the recommendations of the Jameson

Report concerning the recruitment, the training, and the proper field of work for health visitors. It was urged that the local authorities take such action as seemed to them appropriate to improve the health visiting service.[17]

The British Medical Association recognized the complementary nature of the work done by health visitors and by general practitioners. In the Annual Representative Meetings for 1956 and 1957, kind words were uttered about health visiting and examples of co-operative effort were cited.[18] In 1954, the British Medical Association and the Society of Medical Officers of Health jointly issued a circular that set forth certain objectives designed to produce a more harmonious relationship between the family physician and the health visitor. Discussions were advised between all parties involved.

The Jameson Committee discovered that co-operation was "developing reasonably well." It was "apathy" and not "antipathy" that slowed it up, but the encouraging aspect was a growing will to co-operate. When doctors and health visitors got together, misunderstandings seemed to dissolve. Birmingham demonstrated what could be done in fostering a spirit of mutual helpfulness. The practitioners in that city found health visitors to be very useful to them in maternity and child welfare work and in dealing with the aged. In the local authority clinic and the William Budd Health Center at Bristol, it was the care of mothers and children that brought the family physician and the health visitor together.[19] If it were true that the general practitioner was the clinical leader of the domiciliary team, as various Ministers of Health had so frequently reiterated, then he would certainly want the fullest co-operation of the team members. Among these, none had more to contribute to preventive medicine than the health visitor, because of her general knowledge of family health and welfare.

Another important member of the domiciliary team was the district nurse, whose services from the very beginning were understood and appreciated by the family doctor. Relations were good because the home nurse's work was usually done under the doctor's orders, and he was aware of the useful role she played in the lives of his patients. Before 1948, home nursing was given principally to small children, expectant and nursing mothers, and patients suffering from infectious diseases. Under the Health Service, it was made available to all persons who needed nursing in their homes. Only the recommendation of the family physician was required, the service being free to all.

Before the appointed day, home nursing was left mostly to voluntary organizations which received financial support from the local government. In 1948, about one-half of the local health authorities decided to provide the service directly; by 1960, four-fifths were doing so. The others shared the service with or left it exclusively to voluntary associations, with whom agreements were negotiated.[20]

When the county or county-borough council decided to assume direct responsibility for the home nursing service, the change was usually made only after discussion with the local institute of district nursing. The actual transfer of responsibility was done gradually and with a minimum of ill will. Contrary to this pattern, the London County Council without such consultation announced rather abruptly in 1959 its intention of taking over the home nursing service. The proposed change was designed to combine home nursing and midwifery under the direction of one supervisory body and was expected to result in a substantial saving to the local government. The London local medical committee was agreeable to the proposed action, but not the Voluntary District Nursing Association, which for years had supplied the service. Considerable resentment developed, much of which could have been avoided if different methods and better timing had characterized the procedure.[21]

The popularity of home nursing was demonstrated by its vigorous growth. Within 8 years (1949-57), the annual number of visits reached 25 million—a rise of 44 per cent. Although a decline occurred during the next three years, the total for 1960 remained above 23 million. Much of the over-all increase was attributed to aged patients, who accounted for 60 per cent of the visits in 1958. Fifty per cent more elderly persons were attended by district nurses in that year than five years previously.

The additional demands upon the service during the first twelve years were met by a growth of one-third in the nursing staff. In 1960, there were 10,300 district nurses, of whom approximately one-half were whole-time and one-fifth were employed by voluntary organizations. Nurses classified as part-time were mostly full-time employees who did health visiting or midwifery work as well as home nursing. In spite of the steady improvement in the recruitment of district nurses, some areas still remained understaffed at the end of the first decade.[22]

Registered nurses who desired to become district nurses had to undergo several months of additional training. Since requirements were not uniform, a working party was set up to make recommendations. Reporting in 1955, it favored a four-month period of training and the appointment of a committee that would issue a syllabus, supervise the examinations, and advise the Minister on matters concerning district nursing. That advisory body was subsequently set up and formulated specific proposals designed to ensure the maintenance of adequate standards of training for all district nurses.

The work done by home nurses covered a broad range of duties, including general nursing, ante- and post-operative treatment, the preparation of patients for X-ray examinations, and other nursing services. As home care was recognized as being appropriate for more types of illness, the usefulness of the district nurses expanded. The trend was to discharge inpatients earlier and to keep those not seriously ill out of the wards altogether, leaving the space for persons who urgently needed a hospital bed. The aged sick who did not require specialized treatment were more contented and better off at home, and so were sick children who would thus escape exposure to cross-infection—a common hospital hazard.[23]

Home nursing and health visiting leaned heavily upon the domestic help service. Originally established in 1918, this service at first was limited to maternity and child welfare cases, but during World War II, it was extended to include the sick and the infirm. The National Health Service Act left the home help service to the local authorities as an optional responsibility, yet so vital was home help that without exception the local authorities offered the service on a broad basis. Within twelve years, the number of cases yearly in which domestic help was employed increased to 312,000, or 170 per cent. The size of the home help staff underwent an even more phenomenal growth. In 1948, there were 12,000 domestic helpers; by 1960, the total was four times as large. The great majority were part-time employees, because most of them, being married women, could work only on that basis. Since the demands upon the service fluctuated, a large reservoir of part-time workers was considered the most desirable arrangement. In an emergency, most of the home helpers were willing to work extra hours. The standards of the service varied between counties, but they were generally better in the urban areas.

Most of the local authorities administered the service directly, although a few co-operated with voluntary bodies. The domestic help program was usually separated from the other health services and in some counties was decentralized. The local authorities as a rule appointed at least one full-time home help organizer and in many cases deputy and divisional organizers. In areas far removed from headquarters, it was not exceptional for the health visitor, district nurse, or welfare officer to be in charge locally. Some of the organizers did not have sufficient clerical assistance and transportation facilities to supervise the domestic helpers adequately.

The spirit among the domestic employees nevertheless was good, and many of them took what was professional pride in their labor. It was not at all uncommon for them to work overtime without pay. They often helped with the shopping and did other small favors in their off-duty hours. Some of the authorities furnished uniforms, and in the case of at least one county, good conduct badges were awarded at the end of ten years of satisfactory service. Upon being selected for home help work, the applicant was usually given several months of instruction in domestic subjects. Film strips were sometimes used to show prevention of the spread of infection, care of children and invalids, first-aid techniques, and welfare services for the aged.[24]

The character of the work done by the home help service underwent a considerable change. Maternity work, which at one time monopolized this service, no longer did so. In 1950, only 26 per cent of the cases attended by domestic workers were in that category, and nine years later the percentage had fallen to 11. The service became essentially one for the elderly or chronically sick, who accounted for over half of the cases in 1953, and three-fourths six years later. Although it was yet a small minority, a rising group of cases concerned problem families. A family unit on the verge of breaking up because of a sick or maladjusted mother might be assigned a full-time domestic worker, for instance, and as the situation improved, she would gradually reduce her working schedule until the family was finally on its own again. One of the pioneers in this kind of service was London, which initiated it in the mid-1950's.

The home help service was one of the few local health services for which a charge could be made, but the amount was based upon the ability to pay. Only a small part of the cost of the program was actually recovered, since the aged and chronic sick, who were the chief beneficiaries, could seldom contribute much. By enabling people to remain in their homes, this service saved the expense of institutional care. Domestic workers often were assigned to old people for periods ranging up to five, and in some cases as many as ten, years. Night attendance, early morning and late evening visits, and even laundry service were among the special features of the program. From a humanitarian point of view, it helped to sustain the morale of the elderly, and to that extent prevented or retarded the mental deterioration that resulted from loneliness and a feeling of helplessness. The home helpers were more than housekeepers; they were frequently angels of mercy, brightening the hours of bedridden, feeble, and confused persons.[25]

The domiciliary midwifery service was well rooted in the pattern of local health duties before 1948. The statutory basis of the service was not changed by the National Health Service Act, but the charges were abolished and the local health authorities were permitted to provide the service either directly or by arrangement with hospitals or voluntary organizations. At the outset, 70 per cent of the authorities furnished the midwifery service directly, and more than 80 per cent did so ten years later. Ninety per cent of the domiciliary midwives were employed by the local health authorities in 1958.

There was some uncertainty as to what effect the National Health Service would have upon the local authority maternity program. Both the hospital and the general practitioner services were expected to play a major role in this field of medicine. It was reasonable to assume that the role of the domiciliary midwifery service as well as that of the local authority clinics would be correspondingly diminished. While in general this was true, the part which the local authorities continued to play remained important.

The domiciliary midwife, who at first was apprehensive about her status, soon discovered that she had nothing to fear from the obstetrical work of the general practitioner. She attended virtually all of the domiciliary confinements and in a large proportion of cases conducted the delivery without a doctor's being present. The practitioner who had been booked by the expectant mother made examinations before and after birth, performed the delivery when necessary, and otherwise assumed full responsibility for the mother and child. The midwife and the obstetrician each had a special job to do and they were paid for it. Since their work was complementary instead of competitive, the Health Service inaugurated an era of better relations and co-operation between these former rivals.

While the number of domiciliary confinements came to represent not much over 35 per cent of the total, the domiciliary midwives for the most part were reasonably busy. With the rising birth rate after 1955, they were even hard pressed in certain areas to cope with the work. The 7,590 domiciliary midwives in 1960 represented a somewhat smaller number than existed when the Health Service began. As noted elsewhere, quite a few of the domiciliary midwives did part-time health visiting or home nursing as well. In a confinement case, the responsibility of the midwife continued at least two weeks after delivery, and during that time she made periodic visits to the mother. The 276,000 births attended by the domiciliary midwives in 1960 were in view of their divided and extended responsibilities no mean achievement. The standards of training were high, and virtually all of the midwives were well qualified to administer inhalational analgesics.[26]

The role of the midwife was considerably enhanced in the prenatal clinics. As expected, the maternity clinics were adversely affected by the Health Service, which made the hospital and general practitioner services available to expectant mothers as alternative sources of free medical care. Although the total number of local authority prenatal clinics was enlarged to nearly 2,000 during the first decade of the Health Service, a rise of 10 per cent, the number of women who attended these clinics between 1949 and 1955 declined nearly one-fourth. During the next five years, the trend was generally upward. This was attributable in part to the higher birth rate, but apparently more mothers were obtaining maternity medical care from their own family physician and also from the midwife (as distinct from the Medical Officer) at the prenatal clinic. Although the Medical Officers' clinics accounted for the greater part of the total attendance at local authority prenatal clinics, the impressive increase occurred at the sessions held by midwives.[27]

The sharp drop in attendance during the first half of the 1950's was disturbing to both the Guillebaud Committee and the Cranbrook Committee,[28] which were afraid that fewer women were receiving adequate prenatal instruction. The facilities for giving such instruction were not always available in the hospitals or the offices of the general practitioner obstetrician. Those who attended prenatal clinics in 1960 gave birth to less than half of the babies in that year.

The local authority clinics often shared with other local authority services the same premises. In some cases, even church halls were used on certain days of the week, but a building program was furnishing modern quarters in many areas. The prenatal clinics were staffed with midwives, health visitors, and Medical Officers. In addition to giving medical advice, the local authority doctors were prepared to carry out the prenatal and postnatal examination of women who had booked only a midwife or who had been referred to them by the family physician. In a few cases, they accepted women who had arranged for a hospital confinement. The fact that the local authority doctor did not attend deliveries may explain why his influence in the prenatal clinics, while still important, had suffered a steady decline under the Health Service. The midwife, who delivered virtually all of the domiciliary babies, and the general practitioner obstetrician, who was booked in well over 80 per cent of these births (89 per cent in 1960), had acquired new stature. The Cranbrook Committee was of the opinion that prenatal and postnatal care should not be given by doctors who did not undertake deliveries. It was felt that the general practitioner obstetrician should eventually replace the local authority doctor in providing maternity care in the local authority prenatal clinics.[29]

The postnatal clinics, which fulfilled a much less dramatic role in maternity care, suffered a substantial decline under the Health Service. In 1960, only 13 per cent of those who attended prenatal clinics utilized the postnatal clinic service. Thirty-seven per cent fewer women used the postnatal clinic in that year than during the initial year of the service. Although there was a very noticeable reduction in the number of postnatal clinics, this loss in some measure was recouped by using prenatal clinics jointly for postnatal work. The reason for the trend away from postnatal clinics was to be found largely in the postnatal examination which the Health Service required that all general practitioner obstetricians give their patients.[30]

The Cranbrook Committee was convinced from the evidence that the prenatal clinic would always serve a vital role in the field of health education. Among the witnesses that appeared before this committee there was general agreement concerning the value of "mothercraft" instruction to expectant mothers. The prenatal clinics were accessible and well prepared for this phase of maternity care. Breast feeding and the care of breasts, the use of analgesic apparatus, the physiology of pregnancy and labor, and relaxation exercises were among the subjects deemed particularly appropriate for instruction by local authority prenatal clinics, which were also expected to disseminate information about the child welfare services. The Cranbrook Committee recommended that it become the duty of the local health authorities to furnish instructors in health education and mothercraft for their own clinics and to make the services of such instructors available, when the need existed, in hospital clinics and in the offices of the general practitioner obstetricians.[31]

The local authority clinics were used for other purposes—the priority dental services, the distribution of welfare foods, and the care of young children. England showed tremendous concern with the health of its children, and this attitude was reflected in the growth of the child welfare clinics. In 1960, there were over 5,900 such clinics—an increase of more than 1,000 since the inception of the Health Service. In 1960, there were 3,500 more sessions per month than in 1949. Many of the more unsuitable premises were replaced, and mobile clinics were sent to communities where the population size did not warrant permanent installations. The total attendances by children under five at the child welfare clinics (roughly 10 million per year) varied little during the first twelve years of the Service. Approximately 42 per cent of all children under five made use of these clinics in 1960. The primary purpose of the child welfare clinics was preventive and advisory. Only the simplest treatment was given, and if anything more were required, the child was referred to the family doctor. The opportunity for mothers to discuss with each other the problems they shared in common gave the clinics an added value.   Recognizing the significance of this aspect, many of the local health authorities took the initiative in organizing discussion groups, sewing classes, and mothers' clubs.[32]

In a study of local authority child welfare clinics at Coseley and Birmingham in 1951-52, it was discovered that among the reasons why mothers attended the clinic were to have their children weighed, to secure advice about the feeding and care of infants, and to obtain welfare foods.   But most important of all was the medical examination.   In many cases it was routine, but one-fourth of the children examined were treated for some minor ailment—mild respiratory infections, teething rashes, umbilical hernia, and phimosis.   About 13 per cent of the children were referred to their general practitioner, and a few were sent directly to the hospital or to the dental or remedial clinics of the local health authority.[33]

The Welfare Foods Scheme was established early in World War II for the purpose of ensuring that certain important nutrients would not be denied young children and expectant and nursing mothers.   So successful was the program that the government decided to continue it after the war.   When rationing ended in 1954, the Minister of Health became responsible for the distribution of the welfare foods, although the Ministry of Agriculture still bought, processed, and stored most of the foods.   The local authority clinics, as before, assisted in their distribution.   Children under five years of age and expectant and nursing mothers continued to be the beneficiaries of the program.   The cod liver oil and the vitamin A and D tablets were free,[34] but the daily pint of milk (or its equivalent in powdered milk) and the orange juice carried a small charge.   In accordance with the recommendation of the Joint Sub-Committee on Welfare Foods in 1957, orange juice was discontinued for children above two years of age.   There was no evidence, affirmed the report, that a vitamin C deficiency existed after that age, presumably because of the more varied diet.[35]

Whether because of the improved economic conditions or some change in the dietary pattern, the consumption of welfare foods under the Health Service was considerably below expectation.   The sharp reduction in the amount of cod liver oil was particularly disappointing, in view of the importance of vitamin D.   By posters, booklets, and other means, the Ministry of Health did what it could to combat the popular apathy in the matter.   With the exception of milk, the consumption of welfare foods almost every year was not more than a third of what it would have been if all potential beneficiaries had taken their full quota.[36]   The apathy was all the more disturbing in view of the results of a national survey published in 1958. It covered 5,000 children from all social classes born in 1946. The report showed that one-fourth of all families with children under the age of five in 1950 may not have been financially able to purchase a proper diet for the children. In editorializing on the report, the *Manchester Guardian* declared that those "who are suggesting that the welfare provisions for smaller children are no longer needed clearly must think again."[37]

Since the general health of pre-school children and expectant and nursing mothers involved dental health, the local health authorities were required to provide a dental service for such persons. In seeking to discharge this duty, the local health service was faced by a chronic shortage of dentists. While the exodus of dental officers from the priority and school dental services during the initial years was reversed before the mid-1950's, the shortage of personnel in all branches of dentistry seemed likely to remain a serious challenge to the Ministry of Health and the dental profession for some years.

Much progress was nevertheless achieved. During the six-year period ending in 1958, the number of dental clinics rose to nearly 1,275, which represented a 40 per cent increase. Each year saw more new and modern clinics put into operation that were equipped with efficient lights, modern dental chairs, and the facilities for radiographic examinations. In 1959, for example, 36 clinics with dental facilities were built and five other premises were adapted for priority dental work. Comparatively few ill-equipped dental offices remained. Although the number of sessions showed a steady growth almost every year, the priority dental service suffered from inadequate staffing and was unable to treat all of the patients.

It was obvious that not all the priority patients could be put into a state of dental fitness without the co-operation of the general dental service. Although the amount of conservative treatment was increasing, a large part of the work was the extraction of teeth and the provision of dentures. There was no fee for work done in the priority service, but in the general dental service the charge for dentures was applied to all patients until 1961, when expectant and nursing mothers and school children were provided with free dentures. As before, they paid nothing for conservative treatment.

Whereas dentists in the priority service were paid on a salaried or sessional basis, those in general dentistry were compensated on a fee basis and did not normally receive payment from the Executive Council until the course of treatment was completed and the patient was put into a state of dental fitness. Consequently, the regular dentists were somewhat reluctant to accept an expectant mother as a patient if there were an extended amount of work to do, since they knew that it might not be completed before confinement occurred. All of this tended to hamper the most effective co-operation between the priority and general dental services—a situation with which the Cranbrook Committee in 1959 expressed its concern.[38] Despite the man-power shortage, which the establishment of more dental schools would doubtlessly solve, and despite certain other anomalies, which also could be adjusted, the basis was being laid for an increasingly effective priority dental service.

Day nurseries, which represented one of the less important activities of the local health authorities, had functioned on a much larger scale during World War II. Then the Exchequer provided a grant covering all expenses, but after 1945 the grant was reduced to 50 per cent of the operating expenses. During the postwar years, the number of day nurseries operated by the local authorities declined appreciably, and the downward trend continued under the Health Service. In 1960, there were less than 475 day nurseries, or one-third as many as in 1944. The number of children registered at these nurseries in 1960 was 22,000, compared with almost twice that many during the first year of the Health Service.

The day nursery was primarily for the benefit of mothers who had to work to support their families or who were too ill to care for the children. Where home conditions were unsatisfactory from a health standpoint, the children were also accepted at the nursery. At first there was a small fee for food, and after 1952 the charge was increased for those able to pay. Parents who could make other suitable arrangements for their children were generally encouraged to do so, with the result that the day nurseries came to serve primarily the children of poor parents, who were unable to make more than a small contribution toward the cost. Whenever the demand was too small to justify continuation of the nursery, it was closed and registered child-minders were employed to take care of the children who still needed the service. Private nurseries were also playing a bigger role in this field of activity. In 1960, more children were accommodated by non-governmental agencies than were served by the local authority day nurseries.[39]

The Ministry of Education had the general responsibility for the medical program in the schools. Under the Education Act of 1944, the medical inspection of all students from the nursery level through the secondary schools was made compulsory. School health officers, usually employed on a full-time basis by the local authorities, normally gave every student a routine examination at least three times during his enrollment in the public schools. Whenever it appeared that a pupil was suffering from a defect or illness, a special examination was arranged. The school medical officer as a rule sought the concurrence of the child's family physician if there were need for the services of a specialist. Treatment usually was left to the general practitioner, but other branches of the Health Service stood ready to help. Faulty vision seldom escaped the observation of the school doctor, but a congenital weakness of the heart or similar ailment was not always discovered. While the examination procedure in the public schools could not very well uncover all of the diseases, a large proportion were identified and treated.[40]

In the school program and elsewhere, recognition was given to the importance of the prevention of illness. In the opinion of some observers, however, too much emphasis was still being placed on cure and too little on prevention. The Guillebaud Committee received considerable testimony to the effect that the chest physicians, for instance, were more interested in the curative measures for tuberculosis than in the preventive measures and that the clinicians in the hospitals showed too little concern about preventive medicine. Some witnesses pointed to the disproportionately small part of the Health Service budget that was allocated to the preventive services. In evaluating the evidence, the Guillebaud Committee recognized that preventive health measures took many forms. Some, such as good housing, efficient sewerage, and clean food, were outside the scope of the National Health Service. Combating the progress of a disease represented another type of preventive medicine, which involved early diagnosis and treatment. Such work was primarily the concern of the general practitioner, who utilized the diagnostic and specialist services of the hospital. No less important was the prevention of disease and injury—a broad field of activity which belonged largely to the local health authority. The main instruments employed in it were vaccination, immunization, and health education.

Looking into the future, the Guillebaud Committee could see that preventive health measures would tend to follow a somewhat different course than the one followed in the past. While noting that immunization would continue to be a "promising field," the report nevertheless held that "bacteriology has now ceased to be the happy hunting ground of preventive medicine." "Increasingly," declared the document, "it is the home, the family and the everyday way of life, where we may have to look for the basic deficiencies which are leading to ill-health, and particularly to mental ill-health in the community." The Committee was not prepared to designate within the Health Service any "wide fields" in which large amounts of money could be expended to advantage on preventive health measures. It did propose an expanded chiropody service, but otherwise was content to recommend the more effective development of the home health services and better co-ordination between all branches of the Health Service. Inquiries would have to be made to ascertain in what areas preventive medicine could most profitably be pursued in the future.[41]

The great success the public health service had achieved in the prevention of smallpox, scarlet fever, diphtheria, paratyphoid, and typhoid was proof enough to many that the preventive phase offered the greatest hope. Most writers did not appear to be overly pessimistic about what had been accomplished, but they felt more could be done. A prize-winning essayist in the early 1950's set forth a number of suggestions. The first requisite was greater resources, without which the preventive phase could not be made fully effective. There was need for foot clinics and old people's clinics and more health centers. Home nursing and health visiting should be strengthened. Health education, in the widest sense of the term, was necessary, and medical students should be trained in social and preventive medicine. Factories should introduce preventive measures, and there should be more research in foodstuffs and household products. The use of fluorine in water to retard teeth decay and the abatement of the smoke evil in the cities were steps deemed worthwhile. In the field of mental health, greater emphasis should be put on the preventive phase during the childhood period.[42]

What this observer said was well known to public health authorities, most of whom favored all or the great majority of the proposals. But in the realization of these objectives, more than money was required; an enlightened and co-operative public was also essential. Mass education proceeded slowly, and the implementation of such a program would therefore take time. The relative importance of each measure tended to change in the light of experience and expediency. Health centers, once considered urgent, had lost much of their popular appeal. Some of the suggestions, such as preventive health instruction for medical students or the creation of a medical service in each factory, were more or less beyond the jurisdiction of public officials. But if a need were established, neither the universities nor industry would remain unresponsive. Indeed, the medical school curriculums were giving added emphasis to the importance of preventive medicine. And among factory owners there appeared to be a growing awareness of the value of having an in-factory medical and nursing service, not only for first-aid treatments, but to safeguard the general health of the workers.

The Ford plant at Dagenham was a good example of what could be done in the field of preventive medicine by a large industrial concern. Its medical department in 1956 included four doctors and a nursing staff of eighteen, plus thirteen trained assistants. X-ray, electrocardiograph, and audiometer equipment was available, as well as a physiotheraphy center and a pathological unit. Regular physical examinations were standard procedure. Patients deemed unfit for heavy work were recommended for lighter jobs, and such recommendations were almost invariably honored by the foremen. All employees were urged to have their eyes tested frequently and to use safety glasses and face masks when the work necessitated such protective devices. In this and many other ways, the medical service of the plant sought to protect the health and well-being of the employees.[43]

How far the Ministry of Health should go in preventive medicine was a subject which elicited divergent opinions. The Socialist Medical Association advocated regular medical examinations for everybody, sufficient rest and convalescent homes for general use, and a full-time salaried staff in the preventive services. It also supported the creation of a special council that would be responsible for "planning campaigns for the prevention of disease."[44] While the British Medical Association was unprepared to go that far, it favored a more vigorous policy of health education. The Representative Assembly in 1956 deplored "the failure of the Ministry of Health to carry out its proper duty in educating the public in everyday methods of health." The Council of the Medical Association, however, took no immediate action in the matter because the financial restrictions at that time precluded an "extensive propaganda campaign" by the Ministry of Health.[45]

The failure of the Minister to follow a more comprehensive course of action did not involve any lack of awareness on his part of the importance of preventive health. In an address to the representatives of the county and county-borough welfare departments in 1957, he lamented that fact that, though the hospital service took 57 per cent of the budget and the general medical and allied services 30 per cent, the local health authorities, whose primary job was preventive medicine, received only 8 per cent. "This," he protested, "is not commensurate with the importance of preventive health and welfare measures." In spite of the financial demands of the other services, which he feared would not diminish, he assured his audience that the policy of the government would be to encourage the local health services, since, from a long range view, it was to the monetary interest of the central government to do so.[46]

It was the responsibility of the Minister to formulate the general policy on health education and to co-ordinate the program for the nation as a whole.   In discharging his duty in this matter, he was assisted by the Central Council for Health Education—an organization to which the local authorities also turned for advice and guidance.   In the campaign for the prevention of illness, the emphasis shifted during the first ten years of the Service.   The publicity at first was directed, as it had been during the war years, against tuberculosis, diphtheria, venereal disease, and cough- and sneeze-spread viruses.   Because of a decline in the incidence of some of these diseases, the Ministry within a few years shifted the emphasis to such matters as mental health, poliomyelitis vaccination, home accidents, welfare foods, dental health, and food hygiene.

The methods of publicity also underwent change.   The chief reliance at first was upon large posters, national advertising, and "filmlets" attached to newsreels for use in the cinemas.   A score of films designed primarily for invited audiences were also made available from the central film library on such subjects as droplet infection, venereal disease, mental health, smallpox, general health, child health, child welfare, food poisoning, and accidents from fire.   These films were very much in demand all through the 1950's.   But cinemas were no longer willing to show official filmlets—a service they had been willing to perform during the war years.   A noticeable reaction against any form of official propaganda was also a factor in the new approach the Minister deemed necessary.

Press and poster advertising on a national scale was still used when circumstances required and press relations were maintained with feature writers and reporters, but the local health authorities became the chief agents for disseminating health information.   Small posters, cards, leaflets, and wall sheets were supplied to the local health authorities for use in their own offices and for distribution to public libraries and clinics.   It was generally recognized that the most effective agents for health education were those who worked directly with the people—the family doctors, midwives, social workers, health visitors, home nurses, and public health inspectors.   Television, however, was not excluded as an important means of education.   Informative discussions on health matters were presented, and filmlets taking between fifteen and ninety seconds were also produced for television on such subjects as home accidents, food hygiene, dental health education, and diphtheria immunization.[47]

The successful campaign against tuberculosis waged by the mobile X-ray units of the regional hospital boards has already been discussed. The fight against this disease was a co-operative venture in which the local health authorities played an active role through their tuberculosis care committees.   Tuberculosis visitors called upon the patients in their homes and made every effort to work closely with the chest clinics. Home nursing equipment and extra nourishment were furnished, and in other ways care and after-care were provided for such patients. Their rehabilitation included occupational resettlement. Some of the local authorities established workshops where gardening, poultry farming, handicrafts, cabinet-making, and wood-working of various types were taught with a view toward the subsequent re-employment of the patients. In some localities, arrangements were made to maintain tuberculous patients in colonies run by voluntary associations. In the case of the London County Council, three hostels were in operation by 1958 for chronically tuberculous men who were homeless but could work.

The rapidly declining incidence of tuberculosis led to a shift in the emphasis from curative to preventive measures. While miniature X-rays remained an important weapon, vaccination became the most effective deterrent of all. Every effort was made to inoculate adults who had any contact with tuberculous infection. By the end of 1959, nearly a half million such persons and more than twice that many school children had been vaccinated by the local health authorities.[48]

In the campaign to encourage immunization against diphtheria, every medium of publicity was pressed into service. As a result, nearly one-half of the children under fifteen years of age acquired immunity during the 1950's. In 1958, eight deaths were attributed to that disease, which in 1941 took over 2,500 lives. Much was done to educate the public about cough- and sneeze-spread viruses. Virtually all of the local authorities offered vaccination against whooping cough, and 625,000 children in 1960 were inoculated. A growing number of local governments (over one-third in 1959) made provision for tetanus immunization, but all of them offered vaccination against smallpox. While only adults who ran the risk of exposure or who planned to travel abroad were vaccinated, every effort was made to have infants inoculated. In 1960, as in the preceding years, over 40 per cent of the live births were vaccinated for smallpox. One death in 1957 and one in 1958 were enough to keep this dreadful disease before the people and to encourage parents to seek protection for their children. Immunization and vaccination were free and voluntary and were usually given at school clinics and child welfare centers, although family physicians were prepared to provide individual inoculation.

The poliomyelitis vaccination program was much more dramatic than any of the others. A joint committee was appointed by the Central and Scottish Health Services Council in the mid-1950's to determine who should have priority in being vaccinated. Children between the ages of two and nine and hospital employees who might be exposed to the disease were originally accepted for inoculation. As more vaccine became available, the age group was enlarged, and by February, 1960, every person under the age of forty had become eligible. By the end of 1959, more than 11 million people in England and Wales had received two injections. Approximately 75 per cent of all children under the age of sixteen years were then registered for and had received or were in the process of receiving the three injections deemed essential.[49]

Not before the end of 1959 was the British source of supply for poliomyelitis vaccine adequate to meet the greater part of the demand, and until then the Ministry of Health was compelled to import large quantities from Canada and the United States. Shortly after the Salk vaccine was announced, the British revealed that they had their own vaccine, believed to be superior, which was being tested for potency and safety by the Medical Research Council. When it became evident that the English pharmaceutical firms could not produce this vaccine in sufficient quantities, the Ministry of Health reluctantly began to import vaccine from abroad that had to be tested for safety by the Medical Research Council. The effect was to create a bottleneck in a program that, to the popular mind, had become extremely urgent. The Ministry became the target for critical comment. Advised by the Medical Research Council, the Ministry decided, as a temporary measure, that vaccine tested and licensed in America need not undergo the time-consuming "check-tests" in England. But even after this more liberal policy was put into effect there were times that the vaccine was in short supply.

By spring, 1959, the Department of Health had distributed more than 25,000,000 doses of vaccine, of which roughly 60 per cent had been imported. The cost paid by the government for three injections of the vaccine averaged between 10s ($1.40) and 12s ($1.68). The 1959 record of 86 deaths from this disease, one of the lowest for some years, was a hopeful sign that the monetary investment in the preventive measures against poliomyelitis—£7.5 million ($21 million) through 1960—had been wisely spent.[50]

While there was reason to believe that poliomyelitis could be eliminated as a threat to human life, no such hope was held for cancer in the foreseeable future. The growing incidence of lung cancer and the part played in it by smoking had been the subjects of careful research by the Medical Research Council. Although cancer-producing agents had been found in tobacco smoke, it could not be directly demonstrated that they produced lung cancer. The statistical association between lung cancer and cigarette smoking was, however, extremely convincing. On the basis of the evidence, both the Standing Medical Advisory Committee and the Central Health Services Council finally decided that the situation warranted a "national publicity campaign." The Minister of Health endeavored to publicize such information as was available, and in circulars to the local health authorities, he urged that the facts be disseminated by them as well. It was generally recognized that the best approach was to demonstrate the danger to adolescents and others who had not formed the smoking habit. The older school children thus became the primary objective of a campaign to combat the growing menace of lung cancer, which in 1958 accounted for one-fifth of all deaths from malignant diseases.[51]

Mass miniature radiography revealed many cases of malignant thoracic tumors, but it had become increasingly obvious that only through education, conducted preferably on the local level, could the most effective kind of preventive campaign be waged against cancer. The local health authorities were advised to take appropriate action in their program on health education. The response was not satisfactory, owing mostly, it appeared, to divided sentiment in the medical profession. Many physicians seemed to doubt the value of educating the public about cancer. They felt that such information would only serve to cause unnecessary fears about the disease and to encourage hypochondria.

Such misgivings, however, were largely proved groundless in an experiment conducted between 1951 and 1954 in Lancashire by a voluntary organization known as the Manchester Committee on Cancer. The Committee saturated the area with pamphlets, lectures, and newspaper articles on cancer and then observed the effects of its campaign. Hospital doctors, general medical practitioners, and Medical Officers of Health participated in the massive publicity program designed to set forth the facts about the disease. People were urged not to ignore the warning signs of cancer—a sore that would not heal or unexpected bleeding or a painless lump. No false claims were made, but the people were informed that many cases of cancer, if treated in the early stages, could be cured. The response was reassuring. Needless fears were not aroused, and the doctors in the area were not subject to any unnecessary work. An inquiry among 1,200 women in Manchester showed a three-fourth's majority favorable to such a frank and open discussion on cancer. Most significant was the increased number of women who sought early treatment for the cure of breast cancer.[52]

The prevention of food poisoning ranked high among the publicity programs of the Health Service. Housewives and those who handled or processed food in factories, restaurants, canteens, and stores were reminded through virtually every medium of education about the importance of certain basic principles of hygiene. Emphasis was placed upon the necessity for personal cleanliness and of keeping food from contamination.

The local authorities were active in the prevention of venereal disease, but they were not as effective as they should have been, for the incidence of gonorrhea showed a gradual rise during the 1950's. A circular issued by the Ministry of Health in spring, 1959, urged the local authorities to review their arrangements for the prevention of this disease. More publicity was suggested, as well as greater co-operation between the hospitals, the general practitioners, and the Medical Officers of Health, in an effort to reverse the trend.

The high rate of deaths and injuries in the homes led to a nation-wide campaign involving films, cinema or television slides, leaflets, press releases, and display material. A set of pictures, "Death Traps in the Home," was considered so effective that it was reproduced in a leaflet, and over 800,000 copies in 1958 were sent to local authorities and voluntary associations for distribution.[53]

The prevention of illness was closely associated with the care and after-care of those who were sick. The part played by home nursing, health visiting, the home help service, and the domiciliary consultant and general practitioner services has been noted, but there were other types of assistance. Although the pattern varied between areas, milk or other nutrients were generally supplied, and nursing equipment and other apparatus were furnished on a loan basis. Such items included walking aids, invalid chairs, bed pans, hoists for lifting patients, and special beds or mattresses. In some cases, a mobile meals service, a night attendant service, a laundry service, a chiropody service, and facilities for holiday convalescence were also made available.

In the care and after-care program, no group commanded more attention from the local health authorities than the elderly and chronic sick, and the statistical trend emphasized how much greater, even, the problem would be in future years. In 1948 there were about 4.5 million persons 65 years of age and over; ten years later, the number had increased by more than 14 per cent. The Government Actuary's Department predicted a total of nearly 7 million in 1974. An increasing proportion of the aged were women, who represented 58 per cent in 1959.[54] It was apparent that an aging population would impose heavier demands upon the residential accommodations as well as all services that were useful to elderly people. What the hospital service did to meet the problem of chronic illness has been covered. The role of the local health authority in mental health for the aged has likewise been scrutinized. The scope of the domiciliary services also has been surveyed, but certain aspects of old-age care on the local level remain to be treated.

Ninety-five per cent of the people of pensionable age resided in their homes or were otherwise taken care of in the community. The great majority lived on a very meager income. An inquiry in East London at Bethnal Green in the mid-1950's revealed that, upon retirement, the incomes of married people dropped over one-half and the incomes of single or widowed persons declined 68 per cent. One-third of those retired possessed savings, but only 13 per cent had more than £100 ($280). Forty-two per cent received assistance grants that supplemented their pensions. Another 20 to 25 per cent were entitled to supplementary assistance, but they either did not wish to apply for it (perhaps because of a prejudice against "charity") or were unaware they could get it.[55] While the situation at Bethnal Green may not have been quite the same as in all other areas, it was apparent that, without the National Health Service Act of 1946 and the National Assistance Act of 1948, the plight of some members of the elderly population in England and Wales would have been desperate.

The approach to the problem of care for the aged was more or less experimental. There were, however, certain fundamental considerations, most important of which was the desire of elderly persons to retain their individuality, their social contacts, and their independence as long as possible. They much preferred to reside at home rather than in an institution. They wanted to enjoy privacy, to remain in familiar surroundings, and to be a part of the community where they had lived during their productive years. The domiciliary services and the financial assistance program were primarily designed to keep the aged in their homes as long as possible, and all but a small minority were able to remain there. At least one million lived alone. For some, residential accommodations had to be provided. During the eleven-year period ending in 1960, the number of such residents increased from 46,000 to 85,000—an average annual growth of over 3,500. The waiting list indicated that the number would have been larger if more residential facilities had existed.

When the Health Service began, the old spirit of the Poor Law institutions was still very much alive, but within ten years a great transformation had occurred. The welfare authorities recognized that institutional living would be more attractive for the aged if the atmosphere was informal and inviting. The individuality and dignity of the resident could be safeguarded much better in small homes with single and double bedrooms than in large, overcrowded institutions where there was little privacy. The demand for more institutional space by an aging population, together with the restrictions on government spending, made it necessary to use the former institutions much longer than the authorities would have liked. In many cases, however, these buildings were modernized, the large day-rooms and dormitories being broken up into smaller units. The floors were relaid, the walls were plastered, and the lavatories and kitchens were re-equipped. But overcrowding remained a problem; and a few obsolete institutions, which the officials had hoped to relinquish soon, remained unimproved and were still in use at the end of the first decade.

In July, 1948, only 63 small homes for the aged and handicapped were owned by the local authorities, but a steadily expanding program brought the number to over 1,100 at the close of 1959. Such facilities then accommodated 43 per cent of all welfare residents, while an additional 15 per cent were housed by voluntary organizations on behalf of the local authorities. Initially, the great majority of small homes were former hotels or private houses serving groups of about 30 to 40 residents. By installing elevators and otherwise remodeling these buildings to meet the needs of aged occupants, the welfare authorities were able to provide accommodations that were superior to those offered by the old type of institution.

Even more desirable were the newly erected and specially designed homes. Increased funds from the Exchequer made it possible to finance a larger number of them toward the end of the first decade of the Health Service. One-half of those homes opened for use in 1959 were new structures, though, owing to the greater demand for beds, it became the policy to accommodate about sixty people per dwelling. Every effort was made to retain all the advantages of smaller homes, however. Instead of one large sitting room, four or more smaller ones seemed to serve better the divergent interests of the residents. The Minister advised that the local authorities permit the residents to bring with them some of their own furniture. "While this may entail some sacrifice in uniformity," he explained in a circular, "it gives immense pleasure to old people to be able to keep with them some small part of their former home and to retain something which is their own property."[56]

The greater interest in residential care for the aged was reflected in the larger amount of housing erected by the local authorities that was specifically intended for old people. In 1949, the proportion was only 7 per cent, while ten years later it was 22 per cent, and in future years it promised to approach an even higher figure.[57] Quite a few of the aged persons who sought admission to a welfare home could have lived independently if suitable housing were available and certain services could have been provided. Many local governments accordingly built special one-bedroom flats or bungalows where the tenants could be looked after by a caretaker or warden. In some of the schemes, units of small houses were erected in proximity to a welfare home. During illness, meals were brought from the home, and its amenities were always accessible to the residents of the small bungalows. Close acquaintance with the staff of the home made it easier for the individual to move into the home when the infirmities of old age necessitated that course. Whether living in a bungalow or a welfare home, however, each person was free to come and go as he pleased and to maintain whatever links he chose with the community.

Every resident had to pay for his accommodation. In the case of the welfare home, the charge was based upon the operating costs, but adjustment was made according to the patient's means. There was, however, a minimum charge, which in the spring, 1958, was increased to £2 ($5.60) per week. If the person could not from his own resources pay that amount, the National Assistance Board, through a grant, made it possible for him to do so and still to have spending money to meet small personal expenses.

A few of the welfare authorities adopted the policy of boarding out some of the aged persons in carefully selected private homes. Whether on a short-term or permanent basis, it was necessary that the elderly guests be treated more or less as members of the family. There were obvious risks, and only a small number of individuals could be accommodated in this manner, but where properly handled, the arrangement worked very well.

Only 4 per cent of persons over 65 years of age were in hospitals or residential homes in 1959. The great majority of the aged lived with their children or relatives or were visited by them, but a significant minority, between 10 and 20 per cent, were out of touch with relatives or had outlived their contemporaries. They were in danger of being isolated. For these people, more than any others, the domiciliary services assumed a very special importance. The local authorities gave increased attention to this group, providing them with leaflets or booklets describing all the services that were available to them. Precautionary measures were taken in some areas to make sure that no person lacked social or medical care. In Southeast London, for example, several family doctors initiated a scheme whereby in each street a steward was designated to whom the elderly people could turn for help.[58]

Voluntary activity was important in helping the aged. Nearly 1,300 local old people's welfare committees flourished in 1959. Organized and co-ordinated by the National Old People's Welfare Council, these local groups were primarily concerned with the physical and mental well-being of elderly people. The National Council offered refresher and training courses for voluntary workers and a training program for those who wished to become matrons or assistant matrons in homes for the aged. The British Red Cross and the Women's Voluntary Services also gave help to elderly persons. Giving assistance in the home, arranging holiday outings, providing hot meals, and organizing clubs were some of the types of work done by the voluntary organizations.

The recreational needs of many elderly persons were satisfied through membership in clubs at the new day centers that were established in various parts of England. Hot lunches were served and part-time employment could be obtained at these centers. As an example of the progress achieved in this field, in Essex County there were no day centers for the aged in 1948 and 27 ten years later, and during that period the number of old people's clubs grew from 50 to over 300.[59]

The importance of an adequate diet was recognized by all, but many aged people lacked the inclination, the strength, or the money to prepare proper meals. While the home helpers were useful in this respect, not all persons made use of this service. For such individuals, the meals-on-wheels program proved popular in the few localities in which it was employed. Although financed by the local government, the service was usually handled by a voluntary organization, which distributed at least three hot meals a week. Sheffield, for instance, launched a scheme in 1959 that provided for the daily distribution of 2,000 meals from a vehicle especially designed for the purpose. The significance of this service was acclaimed in Parliament, and there was every reason to believe that it would expand.[60]

The chiropody service emerged at the end of the first decade as a growing element of the local health program. Crippling ailments of the hands and feet resulted in much suffering among elderly persons and left many of them seriously handicapped. Owing to the lack of funds, the Minister of Health at first refused to sanction local plans for an effective chiropody service, but with the improvement in the financial situation he was prepared to do so. By the end of 1960, over 100 local authorities had had chiropody schemes accepted, and it was apparent many others would be approved. Treatment was provided in the homes for those who were unable to go to the clinic or the office of the chiropodist. Unfortunately, there was an insufficient number of foot specialists, and until more were trained, the service could not accommodate all who needed this type of therapy.[61]

Within certain limits, the local health authorities were free to experiment. Precisely how far the home help service should be carried, for instance, was a matter largely determined on the local level, although ministerial sanction for any plan was necessary. The County Council of Kent, for example, arranged for a trial evening service and night attendant service in one of the areas under its authority. Designed for old people who were bedridden or confined to their homes, the evening service sent a helper to call for a half hour to prepare a meal or a hot beverage or to render some other service to make the individual comfortable for the night. The night attendant service was for elderly persons who were sick and alone. The helper stayed every night until the patient became better or was removed to a residential accommodation. So successful was this service that it was extended to the entire county. Most of the requests for the evening and the night attendant services came from the general practitioners, and there was no evidence of abuse.[62]

The importance of the Health Service as it affected the aged in their homes was made abundantly clear by a survey of households in two metropolitan boroughs in 1950 and in 1956. In the latter year, the inquiry included 483 aged persons, more than half of whom were seventy-five years old or older. Three-fourths of them were women. Although many suffered from chronic diseases, only one was on the waiting list for admission to the hospital. Two had been recently discharged from the hospital. Only 3 per cent were permanently confined to their beds, but 10 per cent were intermittently bedridden. Significantly, the percentage of bedridden patients was lower than in the earlier survey. About 80 per cent were regularly visited by their family physician, but only one-seventh were under the care of a district nurse. The proportion of elderly persons that remained alone at night in 1956 was smaller than in the preceding year of inquiry.

The 1956 survey showed that in nearly one-half of the homes the domestic worker rendered some assistance in preparing the meals, but cleaning was her chief activity. She worked an average of five hours per week per household. Two-thirds of the aged were unable to pay any part of the cost of domestic help. The service, the survey explained, "cannot be measured in terms of hours of work, or domestic duties performed—it goes far beyond that, and no statistical survey can give a complete picture of the assistance companionship it provides both during and after official visiting hours." An improvement had occurred in the general position of the elderly people since the earlier survey. This was attributed to a "better liaison with hospital geriatric departments, a greater emphasis on rehabilitation, an expansion of the home-help service, and closer co-ordination of effort between the statutory and voluntary agencies concerned."[63]

Although much had been done for the chronic sick and elderly, the program did not measure up to the expectations of its critics. If aged persons had been a homogeneous group, the problem could have been met in a more purposeful way, but they were no more similar than the young. Their interests, needs, and aspirations differed greatly, and what was done for them therefore could not be reduced to a pattern. In studying the literature on the care of the aged, it is impossible to escape the realization that in the final analysis the problem of mental and physical deterioration that characterizes the latter years of human life can have only a provisional solution. There is no definitive cure for the frustrations and infirmities of old age— there are only palliatives. But within the limits prescribed by the true nature of the problem, the medico-social services in England and Wales did much to make those years more bearable and pleasant.

The British were alert to the difficulties and the goals of the care of the aged. This was evident from the Guillebaud Report, the Phillips Report, the Younghusband Report, and the debates in Parliament on the subject.[64] The government had provided a multitude of services, but they were not always co-ordinated or adequate. The local domiciliary services were good, but they suffered from a shortage of personnel. The services supplied by the Executive Councils, the hospitals, and the voluntary organizations too often functioned in tight compartments, and this difficulty was compounded by a lack of funds, especially during the early years. In spite of such handicaps, which were in the course of time being reduced, the British program for the care of the aged represented a solid achievement. If the signposts were not wrong, an even better program lay ahead.

Casting its shadow over all phases of the Health Service was the tripartite structure. It was undoubtedly an obstacle to the smooth operation of the Service. Yet the antecedents of the Service had made a decentralized system more or less inevitable. It should be recalled that prior to 1948 there was a multiplicity of authorities with overlapping health functions. The creation of the Health Service was the first nationwide attempt to provide a comprehensive program. Parliament could not very well have scrapped all the health agencies that had developed over many decades. What could be salvaged was incorporated into the new scheme, and a divided administrative system came into existence as a consequence. But even if a unitary plan of organization had been possible, the tremendous scope and size of the Health Service would have posed inevitable problems of co-ordination.

No theme preoccupied the authorities more than how to promote better co-operation between the local health authority, the general medical practitioner, and the hospital and specialist services. The lack of co-ordination made it difficult to serve in the most efficient way those patients who had to make use of the three branches, or even two of them, during an illness. This was especially true in such fields as mental health, care of the aged and chronic sick, tuberculosis, and maternity and child welfare. The lines were not sharply drawn between preventive and curative medicine, and each was very much dependent upon the other.

A small minority believed that the integration of the services could be accomplished through the statutory reorganization of the machinery, but they could not agree on what the form of the reorganization should be. It was suggested that the administration of the hospital services or the Executive Council services or both should be transferred to the local authorities. It was also proposed that a national board or corporation should exercise central administrative functions. The prevailing sentiment rejected any such modification in the machinery.

Ministerial circulars were issued urging co-operation. The membership of the Executive Councils, the hospital boards, and the management committees included representatives from other parts of the Service. There were a number of standing joint liaison committees on the local and regional level designed to deal with matters of mutual interest. Some liaison committees were set up to handle only special subjects—the care of the aged infirm and the chronic sick, for instance. Co-operation was also accomplished through the joint use of facilities and the joint employment of staff by the regional hospital boards and the local health authorities. Certain clinics were jointly operated by local health or education authorities and the regional hospital boards.[65]

The composite picture as viewed by the Central Health Services Council in 1952 was a rather encouraging one, but there was no room for complacency. In many areas a much greater degree of co-operation was necessary. To help achieve it, the Council recommended the creation in each locality of a standing joint consultative committee that would represent the Executive Council, the local medical committee, the hospital management committee, and the county or county-borough council. The consultative committee would discuss local arrangements of joint concern and would stimulate between these agencies the exchange of data, proposals, and other pertinent information.[66]

Only a few regions established such a committee. The general feeling was that neither the creation of new machinery nor a proliferation of committees would help much. The need was for a "change of heart" among the hospital doctors, family physicians, and local health employees in those areas where there had been too little co-operation. "We would emphasize," asserted the Guillebaud Committee, "that co-operation has been achieved successfully in some areas of the country where there has been a determination to see that it should succeed; and we have no doubt that the authorities and individuals in other areas could achieve the same degree of success if they are made aware of the need and are ready to make the effort required."[67] In the opinion of the Cohen Committee, the "present structure of the Service need not prevent fruitful co-operation between the general practitioner and the other parts of the Service." The Committee noted that "where there is a sincere desire to work together in a spirit of service, co-operation exists."[68]

Much depended upon the basic attitude of the medical doctors and other Health Service personnel toward each other. The Social Surveys in 1956 disclosed that the great majority of general medical practitioners believed that, while their relationship with consultants, Medical Officers of Health, district nurses, midwives, and other family doctors could be closer, it was satisfactory. Few could deny that considerable progress had been made, but it was evident that the National Health Service had not achieved the degree of co-ordination among the various divisions that was essential in a first-class service. As it had in the first decade, the same problem, although it was now less crucial, seemed destined in the second to command the careful attention of the health authorities.

CHAPTER XV

The Dental Service

THE GOVERNMENT could not guarantee treatment to all people in the dental service as it could in the medical program. The shortage of dentists was so serious that the dental needs of the nation could be met only partially. Those who planned the National Health Service had envisioned a comprehensive dental service, but expediency forced the government to resort to charges and certain other measures so that children and expectant and nursing mothers would have first claim upon the dental resources of the nation. Yet even this approach was not very successful.

Understaffed local authority dental clinics, an undermanned dental school program, and an insufficient number of dentists in the general dental service constituted important elements in the failure to make adequate provision even for the priority patients. There was also an appalling amount of popular apathy and ignorance about dental health that could not easily be combated. The higher incidence of caries, owing to changing dietary habits as well as to neglect, would have overtaxed a greatly expanded dental service. But what seemed to impress observers most was not so much the obstacles that beset the program as the discouragingly high percentage of children and adults who still had diseased teeth after ten years of the Health Service. What often passed unnoticed was the steady progress made in the conservation of teeth and the large number of patients who benefited from the dental service.

The first decade was thus not devoid of solid achievement in spite of the generally somber picture. There was reason to believe that the foundation was being laid for a more effective dental service. Apart from the lessons that years of experience had taught the authorities, much was learned from investigations of the dental program made during the 1950's. The observations and recommendations of the reports were slowly shaping the course of the dental service. The difference in points of view between the Ministry of Health and the British Dental Association in no way diminished their determination to make the scheme work, and this was perhaps the best guarantee that a more adequately staffed and better integrated service would gradually evolve.

Any dentist who wished to participate in the National Health Service could do so, and all but a very small proportion of the dental practitioners joined. Those who did could still have private patients, but not more than an estimated 5 per cent of the patients of Health Service dentists were in that category.[1] All Health Service dentists were free to practice where they wished and to choose their patients. There was no restriction placed on the number of patients that the individual dentist could treat. Unlike the young medical doctor, a young dentist could buy a practice, but in view of the great need for dentists in almost every area, the value placed on good will was usually not very high. Assistantship with a view toward partnership was another method of entering dental practice, but this avenue was not followed by many. About 80 per cent of the dentists practiced singly. It was easy to open an office anywhere, and so a substantial number of new dentists entered the Health Service directly as principals. The only major problem was to raise the capital to acquire and equip an office.

The number of assistants was not large, and many who started their dental career in that fashion did not serve long in such a role. The terms were worked out by mutual agreement between the assistant and the principal, but owing to the shortage of qualified dental assistants, salaries averaged £1,575 ($4,410) in 1955-56, which was considerably more than assistants could earn in general medical practice. Like medical doctors, general dental practitioners were responsible for the acts and omissions of their assistants.

The Health Service dentist was under contract with the Executive Council and was subject to the jurisdiction of that body. His office could be inspected, and he was required to keep records and make them available to the proper officials whenever the occasion arose. He could leave the service three months after tendering his resignation, although he was expected to make satisfactory arrangements for Health Service patients whose treatment had not been completed at that time.

A roster of the Health Service dentists was available to the public. The individual could make an appointment with any dentist on the roster who was willing to accept him for treatment. The patient did not have to register or get his name on a list, as he did with the general medical practitioner service. The dental patient had only to sign a form indicating that he wanted to be treated under the Health Service. The dentist, in turn, had to give a signed acknowledgment to the patient that he was accepted for treatment. If the individual refused to have all the work done that his dentist recommended, a notation to that effect was made and was signed by the patient. An estimate showing the scope and cost of the work was prepared, and the dentist could then begin treatment as soon as he wished in the great majority of cases. All emergency treatment was given immediately. No delay occurred for normal fillings, root treatment, prophylaxis, ordinary denture repairs, extractions for the relief of pain, and all other extractions that did not make dentures necessary. In the more complicated and expensive operations, which represented less than one-fifth of all courses of treatment, an estimate had to be approved by the Dental Estimates Board before work could begin. In this group were complex X-rays, extractions for and the provision of dentures, oral surgery, orthodontics, prolonged treatment of gums, gold inlays, and certain other types of work.[2]

The Dental Estimates Board comprised a chairman, a vice-chairman, and seven other members, all appointed by the Minister of Health. Only two were not dentists. With headquarters at Eastbourne, this group presided over a staff of some 900 assessors, assistants, and clerks. The Board served two primary purposes: to prevent abuse of the service and to make sure that the dental treatment was not below proper standards. Approving proposed treatments was only a part of its responsibility. What took the largest portion of time was the examination and verification of the estimates the dentists were required to submit covering all the work they had completed. Not until payment was sanctioned by the Dental Estimates Board could the Executive Council compensate the dentist. Such elaborate controls were deemed necessary because of the fee-for-service method of payment.

The work of this Board was in almost every respect efficient. The Board's personnel were highly trained and only occasionally would a matter require the attention of the Board's dental advisors. And only in exceptional cases was payment not promptly authorized. Estimates for dentures submitted for prior approval generally encountered no delay, but if the proposed course of treatment involved gold inlays or bridges or some other expensive work, it was subjected to careful scrutiny. Proposals for work deemed clinically unnecessary were rejected. If there were any doubt concerning the treatment or fees, a full investigation was made. The dental record for each patient, with all previous treatment received by him, was kept at the central office, and this was carefully checked. If necessary, the

Board asked the regional dental officer to examine the patient personally and make a report.

Unable to begin treatment until action was completed on the estimate, the dentist was inclined to view the whole procedure with impatience and even as an unwarranted interference with his professional rights. If he disagreed with the decision of the Dental Estimates Board, he could appeal it to two independent referees who were dentists. One was chosen by the Minister of Health and the other selected from a panel nominated by the British Dental Association. The referees could examine the patient, if they chose, and their decision was final. In the five-year period ending in 1959, there were an average of 400 appeals per year, the majority of which concerned treatment and not fees. Considering the fact that there were each year over 10 million courses of treatment processed by the board, the number of appeals seemed astonishingly low. In more than two-thirds of the cases, the decision of the board was sustained by the referees.[3]

The Guillebaud Committee viewed the Dental Estimates Board as the most appropriate and least expensive method for providing the necessary check on the work done in the dental service. The McNair Committee, which examined critically this particular phase of the dental program, found that the Dental Estimates Board fulfilled the very useful role of ensuring that public funds were properly spent and that it also "saved dentists and local Executive Councils much time and paper work because of the efficiency of [its] system." But there was some question whether all items on the list of treatments requiring prior approval should have been there. Without suggesting which should be removed, the McNair Committee thought that the list should be reviewed periodically "in the light of the circumstances and clinical methods obtaining from time to time." "It must always be the aim," averred the Committee, "to make and keep the list as short as possible and to include only treatments which cannot be prevented from becoming occasions of abuse."[4]

The British Dental Association recognized that if there were fewer items that required prior approval, there would be more freedom of action for the dental practitioner. Since the procedure of obtaining prior approval could mean a frustrating delay, some dentists tended to recommend the form of treatment they knew from experience would be accepted promptly. In this sense, professional freedom for the dental practitioner was inhibited under the Health Service. Eager to have the situation corrected, the Dental Association frequently importuned the government to revise the list. Action came slowly.

The biggest step in the revision of the regulations was taken in

1960, when it was decided to abolish the requirement of prior approval for gold fillings, apicectomy, the provision of one post crown, and certain initial work for dentures. The list of drugs that could be prescribed by dentists was extended, the right to employ dental hygienists in general practice was recognized, and the rules concerning supplementary and revised estimates were clarified. Moreover, the procedure for dealing with appeals from the decisions of the Dental Estimates Board was simplified. More discussions between the Ministry of Health and the Dental Association were scheduled with a view toward achieving a further relaxation of the regulations. Much encouraged by the concessions, the *British Dental Journal* described them as a "step forward," and took a more hopeful view of the future.[5]

Once a dentist began a course of treatment, he was under obligation to complete it. Only in exceptional cases, when the work extended over a period of more than one year, were there interim payments; otherwise, the dentist received no remuneration until the treatment was finished. Under certain conditions the dentist was allowed to abandon treatment and receive payment for what he had done so far, but he could do this only with the consent of the Executive Council. In reaching a decision, this body gave careful consideration to the interests of the patient. There were, for example, during the 1959-60 fiscal year less than 125 cases in London in which permission to discontinue treatment was granted.[6]

Although, as far as could be determined, dentists seldom provided excessive or unnecessary treatment, a regulation was adopted in 1956 to cover any case that might occur. Where the estimates indicated that needless work was being done, the Minister might refer the matter to the local dental committee for consideration. Upon the recommendation of this committee and the Executive Council, the Minister could require that for a specified period the offending dentist must seek from the Dental Estimates Board prior approval for all work except the examination of teeth and emergency treatment. If the Minister or dental practitioner were dissatisfied with the decision of the local dental committee, an appeal could be taken to referees. During the early part of 1959, in the first case to arise under this rule, a dentist was found guilty of providing treatment in excess of what was required to put a patient in a state of dental fitness and was compelled to obtain prior approval for all estimates during a period of twelve months.[7]

The disciplinary machinery in the dental service in most respects was almost identical to that which functioned in the general medical service. Adequate safeguards, involving the right of appeal, were provided to protect the practitioner against false allegations. The

dental profession accepted the basic features of the disciplinary procedure just as the medical profession did. The fact that dentists
served as referees and were represented on the Executive Council,
the dental service committee, the tribunal, and the dental advisory
committee was proof, if any were needed, that the government was
determined that no dentist should be unjustly punished.

The dental advisory committee, which assisted the Minister in
reviewing cases involving disciplinary action, consisted almost entirely of dental practitioners. Three dentists sat in the Executive
Council, and one-half of the membership of the dental service committee was drawn from that profession. It was this committee that
investigated complaints from patients, the Executive Council, and
the Dental Estimates Board against dental practitioners. The defendant was given ample opportunity to clear himself, but if the evidence indicated violation of the terms of service, the matter was
referred to the Executive Council. The final decision in all disciplinary action rested with the tribunal or the Minister himself.

Since about half of the complaints concerned the fit and efficiency
of dentures, provision was made in 1953 for the appointment of
conciliation committees by the Executive Council. Consisting of a
lay chairman and two dentists, these committees investigated complaints and decided whether the denture was properly constructed and
designed and what adjustment could be made to satisfy the patient.
If a satisfactory settlement could not be reached or if it were established that the dentist had been guilty of willful neglect, the dental
service committee then assumed jurisdiction over the case.

About 50 per cent of the complaints involved a breach of the
terms of service. The total number of cases that came before the
Executive Councils was more than twice as high during the early
part of the 1950's than toward the end of that decade. In 1959,
there were 350 cases. In at least half of them, the Minister found
no breach of the terms of service. In only 14 per cent of the cases
was payment withheld from the dentist. In a somewhat larger number of cases, the patient's expenses had to be reimbursed by the practitioner. Warning letters were issued to some. None was expelled
from the dental service by the tribunal between 1956 and 1959,
but in 1960 there were two dismissals. During the first six years, the
average number of dismissals was four per year.[8]

A formal complaint had to be made within six weeks after the
patient became aware that the treatment was unsatisfactory or within
six months after the work had been completed, whichever was sooner.
Only in the case of dismissal from the service were names ever made
public, but it took a very major offense or a series of misdeeds to war-

rant expulsion. In 1949, a dentist was removed from the Health Service list for accepting fees for work that was then free and for not completing treatment. He also canvassed for patients, which was considered a breach of professional etiquette, and he openly asserted that "Government teeth" were unsatisfactory.[9] A dental practitioner dismissed from the Service in 1954 was found guilty of accepting fees without finishing the treatment. He also failed to produce record cards and did not employ the proper degree of technical skill necessary to make patients dentally fit.[10]

Some dentists were merely censured. One in Devonshire was dissatisfied with the fee authorized for denture work by the Dental Estimates Board and he indiscretely discussed the matter with a patient. A sharply worded letter by the patient to the Executive Council in protest of the delay in treatment and the amount of the fee created an unpleasant situation. In the opinion of the Council, such unprofessional conduct on the part of a dentist merited censure. A fine was reserved for the more flagrant offenses. In 1949, a dentist who had grossed £7,257 ($20,319) during the first year of the Health Service was found to be maintaining such low professional standards that they shocked the dental service committee. The Executive Council proposed a fine of £1,000 ($2,800) as well as a severe reprimand and a warning of dismissal if the practitioner did not improve the quality of his work.[11]

A penalty of 175 guineas ($514) was recommended by the Derbyshire Executive Council in 1957 for a dentist who permitted an unqualified assistant to provide a patient with false teeth that did not fit properly. A dental practitioner in West Riding who was careless in filling out forms and was overpaid for work done had to forfeit £200 ($560) from his pay in 1958. No dishonesty was involved—only administrative negligence. A London practitioner in the fall of 1959 was assessed a fine of 100 guineas ($294). Although denying "evil intent" and pleading carelessness, he was found guilty of various discrepancies, such as the submission of two estimates for the extraction of one tooth. Much graver was the case of a Walsall dentist who was charged in 1958 with many irregularities in the submission of claims. Although he protested that many of them were simple errors committed by an inexperienced staff, the Executive Council took a very stern view of the offenses and recommended that £4,095 10s ($11,467) be withheld from his compensation.[12]

Allegations not well founded were promptly rejected by the Executive Council. As an example, in Lancashire during 1957 a dental practitioner was accused of behaving in "an aggressive, bad tempered and brutal manner." A husband charged that his wife's dentures were unsatisfactory and that their child had so much cotton put in her mouth during a treatment that she became sick. The dentist said that he was bitten by the child six times within five minutes while drilling a tooth and that the husband had to be ordered off the premises because of his objectionable conduct. The refusal of the woman to return to the office of the dentist made it impossible for him to make the necessary adjustment in her dentures. The council could find no evidence that the terms of service had been violated.[13]

Only a small proportion of the charges against dentists ended in disciplinary action. Compared with the many million courses of treatment, the complaints were extremely few. In 1959, fewer than 175, or 1.5 per cent, of the practitioners in the dental service were judged guilty of a breach of the terms of service, but only 50 of them were actually fined.[14] Carelessness and negligence rather than deliberate intent to flout the regulations seemed to explain the vast majority of cases. The dental service committee as well as the Executive Council, both heavily representative of the professional groups, recognized that the success of the National Health Service required that those who failed to honor their obligations, regardless of motives, should be called to account.

The most serious problem that faced the dental service was the shortage of practitioners, and as the years passed it became apparent that there was no easy solution. Before the inception of the Health Service, dentists, unlike family physicians, depended almost exclusively upon private patients. Although persons under the Health Insurance scheme were entitled to limited dental benefits, they constituted only a negligible part of the ordinary dentist's practice. The great majority of people seldom visited a dentist and had little knowledge about the importance of dental health or the conservation of teeth. Judging by the demand at that time, there was no apparent need for an appreciable increase in the number of dental practitioners. Then came the Health Service and the rush for dentures. In a few years this pressure eased, but the steady growth in conservative treatment meant no relaxation in the volume of work. It became a matter of great concern to the authorities that the dental service was unable to show the flexibility in staff size that characterized most of the other branches of the National Health Service.

During the twelve-year period ending in 1960, the number of dentists in the Health Service increased by only 11 per cent. In 1949, there were 9,500 general dental practitioners in the service. Four years later, the number was even smaller, but thereafter a slow increase each year carried the total to 10,500 by 1960.[15] This number represented about two-thirds of all the names recorded on the dental register for the United Kingdom. What did the other one-third do? A considerable group retained their British registry while practicing overseas; some practiced in Scotland and Ulster; others were salaried employees in the military, school, and local health authority dental services; and a small proportion remained in private practice, worked in the hospitals, or engaged in teaching, research, and other related fields of activity. And there were those in retirement whose names had not been removed from the dental register.

The geographical distribution of dentists was uneven—a condition that improved little during the 1950's. For England and Wales as a whole, there were approximately 4,000 persons per dental practitioner in the Health Service. In London and the South-Eastern Region, the number was 3,100 in 1959, compared with 3,700 ten years earlier. But in the North Midland, the region which young dentists seemed to shun most, the situation showed a steady deterioration during those years. In 1950, this area had a ratio of one dentist to 5,300 persons; at the end of the decade, the proportion had risen to one to 5,900.

However discouraging, the picture was not without its bright spots. Much has been said about the high proportion of dentists over 55 years of age, but this dangerous imbalance began to show improvement. Forty-two per cent were in that age group in 1953, but only 32 per cent six years later. Thirty-nine per cent were under forty years of age in 1959, compared with 31 per cent six years earlier.[16] The predicted collapse of the dental service from the exodus of aged dentists was no longer imminent.

In planning the role of dentistry in the National Health Service, the government was not oblivious to the inadequacy of the dental resources. A committee was appointed in 1943 under the chairmanship of Lord Teviot for the purpose of considering and reporting upon "the progressive stages by which, having regard to the number of practicing dentists, provision for an adequate and satisfactory dental service should be made available to the population." In its final report in 1946, the committee recommended the establishment at the outset of a comprehensive dental service as an integral part of the Health Service. It recognized, however, that at first there might be "some unavoidable limitations" in the dental program, and that children and expectant and nursing mothers should be given priority in the use of the services that were available.

While the Teviot Committee could not accurately anticipate the demand for dental treatment, it estimated that at least 20,000 dental practitioners would be needed in Great Britain. To achieve this total within twenty years, 900 new dental students would have to be admitted each year—a number which made allowance for the 10 per cent who normally failed to qualify. Previous to 1940, the annual number of new dental students averaged about 340, but during the war it dropped below 300. In view of these figures, the Teviot Committee recognized that the recruitment program which it proposed would involve an effort of considerable magnitude.

The Committee believed that dentistry was not a very popular career because of the cost of training, the inadequate financial rewards, the nature of the work and the strain it involved, and the low status with which the profession seemed to be regarded by many people. To overcome these obstacles to a larger dental service the Committee recommended the effective use of propaganda in the schools and throughout the nation. The importance of dentistry as a career would have to be brought to the attention of parents and students. An "appreciation of dental health and a rising demand for treatment will affect the position of the dentist in the public estimation." Appropriate action would have to be taken in regard to remuneration. Reference was made to the dental schools that were housed "in old and unworthy premises" and to the pressing need for improved and enlarged training facilities. If the proper measures were taken, the Teviot Committee believed that the goals which it envisaged would be reached.[17]

Although the report was well received by the dental profession and the Ministry of Health, nothing was done about the recommendations. In the years that immediately followed the war, attendance at the dental schools in Great Britain reached capacity, and this fact may have caused the authorities to believe that the problem might solve itself. In 1951, however, student enrollment began to drop, and in 1953 there were less than 470 first-year dental students, compared with 650 in the initial year of the Health Service. In 1954, the situation showed virtually no improvement.[18] The growing proportion of elderly dentists served to underscore the need for prompt action. The government proposed another investigation and in spring, 1955, appointed a committee under the chairmanship of Lord McNair to determine why there were not more qualified students seeking admission to the dental schools and what remedies might be sought.

Published in fall, 1956, the McNair Report was similar to the Teviot document in its general approach and conclusions. The failure to take the vigorous measures proposed by the earlier committee was considered unfortunate by the McNair investigators, who found that the problem each year had grown more crucial. There was a tremendous shortage of dentists in the armed services, the local clinics, and the general dental service. In the school dental service, which needed between 2,200 and 2,800 full-time dentists, there were less than half that many in 1955. The examination of the school children in 1954 disclosed that less than one-third were in a state of dental fitness. Except in an emergency, dental patients had to wait a considerable time for treatment in the general dental service. The only solution was to train more dentists. The basic recommendations of the Teviot Report were reaffirmed by the McNair Committee. Twenty thousand dental practitioners remained the ultimate target. Allowing for students who would not complete their training and foreigners who would return to their native country to practice, the number of students admitted to the dental schools in Great Britain, it was held, should be fixed at 1,000 per year.

The shortage of dentists occurred as the result of causes recognized as being "both deep rooted and of long standing." The attitude of people toward dental health too often reflected the old belief that the best remedy for a toothache was to remove the tooth. The importance of dental treatment was not appreciated by large segments of the population—an attitude which contributed to the inferior status of the dental profession in comparison with other professions. The dentists as a group also suffered from poor public relations. During the early years of the Health Service, the large earnings of a few practitioners together with some unfortunate disciplinary cases gave the profession a bad press. Moreover, the dentists themselves were dissatisfied, and many were apparently unwilling to advise young people to choose dentistry as a career.

What was the cause of their dissatisfaction? In the opinion of some who testified before the McNair Committee, clinical freedom had been impaired by requiring prior approval for certain forms of treatment. The Committee, however, believed that the real cause for irritation was not so much prior approval as the piece-rate system of compensation. This method of payment was deemed effective when applied to repetitive work, but dental work was more than simple repetition. "It called for the exercise of personal judgment and individual skill." The system of piecework pay meant maximum remuneration during the early years of a dentist's career and a sharply diminished income during the latter years, when speed and the volume of work were reduced. Although the McNair Committee was not prepared to suggest an alternative basis for compensation, it did favor a reexamination of the method of payment.

Discontent was also voiced over the unilateral reductions in remuneration by the Ministry of Health and its policy of refusing to arbitrate the issue—a subject that will be explored shortly. A feeling of financial uncertainty thus clouded the future. There were other causes of dissatisfaction, as well, among them the lack of opportunities outside general practice. The hospital service and research offered few openings for dentists, and postgraduate training led to consultant status only for a very limited number.

None of the problems was beyond solution. The issue that overshadowed all others was clearly student recruitment. The McNair Committee seemed confident that through education and publicity the Ministry of Health and the British Dental Association could arouse a lively interest in dentistry as a career. It was suggested that pamphlets, films, and visits to the schools by dentists should be fully utilized for this purpose, and that dental scholarships should be awarded, in addition. Most important was the establishment of an adequate number of modern dental schools, fully staffed, to accommodate the proposed rise in student enrollment.[19]

The publication of the report was not needed to reverse the enrollment trend among dental students. Even before the McNair Committee finished its labors, enrollment in the dental schools reached capacity, and it was to remain that way in the ensuing years. The schools were now overcrowded and students were turned away. But the need for more and better dental schools was apparent to all. In Parliament and in the lay and professional press, the demand for the training of more dentists grew louder and louder.[20]

In turning its attention to the problem of increasing the number and size of the dental schools, the government moved with such deliberation that misgivings were aroused in dental circles. Yet the Ministry was exploring all possibilities. Details had to be worked out with the University Grants Committee. Not until 1959 did the plans take shape. It was then announced that Wales, which had no training facilities, would get a dental school at Cardiff, and that new institutions would also be built at Birmingham and the University College Hospital. Moreover, new buildings or extensions to existing ones were planned that would increase the size of the dental schools at the London Hospital, King's College Hospital, Leeds, Bristol, Manchester, Newcastle, and possibly Liverpool.[21]

Many years would pass before the goal of 20,000 dental practitioners could be achieved, and even this number would be insufficient to meet the needs of all the people. An average dentist could treat no more than 800 patients a year. Children and expectant mothers should be examined by a dentist more than once a year; persons with dentures require the services of a dental practitioner less frequently. Taking the population as a whole, an estimated four or five times the number of practicing dentists in 1960 would be necessary to keep all

the people dentally fit.[22]   But between need and demand there was
a wide gulf.   The goal set by the Teviot and McNair Committees was
based upon the anticipated demand for dental treatment.   Precisely
how many people in the next decade or so would be taught to visit
the dentists regularly could not very well be plotted on a graph.
Much depended upon the success of dental health education.

A standing Committee on Dental Publicity was set up in 1958
to disseminate information about dental health.   By 1960, there was
evidence of a more purposeful approach in dental health education
and a greater awareness of its value among the general public.   Pamphlets, posters, picture sets, and the press, radio, and television were
being used on a somewhat more extensive scale.   Script writers were
invited to stress the importance of dental care as a health measure
in programs that were intended primarily for parents.   In 1959, two
new filmlets on the care of the teeth were produced, and in 1960 a
new dental film, "Guilty or Not," was released.   Eight new leaflets
were in preparation, each treating a phase of dental care.   They were
designed primarily for distribution by dental practitioners.[23]

The growing importance of dentistry was reflected in the Dentist
Law of 1956.   For many years the supervisory agency for the dental
profession had been the Dental Board, which was subordinate in
many respects to the General Medical Council.   Under the new law,
the Board was replaced by the General Dental Council—an administrative agency which raised the profession to the status of a self-
governing body.   Other significant changes were initiated by the law.
It was now easier for dentists with Commonwealth or foreign qualifications to practice in England.   Oral hygienists, who cleaned, scaled,
and polished teeth in the hospitals and local clinics, could be employed in general practice under the supervision of dentists.   Even
more significant was the provision for the experimental use in the
priority dental services of ancillary workers who would fill teeth and
extract deciduous teeth.[24]

The Teviot Committee favored the use of oral hygienists, but was
reluctant to recommend the training of any other ancillary helpers.
The Guillebaud and McNair Committees accepted the need for a
new class of dental operative assistants who could be used in the
school and the local authority dental clinics.[25]   By performing the
more routine types of work, such assistants would release the fully
trained dentists for the more highly skilled operations.   The dental
profession opposed the idea, realizing that if these ancillary employees should prove successful in the local clinics, as they did in
New Zealand, they might be made available in the general dental
service.   There was fear that the standards of the profession might

be lowered by the use of personnel with such limited training and that eventually the economic status of the regular dentists might be adversely affected. Learning how to fill teeth and to perform other elementary operations would require only two years of training, compared with five years to qualify for general dental practice. The two-year program, it was argued, would attract candidates who might otherwise become dentists.[26]

The Minister of Health was unimpressed by such reasoning. He held that in a profession so understaffed, it was common sense for dental practitioners not to do work that could be done competently by assistants with only two years of training. Assurance was given that the facilities required by regular dental students would not be used in training these special assistants. Plans for the commencement of the experimental training program were not completed before 1960, and in the fall of that year sixty carefully selected young people began their training as dental operative assistants.[27]

The Ministry of Health was not content to increase the number on the dental register; it was also eager to keep dental practitioners abreast of the latest developments. Postgraduate refresher courses were offered by the universities in such fields as children's dentistry, orthodontics, prosthetics, general oral surgery, and conservative dentistry. Largely financed by the government, with an expense allowance for the dentists who attended, these courses more than quadrupled in number between 1954 and 1960. Enrollment increased 260 per cent, with 2,350 dentists taking courses during this period.[28]

In the field of dental research there was progress, but not as much as the Ministry of Health or the dental profession desired. Financial restrictions proved a serious handicap in the earlier years, but toward the end of the decade, when more funds were available, there seemed to be a scarcity of dental research graduates. In 1958, about £53,550 ($150,000) was spent on dental research. The Medical Research Council did what it could to encourage more dental graduates to take training in research methods. A survey by the British Dental Association found that there had been a gradual improvement in the research facilities, although a shortage of laboratory accommodations still existed. An indication of the growing interest in this field of activity was the establishment in 1959 of a Nuffield Research Chair in Dental Science in the Department of Dental Science of the Royal College of Surgeons in England.[29]

Between the British Dental Association and the Ministry of Health there was frequent consultation on many issues, and for the most part a friendly spirit seemed to prevail, despite sharp differences. They seemed to agree, at least in principle, on such matters as dental health education, experimentation in fluoridation, the importance of dental research, and the need to build more dental schools and train more dental practitioners. On other matters, such as the charges imposed upon patients in the general dental service, there appeared to be no agreement. The profession wanted them abolished, or at least eliminated for persons who visited the dentist regularly. There was a difference of opinion as to what items should be subject to prior approval but, as already noted, a reduction of the list in 1960, along with certain other changes in the regulations, showed that both parties through negotiation could reach adjustment of their differences. In 1954, the Minister of Health paid tribute to the British Dental Association "for the constructive way in which the problems have been faced." "I should also like to add," he asserted, "that my personal relationship and those of my Ministry with the dental profession are closer and friendlier than ever before."[30]

However co-operative the Ministry and the dental profession may have been in reaching an accommodation on certain issues, the fact remains that in the most vital field of all, remuneration, there was often a deep cleavage of opinion. It was in this area that the opposing sides experienced their greatest failure, primarily because of the absence of arbitration or some other effective means for reaching a mutually acceptable agreement. In some respects, there was a parallel to the experience of the medical profession, and in both cases a possible solution to the problem seemed to have been found in 1960.

The negotiating body of the dental profession was the General Dental Services Committee. Comprising 70 members, it was elected partly by the British Dental Association's Representative Board and partly by the local dental committees. Its democratic basis was thus even broader than that of the Association itself. Founded in 1880, the Dental Association at first grew slowly, but in 1949 it was able to absorb two smaller dental organizations. By 1958, its membership had reached 11,000, or about four-fifths of those in active practice. Its moderate tactics and policies, however, resulted in the establishment of a splinter group known as the General Dental Practitioners' Association. With a membership of 1,100, this dissident organization favored militant, trade-union methods in the fight for improved terms under the National Health Service. Since the Dental Practitioners' Association was not recognized by the Ministry and was not on amicable terms with the British Dental Association, its influence appeared to be negligible.[31]

In seeking to establish a fair basis for the compensation of dentists, the Minister of Health in 1946 set up the Spens Committee on the Remuneration of General Dental Practitioners. Its report, published two years later, revealed the discouragingly slow progress that had characterized recruitment in the dental profession during the preceding twenty years. In a profession that was "exceptionally arduous," involving "intricate manual work," most of the practitioners, it was shown, made "net incomes of less than enough to meet minimum middle-class expenditure," and one-fourth of them lived below this standard. Recognizing that substantially more money would have to be paid to dental practitioners, the Spens Committee recommended average net earnings of £1,600 ($4,480) per year for a dentist. This was in terms of 1939 values.

The suggested compensation was for a working week of 33 chairside hours for 46 weeks, or a total of 1,500 chairside hours a year. Including non-chairside hours, the number of office hours per week would be 42. Owing to the strain from dental work, it was believed that a longer working week would normally result in the loss of efficiency; but for those who could work a greater number of hours, the remuneration should be proportionately larger.[32]

There was very little time for a scale of fees to be drawn up before the appointed day. Working under great pressure, the dental profession and the Ministry formulated rates designed to implement the Spens Report that both parties had earlier accepted. A 20 per cent betterment of the Spens figures was allowed by the government to offset the rise in living costs since 1939. The average net income per year was now fixed at £1,920 ($5,376), which included the Exchequer superannuation contribution. Although the profession did not have the chance to approve formally the scale of fees because it was made effective on such short notice, the overwhelming majority of dentists entered the Health Service.

The dental profession, like the British Medical Association and for the same reasons, refused to join the Whitley Council system. It was felt that more could be gained by direct negotiation, and if this were unsuccessful, then by arbitration. The Ministry, however, was reluctant to accept arbitral procedure at all, since the awards made might cost the Exchequer a large sum of money at a time when England was faced by a serious budgetary problem.

The tremendous rush for dentures and dental treatment was unexpected. The cost of the dental service soared. By working long hours and completing treatment more quickly, many dentists were able to earn larger sums than were contemplated by the Spens Committee. The newspapers publicized cases of excessive earnings, and while these were exceptional and were the result of long hours of hard work, the profession was nevertheless subjected to much critical comment. Confronted by a situation that seemed to call for drastic measures, the Ministry announced that, effective in January, 1949, the government would retain one-half of the gross earnings of any dentist above £400 ($1,120) per month.

In fixing the dental rates, it was necessary to know the average time required to complete each type of dental treatment. With the co-operation of the dental profession, the Minister early in 1949 set up a working party under the chairmanship of William Penman to make a report on the matter. But without waiting for its findings, the Minister decided to order a 20 per cent reduction in the scale of fees on June 1. The earlier action for curbing larger incomes was simultaneously abandoned.[33] The dental profession was very disturbed by this unilateral policy, particularly because it was taken without regard to the Penman Report, which was to be finished within a few weeks.

The Times (London) took the position that in view of the evidence submitted to Parliament the Minister of Health had no choice but to scale down the fees. Fifty-nine per cent of the dental practitioners, it was pointed out, were earning more than was ever intended for a 33 hour chairside week. Some were receiving exorbitant amounts. While viewing the methods used by the government in slashing dentists' earnings as "clumsy" and the alteration of the scale without agreement as unfortunate, the editorial was of the opinion that the dental profession could not escape responsibility since it had refused to discuss the matter of excessive earnings with the Minister.[34]

The British Dental Association did not believe that the dentists were earning sums in excess of what the Spens Committee had recommended for a working week of 33 chairside hours. It was claimed that the larger sums were the result of longer hours. For proof, the Association awaited the Penman Report.[35] Completed early in August, 1949, the document was based upon a careful inquiry under the watchful eye of an eminent actuary. The evidence showed that nearly two-thirds of the dental practitioners were working 25 per cent in excess of the chairside hours recommended in the Spens Report, and that, prior to the reduction in rates, the average earnings of dentists were 19 per cent above the Spens standard. Eleven per cent of this amount was earned by hours in excess of those prescribed by Spens and 8 per cent by speed. It was explained that there were legitimate ways by which chairside time could be reduced—a second dental chair, a more systematic routine, and chairside assistance. The investigation disclosed that most dentists were working "more quickly than they worked normally." While a comparatively small minority were working "too long, too quickly and with an eye fixed too closely on the monetary reward for their labours," this was not true of the great majority, who, it was observed, had "been trying to cope with the difficult problem of keeping pace with demand without loss of efficiency. . . . They should have received more gratitude and less adverse criticism than has actually been the case."[36]

Based upon the average time for each type of dental work as established by the Penman Report, the Ministry of Health and the dental profession early in 1950 began to negotiate a new scale of rates. In the meantime, the Ministry felt justified in instituting an additional 10 per cent reduction in the 1949 scale—an action that evoked a sharp protest from the British Dental Association. The Ministry did not believe that the longer hours dentists worked warranted the earnings they received. The 1949-50 budget showed that the dental service, with one-half as many practitioners, cost the nation more than did the general medical service. The need to check the rising dental costs as well as to protect the priority dental services led to the abandonment of a completely free service. In the general dental service during spring, 1951, charges for dentures were imposed, and one year later charges were assessed for conservative treatment. The immediate effect, which proved to be temporary, was a decline in the demand for the dental services. The earnings of dentists suffered, and this made the British Dental Association more determined to have the 10 per cent reduction canceled. Inquiries conducted by the Inland Revenue and the dental profession itself proved that the gross as well as the net incomes of dentists had declined substantially between 1949 and 1953. On May 1, 1955, the Ministry accordingly restored the 10 per cent cut which had been imposed five years previous.[37]

The way was now cleared for the Association to co-operate in producing a revised scale of fees. The scale was completed and was made effective in April, 1957. Under the new schedule, the gross fee the dentists would receive from the government for scaling was 12/6d ($1.75). The amount for filling one surface of a tooth was £1 2/6d ($3.15), and for the extraction of one or two teeth, 8/6d ($1.19). The sum allowed for full upper and lower dentures was £9 9s ($26.46).[38]

Even before the new scale became effective, the British Dental Association pressed for an increase in remuneration to counteract the depreciation in the purchasing value of the pound. The Ministry resisted the claim because of economic conditions, but agreed to submit the whole issue of remuneration to a Royal Commission. Owing to the determined fight the medical profession had been waging for a substantial betterment of its income, a crisis had arisen that the government felt provided an opportune time for a comprehensive review of medical and dental compensation. While the dental profession was not enthusiastic about the proposed investigation, it took the position that co-operation was the only sensible policy.[39]

Before the report of the Royal Commission was completed, the government gave two interim increases to dentists, one in May, 1957, and the other in January, 1959. The first was 5 per cent on net remuneration, and the second was 4 per cent.

Contrary to the contention of the British Dental Association, the Pilkington Report showed that between 1952 and 1956 there had been no increase in the number of hours worked by dentists. The number of dental practitioners changed little during this period, yet the volume of work they were able to do had expanded substantially, owing largely to new techniques and improved equipment. While the average gross earnings per dentist remained about the same during the first half of the 1950's, they increased 30 per cent during the last five years of that decade. In 1959-60, the average gross receipts of a dental practitioner were estimated at £5,300 ($14,840), of which 52 per cent represented practice expenses. The earnings of dentists had improved so much after 1957 that the Pilkington Report did not recommend any retroactive pay for them.

A study of comparative earnings for 1955-56 revealed that general dental practitioners averaged larger incomes than general medical practitioners and were surpassed in earnings only by consultants and actuaries. Among individual dentists, there was a substantial spread of income, owing to differences in skill, hours of work, and age. Because of the nervous and physical strain of dental work, the thirty-five to fifty-five age group enjoyed the largest net income. Thereafter, earnings dropped sharply. Dentists sixty-five and over in that year averaged little more than £1,100 ($3,080) per year, compared with £2,781 ($7,786) for the forty to forty-four age category, the highest income group of all. The average net income in England and Wales for all dental practitioners in that year was nearly £2,290 ($6,412) per dentist.

The Pilkington Commission found no objection to the spread in earnings and did not feel that any special arrangement should be made for elderly dentists. The individual dentist, knowing the nature of the work, should make appropriate provision for the decline in his earnings. It was held that the same rates for items of service should apply to all dental practitioners irrespective of age, although a special financial inducement, comparable to that in the medical service, should be used to encourage dentists to practice in the more remote and less desirable areas.[40]

The Pilkington Commission had no doubt that the items-of-service method of compensation should continue as the basis for remuneration.   Since new and better techniques would continue to affect the volume of work, the Report favored linking the general level of compensation to the number of hours worked rather than the number of treatments given.   This, of course, would require an effective method of fixing rates and times for each phase of dental work.   It was suggested that a Dental Rates Study Group be appointed to fix the amount of time required for each dental operation, to decide what the gross fee should be for each type of work, and to determine how many hours per year were worked by the average dentist.   Instead of seeking information from the dentists, as the Penman Working Party did, the Study Group should employ work study techniques.   Two work study technicians should thus be appointed to the Study Group, which would consist, in addition, of representatives from the Ministry of Health and the dental profession.   The times affected by changing dental techniques would be reviewed constantly, and they, together with the number of hours worked, would be used by the Study Group to arrive at the level of remuneration that at infrequent intervals the Review Body would recommend.

The Pilkington Report suggested that, exclusive of the Exchequer superannuation contribution, the current average annual net remuneration for general dental practitioners should be £2,500 ($7,000), representing a total of between 2,050 and 2,200 hours of work per year, or roughly 46 hours per week.[41]

The British Dental Association was disappointed that its remuneration claim of £2,950 ($8,460) had been rejected and that there would be no retroactive payment for dentists.   Certain other aspects aroused mixed feelings.   The proposed machinery to review rates and earnings was acceptable and seemed to promise smoother relations and more security for the general dental practitioners.   From a long-range view, the Pilkington Report had much to offer to all concerned. Although cautious about subscribing to all parts, the dental profession finally indicated on March 4, 1961, after certain provisions had been clarified through negotiations, that it would do so.[42]

It will be recalled that the charges imposed upon patients were designed primarily to protect the priority services, but were also intended to check abuses and to furnish revenue.   Dentures bore the heaviest charge, which, prior to 1961, ranged from £2 ($5.60) for one, two, or three teeth to £4 5s ($11.90) for a full upper and lower set of teeth.   In that year, the minimum charge was increased to £2 5s ($6.30) and the maximum to £5 ($14).   The government derived from this source approximately 45 per cent of the total cost of dentures.   The charge for a course of conservative treatment was only £1 ($2.80), but if the work cost less than that sum, the patient paid whatever the actual cost was. Since the amount collected from patients for conservative work represented only one-tenth of the cost to the Exchequer, it was apparent that there was no desire to discourage conservative treatment, beyond, of course, giving preference to persons under twenty-one and expectant and nursing mothers. For these latter two groups, conservative treatment was free. There was no charge to any person for a domiciliary visit, for the arrest of bleeding, for a dental examination, or for repairs to dentures. The patient, however, was required to pay all or a part of the cost of dentures that had to be replaced because of carelessness. Should the patient deny carelessness when the evidence indicated otherwise, the Dental Estimates Board would ask the Executive Council to investigate and determine what part of the cost, if any, the patient should have to pay. For work not clinically necessary, the patient had to pay the extra cost. In 1960, less than one-fifth of the expenditures on the dental service were recovered from the patients.[43]

As intended, the charges restricted the amount of work for adults in favor of treatment for children. During the first decade of the Health Service, the courses of treatment for individuals under twenty-one years of age in the general dental service increased fourfold, reaching 5 million in 1959. Among adults, the number of courses at the end of that period was about the same as in the beginning— about 5.5 million. In 1949, only 16 per cent of the patients treated in the general dental service were twenty or under, whereas ten years later the proportion was 45 per cent. This trend was hailed as a very important one, since the conservation of teeth depended ultimately upon the dental habits of adolescents.

The over-all growth in the volume of work was encouraging. In 1960, over 13.5 million patients were treated in the general dental service—74 per cent more than twelve years previous. Since the number of dentists increased by only 11 per cent during this period, it was obvious that the amount of work per dentist had risen appreciably. No less significant was the ratio between the provision of dentures and other types of dental work. In 1949, 36 per cent of the patients were supplied with dentures, compared with only 11 per cent in 1960. In the latter year, fillings in permanent teeth accounted for 47 per cent of the fees paid to dentists. Dentures, once the largest item, represented only 25 per cent of the fees in that year. Examination of teeth absorbed 6 per cent; scaling and gum treatment for adults, 5 per cent; and the extraction of permanent teeth, 4 per cent.

Owing to the uneven distribution of dental practitioners, the proportion of persons treated varied greatly between regions. In 1958, London and the South-Eastern area averaged 300 courses of treatment per 1,000 population, compared with only 130 in Wales. Moreover, for every tooth extracted in that year in the London area, three were filled; but in Wales slightly more teeth were extracted than were filled. These represented extreme examples, but they showed the effects of social habits and dental health education, as well as the ratio of dentists to the population.

The patients accepted for a full course of treatment were made dentally fit in all but a small fraction of cases, which in 1959 was slightly over 7 per cent. Another encouraging aspect was the fact that there were fewer patients who required emergency treatment in 1959 and 1960 than during the early years of the decade. Emergency treatment involved extraction of not more than two teeth, arrest of bleeding, inexpensive repairs to dentures, administration of a general anesthetic, and a few other items. The decline in the number of emergency patients was construed as evidence that more patients were seeking regular treatment.[44]

In the priority dental services, the progress in some respects was disappointing. At no time were there more than half enough dentists to cope with the work. The local authority dental service, which served pre-school children and expectant and nursing mothers, was able to treat a record 110,000 patients in 1956, but during the next two years a 10 per cent decline in the number occurred. Conservative work in the general dental service was also free to these patients, and at least seven times more patients were treated there than in the maternity and child welfare clinics. As in the general service, in the local authority service there was a sharp rise in the number of fillings during the first decade, and in the case of pre-school children, fillings and conservations by 1957 overtook the number of extractions. Of those treated in the local authority dental clinics, 70 per cent of the mothers and 80 per cent of the children were made dentally fit in 1958.

But there was also a dark side to the picture. The incidence of decayed teeth was shockingly high among pre-school children. A study made by the dental staff of Staffordshire in 1954 revealed that among school entrants aged five, only 17 per cent had sound dentitions. Over half the children had four or more carious teeth. The evidence seemed to indicate from this survey, which covered 1,000 children, that the caries rate was increasing. While these were deciduous teeth, their preservation, until replaced by the permanent teeth, was considered important in the health of the child.[45]

The deterioration in the teeth of children seemed to be a rather general phenomenon in England and Wales after the abandonment of rationing at the end of World War II. A comparison of a series of detailed studies in London from 1929 to 1957 showed a very definite rise in caries among five-year-old children after 1947. The cause of this increase was not ascribed to any dereliction on the part of the local health authority dentists but to the diet. During the war and the rationing period, the nutrition of infants and expectant mothers was more scientifically controlled, with an increase of the calcifying properties of the diet. But afterwards, there was a freer choice of foods, and the consumption of cod liver oil and milk declined. The popularity of confections and iced lollipops may have also contributed to the higher incidence of decayed teeth.[46] Meeting this problem quite obviously involved much more than increasing the number of dental practitioners.

The situation among school children was somewhat analogous to that among children of pre-school age—too few dentists to cope with a steady growth in the volume of work caused by a rising birth rate and a higher incidence of carious teeth. An increasing proportion of school children turned to the general dental service, which in 1957 treated 2.3 million children from five to fourteen years of age, filling 1.8 million teeth. This was a larger number than were treated in the school dental service. But all the dental resources combined could not begin to do the job. The president of the General Dental Council in 1957 declared that, in spite of every effort on the part of the profession, only one-third of the children received dental treatment in any one year.[47] While the ratio of fillings to extractions improved greatly, the inspection of school children disclosed that an appallingly large number of adolescents were not dentally fit.[48] The lack of hygiene and unsuitable diets were the real enemies and in many ways constituted a more serious problem than understaffed dental clinics.

Many articles in the professional journals as well as the lay press and a considerable amount of comment in Parliament attested to a growing awareness of what should be done. The training of a larger number of dentists and a more effective program of health education were matters about which concrete action was being taken. A proper diet and the adequate care of teeth were receiving greater emphasis. The importance of research was not overlooked, and it promised more than an illusory hope. The fluoridation of water supplies seemed to offer something very significant in checking dental caries.

As a result of successful experiments in Canada and the United States, England became interested in fluoridation as a preventive dental health measure. By adding a small amount of fluoride to public water supplies, the teeth developed a resistance to caries that was claimed to reduce the amount of teeth decay by 50 per cent. Limited experiments were conducted in 1949 and 1950 that seemed to justify a more thorough investigation.   A mission sent to the United States to study fluoridation recommended its introduction in a few selected areas.   With the full support of the Medical Research Council, four communities agreed in the mid-1950's to accept fluoride in their water on an experimental basis.   So much opposition developed from those who contended that flouridated water was harmful that one of the boroughs withdrew from the scheme.   Although the evidence was all to the contrary, fluoridation became a controversial issue throughout the nation.   There was, however, solid support for it from the British Medical and Dental Associations.   The results from the test areas would not be known before 1962, but it was expected that the data would then establish an irrefutable case for the general use of fluoride in drinking water.[49]

In surveying the dental service, it is not easy to strike a balance. In view of the limited resources and the tremendous need for treatment, the dental profession was faced from the outset by an impossible situation.   The dentists rose to meet it as well as circumstances permitted, and each year they were able to turn out a greater volume of work.   The heavy pressure of work tended to make the service utilitarian, but the quality of work was generally good and the relationship between the practitioner and patient remained friendly.

Many practitioners had difficulty adjusting themselves to the new scheme.   The older dentists, accustomed to the freedom associated with private practice, found it irksome to get permission before doing certain types of work.   Filling out forms and otherwise complying with regulations were viewed by some as a threat to the dentist-patient relationship.   Although the Minister of Health scrupulously sought to preserve clinical freedom, some of the dentists complained that they were needlessly restricted.   Wherever large sums of public money were involved, it was essential to establish safeguards which the older dentists, more than others, equated with bureaucratic interference.

The younger dentists, many of whom had served in the armed services, entered the National Health Service with much less antipathy toward it than the more elderly dentists.   The younger practitioners seemed to appreciate better the humanitarian aspects of the service and the tremendous benefits it bestowed upon the people.   They also could see more clearly the personal advantages inherent in the program.   There was no worry about having to collect private fees. It was easy to start a practice and to have a full quota of patients within a very short time.   Earnings were good, and the government was a prompt paymaster.   Few vocations yielded a better income. Certainly from the standpoint of remuneration, the dental profession was infinitely better off than it had ever been before.   The trend toward conservative work gave the dental practitioners a greater opportunity to employ some of the more refined techniques associated with good dentistry.

As a profession, the dentists were critical of certain aspects of the dental service, but years of agitation brought major concessions, the more important of which have already been mentioned. A speedier and more simplified procedure for handling appeals from the Dental Estimates Board was very much desired, and here also the Ministry of Health largely yielded to the wishes of the profession. While the government refused to accede to the arbitration of remuneration disputes, it did agree to the creation of machinery to review the income of dentists and doctors periodically. This was viewed as a major step toward ensuring adequate earnings at all times.

More dental schools and greater emphasis on dental health education were other pledges made. There were many things the profession did not want changed, such as the method of remuneration or the pattern which permitted the younger dentists to earn more than the older ones. The first decade with its acute man-power shortage, its fiscal difficulties and remuneration crises, and its failure to provide dental care for everybody left a picture of frustration; but the second decade, with its more auspicious beginning, appeared to presage a much more hopeful future for the dental practitioner.

To the patient, the dental service was a tremendous boon. The availability of dentures and dental care proved of inestimable value to millions of people. While it was true that only a fourth or a third of the population was treated in any year by the dental service, that was considerably more than before the appointed day. Professor Ross, in his survey of a factory town in 1952, found that since the beginning of the Health Service 43 per cent of the people had received dental treatment, and that each year there was a steady increase in the use of the service.[50] English teeth, bad as they were, had improved, and more and more people were becoming alert to the need for taking care of their teeth. Real progress had been achieved, and there was reason to believe that the trend would be accelerated during the second decade of the National Health Service. Indeed, everything pointed to a greatly expanded service and a more dentally conscious people as new and larger training facilities reduced the shortage of dentists in the priority as well as the general dental service.

CHAPTER XVI

The Ophthalmic Service

THE OPHTHALMIC SERVICE seemed to experience less difficulty than any other branch of the Health Program and was among the most popular. From the very beginning, it had the sympathetic support of the ophthalmic opticians. It was comparatively free of abuse and for the most part operated efficiently. Few complaints were raised against this service, and critics found little to condemn about it. Although problems arose, none seemed to create any deep anxiety among the opticians or the officials at Savile Row.

The future pattern of the ophthalmic service at first aroused the apprehension of the opticians, but as the years passed the issue seemed to become academic. The Minister of Health was authorized under the National Health Service Act to establish, when conditions permitted, the ophthalmic service as a part of the hospital program. It was intended that eye clinics, under the jurisdiction of the regional hospital boards, would eventually prescribe all the Health Service glasses as well as provide whatever treatment was required for the eyes. But until such time as the necessary facilities could be furnished by the hospitals and the Minister should deem such a course advisable, the prescribing and dispensing of spectacles was to be done by the supplementary ophthalmic service under the Executive Councils.[1]

Since this arrangement was considered only temporary, the optical profession was allowed no representation on the Executive Council. Opticians were nevertheless given a major role in the administration of the service. The Executive Council appointed a committee, usually of sixteen members, known as the ophthalmic services committee, seven members of which had to be from and approved by the ophthalmic profession. This committee was responsible for supervising the arrangements for testing sight and providing optical appliances. Opticians were also liberally represented on the ophthalmic investigation committee, which was set up by the Executive Council to assist in handling complaints that arose. There was also a local optical committee elected by the profession to advise the ophthalmic services committee, to protect the interests of the opticians, and to seek improvement of the service. Unlike the dental, medical, and pharmaceutical committees, the local optical committees were not authorized by the Health Service Act of 1946, but they were established anyway and became so useful that they were subsequently given a statutory basis.[2]

The supplementary ophthalmic service functioned so smoothly and suited the opticians so well that the Ministry of Health appeared to accept the arrangement as something that should be continued for many years to come. No steps were taken to curtail this phase of the service, and the optical profession was left with the impression that the supplementary ophthalmic service would not be abolished within the lifetime of its members, if then. It could very possibly become a permanent part of the Health Service.[3]

Public opinion favored the retention of this service essentially as it was, and the Ministry of Health seemed to be in accord with such a policy. The Guillebaud Committee strongly urged such a course. In examining the evidence, this Committee could see no reason for extending the function of the existing hospital eye service beyond its present role of providing contact lenses, supplying artificial eyes, dealing with pathological cases, and performing minor operations. Under the supplementary ophthalmic service, more than 7,000 establishments tested eyes and supplied glasses, but if hospital clinics were to do this work, the public, it was argued, would find the arrangement much less convenient. The estimated 450 hospital clinics that would be required to furnish a comprehensive eye service would be widely separated and not as readily accessible to the public. The government would incur much greater expense in providing space and equipment for these clinics, and the people would have little freedom of choice among ophthalmic opticians in the hospital clinics.[4]

The supplementary ophthalmic service recognized three professional groups: the ophthalmic opticians, the dispensing opticians, and the ophthalmic medical practitioners. The last were doctors with special qualifications and, as part of their work, they tested sight and prescribed glasses, but they did not supply them. The ophthalmic opticians did all three of these things, while the dispensing opticians were qualified only to fill prescriptions. By far the most important of the groups was the ophthalmic opticians, who examined 80 per cent of the eyes and who represented more than three-fourths of the total personnel in the supplementary ophthalmic service. In 1960, they numbered 6,367, or 11 per cent more than when the Health Service began. While the dispensing opticians enjoyed a more rapid rate of growth, they did not exceed 986 in 1960. The ophthalmic medical practitioners were slightly fewer, having suffered a small decline in numbers since the beginning of the service.[5]

Under the Health Insurance Law, only those gainfully employed and not the members of their families were beneficiaries. The amount of money which the Approved Societies were able to contribute toward the cost of sight testing and spectacles depended upon their financial condition. Viewed as an additional benefit, the ophthalmic service was administered by the Ophthalmic Benefit Approved Committee, which represented the Approved Societies as well as the various optical organizations. The scale of fees, which was determined by this committee, was based upon the classes of frames that were selected for use. The grant which the insured received toward the cost of the eye examination and the spectacles was deducted by the optician from the fixed charges which the individual had to pay.

The supplementary ophthalmic service continued the arrangement used by the Health Insurance, in which sight testing and the prescribing and supplying of spectacles were carried out by opticians in their own consulting rooms. But the administrative machinery was different under the National Health Service. The ophthalmic profession, as indicated, still retained a major role in shaping policy and supervising the operation of the service on the local level. On the national level, the Central Health Services Council was advised on ophthalmic matters by a standing committee composed entirely of members from the optical profession. In determining policy, the Minister freely consulted with the Joint Committee of Ophthalmic Opticians, which represented the entire profession. The negotiations were amicably conducted, and a satisfactory decision was reached on most matters. A source of disagreement was the question of fees, which had to be ironed out by the Optical Whitley Council.[6] The bitter altercations over remuneration which troubled the medical and dental professions were largely absent from the ophthalmic scene.

The National Health Service made the eye service available to everybody, and until spring, 1951, it was free. The rush for glasses swamped the service, creating an embarrassing backlog of orders and boosting the cost of the service to unexpected heights. Partly to check abuses but mostly to keep expenditures within certain budgetary limits, charges were imposed. Children under sixteen years of age and all students were exempt, but others had to pay 10s ($1.40) per lens and the cost of the frame. In 1961, the charge for lenses was increased to 12/6d ($1.75) each, but even then the total payment which a patient had to make for a pair of spectacles, including a good, strong frame, need not be more than £1 16s ($5.04). There was no fee for examination. If repairs or replacement were necessitated by carelessness, the full cost was borne by the individual; otherwise, a part of it was met by the government.

To what extent the charges affected the ophthalmic service was difficult to measure. The demand for spectacles was already falling before 1951. Charges accelerated the decline, but beginning in 1953 the trend was reversed and each year saw an increasing volume of work. By 1960, the number of sight tests reached 5.5 million which, although below the number in the record year of 1949, was 46 per cent above the lowest number registered under the Service in 1952. There were 4.8 million pairs of spectacles supplied in 1960 (43 per cent above the level for 1952), but this total still fell far short of the 1950 record, which was established by an extraordinary accumulation of prescriptions that had to be filled. During the first decade, over 50 million sight tests were given, only a small portion of which did not reveal the necessity for glasses. Once the pent-up demand from elderly persons was met, some of whom had to have two pairs of spectacles, the proportion of sight tests resulting in spectacles dropped to about 89 per cent.[7]

In spite of the large number of sight examinations, the optometrists[8] believed that it fell short of what was essential to insure the proper care for all people requiring visual aids. The optical profession put the blame on the charges, which the Guillebaud Committee likewise felt were an unfortunate deterrent to the fullest use of the service. Although hardship cases were eligible to receive a refund of charges, it was believed that some who needed glasses did without because they did not wish to receive "charity" from the National Assistance Fund. The over-all figures nevertheless left little doubt that, even with the charges, no branch of the Health Service was more widely used or deeply appreciated than the supplementary ophthalmic service.

Its importance was evident from a Social Survey in 1951 that disclosed that 80 per cent of all persons between 45 and 65 years of age in England and Wales wore spectacles and that among older people well over 90 per cent used them.[9] Ross in his survey of a factory town in 1952 observed that an increasing proportion of people were using the eye service and that one-third of the population had done so during the first four years of the Health Service.[10]

Only a negligible proportion of the opticians failed to join the Health Service. Every optometrist was free to enter the service, and he could leave it after giving the Executive Council three months' advance notice. He could choose his Health Service patients and was privileged to have private patients. He was under contract with the Executive Council; and, like the family doctor, the druggist, and the dentist, he had to keep careful records and to maintain adequate office facilities that were subject to inspection. Every effort was made to safeguard clinical freedom, and in this matter there apparently were no complaints. The paper work was not objectionable, and the *esprit de corps* in the profession remained good.

The individual who for the first time desired a pair of Health Service glasses had to get a recommendation from a medical practitioner or, if the patient were a Christian Scientist, from the clerk of the ophthalmic services committee. There were many who questioned the necessity for this requirement and who urged that the patient be allowed to go directly to the optician. Theoretically, the physician was supposed to determine whether the applicant's symptoms were caused by eye defects or by some other physical condition that might necessitate medical treatment. In practice, the family physician usually issued the recommendation in a routine manner. It was then taken to any ophthalmic medical practitioner or ophthalmic optician whose name was on the Health Service list. If medical treatment were needed, the patient was referred back to his physician. Upon the completion of the sight test, if glasses were required the necessary form was forwarded to the ophthalmic services committee, where it was examined and compared with the records. Unless there were evidence of fraud or misuse of the service, the request was promptly approved and the person was authorized to go to any ophthalmic or dispensing optician on the list to have the prescription filled. With the exception of the early years, when demand greatly exceeded supply, only a few days were usually required to obtain glasses.[11]

For a second or any subsequent pair of spectacles, the individual could approach the optician directly for an examination. If the patient desired safety or plastic lenses, there was an additional charge. Originally there were over forty Health Service frames from which to choose, but several of these were in such small demand that they were later discontinued. The price for a Health Service frame varied from less than 8s ($1.16) to three or four times that amount. If the patient desired some other frame than those provided by the Service, he was permitted to buy it and still have Health Service lenses, providing they could be fitted in the frame.

Health Service frames were sturdy and reasonably attractive, but they tended to be standardized and did not always reflect the latest styles. Modification was made occasionally in their structure and appearance, but younger people, especially, often desired more stylish frames. These could be purchased in a private transaction from opticians, who were happy enough to furnish them in view of the profit involved. Not all Health Service frames for children were free. A number of children preferred to have plastic Health Service frames, for which there was a charge, or to obtain frames and even lenses that were supplied privately. Disturbed about the trend and eager to gather other data about sight tests, the kind of frames used, and the type of glasses prescribed, the Ministry of Health undertook in 1959 and 1960 a special survey.

The results indicated that 60 per cent of all sight tests in 1959 were given to persons 45 years and older. The proportion of sight tests that did not result in a prescription was 13 per cent for all age groups, 14 per cent for the aged, and 28 per cent for children under fifteen. Two-thirds of the lenses prescribed in 1959 for children in that age group were furnished with new Health Service frames, but for the fifteen to forty-five age group, only 18 per cent of the frames supplied were in that category. Information gathered since the survey revealed that in 1960, 14 per cent of glasses prescribed under the supplementary ophthalmic service were not dispensed by the service. Thirty-two per cent were fitted with new National Health Service frames, 17 per cent with old frames reglazed, and 37 per cent with new private frames.[12]

School clinics examined the eyes of pupils and provided glasses prior to 1948. With the inception of the Health Service, it was decided that for the time being these clinics would continue under the control of the local school authorities, but that ultimately the regional hospital boards would assume jurisdiction. Prescriptions issued in the school clinics or elsewhere by Health Service opticians were filled under the supplementary ophthalmic service by very much the same procedure employed for adults. Approximately one-third of the sight tests for children took place in the school clinics, and all but a small portion of the remainder occurred in the supplementary ophthalmic service. A few were obtained privately.

In view of the millions of spectacles prescribed annually, it would seem that the ophthalmic service might have been burdened with an inordinate number of complaints. The ophthalmic services committee was prepared to act upon any grievance, but the number of complaints was surprisingly small. During the five-year period ending in 1959, the average annual number of disciplinary cases was 25, and in 1960 the total was only 15. No optician was dismissed from the service in those years. The handling of disciplinary cases followed very much the same procedure as that used in the dental and medical services.[13]

In the early part of 1960, a member of Parliament accused the optometrists of attempting to persuade their patients to purchase private frames. He alleged that some of them failed to display the full range of Health Service frames. He also claimed that the official notice showing the scale of charges was not adequately displayed in many of the offices. An investigation in London and elsewhere disclosed, however, that the great majority of the optometrists exhibited the notice and that those that did not were willing to do so upon receipt of another copy to replace the one that they had lost. There seemed to be little evidence to sustain the allegations of abuses in the eye service, although it was recognized that in any group there would always be some infractions. The Executive Councils received few complaints about abuses. The feeling appeared to be general that there was much to commend in the ophthalmic service and little to condemn.[14]

The fees the opticians were allowed for sight testing and the dispensing of glasses were determined by the Whitley Council. In so far as the frames and lenses were concerned, the optometrist was permitted to recover only the wholesale cost, with some small addition for the risk of breakage. The dispensing fee at first was based upon the amount provided under the Health Insurance scheme— £1 5s ($3.50) for each pair of spectacles. The optical profession favored a higher rate, in view of the loss of private practice that was expected from a free service. The increased volume of work, however, more than offset this loss and even resulted in earnings for many optometrists that seemed excessive. This led to a 15 per cent reduction in the fees, which was accepted only as a temporary arrangement pending an inquiry into the whole question of remuneration. Once the accumulated demand for spectacles was met, the amount of work declined. The income of opticians fell and this, combined with an inflationary trend, caused the profession in 1952 to demand a restoration of the fee cuts, plus a 20 per cent cost-of-living increase.[15]

The Optical Whitley Council moved slowly in making adjustment in the scale of fees. Several years elapsed before the average level approximated that which prevailed in 1949. By 1959, the fees were 5 per cent higher. A rising demand for spectacles and a growing number of sight-tests contributed to an improved situation. There were other factors which influenced the Whitley Council in fixing the fees—the profit opticians realized from the sale of private frames, for instance. So important was this item that the Whitley Council granted the government's demand that the dispensing fee effective in January, 1960, should be reduced by 20 per cent if the lenses were fitted in private frames.[16]

The dispensing fee in force during the early part of 1960 was £1 4s ($3.36) for the first pair of glasses with single-vision lenses or £1 11/6d ($4.41) for the first pair with bifocal lenses. The dispensing fee for an additional pair of spectacles of any type was 10s ($1.40). If non-Health Service frames were used, these amounts were reduced by approximately one-fifth. The fee paid to an ophthalmic medical practitioner for sight testing was £1 1/3d ($2.98). An ophthalmic optician received 18s ($2.52) for this work if he considered it unnecessary to prescribe; otherwise, he got 16s ($2.24). The optician collected the full cost of the frame from the patient. The Executive Council reimbursed the optometrist for the difference between the cost of each lens and the amount paid by the patient. The sight testing and dispensing fees, as well as all other payments, were remitted to the optician monthly. Unlike most other Health Service personnel, opticians were not included in the superannuation scheme of the National Health Service.[17]

It may be recalled that over a third of the cost of the ophthalmic service was financed by charges, the balance coming from the National Treasury. Of the total cost of the service in the 1960 fiscal year— £15 million ($43 million)—29 per cent was spent for sight testing, 35 per cent for dispensing fees, 35 per cent for lenses, frames and cases, and less than 1 per cent for replacements and repairs. Thus, roughly two-thirds of the ophthalmic service budget constituted remuneration for the opticians. This amount did not represent total earnings, since private frames and lenses yielded an additional source of income; and in the case of the ophthalmic medical practitioner, the medical phase of his practice was a source of income.[18]

The ophthalmic profession had ample reasons to be grateful for the National Health Service. It brought a substantial increase in the distribution of glasses. At no time in English history had there been more or better protection for the eyes of those who required spectacles or other visual aids. No longer were impecunious persons, especially among the aged, compelled to do without spectacles or to seek cheap, ill-fitting frames and badly adjusted lenses from chain stores. The Health Service Act also promoted closer ties between the opticians and the medical doctors—an important development in view of the dependence upon both professions by patients with weak and diseased eyes.

The National Health Service enhanced the professional standing of the ophthalmic and dispensing opticians. A consequence of their improved status was the adoption of the Opticians' Act of 1958.

Under this enactment, the optician, like the pharmacist, doctor and dentist, acquired the privilege of statutory registration. A General Optical Council was set up, comprising representatives from the optical and medical professions and the optical examining bodies, as well as nominees of the Privy Council. The General Optical Council was given extensive power to determine such matters as professional conduct, discipline, qualifications, and standards of training. The act specifically prohibited the sale of ready-made glasses by chain stores and street vendors. Sight-testing and the prescribing of spectacles were functions that only registered ophthalmic medical practitioners and opticians could now legally exercise. The measure also emphasized the clinical relationship between the ophthalmic optician and the medical practitioner. Signed on the tenth anniversary of the appointed day, this legislation not only underscored the progress that had been achieved by the optical profession but laid the basis for even more productive years ahead.[19]

CHAPTER XVII

The Pharmaceutical Service

THE EXTRAORDINARY COST of the pharmaceutical service has already been the subject of comment. During the first decade, the cost of drugs more than doubled. At the outset, 8 per cent of the total gross Health Service expenditures went for drugs; by 1959-60, the proportion had risen to 10.5 per cent. In that year, as in some of the others, the pharmaceutical service was more expensive than the general medical service. The government tried hard to keep the rising drug bill within more manageable limits.

Until the middle of 1952 all drugs were free. At that time, a shilling charge was imposed on each prescription, and four years later this sum was collected on each item prescribed. In spring, 1961, the amount was increased to 2s (28 cents) per item. The charge had the effect of curtailing the number of prescriptions issued, but it did not check the rising cost of the pharmaceutical service. It should be observed, however, that the price of pharmaceutical products had risen sharply in all nations and in most of them at a more rapid rate than in England. The mounting costs were thus a universal phenomenon, attributable largely to the new and expensive proprietary drugs that had come out of the research laboratories. There was a tremendous demand for them because of their miraculous power to save human life. How to make them available to everybody was largely a problem of finance, and that problem confronted the many national schemes throughout the world that provided medical care.

Countries with health programs less ambitious than the one in England and Wales were often compelled to adopt stringent countermeasures, such as reducing the list of free drugs.[1] The sentiment in Great Britain strongly opposed any limitation of the pharmaceutical service. While the Ministry of Health urged economy, it would not go beyond a very modest charge in seeking to regulate prescribing. In the 1959-60 fiscal year, only one-seventh of the pharmaceutical cost was recovered in this manner from the patients. Although objectionable to pharmacists and doctors, the charges did not seem to hamper the effective distribution of drugs where they were needed.

Under the Health Insurance Act, drugs were provided to all workers as a part of the medical program, but no provision was made for members of the families. Although limited in scope, the scheme worked so well that many of the regulations were continued under the National Health Service. Insurance Committees, which had served as administrative agencies, were replaced by Executive Councils, but the same personnel were retained to do the work. The staff, of course, had to be enlarged, since the pharmaceutical service, like the other health services, was now available to the entire population.

The dispensing of drugs prior to 1948 was largely done by the family physician, but thereafter this work was delegated to pharmacists, except in the rural areas where they were not easily accessible. There the general practitioner was expected to supply the medicine, but only a small proportion of the doctors had to do so. All but 6 per cent of the population obtained their drugs from registered pharmacists.

By enlarging their dispensaries, the druggists were able to meet the increased volume of business without any difficulty. Little delay was experienced by patients in getting their prescriptions filled, and there was an almost complete absence of public complaints. The dispensing of private drugs dwindled to less than 10 per cent of the total volume of prescriptions. Since the services of the family physician were free, there was no longer need for a mother to seek furtive advice from the druggist about what nostrum might help her sick child. Prescriptions revolutionized this phase of pharmacy and put it on a much sounder basis. The public could now get the proper drugs when they were needed and regardless of price, and the role of the pharmacist took on a greater importance than at any time previous. Relations with the medical profession so improved under the new scheme that the secretary of the British Pharmaceutical Society described them as "cordial."[2]

Almost all of the 14,300 pharmacists joined the Health Service. By the mid-1950's, the number approached 16,000 (a rise of 11 per cent) and then leveled off at a slightly lower figure during the remaining years of that decade. By 1956, the volume of prescriptions had increased 13 per cent. Within two years, however, the shilling charge decreased the number to 203 million, or about the same level as in the initial year. A 7 per cent rise in 1959 and 1960 seemed to presage a reversal of the downward trend.[3]

Like the dentist, optician, and medical practitioner, the pharmacist was under contract with the Executive Council and was subject to certain regulations. He was privileged to withdraw from the scheme by giving sufficient notice, but with very few exceptions he could not afford to withdraw, since few druggists were able to operate on an exclusively private basis. The pharmacist in the Health Service displayed a "form notice" in the window, and his name and address appeared on a list available at the post office and the Executive Council office. No druggist was permitted to capitalize on Health Service membership in any advertisement, beyond using the precise wording in the "form notice." In addition to the regular hours that he served the public, he was expected to enter into a rota arrangement so that one or more pharmacies within a given area would be open for a short period in the evening, on Sundays and on public holidays. Most druggists who lived in or near their premises dispensed a prescription at any time if it were marked urgent by the doctor or dentist. For this service and rota work there was extra payment.

Like other professions in the Health Service, the pharmacists played a significant role in policy-making and administration. On the national level, there was the Standing Pharmaceutical Advisory Committee, which gave technical advice to the Minister of Health. Two druggists were on the Central Health Services Council. In each Executive Council area, the Health Service pharmacists elected a local pharmaceutical committee, comprising ten or more members, who looked after the interests of the profession and co-operated with the Executive Council in various matters. The local pharmaceutical committee chose two members of the Executive Council and also selected one-half of the pharmaceutical service committee. It was this latter agency that investigated complaints and otherwise assisted the Executive Council in insuring compliance with the terms of service.[4]

The Ministry of Health was careful to consult the pharmaceutical profession on all matters of mutual interest. The contractors' committee, sponsored by the National Pharmaceutical Union, represented the profession as a whole in negotiations over the terms and conditions of service. Although discussions did not always go smoothly, they never collapsed. On fiscal matters there were sharp differences of opinion, but a satisfactory agreement was usually reached. When it entered the Health Service, the profession labored under serious misgivings, but before long these had largely disappeared. There seemed to be little doubt that the new service strengthened the economic standing of the pharmacists and improved their status in general.[5]

In order to make sure that drugs and appliances measured up to the accepted standards, each Executive Council, with the approval of the Minister, adopted a scheme to test samples. A pharmacist normally received a test prescription once every two years. Subject to the guidance of the chairman of the pharmaceutical service committee, the clerk of the Executive Council would select the pharmacists to be visited and the drugs or appliances to be examined. A prescription in duplicate would be obtained from a medical practitioner without disclosing to him the name of the druggist to whom it would be given. An agent, after getting the prescription filled, notified the pharmacist concerned that it was a test prescription. The pharmacist then divided the dispensed medicine into three parts, one of which he retained. One sample went to an analyst under contract with the Executive Councils. Dressings and other appliances were sent to the Testing House of the Manchester Chamber of Commerce.

All certificates of analysis were scrutinized by the chairman and a druggist member of the pharmaceutical service committee, and if they found that an appliance or drug were deficient in quantity or quality, they could refer the matter to the pharmaceutical service committee for investigation. The pharmacist had the right to have his sample tested by an analyst selected by himself. In case of a dispute over the accuracy of the first analysis, the third specimen was examined by a referee appointed by the Minister. Although some pharmacists, especially at the outset, viewed the scheme as a "personal reproach to [their] professional integrity," the arrangement had the support of the profession as a whole, which recognized the need for some type of inspection. It was in co-operation with the National Pharmaceutical Union that the Ministry of Health worked out the broad aspects of the plan.[6]

If a druggist failed to comply with the terms of service, he was subject to disciplinary action. Only a small proportion of the certificates of analysis were unsatisfactory. During 1952, 8.6 per cent of the samples required further investigation; in 1959, only 5.1 per cent required such investigation. There were more than 7,000 samples tested that year, and less than 375 seemed to warrant formal investigation. Acting upon the recommendation of the pharmaceutical service committee, the Executive Council decided what action should be taken. The disciplinary procedure was the same as for the dental and general medical services. Two hundred and seven pharmacists were warned in 1959, but only 96 had money deducted from their remuneration. The drug-testing program furnished proof in that year, as in the others, that dispensing standards were high.[7]

The right of a general practitioner to prescribe any drug that he deemed necessary for the treatment of his patients was a fundamental feature of the National Health Service. Expounded by the Joint Committee on Prescribing and made an integral part of the law, this principle stood in no danger of being scrapped. It was identified with clinical freedom and considered indispensable in medical practice. The doctors, it was felt, should be the sole judge of the medicaments that would most effectively serve the needs of his patients. If a free and a restricted list of drugs had been employed, two standards of medicine would undoubtedly have resulted. A second-class service would have been provided those who could not afford the drugs that had to be purchased. A financial barrier would have arisen between the physician and the patient, and the doctor's effectiveness would have suffered. Such was the thinking of the Hinchliffe Commission, and such was the view of Parliament, the Ministry of Health, and the medical profession. All were opposed to any interference in the absolute freedom of the doctor to write medical prescriptions.

The duty of the physician to prescribe whatever medicine the case required did not, however, warrant waste or extravagance. While the Minister had no authority to direct or in any way to circumscribe the doctor's right to prescribe, he was permitted to furnish guidance. The Minister, for example, might urge the physician not to prescribe excessive amounts and not to prescribe expensive drugs when there were other preparations known to be as effective. The doctor could disregard such advice, but if the cost of his prescriptions were far above the average, his colleagues in the local medical committee had the right to call upon him to justify the additional expenditures. If he were unable to do so, he faced disciplinary action. This policy had the full approval of the medical profession and was not regarded as a threat to clinical freedom or the physician's right to prescribe.[8] There is no evidence that the practitioner felt inhibited in writing prescriptions. The inquiry of the Social Surveys in 1956 indicated that three-fourths of the doctors did not feel that they were restricted in their right to prescribe freely.

The pattern of prescribing varied greatly between some areas. In 1957, for example, the county-borough of Tynemouth had an average of less than 4 prescriptions per person, compared with twice that many for Wigan. The average cost of prescriptions per person in that year was £1 4/6d ($3.43) for Tynemouth and £2 2/7d ($5.96) for the other county-borough. The cost for the great majority of counties and county-boroughs were midway between these more extreme cases.[9]

In an investigation of the social aspects of prescribing, J. P. Martin found that the cost and frequency of prescribing were influenced by such factors as morbidity, geography, climate, occupation, and local customs. He discovered that local attitudes varied considerably between regions, contributing, for example, to low frequencies of prescribing in the Midlands and the North-East and to high frequencies in Lancashire. He observed that expensive drugs were more frequently prescribed in wealthy areas and cheap ones in the poorer regions where the physicians had longer lists of patients and more sickness. He also noted that partnerships tended to have a lower frequency of prescriptions than single doctors. Differences in the age composition of the population did not seem to have an appreciable effect upon the average frequency of prescribing per patient.[10]

The average number of prescriptions per person in England and Wales rose from 5 in 1949 to 5.5 in 1956, but by 1958 it was again 5 or even a trifle below that figure. None of the studies on the subject disclosed the existence of much waste or other serious abuse in prescribing. The most thorough investigation of all, that of the Hinchliffe Commission, 1957-59, found no proof of "widespread and irresponsible extravagance." There was evidence, however, that some doctors could have practiced more economy in the amounts which they prescribed and could have made greater use of standard preparations.

Increasingly, doctors prescribed proprietary preparations, which were usually more expensive than standard drugs not sold under brand names. In 1947, only 7 per cent of the prescriptions were for proprietary medicine; by 1959, the proportion had risen to 55 per cent. The value of proprietaries rose during this period from less than one-fourth of the total ingredient cost of prescriptions to more than three-fourths. Antibiotics and hormones alone accounted for nearly 30 per cent of the ingredient cost of drugs in 1959. The Ministry of Health was unsuccessful in checking the trend toward more proprietary medicines largely because a growing number of them, often the most expensive, were unavailable in any other form. But there were many proprietary drugs which had their equivalent in a standard preparation that was just as good and cost less. Getting physicians to prescribe the standard preparations was difficult, since busy doctors found it more convenient to use medicaments that were known through their widely advertised trade names. The greater use of proprietary drugs was by no means peculiar to England; it was even more pronounced in other countries. In Germany and Italy, for example, the proportion was 85 per cent or more.[11]

The remuneration of the pharmacists was complicated because of the vast number of prescriptions that had to be priced and the nature of the work involved. This phase was handled by pricing offices, most of which had been established by the Insurance Committees or groups of committees under the Health Insurance scheme. In the National Health Service, the pricing bureaus were placed under the central jurisdiction of the Joint Pricing Committee, which was chosen chiefly by the Executive Councils with a few additional members being nominated by the Minister of Health. There were over fifteen of these offices, with a total staff of at least 1,400. In view of the amount of paper work required of the pharamcists and doctors who dispensed drugs, the elaborate methods of the pricing bureaus, and the large number of regulations necessary to insure the efficient operation of the remuneration scheme, the process of providing payment for drugs was complex. Efforts were made to simplify the procedure, but there was no easy way to price accurately over 200 million prescriptions that varied so much. Significantly, neither the Guillebaud or Hinchliffe committees had any serious criticism of the machinery or how it functioned.

The druggists were paid for each prescription dispensed. Payment was made in accordance with the Drug Tariff, which specified the quality of the materials and their prices or the methods of computing them. The Minister of Health prepared the Tariff and revised it frequently. The pharmacist was allowed the wholesale cost of the appliance or ingredient, as provided by the Drug Tariff, and in addition an on-cost allowance of 25 per cent to cover all overhead expenses and to provide a modest profit margin. For professional services, a dispensing fee was also allowed, which ranged from 5d (6 cents) to more than 7s (98 cents) per prescription, depending on the work required on the part of the druggist. A small flat-rate allowance was made for the container. Such elements as the dispensing fee and the container and on-cost allowances were determined by negotiation between the Ministry of Health and the contractors' committee of the National Pharmaceutical Union, but this negotiation was carried on within the framework of the Whitley Council.

The first complete revision in the range of dispensing fees did not come before 1958, and then the schedule was simplified with the hope that the work of the pricing bureaus would thereby be expedited. A slight increase in the container allowance also occurred in that year. But there had been previous adjustments in the container allowance, as there had been in the dispensing fee for each prescription. On the question of remuneration there seemed to be no sharp division at any time between the pharmaceutical profession and the Ministry of Health, and the agreements reached appeared to be mutually satisfactory. Always mindful of the taxpayer, the Ministry endeavored to keep drug prices within reasonable limits. The Hinchliffe Committee found that, in almost all cases, what the government paid to the pharmacists for the medicine dispensed was less than the price would have been if the medicine had been sold privately over the counter.[12]

There was some criticism about the manner of pricing of prescriptions, but a satisfactory adjustment was finally reached. Partial pricing, or what was known as "averaging," was the issue. Under the Health Insurance program, it was the policy to price each prescription individually, but after the war, because of a shortage of personnel, it was no longer possible to do this, and a system of partial pricing was adopted. The National Health Service had to continue this arrangement, owing to the greatly increased volume of prescriptions and the lack of a skilled staff. The pricing offices even fell badly in arrears, and it was not until June, 1954, that they were able to keep abreast of the work. Partial pricing had to be continued, but it was done less extensively, and by 1958 about 70 per cent of all prescriptions were fully priced. Full pricing was the rule for the druggists who did not dispense over 500 prescriptions per month. Every prescription with an ingredient cost of 5s (70 cents) or more was likewise priced. All regions in turn received full pricing three months in every year. Otherwise, only 20 per cent of the prescriptions, selected at random, were priced, while the others were averaged on the basis of those that were priced.

The margin of error in such an arrangement was found to be not more than 3 and usually less than 2 per cent. The Guillebaud Committee did not feel that under the circumstances there was justification for any change in the system, but the Hinchliffe Commision urged that the matter be explored with a view toward adopting a policy of full pricing. Such a course was desired by the pharmaceutical profession, on the grounds that it would produce more accurate remuneration.[13] Acting upon this suggestion, the Ministry of Health investigated the matter and, after consultation with the spokesmen for the pharmaceutical profession and the Joint Pricing Committee, decided upon the introduction of full pricing in three stages, beginning in spring, 1959. One year later the last stage was reached, and all prescriptions were then fully priced.[14]

A general medical practitioner who dispensed drugs could choose to be paid on the same basis that was used for the pharmacists or he could accept a capitation fee and receive additional payment for certain expensive drugs and appliances. Prescriptions dispensed were sent to the pricing bureau every month, and when the pricing was done, the amount was certified to the Executive Council, which paid the pharmacist and the dispensing doctor. The latter surrendered the charge collected from the patient, but the druggist retained this money, which was deducted from the total sum due him. Payment was made monthly even when the pricing offices were in arrears with their work, but it was then done on account, based on the average cost of the pharmacist's prescriptions for an earlier month. Final settlement occurred when the pricing or averaging was completed.[15]

In the 1959-60 fiscal year, 65 per cent of the gross payments to the pharmacists covered the cost of ingredients and containers. Overhead expenses and profits claimed 16 per cent, and dispensing fees took the remaining 19 per cent. The gross payments to medical practitioners in that year for dispensing drugs were less than 4 per cent of the amount received by druggists.[16]

Other branches of the Health Service experienced a substantial rise in cost, but very few, and none of the major ones, could show a relatively greater increase than the pharmaceutical branch. During the first twelve years of the Health Service, expenditures on drugs rose 145 per cent, compared with 100 per cent for the hospital service. During this period the average cost of a prescription moved steadily up—from 2/9d (38 cents) to 7/3d ($1.01). Inflation accounted for at least half of this increase. As noted elsewhere, the use of more proprietary drugs and the prescribing of larger quantities were factors, but the most important element was the new and expensive preparations—antibiotics, cortisone, and other corticosteroids. The fact that other nations were experiencing the problem of higher pharmaceutical costs to a much greater degree was of little consolation to the Exchequer. Too often the authorities were unmindful of the fact that the growing expenditures on drugs were counterbalanced by a healthier population and a declining death rate. The matter of primary concern to the government was how to check the rising costs without restricting the use of drugs.[17]

Much thought was given to the matter, but the most purposeful effort was the appointment of a commission of twelve, mostly medical doctors, under the chairmanship of Sir Henry Hinchliffe. For two years it studied the problem. An interim report was issued in 1958, and the final report followed a year later. Before considering the recommendations of this committee, the measures already taken to effect greater economy should be surveyed.

Early in the history of the Health Insurance scheme, a special committee was appointed to advise on the items that should be classified as drugs. A National Formulary was furnished to the doctors with suggestions for their guidance. A list of proprietary preparations with their chemical equivalents was made available, and a special memorandum was issued to advise the physicians on such matters as the choice of medicaments and the quantities to be prescribed. The Drug Tariff was likewise put into the hands of the doctors as a source of general information. And measures were taken in the Health Insurance program to discourage excessive prescribing by deducting money from the remuneration of those found guilty of this offense.

From almost the very inception of the Health Service every effort was made to put prescribing on an economical basis. The Standing Medical Advisory Committee in 1949 suggested that a committee be set up to investigate drugs of "doubtful value" and the "unnecessarily expensive brands of standard drugs." Known as the Joint Committee on Prescribing, this body promptly urged doctors whenever possible to use standard drugs in the place of proprietary brands. It was recommended that publicly advertised proprietary preparations should not be prescribed. All other proprietary preparations were to be classified in such a manner as to encourage the prescribing of some and to discourage the use of others, depending upon such factors as their proved therapeutic value, the price arrangement, and their availability in standard form. Six categories were created. Physicians were called upon to co-operate. By 1953, some 5,000 proprietary preparations were classified, and as new drugs became available, each was designated by category as to its desirability for use by Health Service doctors. In 1958, the system was revised and simplified with a view toward making it more effective.[18]

Early in the service it was apparent that some physicians were prescribing substances that were not drugs. A Joint Sub-Committee of the English and Scottish Medical and Pharmaceutical Advisory Committees was accordingly set up to study the matter. Certain regulations were laid down governing the use of food, disinfectants, and toilet preparations. Whether some of the products should be prescribed or not depended, according to the Sub-Committee, upon their nature and the purpose for which they were used. It was recommended, for example, that nutritional substances which supplemented the diet of healthy persons, even when used for medical purposes, should be classified as foods. But nutritional preparations manufactured primarily for the treatment of disease should be considered drugs. Medicated soaps, it was held, normally should not be prescribed if they might be used for regular toilet purposes. Disinfectants, if intended for general hygienic purposes, were not to be considered drugs; but if they were for the treatment of a patient, externally or internally, they should be regarded as drugs. The Joint Sub-Committee classified a large number of substances in accordance with these principles.[19]

A standing joint committee was subsequently created to keep the principles under review and to revise the lists. Preparations not classified as drugs in 1960 covered several pages and included such items as cereal, milk foods, homogenized foods, ovaltine, malt extract, dextrin maltose, saccharine tablets, and lactose. Preparations such as hair tonics, skin lotions, tooth pastes, talcum powders, vanishing creams, and shampoos were normally not to be prescribed. If a preparation not classified as a drug should be prescribed, the cost of the preparation could be recovered from the doctor. There was no hard and fast rule, and the same substance might be considered a drug for one patient and a toilet article or a food for someone else. If a physician challenged the judgment of the Executive Council, the matter was referred to the local medical committee, and its decision could be appealed to referees. In 1960, for instance, a case arose involving "neutrogena" soap, which had been prescribed for a patient with a skin disease. The referees, overruling the local medical committee, held that it was medically necessary and was therefore a drug.[20]

Mention was made in an earlier chapter of two of the informative publications for guidance in prescribing—*The British National Formulary* and the *Prescribers' Notes*. The latter dealt with the cost of prescribing. Issued several times during the year, it brought to the attention of the physician pertinent clinical information about drugs. The *Formulary*, of pocket size, carried a comprehensive list of drugs and compound preparations which could be obtained by short title. Price lists showed the comparative prices between standard and certain proprietary preparations.

Because many doctors regarded *Prescribers' Notes* as not being sufficiently independent in its point of view, the Hinchliffe Committee proposed that it be replaced by a publication that might be called *Prescribers' Journal*. The new journal would be managed by a small council representing the appropriate professions. It would be independent of the pharmaceutical industry as well as the Ministry of Health, although the latter would help to finance it as far as the editorial organization was concerned. The Ministry would distribute it to senior medical students and all Health Service doctors. The journal would include editorial comment, the results of clinical trials, and information about new drugs.

The oldest publication was *The British Pharmacopoeia*—a voluminous publication issued under the direction of the General Medical Council every five years and followed by a supplement two and one-half years later. More useful to pharmacists than doctors, the *Pharmacopoeia* was a manual of practice which contained a list of drugs and compounds and directions on how to prepare them. It also included methods of testing and much factual information on doses and preparations used in medical practice. Another reference book, *The British Pharmaceutical Codex,* was issued by the Council of the Pharmaceutical Society. Intended for the use of physician as well as pharmacist, it described all new drugs that had been demonstrated to be clinically useful.[21]

Following the recommendation of the Hinchliffe Committee, the Ministry of Health published in 1960 a loose-leaf handbook designed to furnish the most recent comparative drug prices. Up-to-date information from various sources was brought together in this volume for the purpose of furnishing quick and accurate aid in economical prescribing. There was a pocket in the back cover of the handbook to accommodate *The British National Formulary.* All medical students as well as doctors received a copy of the handbook on prescribing; and in spring, 1961, they also were sent the *Prescribers' Journal,* the new bimonthly publication that superseded *Prescribers' Notes.*[22]

Medical practitioners certainly did not lack guidance; and with the new, compact handbook, it was hoped that they would be in a position to prescribe more prudently. Although the Hinchliffe Committee found little evidence of irresponsible prescribing among Health Service physicians, it did observe that expensive drugs were prescribed when less costly ones would do as well and that the quantity prescribed was often larger than the patient really needed. The most effective way to meet this situation, in the opinion of the Committee, was to supply the doctors with full information on the cost and therapeutic value of drugs. The handbook and other guides would help, but they were not enough. It was necessary to educate the doctor on the importance of careful prescribing. The place to begin was in the medical schools. Without making it mandatory, the Hinchliffe Committee suggested that these institutions should familiarize the students with pharmacuetical costs and methods of economical prescribing. It was evident that the medical colleges could do much more along such lines than they had been doing. But the education of the doctors should not stop there. As junior staff members in the hospitals, as trainee-assistants, and as family practitioners enrolled in refresher or postgraduate courses, they should be indoctrinated with the importance of careful and economical prescribing.[23]

The Select Committee on Estimates in 1956-1957 urged that medical students, before qualifying as doctors, should statisfy their examiners that they had "a proper knowledge of the financial structure of the National Health Service, and of the costs of treatment for which they may be responsible." In compliance with this recommendation, the Minister consulted with the deans of the medical schools and arranged that the *National Formulary* and the *Prescribers' Notes* should be distributed among medical students, but he was unwilling to interfere in their curricular or examination policies.[24]

The rising cost of the drug bill could be attributed partly to excessive prescribing, and this could be traced in some measure to pressure applied by patients. While all doctors experienced it, the Hinchliffe Committee could not determine the extent of it. There was evidence that the older, more experienced physicians and those in partnerships were able to resist the pressure better than the younger, single-practice doctors who were trying to attract new patients. The fear of losing patients to another physician may have influenced some doctors in prescribing unnecessarily. The Committee believed that moral suasion and the use of notices and posters would be more satisfactory in discouraging the importunities of patients in this matter than new regulations designed to curtail the right of transfer to another doctor.

The tendency to prescribe larger quantities was stimulated by the existence of the item charge. Precisely how to cope with this problem baffled the authorities. Disciplinary measures were used only against those who were grossly guilty of over-prescribing. The policy was to refer a case to the local medical committee for investigation only if the doctor's prescribing costs per patient were twice the average for his area. As the reader will recall, few practitioners were actually disciplined for excessive prescribing. The Hinchliffe Committee was of the opinion that the penalties should be more severe, and that, if a physician exceeded the local average by 50 per cent, he should be investigated by the local medical committee.

While disciplinary measures were considered necessary in dealing with the more flagrant cases, such a policy could not solve the larger problem of moderate over-prescribing which involved a substantial proportion of doctors. The Hinchliffe Committee felt that the matter could be handled effectively on a voluntary basis. Since the charge was resented by doctor and patient alike as a tax on illness and since it encouraged wasteful habits of prescribing, the Committee felt that the advisability of retaining it should be reviewed. It was proposed that the Minister and the medical profession enter into an agreement by which the physician would voluntarily limit the amount of a drug that he prescribed to one week's supply, except for special cases, such as chronic patients. *The British National Formulary* would have to give more extensive information in an alternate edition on what would constitute reasonable quantities to be prescribed. If, after a trial period of two years, such a voluntary approach should prove successful in controlling drug expenditures, then the Ministry of Health, it was suggested, might consider it expedient to eliminate the prescription charge.[25] The Minister accepted the proposal, promising that if the scheme were effective in achieving its objective, he would consider whether the situation justified the abolition of the charge.[26]

It was recognized that economy in prescribing bore some relationship to the sales propaganda of the drug companies. In a highly competitive field, pharmaceutical firms resorted to various promotional techniques. The medical journals were utilized extensively as an advertising medium, and in addition, literature and samples of drugs flooded the doctors' offices. More effective, perhaps, were the representatives of the drug firms that visited physicians periodically. Not only were these sales efforts expensive (producing higher drug prices), but the information provided about the therapeutic value of the preparations was sometimes misleading. In many cases, prices were not given and the physician did not always know how expensive were the drugs that he prescribed.

Although willing to see representatives of pharmaceutical houses if they did not call too often, the doctors decried the vast quantity of reading matter and the many samples that came in the mail. In 1957, the Annual Representative Meeting of the British Medical Association adopted resolutions to the effect that "standardized literature of a concise nature" be used to publicize drugs, that the amount of pharmaceutical advertisement be limited, and that unsolicited samples be banned.[27] The Hinchliffe Committee was convinced that the more extreme forms of advertising should be curbed and that prices should always be listed. So vital was the latter phase considered that the Committee even recommended that the drug houses be compelled by law, if necessary, to quote retail prices of their products in the quantities likely to be prescribed in daily practice. Some of the Executive Councils furnished drug companies with the names and addresses of Health Service doctors—a practice the Hinchliffe Committee felt should be discontinued so as not to give official encouragement to the advertising campaigns of the pharmaceutical firms. The Ministry of Health notified the Executive Councils to stop this practice,[28] but in implementing some of the other recommendations, it sought the voluntary co-operation of the drug companies.

The Association of British Pharmaceutical Industry was aware of the need for action. In spring, 1959, this organization announced the adoption by its members of a marketing code. Promotional campaigns were to be appropriate to the professional status of doctors. Statements based on pharmacological and clinical data were to be distinguished from those resting on theory or speculation, and no extravagant or deceptive claims were to be made. Sensible restraint would determine the frequency with which literature and samples were mailed to physicians, and the price of all drugs would be disclosed in the advertisement. Firms that refused to comply with the provisions of the code faced expulsion from the Association.[29]

It was a source of frustration to the practitioner that among the five thousand proprietary drugs there were various trade names and different prices for identical preparations. The Hinchliffe Commission believed that if simple, approved names were given by the British Pharmacopoeia Commission to new products, much of this confusion could be avoided and greater economy achieved. Drug manufacturers were urged to apply for an approved name before putting a new product on the market. Under existing conditions, the British Pharmacopoeia Commission usually had delayed one or two years in designating drugs with an approved name. In the meantime, the physician, in prescribing a drug, got the habit of using the trade name which, owing to persuasive salesmanship, had become familiar to him. In order to assist the practitioner to prescribe what was often the cheaper version of a new preparation, the Hinchliffe Commission suggested that the approved name should appear on the label and in the advertising literature along with the trade name. It would be the function of the loose-leaf handbook to supply the physician with timely information concerning the price of the standard preparations which were the equivalent of the new proprietary drug.

Often there was no equivalent, or if there were, it was an inferior preparation. Among 430 frequently prescribed proprietaries in 1958, one-fourth had equivalents costing less, and 15 per cent had equivalents available at the same price. For less than 4 per cent, the equivalent cost more; and for the remaining 57 per cent, there was no equivalent at all available or no equivalent in standard preparation.[30]

The pharmacists purchased their pharmaceutical products directly from drug houses or wholesale dealers, usually at a discount, and this procedure led to a reduction in the Drug Tariff prices for 1960.[31] The Drug Tariff served as the basis for determining the payments made to pharmacists. The government was naturally very much concerned about the cost of drugs and kept a sharp eye upon it. An investigation of wholesale prices for unbranded standard drugs concluded early in 1955 did not suggest that the level of prices was excessive.[32] More important as a cost factor were proprietary drugs, and for two and one-half years the Ministry of Health negotiated the matter with the Association of British Pharmaceutical Industry. In

1957, an agreement was reached designed to embrace over 4,000 pharmaceutical products and to run on a trial basis for three years.

The scheme provided that the home price would not exceed the export price for those preparations that had a good market abroad. For those that were unimportant in the export field and had an exact standard equivalent, the price would be no more than that of the equivalent preparation. For the others, the maximum price would be computed by a trade price formula related to such cost factors as ingredients, processing, packaging, and the wholesaler's discount. If the price formula were considered unsuitable for any drug, the manufacturer was privileged to negotiate a price separately with the Ministry of Health. The scheme did not apply to new drugs during their first three years on the market. The price of such preparations was left entirely to the discretion of the manufacturers who, it was felt, had every right to recover the cost of research. By 1959, all but a small fraction of the proprietary drugs had been brought under the scheme.[33]

The success of the scheme was not conclusively demonstrated. In the opinion of the Comptroller and the Auditor General, the profits of the pharmaceutical companies during the trial period were too high, largely because of the exemption of the new drugs from price regulation. Instead of the £714,500 ($2 million) in savings that was expected, the government realized little more than half that amount, or only 3.2 per cent of the cost of proprietary preparations. The Comptroller and the Auditor General questioned the efficacy of the arrangement, but the Minister of Health seemed satisfied that it had imposed restraint on prices and had even contributed to some reductions. It was pointed out that the prices of Health Service drugs were lower than the average level of prices in the chief export markets and that the people had benefited tremendously from the progress achieved in the field of pharmaceutical research. Convinced that the Voluntary Price Regulation Scheme should be continued for another trial period, the government, after insisting upon some important modifications, renewed the agreement in 1960 for three more years.

The drug manufacturers appeared to be pleased with the price regulation scheme and with the general status they enjoyed under the Health Service. The spokesmen for the industry felt that prices were reasonable and that profits were sufficient to foster research and to stimulate a healthy expansion of the industry. They could point to the fact that during the first ten years of the Health Service the price index for manufactured products except tobacco, food, and fuel had advanced more than 40 per cent, compared with an increase of less than 7 per cent for pharmaceutical products. Much was being accomplished in the field of research, 90 per cent of which was financed by the drug industry itself. The drug manufacturers spent £5 million ($14 million) on research in 1958, or nearly twice the total expended four years previously. No less spectacular was the achievement in the field of exports. In 1959, £40 million ($112 million) worth of drugs were marketed abroad—six times more than in 1945. Drug imports in 1959 for the United Kingdom had fallen to £4,275,000 ($12 million), the lowest figure since 1950.[34]

One-third of the output of the pharmaceutical industry was absorbed by the National Health Service, one-third was exported, and the other third, mostly of a miscellaneous character, was sold privately on the domestic market. All but a small part of the drugs distributed in England and Wales were purchased by the Health Service, and it was this assured market which apparently attracted a number of branch factories of foreign pharmaceutical companies to Great Britain.

There were many criteria by which the viability of the pharmaceutical industry could be measured, but perhaps the most significant was the number of effective drugs introduced during recent years— poliomyelitis vaccine, antibiotics, diuretics, hypotensives, and drugs for mental illness. Not all the research was done in the modern laboratories of the drug companies; some was accomplished by the Medical Research Council and by academic research institutions. But the production and marketing of the new products, often a very expensive operation, was the responsibility of the drug industry.[35]

The Hinchliffe Committee was not satisfied with the way clinical tests for new drugs were handled or interpreted or the arrangements of publishing the data obtained. The Committee suggested that an impartial committee be set up by the appropriate professional bodies for the purpose of organizing clinical trials of new preparations and evaluating the results. The cost of such trials would be financed by the manufacturers. The hospitals should encourage the testing program by offering facilities for this work, but the doctors who participated would not be compensated by the pharmaceutical firms. The findings would be publicized in the new *Prescribers' Journal*. Acting upon this suggestion, the Minister of Health, after discussing the matter with the professional bodies, decided to broaden the authority of the Standing Joint Committee on the Classification of Proprietary Preparations in order to permit the Committee to advise on clinical trials.

The need to deal scientifically with the problem of pharmaceutical costs prompted the Hinchliffe Committee to propose the appointment of a permanent body, to include a statistician, an economist, and men with business experience, to advise the Minister on all aspects of the cost of the pharmaceutical service.[36]   The Central Health Services Council endorsed the suggestion and cleared the way in December, 1959, for the creation of a Committee on Prescribing to help avoid unnecessary expenditures.   The Committee would approach the problem in a very methodical manner, collecting and interpreting all pertinent socio-medical, economic, and statistical data.[37]

It was obvious to careful observers that if the cost of the pharmaceutical service seemed high, it returned large dividends in better health.   In reality, this phase of the Health Service was one of the most economical.   Drugs lowered the mortality rate, eased suffering, and shortened recovery periods.   Many patients who in a previous decade would have been sent to the hospital were now treated at home, and inpatients were released much earlier.

The most casual student of medical science could not remain indifferent to the wonder-working powers of the new drugs.   Thanks largely to chemotherapy, tuberculosis mortality declined sharply, and the hospital waiting list for tuberculous patients disappeared.   Owing to sulfonamides and certain antibiotics, the shortage of beds for infectious diseases was transformed into a surplus.   Pneumonia patients, who once spent many days and even weeks in the hospital, could now remain at home and expect recovery within a much shorter period.   In the treatment of acute mastoid infections, surgery now could be avoided by the administration of sulpha drugs and antibiotics in the home.   The use of tranquilizing drugs for mental patients had marked the beginning of a new era in dealing with mental disorders. In noting the "compensating benefits from present expenditures on drugs," the Hinchliffe Committee deplored "the totally inadequate publicity given to the remarkable saving in life, improvement in health, increase in efficiency and saving on expensive institutional treatment which all stem from, among other things, the use of new drugs."[38]

In England and Wales these life-saving drugs, as well as the more prosaic medicaments, were available to all.   They were all available for a token charge.   They were prescribed on the basis of need, and those who required them most and could afford them least got them, as did all other patients.   Without such a program, the general medical practitioner service would have been seriously crippled and the Health Service would have lost its most effective weapon against illness.

CHAPTER XVIII

An Appraisal of the National Health Service

MORE THAN A THIRD of a century separated the establishment of the National Health Insurance and the foundation of the National Health Service. Adopted in the face of opposition from the medical profession, the earlier program provided free drugs and the care of a physician to workers, but not to members of their families. There was no provision for hospitalization or the services of a specialist. At least one-half of the population, including all of the middle class, was entirely excluded. The medical needs of many people were neglected. For some, especially the aged sick, the only recourse was charity. But charity was lamentably inadequate because of financially starved hospitals, underpaid doctors, a chaotic ambulance service, and a distressing lack of nurses, dentists, and specialists. Voluntary non-profit contributing schemes did little to solve the financial crisis from which the hospitals were unable to escape. The hospital survey of 1945 depicted a situation that called for drastic action.

England had long been conscious of the need to reform her medical program. Various studies were made. In 1919, the Dawson Report recognized that the coverage of Health Insurance should be broadened. In 1926, a Royal Commission favored a more effective co-ordination of the health services and protection for the wives and children of the insured. The report even suggested that public funds, not insurance, would ultimately have to finance medical benefits. The British Medical Association, by then a staunch supporter of Health Insurance, urged in two reports, in 1938 and 1942, that protection be extended to 90 per cent of the population and that such additional benefits as dental, eye, and specialist care be included in the program. In 1942, the Beveridge Report expressed strong support of a comprehensive medical scheme for everybody—to be financed mostly by Exchequer funds. The White Paper of 1944 spelled out many of the details, and two years later Parliament enacted the National Health Service Act.

Unprepared for such a sweeping program, the British Medical Association opposed it. But, as in 1912, the Association, after a show of force, bowed to the popular will. The Ministry of Health made some concessions and gave certain assurances which made the scheme more palatable to many doctors. Among other things, the Ministry agreed that there would be no whole-time salaried service for general practitioners. The physicians would continue to enjoy complete clinical freedom and would have the right to choose their patients and practice wherever they wished, except in over-doctored areas. Although troubled by misgivings about the future course of medicine, the profession could not overlook the fact that relations with the Ministry of Health had been friendly and quite satisfactory under the Health Insurance program.

The National Health Service, then, was not hastily foisted upon the nation by a Labor Government in the excitement of the postwar years. It was the evolutionary result of many years of planning, and it had the broadest sort of bipartisan support. The framework of the Health Service was carefully constructed, with due regard to salvaging what was worthy in the old arrangements. Some features were borrowed from the Health Insurance scheme. The local health authorities could not be ignored and the professional groups exerted their share of influence. The new program was thus a compromise among the realities of the past, the imperatives of the present, and the hopes of the future.

The tripartite system, however cumbersome, seemed quite logical to the planners who recognized that the disorganized hospital service had to be integrated and administered on a regional basis. They could see no reason why local health authorities should not continue to be responsible for preventive health functions or why the Insurance Committees, revitalized as Executive Councils, should not administer the dental, ophthalmic, pharmaceutical, and medical practitioner services. It was inevitable that the services of these three divisions would overlap. If the scheme seemed unwieldy, it had the authority of usage. It posed problems, but they did not appear to be insolvable. The performance of the new Health Service did not disappoint its founders. And none of the surveys during the first twelve years saw the need for any major modification of the administrative machinery.

The basic conception of the administration of the National Health Service is to decentralize as much authority as possible. The division of duties between the local and national authorities and between elective and appointive bodies has worked surprisingly well. What the Health Service lacks in flexibility it has gained in the popular support which comes from the participation of thousands of voluntary workers. Through the Executive Councils, the regional hospital boards, the hospital management committees, and the local health authorities, the National Health Service has achieved a democracy that is perhaps its unique characteristic. Considering the scope of the hospital service, its administration by a partnership between the state and the voluntary bodies can very aptly be described as "a courageous and imaginative experiment."

The three-tier system of hospital administration represents an innovation that required considerable adjustment on the part of the hospitals. The transition was not easy, but it was accomplished with a minimum of confusion. By virtue of interlocking membership between the hospital boards and the management committees and between the management committees and the house committees, the relations between all levels for the most part have been good. The many conferences between the chairmen and staff officers have been helpful. The easing of fiscal controls and the elimination of staffing restrictions did much to foster a more harmonious spirit. The delegated powers of the hospital authorities are large, and the Minister has sought to prevent any encroachment upon them. Periodic consultations between Savile Row and regional officials have promoted more effective co-operation, but in the opinion of some observers, more can be done to improve the liaison with the subordinate bodies.

In hospital management, as elsewhere, the general policy is to put trained lay administrators in authority. Only in the mental hospitals and a few other specialized institutions have medical superintendents been retained. But whoever serves as chief administrator, clinical freedom in no way is disturbed. The nursing and medical staffs have been left in complete control of their own areas of activity, and relations between them and the lay staffs remain friendly.

The influence exerted by government organizations has proved beneficial. Such Parliamentary agencies as the Public Accounts Committee and the Select Committee on Estimates keep a sharp eye on the hospitals. The primary concerns of these committees are to eradicate waste, to promote efficiency, and to improve standards. Their contribution in such matters has been noteworthy, but any effort on their part to foster greater centralization in hospital control has been resisted by the Ministry of Health. The interest of both houses of Parliament in the Health Service is disclosed in high-level debates and, more frequently, in the question-and-answer periods. Numerous investigations have been sponsored by the Ministry and its agencies. Few phases of the Health Program have escaped scrutiny or lacked suggestions for improvement. No Minister of Health can remain indifferent to the manifold efforts to better the Service, but, in practice, the Minister has not always furnished the dynamic leadership required to implement the proposed changes. Although he can exert pressure and invoke his authority in seeking to initiate certain policies, it is apparent that moral suasion is the more prudent course in dealing with voluntary bodies. Time is required to make innovations or to modify existing procedures in an organization so vast and varied, and so decentralized, as the Health Service.

The policy of the Minister has been to keep the regional hospital boards free of partisan influence. While some of the appointments to the boards may have been influenced by political considerations, there is little evidence that they have been a factor of significance. There is scant testimony that bureaucracy has worked to the serious detriment of the hospital service or that hospital efficiency has been much impaired by political pressures.

The allegation that the National Health Service has suffered from the influence of party politics has not been taken seriously by any responsible report on the workings of the program. Precisely what hostile critics mean by "the intrusion of party politics into medicine" has never been clearly defined, but they could not have had in mind clinical freedom or the right of the doctor to practice his skill as he wishes. These remain untouched by politics. As part of a great system supervised and financed by the government, the physician must, of course, submit to certain regulations. His own profession has helped to make them, however, and that he must obey them does not mean he is subservient to politicans or that his professional freedom is in jeopardy. The fact that an American specialist entertained such a distorted conception of the status of the British medical practitioner caused a member of the House of Commons to make this statement in 1958:

During my visit to the United States I was flabbergasted at the appalling ignorance about our National Health Service revealed in circles where one would not expect to find it. . . . I met a consultant, attached to a large city hospital and a large medical school in a university, who believed that all the doctors in this country are directed by Whitehall, exactly like soldiers in the army. He had other strange ideas about our Health Service and it gave me great pleasure to disabuse the mind of this eminent medical gentleman of them. A useful service would be performed by our Foreign Office, or the Ministry of Health, or by both acting together, if they did something to inform American people about what our Service is, what it does, and what we wish it to do in the future.[1]

In seeking more remuneration, the medical profession had to bargain with the government, whose position was influenced by the condition of the national economy. Here political considerations were a factor, and in the absence of arbitral machinery this could not very well be avoided. But with the creation in 1960 of the Review Body for doctors' and dentists' remuneration, there is reason to believe that the most disturbing issue of all has been removed from the arena of political deliberation.

Some critics of the Health Service have denied that the relationship between the medical profession and the government is a partnership; they claim that it more closely resembles the employee-employer relation. While the controversies over remuneration have lent some support to that view, it ignores the administrative and policy-making role of the medical profession. The influence of the British Medical Association often has proved so decisive that there seems to be some foundation to the charge that control of the Health Service is weighted in favor of the doctors. Their prestige is constantly felt through numerous bodies. Reference need only be made to the Central Health Services Council and the Executive Councils, with their heavy professional representation, or the groups concerned with the medical practitioner service, such as the local medical committees, the Medical Service Committee, and the Medical Practices Committee. Many doctors are members of the hospital boards and management committees. Virtually every phase of the Health Service that concerns the medical profession has been the subject of discussion between the Ministry of Health and the General Medical Services Committee, which functions as the negotiating agency for the British Medical Association. The other professions are served in similar fashion by committees and negotiating bodies. The Minister of Health has often acknowledged his complete dependence upon the professions in the successful operation of the Health Service.

If England seems to be content with the general framework of the Health Service, that does not mean that country is completely satisfied with the actual workings of the program, either qualitatively or quantitatively. In many areas, performance has not measured up to expectations. It is recognized that, however sound are the basic concepts, their translation into a highly efficient system will require years of effort and careful planning. An examination of the voluminous literature covering almost every facet of the scheme leaves one impressed with the investigative zeal of the British and the many suggestions to diminish or remove deficiencies. It is generally accepted that only through experimentation and the application of improved techniques can the Health Service remain a dynamic force. Proof of this spirit is to be found in the reports covering such phases as internal hospital administration, general medical practice, hospital staffing, drug prescription, convalescence, treatment of the chronic sick and the aged, rehabilitation of the physically handicapped, welfare of inpatients, health visiting, maternity care, and mental health. Such studies contribute to a better understanding of the program and in some cases have resulted in a more effective approach.

Although substantial progress has been made toward a better Service during the first twelve years, some problems do not easily yield to corrective action. The most troublesome one arises out of the tripartite system. No subject has been discussed more avidly than how to achieve better co-ordination between the hospitals, the general practitioners, and the local health authorities. Before 1948, these services were locked in comparatively tight compartments, and in some cases there was even unfriendly rivalry between them. Under the Health Service, a new climate of mutual helpfulness has slowly begun to emerge.

It has been clearly demonstrated that the tripartite system does not preclude co-operation where there is a real desire to work together. In some regions a high degree of co-ordination has been achieved through liaison committees, the joint use of facilities, and the joint employment of staff. More often, it is accomplished informally. As leader of the domiciliary team, the general practitioner has found it advantageous to work closely with the home nurse, the midwife, and the health visitor. In such fields as maternity care, chronic illness, and mental health, the need for effective co-operation on the part of all branches of the Health Service is most apparent. Considerable emphasis has been given to this matter in specialized reports and memorandums issued by the Ministry of Health. Noteworthy gains have been made, with the problem largely disappearing in some areas, but the over-all picture leaves no room for complacency.

One of the most satisfying aspects of the Health Service is the vigorous part played by voluntary workers. Thousands of men and women have, without compensation, been willing to accept appointment to bodies that administer the vast hospital empire and the services of the Executive Councils. There seems to be no lack of competent people who welcome the opportunity to serve gratuitously in a program which they look upon as their own. In the local clinics, in the domiciliary service, and in the hospitals, voluntary workers are active. It was gloomily predicted at the outset of the Health Service that if the hospitals were nationalized the great reservoir of voluntary help would dry up. On the contrary, more persons than ever have offered their services. The Leagues of Friends, the British Red Cross, the Order of St. John, and the Woman's Voluntary Services are among the better known organizations that have contributed so much to the viability of the Health Service.   By assisting patients in many useful ways, the voluntary workers have helped to give the Health Service a humanitarianism that is one of its distinguishing characteristics.

In spite of the trend toward specialization, the National Health Service has never lost sight of the importance of the general medical practitioner.   Every effort has been made to strengthen this phase of the program.   Through financial inducements and the use of negative direction, the government has been able greatly to improve the distribution of physicians.   In 1952, the number of people residing in under-doctored areas represented more than one-half of the population; six years later, it was less than one-fifth.   This improved distribution of doctors was accomplished without coercion and without restriction upon general freedom of movement.   A few areas have been closed from time to time, but since there is little incentive to practice where there are too many doctors anyway, the procedure has been strongly endorsed by the medical profession.

Although entrance into general medical practice is not easy, the situation has improved through Initial Practice Allowances and a special "loading" arrangement in remuneration that encourages the establishment of partnerships.   The great majority of those entering practice do so as partners.   The medical schools have overflowed with students, many of whom are the sons of doctors, and each year has witnessed a healthy growth in the number of physicians.   The trainee general practitioner scheme makes the transition into medical practice easier for hundreds of inexperienced doctors.   While competition is keen for those vacancies that are advertised, only a negligible number of practitioners are unable to secure employment in the Health Service.   Not all doctors find the type of work they most want, and for older physicians it is especially difficult to make a change.   Yet the general picture is one of greater opportunity for physicians to practice their skill—and under conditions immeasurably better than England has ever known before.   The very small proportion of emigrating doctors suggests that the Health Service offers advantages that make medical practice in England especially attractive.

While there is competition among physicians for patients (for there is freedom of choice for both doctor and patient), the Health Service has done much to foster professional co-operation.   This has been achieved primarily through partnerships, which now embrace more than two-thirds of all principals.   Rota schemes, to which over one-half of all family doctors belong, provide more off-duty hours.   Group practice, however, has the most to offer in co-operative medicine.   Through interest-free loans, the government encourages the establishment of communal premises, so that several doctors can work together as a clinical team. This approach holds great appeal for many physicians, but the funds available have never been great enough to meet the demand. Both the partnership arrangement and group practice make possible more ancillary help, more leisure, and, generally, higher standards of practice.

Health centers, which originally appeared to hold such great promise in uniting curative and preventive medicine, have proved a disappointment. The few that have been established provide a poor image of what the founders had envisaged. Opposed by most doctors, the health center has made limited headway only in the new housing areas. Group practice, much more than health centers, seems to represent the future pattern of medical practice.

Not only is there greater co-operation under the Health Service, but more professional interest has been shown by doctors. This is evident in the growing number of doctors who take postgraduate work and refresher courses. The rapid expansion in the membership of the College of General Practitioners suggests a wholesome interest in professional advancement. Doctors' pride in their work is reflected in an improvement in the condition of their premises. While some doctors' offices remain barely satisfactory, many have attained a high level of excellence, and the trend is toward better facilities.

Whatever apprehension the practitioner may have had about security in his job soon vanished as it became clear that the disciplinary machinery, if anything, was weighted in his favor. A doctor accused of violating the terms of service is given every opportunity to defend himself in secrecy and without jeopardy to his professional standing. So much does the medical profession like the arrangement, including the tribunal and the appellant jurisdiction of the Minister, that any proposed change has been strongly resisted. Few medical practitioners are ever disciplined.

The doctors have attained a large measure of financial security, which includes a generous pension. Compared with their economic status before World War II, they have done significantly better under the Health Service. They are one of the most highly paid groups in England. When their position has shown evidence of slipping, as it did in the early years of the Service and again in 1956, they pressed for an increase, and after a struggle won substantially what they demanded. The two controversies engendered a considerable heat, which disappeared as soon as the awards were made. The absence of suitable machinery to adjudicate differences over remuneration was a major weakness in the Health Service which the Pilkington Commission in 1960 sought to remedy through the creation of the

Review Body. This agency has been authorized to survey periodically the remuneration of doctors and dentists and to propose an adjustment whenever circumstances require it.

The medical profession realized that the straight capitation system of payment encourages work based on quantity rather than quality. This method was accordingly modified by providing an additional payment, or loading fee, for each patient within a fixed medium range. Large lists were discouraged in this way, and doctors with small lists were benefited. Even so, physicians with few patients remain at a disadvantage, although they are usually eligible for special financial assistance. The capitation system does not reward merit unless list size can be equated with ability. To remedy this shortcoming, the Pilkington Commission proposed that a system of awards be set up to recognize distinguished work among general medical practitioners. Still, the capitation system has worked reasonably well and is preferred to either the salaried or item-of-service methods of remuneration, neither of which ever appeared to have much support.

Owing to the more equitable distribution of general practitioners and to the loading arrangement, the size of the doctors' lists diminished. In 1958, the national average stood below 2,275 patients per doctor. Many physicians have fewer patients, but one-fourth of the doctors still have lists of over 3,000. That number is considered too large by some, but not by all. Physicians disagree about how many patients can be adequately attended by a doctor, but there is growing support for a reduction of the maximum to 2,500. Since most practitioners have fewer than that number, the average physician does not seem to be overworked. The evidence would indeed sustain this assumption, since the rate of consultations, home visits, and night calls is no greater and is sometimes smaller than existed during the pre-Health Service era. Paper work, involving certification, medical records, prescription forms, and so forth, is not viewed as burdensome by most doctors. Secretarial help eases the clerical burden, and the rota system increases the free time of family doctors. Many of them seldom keep their patients waiting in the reception room more than thirty minutes.

While the physician is free to prescribe any drugs deemed necessary, the Ministry by moral suasion seeks to discourage over-prescribing and the use of expensive proprietary preparations when the equivalent in standard drugs is available. Although none of the studies discloses the existence of serious abuse or any great amount of waste, it is evident that many practitioners could exercise more prudence in prescribing. Overshadowing all factors, however, are the tremendous benefits derived from drugs. These more than offset the cost and in reality represent a very good investment in health.

The exclusion of the general practitioner from the hospital is often listed as a weakness of the Health Service, but, like so many other trends, it began long before 1948 and can be observed in most countries of the world. Increased specialization has diminished the role of the family doctor in hospital work. The great majority of general practitioners have no desire for hospital work, but for those who do, the Ministry of Health has urged hospitals to make some provision. A small but increasing number of beds and hospital appointments accordingly have been made available to family physicians. Some of the normal maternity patients and some of the other more ordinary hospital cases can be attended by general practitioners.

If it is true that a widening gulf has separated the family doctor from the specialist, the Health Service may have contributed to it. Before 1948, the specialist cultivated the practitioner as a source for patients. Under the Health Service, this has been unnecessary, since the hospital service is free and the consultant is paid by the state. While the old relationship no longer exists, the general practitioner has made far greater use of the services of the specialists, both in the domiciliary consultant service and in the outpatient departments. The family physician has even been accused of sending more patients to the hospital than is really necessary, and this may be true, although a second opinion in a doubtful case occasionally reveals an illness that is serious. As for minor surgery, the hospitals are better equipped to handle it than the practitioner, who has no desire to incur the risk of a liability suit.

The denial of direct access to the radiological and X-ray departments, also listed as a weakness of the Service, is largely an inherited situation. The National Health Service has done much to correct the matter through the intercession of the Minister of Health. By 1958, the overwhelming majority of hospitals had made their diagnostic facilities directly accessible to the family doctor who, in spite of all the agitation, has not made extensive use of them. He generally prefers to send the patient to the outpatient department, which furnishes much of the work done by the diagnostic division.

There is no very accurate way to measure the effects which the Health Service has had upon the doctor-patient relationship. The very vagueness of the term makes for confused thinking, since it means so many different things to people. To one person, bedside manners and leisurely treatment are the main criteria for judging the doctor-patient relationship; to another, the test is effective treatment without any frills. If the former is accepted as the standard, then it can be argued that there has been some deterioration under the Health Service, since the physician's approach by necessity has become more utilitarian. He is not likely to give as much time to a Health Service patient as he would to a private one who is willing to pay for a prolonged consultation. But the quality and adequacy of the treatment have not suffered under the health program, nor has there been any decline in the doctor's professional or even friendly interest in his patients. Indeed, the practitioner, who can now offer so much more in the way of complete medical treatment, is able to put his relationship with the patient upon a more enduring foundation.

The physician is far more effective clinically because he can minister to all patients, irrespective of their economic status, and he can give them whatever treatment is required. No longer does he ask himself, as he once did, whether a patient can afford to go to the hospital or purchase certain very expensive but vital drugs. No longer does he hesitate to visit a patient for fear his visit may be interpreted as an excuse to collect an additional fee. Under the Health Service, need determines treatment and there is no means test.

The elimination of the financial barrier between doctor and patient has been construed by many observers as putting medicine upon a much more wholesome basis. The high cost of treatment left England no alternative but to nationalize the medical services. The implications of the change were the subject of comment on the tenth anniversary of the Health Service. The *Daily Telegraph and Morning Post* observed that, in view of the high cost of drugs and hospital care, a long illness could be ruinous were it not for the Health Service. "The public," it acknowledged, "has good cause for gratitude."[2] Writing in *The New Statesman,* an eminent lay authority on the Health Program declared, "Before 1948 medical bills were a source of anxiety for the middle class, and the cost of professional services kept many a working class woman from going to the doctor. This fear has been banished from England."[3] A doctor in *The Spectator* said, "The sharpest critics of the National Health Service have got to admit that the service provided for the ordinary citizen is better than it has ever been. The man who earns his living has been relieved of the fear that grave illness in one of his family may eat into his savings. He knows that he, and his dependents, can have a consultant opinion, and any treatment they may need, in hospital, or out-patient clinic, not as charity, but as a public service to which they have contributed by tax payments."[4]

"What the Health Service has done," proclaimed *The Times* (London), "is to ensure that the discoveries of the research laboratories and institutions of the world are made freely available to every citizen of these islands to an extent that was not possible under the pre-1948 system."⁵   And in Parliament, a member made this observation:

One of the things that the Health Service has done, and a very important thing it is, is to eliminate the fear of the economic consequences of serious or protracted illness, the fear of the doctor's bill. Anybody who goes across the Atlantic, as I did for a fairly brief period last autumn, can see very quickly what a real fear this is in Canada and the United States.   The knowledge that a serious illness can run away with one's life savings, and probably put one into debt in no time at all, constitutes a neurosis in itself. That is something, thank heaven, that we have been able to eliminate here once and for all.⁶

Under the Health Service the proportion of families having a family doctor has increased to possibly three-fourths.   This is because the children and mother are now eligible for medical care as well as the breadwinner.   Although a patient can easily change doctors, he rarely does so.   While some patients abuse the Service, the vast majority do not.   Most patients show a co-operative and understanding spirit.   There is little evidence that the Health Service has fostered more hypochondriacs than would normally be found under any other system of medicine; it may have produced fewer.   The privacy of the doctor-patient relationship in no way has been imperiled by the new service.   Aneurin Bevan, the chief architect of the National Health Service, firmly asserted that the "consulting room is inviolable and no sensible person would have it otherwise."⁷   Not even the most probing critic has been able to challenge convincingly the effective application of that principle.

Opinion differs as to the effect which the Health Service may have upon the future of general medical practice in Britain.   But there are many who believe that it has opened new vistas for the family physician.   One doctor whose articles in the medical journals have been well received wrote in 1958 that "It is felt by many that 1948 marked the turning point in a renaissance in general practice."⁸   A lay authority of repute observed in the same year that the Health Service "has made a beginning in the process of establishing a social framework in which the great majority of general practitioners, gradually assimilating the benefits of scientific medicine, may find a more assured and satisfying role than was their lot before 1948."⁹

General acceptance of the Health Service by the medical practitioners was clearly shown by the Social Surveys' poll of 1956, in which over two-thirds of the respondent practitioners indicated that if they had a chance to go back ten years they would vote in favor of the establishment of the Service.   In a program of this character, it is understandable that there can never be complete unanimity.

Criticisms of various features were rife from the beginning, but they were mostly about the less important aspects. While many doctors exercise their "natural prerogative to grumble on all occasions," only a few have noisily proclaimed their distaste for the Health Service. The great majority accept it as basically sound, while seeking to improve it. No one knows this better than the General Secretary of the Medical Practitioners' Union—an organization of some 5,000 doctors. In 1957, he disclosed to me that, apart from the remuneration issue which was then preoccupying the profession, the general practitioners were reasonably satisfied with the Service. "If certain modifications were made, largely of a minor character," he averred, "I would say they would be as satisfied as any professional group of men are likely to be in a modern, highly taxed society."

The editor of the *Medical World Newsletter* suggested in the columns of that publication that to really understand what the doctors as a body were saying about the Service, one should read the Report of the Annual Conference of Local Medical Committees. "This is," he explained, "a remarkably dull document and is concerned with putting right a lot of minor, but, to doctors, important questions regarding the regulations and details of the National Health Service generally. I have attended the last six of these conferences and of recent years I can hardly remember on any occasion hearing a speech which condemned participation in the National Health Service and calling for a return to pre-Health Service conditions."[10]

By 1960, the family physician was in a much more favorable position, with many of the irritations having been reduced or largely eliminated. In general, what does the picture show? There is still too much variation in the size of lists. The permissible maximum is too large. The immobility of elderly doctors continues to plague the service. Small-list doctors seem to be inadequately rewarded. Excessive prescribing is difficult to control.

Many aspects, however, are encouraging. Most important has been the satisfactory adjustment of remuneration and the provision for a Review Body. The bulk of the practitioners have gained direct access to diagnostic facilities, and there has been some increase in hospital beds and hospital appointments for family doctors. The distribution of physicians has greatly improved, and the average doctor's list has been reduced to manageable proportions. Reduction in list size and the growth of partnerships, group practice, and the rota system have left a substantial proportion of the practitioners with more time for other activities. The trend has favored more co-operation among doctors, which improves the tone of medical practice. Clinical freedom remains inviolable, and the doctor-patient relationship has improved, since the practitioner can offer every patient better and more complete treatment. The physician has security in his job and an adequate superannuation allowance after retirement. The Health Service has not dealt unkindly with him.

In no branch of the Health Program is progress more easily measured than in the hospital service. In matters relating to staff, beds, inpatients, outpatients, new and renovated buildings, and the growth of hospital departments, data is available that permits clear comparison. Not all factors are favorable, but as a whole the picture is one from which the British people draw great satisfaction.

Most lamentable has been the failure to replace obsolete buildings with new ones. Although conscious of the need to do this, the authorities were at first handicapped by budgetary restrictions, material shortages, and inflation. Not until the latter part of the 1950's did the government begin to tackle the problem seriously. The way was then cleared for an expanded building program that would give England and Wales the modern hospitals that are needed.

An achievement of magnitude was the reorganization and integration of the heterogeneous hospital system. The Ministry of Health has sponsored a policy of renovation, equipment modernization, and proper staffing. Even remote hospitals are not neglected. They are more adequately provided with specialists and other trained personnel and are furnished with diagnostic facilities, operating rooms, and whatever apparatus is necessary to deal effectively with all but the more unusual and specialized cases. These are transferred to the hospitals that can accommodate them.

The improvement of all hospitals is reflected in the greatly improved ratio of treatment to beds, the substantial increase in the number of inpatients and outpatients, the drop in the size of the waiting list, and the drastic reduction in the shortage of hospital personnel. It mattered not who scrutinized the hospital service—whether it was the Acton Society Trust, the Guillebaud Committee, the Select Committee on Estimates, or the King Edward's Hospital Fund—the verdict was one of unrestrained praise for the rising standards and the increased efficiency. While there is ample room for more improvement, it is evident that the gloomy forecasts about the irreparable harm that would engulf the hospitals under a nationalized program could not have been more mistaken.

Making the hospital service more effective is a continuing operation that has absorbed the attention of the Ministry, the hospital authorities, and numerous investigating committees. One cannot avoid being impressed with the constant effort made to promote more economy and better performance. While there has been no obvious waste, it is clear that new and improved techniques save both time and money. Introducing departmental costing was a major step. Under this system, expenditures are broken down by departments and services, and ward costs are even classified on the basis of the various specialties. From such information, comparative studies suggest where inquiries most appropriately can be made to reduce expenses. Other measures have been taken, some very helpful, such as the institution of the Advisory Service to help raise the level of performance in the various fields of hospital activity. One of the most widely publicized efforts is the Hospital Organization and Methods Service, which sends efficiency experts to any hospital that desires them. Trained industrial consultants are also used, as well as work study engineers.

The competitive pattern which so completely characterized the hospital world prior to 1948 has yielded to a more co-operative approach. This has been most graphically demonstrated in the purchase of hospital supplies through group and joint-group endeavor. It is by such effort, rather than by procurement on a national or purely local basis, that the great bulk of the purchases are now made. Substantial savings are thus effected and quality assured, but the individual hospital always determines its own needs. Inter-group co-operative ventures have also been developed in other fields of activity.

By utilizing most of the unstaffed beds and by shortening the stay for patients, the hospitals were able to accommodate 30 per cent more inpatients at the end of the first decennium. Although waiting lists have declined, they remain noticeably high. Their size, however, is deceptive since the figures appear to be greatly inflated. Some hospitals periodically revise their lists, but others fail to do so. There is no period of waiting for an emergency patient, and in London rarely does it take more than thirty minutes to find a bed for a person who requires immediate hospitalization. Admission for non-emergency patients depends upon the department and varies from almost no delay to a delay of several months. In dealing with waiting lists, the view of the experts seems to be that, instead of more beds, the need is for better distribution of the existing number in modern hospitals and the further development of the local health authority services.

The Ministry of Health recognizes that the outpatient service is indispensable to good doctoring and has encouraged its expansion. Within ten years, the number of specialists increased more than one-third, thus permitting many more outpatients to be treated. Free access to the outpatient service is a vital part of the medical edifice, greatly strengthening the effectiveness of the general practitioner, who can always get the opinion of a consultant for any patient. The use of specialists in the domiciliary service is likewise praiseworthy and has won the commendation of even the sharpest critics of the Health Service. The number of such visits has increased impressively, with virtually every speciality being represented. There is no charge and need alone determines who may use the service. A request from the family physician brings the specialist to the home of the patient.

A phase of the hospital program that deserves special credit is rehabilitation. Increasing use has been made of physiotherapy and occupational therapy in an effort to restore the functional activity of the patient, to teach him to live with his disability and to do useful work. Remedial gymnasts, almoners, and psychiatric social workers are also used in rehabilitation. Some hospitals operate resettlement clinics which help the individual to adjust to home life. Although not a part of the hospital service, the Retraining Program, which simulates conditions existing in industry, assists in the annual rehabilitation of thousands of patients, most of whom are able to find employment.

Medical research enjoyed a healthy expansion after 1948, with larger sums of money being made available for this purpose. The Medical Research Council, an independent agency, co-operates closely with the hospitals in their research effort. A Clinical Research Board in the early 1950's was created to promote and supervise major research schemes in the hospitals. At no time has medical research in England seemed to command more prestige or attract abler medical scientists for lifetime careers.

The hospital service is active in many other areas. A function greatly appreciated by elderly people is the provision of hearing-aids. There is no charge, not even for batteries or maintenance. Other appliances—artificial eyes, arms, and legs, as well as invalid chairs and tricycles—are furnished free. A rapid expansion of the X-ray and pathological facilities ensures that all patients who require a diagnostic examination receive it. Mass radiography by means of mobile units has vastly increased the number of chest X-rays, thereby making it possible for more patients with tuberculosis and other chest diseases to get early treatment. In collecting blood, the hospital service was able to double the number of donations during the first decade.

In the field of mental health, the National Health Service has made some of its greatest progress. Prior to 1948, mental and mentally deficient patients were almost entirely the responsibility of the local authorities. The places of confinement were isolated and dreary, the emphasis being on the custodial function. The Health Service sought to provide a new framework in which physical and mental health are joined under a comprehensive program. Mental disorders are viewed in the same way as other types of illness requiring early treatment; and patients are encouraged to seek such treatment on a voluntary basis. The important role of community care and after-care is likewise stressed, and the local health authorities are urged to provide more clinics, hostels, residential homes, and training and occupation centers. There has been greater insistence upon co-operation between the local health authority, hospital, and practitioner services in mental health.

By the end of the first decade, there was evidence of real progress. Voluntary admission of mental patients increased rapidly, compared with a sharp drop in the number of those who were accepted on a compulsory basis. Substantially more nurses attended the patients. The steady growth of the psychiatric outpatient departments, the greater use of mental health consultants in the domiciliary service, the establishment of day hospitals, and the more active role performed by the local health authorities contributed to a reduction in the number of beds in the mental hospitals. Better facilities, an improved diet, and new types of treatment greatly modified life in the mental institutions.

The new approach involved more than the use of electrical treatments, insulin, or tranquilizing drugs; it embraced social activity and the use of group and occupational therapy. By granting more freedom of movement and by developing in the patient a feeling of responsibility, pride and usefulness, the hospitals noted amazing progress toward recovery. Individuals for whom there once seemed to be no hope were allowed to return home, and for most patients the length of treatment was shortened. The aged, in particular, benefited from the new methods. There was a noticeable decline in the institutional death rate of chronically ill mental patients and a surprising increase in the annual discharge rate of elderly persons.

Parliament in 1959 enacted a new Mental Health Law based upon the recommendations of the Royal Commission on Mental Health. The new legislation marked an almost complete break with traditional concepts and greatly accelerated the trends which the Health Service had been following. Provision was made for more complete integration between the mental and mental deficiency institutions and the other hospitals. Compulsory segregation was completely swept away, and mentally disordered persons were now privileged to enter any hospital for treatment on a voluntary basis. Elaborate safeguards were created to protect the patient against wrongful detention, and only when the interest of the individual or society required it could he be coercively detained. The way was paved for more co-operation among all who had a part in the mental health program, with greater emphasis upon community care and the preventive services.

The proper care of all hospital patients required a greatly expanded staff. By the end of the first decade, the medical and the nursing staff had increased by one-third; and the professional and technical staff, other than doctors and nurses, had grown by 50 per cent. Every effort was made to improve the performance of the hospital personnel. The medical ancillary services—the occupational therapists, dietitians, chiropodists, physiotherapists, radiographers, remedial gymnasts, and medical laboratory technicians—were put on a professional statutory basis. Various schemes have been initiated to help train hospital administrators. An investigation led to the reclassification of the clerical and administrative grades.

The hospital service had reason to be pleased with the rapid growth in the nursing staff. Before the appointed day, the grave shortage in this profession remained a problem which seemed to be without solution. While not all hospitals had a full complement of nurses in 1958, the situation was so much improved that unstaffed beds had shrunk to a negligible number. The reasons why the rapidly increasing supply of nurses could not quite overtake demand were a reduction in nurses' hours, a rise in the number of inpatients, and advances in medical practice that took more of the nurses' time. Nursing had very definitely become more attractive. The growing number of applicants even led to a more selective policy of recruitment. Working conditions underwent improvement, as did nurses' homes, and a higher scale of remuneration was offered. The techniques of nursing remained flexible, there being a growing disposition to experiment. Foreigners were attracted as observers to study the nursing service and what had been accomplished in it.

All medical grades derive substantial benefits from the Health Service, but the one that occupies the most favored position is the consultant. The consultant's improved status is frequently the subject of comment. In the pre-1948 era, it was a serious struggle to become a specialist. Years of penury usually characterized the long climb to the top, and once the doctor reached his coveted goal, his position remained precarious, especially during the latter years of his life. All this has been changed under the Health Service. The lower-ranking hospital posts are now reasonably well paid, and once the doctor becomes a specialist he not only has unlimited security in his job but receives earnings which put him at the head of all professional groups in England. He enjoys the right to work on a part-time basis.   Part-time consultants can have private patients and are granted certain fiscal benefits denied whole-time specialists.   All specialists are eligible to receive merit awards, and all are generously pensioned.

Only a few of the specialties were not fully staffed at the end of the first decade.   Unlimited tenure, complete clinical freedom, and the assistance of a team of skilled workers make the rank of consultant extremely desirable.   Although one-third of the hospital medical staff are of that rank, competition to fill the vacancies is very keen, and some highly trained doctors have been unsuccessful in getting an appointment.   The problem of "time-expired" senior registrars and the anomalous position of the Senior Hospital Medical Officers, having bedeviled the hospital service for years, finally led to some ameliorative action.

Hospitals exist for the patients, and this fact has never been overlooked by the Ministry of Health and the hospital authorities.   While any generalization should be made with caution, the evidence is clear that a continuing effort has been made to improve the well-being of patients.   Yet complaints can be heard about noise, unappetizing meals, inadequate staffing of the wards at night, and the unwillingness of some nurses and doctors to give the patient any information. Although conditions are not ideal in all hospitals, a big improvement has occurred under the Health Service.   In a vast number of institutions, life in the wards has become more pleasant, and the personnel have shown a more sympathetic understanding of the patients' needs. The old attitude toward charity patients has no place in a system in which any person without charge can claim the right to use the full services of the hospital.

Redecoration of wards, improvement in catering, utilization of bed curtains and ear phones, use of heated food trolleys, and mitigation of noise are examples of what is being done to contribute to a more pleasant arrangement for patients.   Procedure varies among hospitals, but many use brochures to help adjust the patients to hospital routine; and an effort is being made to diminish the institutional features of hospital life.   The welfare of children is a special matter of concern.   The voluntary workers have done much to improve the comfort of the inpatients by tending to personal needs that are beyond the scope of the trained nurses.   The middle class seems to have no reluctance to enter the wards—a fact of significance in any evaluation of hospital standards.

As early as 1954, King Edward's Hospital Fund revealed that many "visits have been paid on behalf of the Fund [to hospitals] in the metropolitan area in the last few years and the general picture lends no support to the pessimists.   On almost every hand progress and a spirit of initiative are in evidence."[11]   There were many on the tenth anniversary of the Health Service who spoke in glowing terms of what had been done. Among them was *The Observer,* which recognized that in the "hospitals the average standard of medicine is probably the highest in the world. The genteel poverty of the voluntary hospitals, the Victorian bleakness of the municipal institutions that we knew in the past, both have been transformed by a level of expenditure that is lavish in comparison with the old days. Skill has been spread evenly; diagnostic facilities without which the doctor is often mute and helpless have been provided within every hospital, and treatment of the most complex kind is available in every area close to anyone that needs it."[12]

In summary, what then can be said for the hospital service? In spite of exceptional progress, the authorities are aware that much remains to be done to raise the service to a first-class level. Waiting lists are a disturbing element. Too many hospitals are substandard and only modern buildings can correct the situation. Increased Exchequer funds promise an ultimate solution of this problem, but it will take years to erect the required number of new hospitals. Some believe that the leadership should show greater flexibility in adopting new trends of thought.

The hospital record nevertheless is impressive. Among the gains are the improvement of a vast number of institutions, a more equitable distribution of specialists and other staff workers, a marked increase in virtually every category of hospital employees, a new and more hopeful approach to mental health, substantial progress in the field of geriatrics, the expansion of outpatient departments, the creation of ample diagnostic facilities, the growth of the domiciliary consultant service, and the more efficient use of beds. The integration of such a great array of dissimilar institutions is a feat of no mean proportions. The *esprit de corps* of the personnel is perhaps the most encouraging aspect of all. The hospital service has demonstrated the capacity to move forward on a broad front.

Although associated with the hospitals, the ambulance service is a local authority function. Before 1948 it was disorganized; afterwards it became mandatory for the local authorities and developed into one of the best efforts of the Health Service. The average number of miles per patient was reduced by nearly one-third, and in other ways there has been greater operational efficiency of the ambulances. Among the factors responsible for the improvement are the costing returns and other studies of the ambulance service, the use of radio control, and a more effective liaison between the local and hospital authorities.   Little abuse and few complaints have been associated with this service.

While the prevention of disease and injuries is primarily an activity belonging to the local health authority, much depends upon the co-operation of the general practitioner and hospital services.   The feeling is that the prevention of illness has been unduly subordinated to the curative phase and that the role of the family doctor in preventive medicine has been disappointing.   The Ministry of Health is not indifferent to the matter and through nationwide campaigns has done much to educate the people about dental care, mental health, tuberculosis, respiratory infections, the prevention of home accidents, and the importance of immunization and vaccination.   A determined and successful battle has been waged against tuberculosis. Without charge, the people, especially children, have been rendered immune to several of the communicable diseases.   But there are other preventive phases that should be noted, such as the Welfare Foods Scheme, the effective work done by child welfare clinics, and the periodic medical inspection of school children.   Such factors have contributed to the low mortality rate and the good health of British youth.

Of great usefulness among the domiciliary services are health visiting, home nursing, the domestic help service, and the domiciliary midwifery service.   Whereas the health visitor is concerned with the entire gamut of mental and physical illness, the others are limited in their work, each performing a more specialized function.   So popular are the home nursing and domestic help phases that they have enjoyed a phenomenal expansion, being increasingly utilized in the care of the elderly and chronic sick.   The district nurses are used to administer injections and for general nursing care in the home.   They have proved of inestimable value to the general practitioner.   The domestic worker does routine work in homes that require such help.   Without these two services, many households would have been broken and the patients removed to an institution.   The desire to remain in the community amid familiar surroundings is very strong among the aged.   The Health Service is doing what it can to make this possible.

The care of the chronic sick has taken precedence over many other phases of the Service.   The growing proportion of aged people has dramatized the need to expand some of the health facilities and to adapt them in a more purposeful manner.   Co-operation between the local authority, the hospital, and the general practitioner services has not always been completely successful.   Yet much has been accomplished, and the growing interest in the matter promises a more co-ordinated approach.   Most effective in dealing with the problem of chronic illness are the geriatric outpatient departments and geriatric units in the hospitals. Also day hospitals and short-stay convalescent wards or annexes are of value. Chronic-sick beds have been increased. In London during 1959, only 1 per cent of the aged sick had to wait over two months to gain admittance to the hospital. Improved techniques of treatment greatly expedite the discharge of elderly patients. In that city there are few patients with treatable medical disabilities that go untreated.[13]

The approach to the problem of the elderly and chronic sick involves the local authorities in many different ways. Such activities as meals on wheels, a chiropody service, and an evening and a night attendant service are used in some areas with promising results. Of primary importance are residential accommodations. More housing for old people is being erected by the local authorities, the trend being away from the larger institutional approach. Small homes, some newly erected and others remodeled houses, have been opened to the aged. The Ministry has urged that the residents be permitted to bring some of their own furniture and that they be given as much privacy as possible. Both the local authorities and the hospitals are putting greater emphasis on rehabilitation. Through detailed studies on care for the aged, the British people have grown increasingly alert to the problem. The aged are not forgotten citizens in England and Wales.

All segments of the population can be grateful for the pharmaceutical, the dental, and the ophthalmic services. Subject to a nominal charge, the most expensive drug may be obtained from the pharmacist, and doctors are permitted to prescribe freely whatever most effectively will help the patient. This fact, more than any other, has strengthened the doctor-patient relationship and has given the family physician a weapon of incalculable value in curative and preventive medicine. The rising cost of drugs poses a problem which, however, is less serious in England than in other countries. What the government pays to druggists for medicines dispensed is less than the price would be were they sold privately over the counter. In many ways the pharmaceutical service is one of the most economical of all branches when measured in terms of the amelioration of suffering, speedier recovery, and a lower mortality rate.

The Ministry of Health has kept wholesale drug prices under careful review, seeking to maintain them at the lowest possible level consistent with sound business policy. Allowance is made for the high cost of pharmaceutical research, which has greatly expanded. There is no evidence that the industry has suffered any ill effects from the National Health Service. On the contrary, there seem to be some very definite advantages for the drug manufacturers. The policy of periodically testing the drugs that are dispensed insures the highest quality. There has been an appreciable expansion in production owing to a much larger domestic market and a phenomenal increase in exports. All of this was accomplished with an advance in drug prices considerably less than the advance in the prices of most other manufactured goods. The viability of the industry is best demonstrated by the many new and improved drugs being put on the market.

The benefits that flow out of the ophthalmic service affect the opticians as well as those who need spectacles. Over 50 million sight tests were given during the first ten years, and most of them involved the dispensing of glasses. Few people in need of spectacles have not obtained them from the Health Service. The most satisfying feature is that no longer do impecunious persons, particularly among the aged, have to wear glasses of dubious value obtained from chain-store counters or street vendors. A tremendous step has been taken to protect the eyes of the British people. The Health Service also strengthened the professional standing of the opticians, whose ties with the medical doctors have become closer.

The dental profession likewise gained from the Health Service, although it has been plagued with problems that could not easily be solved. In 1956 the profession was raised to the status of a self-governing body and provision was made for the use of oral hygienists in general dental practice and for the possible use of ancillary helpers in the priority services. All of this was part of the program to deal with a serious shortage of qualified dentists—a condition inherited from an earlier period. Acting upon the recommendation of a commission, the government somewhat tardily decided to expand the student training facilities and thus increase the number of dentists.

The introduction of charges was primarily motivated by a desire to strengthen the priority services, which treated the teeth of children and nursing and expectant mothers. For such persons there is no charge for conservative treatment, not even in the general dental service. In spite of the limited dental facilities, the amount of conservative work has enjoyed a gratifying increase. But the general condition of British teeth remains far from satisfactory. It is in this area that the Health Service has experienced its smallest success, but in no other phase were the odds so great or was the influence of the past so hard to combat.

One important aspect constitutes a tremendous boon to the elderly—the availability of dentures. In the pre-1948 era there were those who, unable to afford artificial teeth, went without or had to use ill-fitting dentures inherited from others. The Health Service made good dentures available to all, at first free and then later subject to a moderate charge. The emphasis on conservative work, however, has been reflected in a decline in the number of patients requiring dentures.

In reviewing the full sweep of the National Health Service, one can only marvel at the way the Beveridge Report of 1942 has become an impressive reality. The test of the first twelve years has not shaken the program, but has instead left it strengthened, causing it to send down deeper roots. Many weaknesses have been eliminated or reduced, and others are being acted upon by a government that has improved its fiscal position. No longer does England have doubts as to whether the economy can afford such a comprehensive scheme. Prudent spending and careful management have produced a service of incalculable value. The program is paying tremendous dividends in a healthier nation. As one observer put it: "The Health Service was not a money-consuming service; it was a wealth-producing service."[14]

The health program is available to everybody without qualifications, and all but a very tiny part of the population share in the benefits. Like education, medical care is viewed as one of the necessities of life that should be the responsibility of the government. The program is financed by taxes except for the 5 per cent from charges, the 5 per cent from superannuation contributions paid by Health Service personnel, and the 14 per cent from weekly Health Service insurance contributions paid by the active members of the population. This was the picture in 1960.

The cost has been surprisingly low considering what the people receive. Including all sources of revenue (charges, insurance payments, local rates, and Exchequer funds), the total gross cost per capita in that year was in the neighborhood of £16 ($45) a year, or 11d (12½ cents) a day. This outlay bought such benefits as full dental, hospital, and medical practitioner care, as well as all necessary drugs, appliances, and spectacles. The amazing thing is that the cost of medical care in England under the Health Service at no time has been more than 4 per cent of the national income. Many other nations spend a larger proportion. Among them is the United States, which in 1959 expended a total of 4.5 per cent of her national income on medical care.[15]

There are many reasons why the British take pride in the Health Service, but perhaps the one that stands out most graphically is the steadily improving health of the nation. While other factors have contributed to this situation, the health program, it is felt, deserves a good share of the credit. The picture in 1959 had never been better. In that year the infant mortality rate had fallen to 22.2 per 1,000 live births, and the maternal mortality rate to 0.32 per 1,000 births—lower than at any previous time. Only in the Netherlands was infant mortality less, but no nation had a smaller rate of mortality for children between one and fourteen years of age than England and Wales. In that year, for the first time, no one died from diphtheria, and deaths from such diseases as acute poliomyelitis, scarlet fever, tuberculosis, whooping cough, syphilis, and acute rheumatism were the lowest ever recorded.[16]

On the tenth anniversary of the Health Program, the *Daily Herald* made this observation: "Here in Britain, before the National Health Service, how many working mothers put up with a pain or a 'lump' for years for fear of costing her husband too dear—and died because urgent aid came too late? We who come from humble homes know they did. You see a lot of people today with glasses and false teeth and hearing aids and artificial limbs. . . . These . . . are people many of whom would have gone about before the National Health Service hard of hearing, short of sight, sore of gum and lame of leg."[17] On the same day, *The Times* (London), in a somewhat more erudite tone, acknowledged that while the program had been criticized in detail "the concept as such has not been seriously challenged. Mistakes have been made, but an impartial review of the past ten years indicates that the nation has good reason to be proud of the Health Service."[18]

At the end of the ten-year period *The Practitioner* had its reservations about the program but philosophically affirmed what everybody knew, that the Health Service had "come to stay," that to oppose it was "futile" and to guide it along the proper course was "statesmanship."[19] Such sentiment has been voiced vigorously on numerous occasions from many different quarters, but none put it more pointedly than a prominent Conservative politician in London. Writing for an American publication, he implied that the Health Service had become sacrosanct. "You can cut defense spending. You can raise taxes. You can even get along with a dose of unemployment. But meddle with National Health? That's political suicide over here."[20]

That the Health Service had won its way into the hearts of the British people was demonstrated in every poll taken. The Ross Survey of 1952 found only 5 per cent opposed to it. Over 80 per cent of the people declared it was a good service with at the most one or two reservations.[21] The Social Surveys in 1956 reported that 90 per cent of the people gave the National Health Service a favorable rating. Seven per cent were undecided and only 3 per cent voted negatively.

The Gemmill Survey of 1956 noted that, while the people were conscious of imperfections in the Health Service, their attitude was one of "restrained optimism," since they knew the Service was worthwhile and they were determined to improve it. A Conservative member of Parliament said to Professor Gemmill: "We do not have a first-class, but only a second-class medical service. However, before 1948 it was only fourth-class. It has been improving ever since, and by and by we shall have a Health Service that is truly first-class."[22]

While the National Health Service is something magnificent in scope and almost breath-taking in its implications, certainly ten or twelve years hardly permits a definitive judgment. As a growing, evolutionary program it will be reappraised from time to time. With its origins deeply imbedded in the past, the Service is giving good performance in spite of blemishes. In the light of past accomplishments and future goals, the Health Service cannot very well be excluded from any list of notable achievements of the twentieth century. So much has it become a part of the British way of life, it is difficult for the average Englishman to imagine what it would be like without those services that have contributed so much to his physical and mental well-being.

The need for the state to maintain health and insure full medical care for all citizens now enjoys the same measure of popular support as education, police and fire protection, and the other essential functions of government. If the man in the street ever thinks about the philosophical aspects, he may even tend to view the Health Service as something that was historically unavoidable—the irresistible unfolding of social forces. Quite possibly it was with that idea in mind that the Newsam Report could say in 1959, "Fifty years hence what is happening to-day and what may happen tomorrow in the National Health Service will seem to have been inevitable."[23]

NOTES

Notes

CHAPTER I

1. Hermann Levy, *National Health Insurance* (London: Cambridge University Press, 1944), pp. 77-78, 86-88.

2. J. R. L. Anderson, "The Quest for Security: Trade Union Policy," *Manchester Guardian*, September 3, 1956.

3. James Mackintosh, *The Nation's Health* (London: The Pilot Press, Ltd., 1944), p. 24.

4. Alfred Cox, "General Practice Fifty Years Ago: Some Reminiscences," *Fifty Years of Medicine: A Symposium* (London: British Medical Association, 1950), pp. 290-91.

5. *A National Health Service* ["White Paper"] (London: His Majesty's Stationery Office, 1944), p. 64; *Manchester Guardian*, February 20, 1957; Levy, pp. 39, 43, 123.

6. Levy, pp. 122, 129, 131.

7. A. Bradford Hill, "The Doctor's Day and Pay: Some Sampling Inquiries Into the Pre-War Status," *Journal of the Royal Statistical Society*, CXIV (1951), 25-26.

8. *Report of the Inter-Departmental Committee on Remuneration of General Practitioners* ["Spens Report on Remuneration of General Practitioners"] (London: His Majesty's Stationery Office, 1946), pp. 4-5.

9. Samuel Leff, *The Health of the People* (London: Victor Gollangz, 1950), pp. 210-11.

10. Levy, pp. 104 ff.

11. Hill, p. 18.

12. Levy, pp. 128-31.

13. "Health Centres: Interim Report by the Council of the B.M.A., July, 1948," *British Medical Journal, Supplement*, September 11, 1948, pp. 112-13.

14. *Report of the Committee of Enquiry Into the Cost of the National Health Service* ["Guillebaud Report"] (London: Her Majesty's Stationery Office, 1956), p. 157; Levy, pp. 47, 207, 332-34.

15. *Brit. Med. J., Suppl.*, December 21, 1912, pp. 682, 684; December 28, 1912, p. 453.

16. *Brit. Med. J., Suppl.*, January 25, 1913, p. 184.

17. Levy, pp. 1-4.

18. *Ibid.*, pp. 215-17, 301; Sir William Beveridge, *Social Insurance and Allied Services* [American edition] (New York: The Macmillan Co., 1942), pp. 23-24.

19. Levy, pp. 13-14, 212-14, 290-300.

20. "Guillebaud Report," pp. 151-52.

21. *Ibid.*, p. 160; Levy, pp. 186 ff.

22. Levy, pp. 26-28, 95-97, 161; G. H. Giles, *The Ophthalmic Services Under the National Health Service Acts, 1946-1952* (London: Hammond, Hammond and Co., Ltd., 1952), pp. 21-24; "Guillebaud Report," p. 184.

23. "White Paper," pp. 64-65; John W. Gilbert, "The Public Dental Service of England and Wales," *International Dental Journal*, II (1951-52), 499; Levy, pp. 153-56.

24. "The Wage-Earner's Teeth," *The Spectator,* Vol. 168 (1942), 416.

25. *Report of the Chief Medical Officer of the Ministry of Health, 1939-45* (London: His Majesty's Stationery Office, 1946), pp. 200-1.

26. *Report of the Ministry of Health For the Year Ended 31st March, 1946* (London: His Majesty's Stationery Office, 1946), p. 90.

27. *Report of the Inter-Departmental Committee on the Remuneration of General Dental Practitioners* ["Spens Report on the Remuneration of General Dental Practitioners"] (London: His Majesty's Stationery Office, 1948), pp. 5-6.

28. "White Paper," pp. 54-55; "Guillebaud Report," pp. 63-64; Sir Herbert Eason *et al., Hospital Survey: The Hospital Services of the Yorkshire Area* (London: His Majesty's Stationery Office, 1945), p. 30.

29. *Brit. Med. J.,* June 11, 1921, p. 870; *Voluntary Service and the State: A Study of the Needs of the Hospital Service* (London: George Barber and Son, Ltd., 1952), pp. 22-23.

30. Levy, pp. 162-64; "Guillebaud Report," p. 64.

31. A. M. H. Gray and A. Topping, *The Hospital Services of London and Surrounding Area* (London: His Majesty's Stationery Office, 1945), p. 5.

32. Sir Hugh Lett and A. E. Quine, *The Hospital Services of the North-Eastern Area* (London: His Majesty's Stationery Office, 1946), p. 13.

33. Gray and Topping, pp. 11-12; V. Zachary Cope *et al., The Hospital Services of the South-Western Area* (London: His Majesty's Stationery Office, 1945), p. 119.

34. Sir Heneage Ogilvie, "The Practitioner and the Hospital Service," *Brit. Med. J.,* September 26, 1953, p. 707.

35. "White Paper," pp. 55-56; A. Trevor Jones *et al., The Hospital Services of South Wales and Monmouthshire* (London: His Majesty's Stationery Office, 1945), p. 3.

36. *Report of the Ministry of Health, 1946,* pp. 64-65; L. G. Parsons *et al., The Hospital Services of the Sheffield and East Midlands Area* (London: His Majesty's Stationery Office, 1945), p. 8; Gray and Topping, p. 12; Cope *et al.,* pp. 119, 124.

37. Parsons *et al.,* p. 11; Jones *et al.,* pp. 8, 10; Lett and Quine, pp. 12, 29.

38. *Report of the Working Party on the Recruitment and Training of Nurses* (London: His Majesty's Stationery Office, 1947), pp. 5-6, 37, 74.

39. Gray and Topping, p. 11.

40. Jones *et al.,* p. 12.

41. Parsons *et al.,* pp. 13-15.

42. "White Paper," p. 57; "Guillebaud Report," p. 65.

43. Sir Ernest R. Carling, "The Chronic Sick: Proper Care for the Aged and Infirm," *The Times* (London), November 25, 1946.

44. *Brit. Med. J., Suppl.,* September 11, 1948, pp. 109-10; "White Paper," p. 62; D. L. Hobman, *The Welfare State* (London: John Murray, 1953), pp. 18-19.

45. "Guillebaud Report," p. 196; Levy, pp. 100-1; "White Paper," pp. 62-63.

46. "White Paper," pp. 59-61, 64-65.

47. General Register Office, *Matters of Life and Death* (London: Her Majesty's Stationery Office, 1956), pp. 9, 23; *The Registrar General's Statistical Review of England and Wales For the Year 1955*, Part I (London: Her Majesty's Stationery Office, 1956), pp. 4-5, 10; *Report of the Ministry of Health, 1955*, Part II, p. 22.

48. S. Mervyn Herbert, *Britain's Health* (Harmondsworth, Middlesex: Penguin Books, Ltd., 1939), pp. 22-23.

49. *The Lancet,* November 21, 1942, p. 623.

CHAPTER II

1. James Sterling Ross, *The National Health Service in Great Britain* (London: Oxford University Press, 1952), pp. 4-5.

2. Peter Self, "The Health Services in Relation to Central and Local Government,"

in Henry Lesser (ed.), *The Health Services: Some of Their Practical Problems* (London: George Allen and Unwin, Ltd., 1951), p. 19.

3. Ffrangcon Roberts, "Where are We Going? Medicine in a Planned Economy," *Brit. Med. J.*, March 13, 1948, pp. 485-86; and *The Cost of Health* (London: Turnstile Press, 1952), pp. 57-58, 63-65.

4. *Proceedings of the Annual Meeting of the British Medical Association, 1948* (London: Butterworth and Co., 1948), pp. 5-6.

5. *Interim Report on the Future Provision of Medical and Allied Services* ["Dawson Report"] (London: His Majesty's Stationery Office, 1920), pp. 5 ff.

6. *The Lancet,* January 24, 1948, p. 150; Levy, p. 28; Ross, pp. 53-56.

7. Ross, pp. 58-59.

8. *A General Medical Service for the Nation* (London: British Medical Association, 1938), pp. 17-18, 50; "Medical Planning Commission Draft Interim Report," *Brit. Med. J.*, June 20, 1942, pp. 744-45, 747-50.

9. *Brit. Med. J.*, June 20, 1942, p. 750; *General Medical Service for the Nation,* pp. 17-22, 31-32, 48.

10. *General Medical Service for the Nation,* pp. 31 ff.; "Medical Planning Commission Draft Interim Report," *Brit. Med. J.*, pp. 744-50.

11. "Medical Planning Research Interim General Report," *The Lancet,* November 21, 1942, pp. 614, 616-17.

12. Beveridge, pp. 2-3, 7-10, 104, 158-63.

13. *Brit. Med. J.*, December 12, 1942, p. 700.

14. Ross, pp. 83-84.

15. "White Paper," pp. 76-77.

16. *Ibid.*, pp. 5-9.

17. *Ibid.*, pp. 11-13, 20-25.

18. *Ibid.*, pp. 11, 26-29, 35-36, 80.

19. *Hansard,* House of Commons, Vol. 398 (1944), cols. 427-32, 633.

20. *Brit. Med. J., Suppl.,* August 5, 1944, pp. 25, 28.

21. *Ibid.*, pp. 26-29; December 16, 1944, p. 153.

22. *Brit. Med. J.,* February 26, 1944, p. 295.

23. *Brit. Med. J., Suppl.,* August 5, 1944, pp. 25-29.

24. *The New Statesman and Nation,* Vol. 31 (1946), 223.

25. *Hansard,* H. of C., Vol. 422 (1946), col. 60.

26. *Ibid.*, cols. 51-56.

27. Aneurin Bevan, *In Place of Fear* (New York: Simon and Schuster, 1952), pp. 78 ff.

28. *Hansard,* H. of C., Vol. 422 (1946), cols. 43 ff.

29. *Ibid.*, Vol. 426 (1946), cols. 392-97.

30. *Brit. Med. J., Suppl.,* February 1, 1947, p. 18; *Brit. Med. J.,* December 21, 1946, pp. 956-57.

31. *Brit. Med. J.,* December 21, 1946, p. 957.

CHAPTER III

1. Ross, pp. 123-24.

2. *Hansard,* H. of C., Vol. 447 (1948), col. 39.

3. *Brit. Med. J.,* January 17, 1948, p. 112.

4. *Ibid.*, January 3, 1948, p. 17.

5. *Ibid.*, May 15, 1948, p. 937; *The Lancet,* January 24, 1948, p. 143.

6. *Hansard,* H. of C., Vol. 447 (1948), col. 59.

7. *The Lancet,* January 24, 1948, p. 149; *Brit. Med. J.,* January 3, 1948, p. 18.

8. *Brit. Med. J.,* January 10, 1948, p. 58.

9. *The Lancet,* January 24, 1948, p. 144.

10. *Brit. Med. J.,* January 10, 1948, pp. 53, 59.

11. *The Lancet,* January 24, 1948, p. 144.

12. *Hansard,* H. of C., Vol. 447 (1948), cols. 39-41.

13. *National Health Service Act, 1946* [9 & 10 Geo. 6, Ch. 81] (London: His Majesty's Stationery Office, 1946), Part IV, secs. 35-36.

14. *Brit. Med. J.*, January 10, 1948, p. 58.

15. *Ibid.*, p. 62.

16. *National Health Service Act, 1946*, Part IV, secs. 31, 42-43.

17. *The Lancet*, January 24, 1948, p. 149.

18. *Ibid.*, p. 150; *Hansard*, H. of C., Vol. 447 (1948), col. 43.

19. *Brit. Med. J.*, January 10, 1948, p. 64; January 17, 1948, p. 112; April 17, 1948, p. 743.

20. *Ibid.*, January 10, 1948, p. 54; January 17, 1948, p. 109.

21. *Hansard*, H. of C., Vol. 447 (1948), col. 34.

22. *Brit. Med. J.*, January 10, 1948, p. 60.

23. *Ibid.*, January 17, 1948, p. 112.

24. *The Lancet*, January 24, 1948, pp. 144-45.

25. *Hansard*, H. of C., Vol. 447 (1948), cols. 35-39.

26. *Brit. Med. J.*, February 21, 1948, pp. 252-53.

27. *Ibid.*, p. 347; March 13, 1948, p. 503.

28. February 19, 1948.

29. February 22, 1948.

30. February 19, 1948.

31. *Brit. Med. J.*, March 6, 1948, p. 464.

32. *Ibid.*, March 27, 1948, p. 604; *Brit. Med. J., Suppl.*, March 27, 1948, pp. 49-54.

33. *Brit. Med. J.*, March 27, 1948, p. 605.

34. *Hansard*, H. of C., Vol. 447 (1948), col. 1309.

35. *Brit. Med. J.*, April 17, 1948, pp. 742-43.

36. *Ibid.*, May 8, 1948, p. 893.

37. *Ibid.*, May 15, 1948, p. 119.

38. *Brit. Med. J., Suppl.*, June 5, 1948, p. 155.

39. "Proceedings of the Special Representative Meeting of the B.M.A.," *Brit. Med. J., Suppl.*, June 5, 1948, pp. 147-54.

40. *Brit. Med. J.*, June 5, 1948, p. 1087.

41. June 18, 1948.

42. *Brit. Med. J.*, July 3, 1948, p. 30.

43. *The Lancet*, July 3, 1948, p. 17.

44. *British Journal of Ophthalmology*, XXXII (1948), 373.

45. Harry H. Eckstein, "The Politics of the British Medical Association," *The Political Quarterly*, XXVI (1955), 357-58; "Annual Report of the Council of the British Medical Association," *Brit. Med. J., Suppl.*, April 13, 1957, p. 187.

46. "Annual Report of the Council," *Brit. Med. J., Suppl.*, April 13, 1957, p. 185; April 19, 1958, pp. 179, 184; March 19, 1960, pp. 141, 146.

47. *The Times* (London), May 21, 1948; July 15, 1949.

48. *Ibid.*, November 15, 1948; *Fellowship For Freedom in Medicine*, October, 1955, pp. 12-13.

49. *Fellowship For Freedom in Medicine*, January, 1957, p. 34.

50. *Ibid.*, December, 1951, p. 5; February, 1958, p. 21; February, 1959, p. 16; January, 1960, p. 22.

51. Information in a letter to the author from the General Secretary of the Socialist Medical Association, April 26, 1957; *Brit. Med. J., Suppl.*, December 14, 1957, p. 193.

52. *Twenty-fifth Anniversary Commemoration Brochure* (London: Socialist Medical Association, 1957), p. 4; "Draft Definitive Policy Statement, No. 2 (Revised), December, 1955" [Socialist Medical Association], p. 2.

53. *Medical World*, March 18, 1949, p. 115; *Medical World Newsletter*, October 31, 1952, pp. 1 ff., October, 1955, pp. 1, 3, and January, 1956, p. 1; Information in a letter to the author from the General Secretary of the Practitioners' Union, March 11, 1955; *Brit. Med. J., Suppl.*, January 25, 1958, p. 31.

54. Allendale Sanderson, "Five Years of the National Health Service," *Twentieth*

Century, CLIV (1953), 123; Information in a letter to the author from the Honorary Secretary of the Joint Committee of Ophthalmic Opticians, August 10, 1956.

55. *The Pharmaceutical Journal,* Vol. 103 (1946), 289.
56. *Ibid.,* Vol. 107 (1948), 431.
57. Ross, p. 257; Sanderson, p. 123.
58. *British Dental Journal,* Vol. 81 (1946), 323.
59. *Ibid.,* Vol. 84 (1948), 273-74, and Vol. 85 (1948), 13; Ross, p. 257.
60. *British Dental Journal,* Vol. 85 (1948), 211.
61. *News Chronicle,* July 5, 1948.
62. *The Lancet,* July 3, 1948, p. 24.
63. *Ibid.*

CHAPTER IV

1. *The Times* (London), Oct. 8, 1948; *Health Services in Britain* (London: Her Majesty's Stationery Office, 1957), pp. 7-8.
2. Ritchie Calder, "Doctors' Parliament," *The New Statesman and Nation,* Vol. 37 (1949), 665.
3. *Brit. Med. J.,* May 8, 1948, p. 885.
4. *The Times* (London), July 21, August 7, 1948; *The Spectator,* Vol. 181 (1948), 99.
5. *Brit. Med. J.,* September 3, 1949, pp. 521-23; October 1, 1949, pp. 746-48.
6. *The Times* (London), October 7, 1949.
7. *The National Health Service Act in Great Britain: A Review of the First Year's Working* (London: The Practitioner, 1949), pp. 1-10.
8. Calder, pp. 665-66.
9. *The National Health Service Act in Great Britain: A Review of the First Year's Working,* pp. 95-96.
10. *The Spectator,* Vol. 184 (1950), 333.
11. Joseph S. Collings, "General Practice in England Today," *The Lancet,* March 25, 1950, pp. 555 ff.
12. Sanderson, p. 124.
13. *The Times* (London), January 25, February 10, 11, 1950.
14. *National Health Service (Amendment) Act, 1949* [12, 13, & 14 Geo. 6, Ch. 93] (London: His Majesty's Stationery Office, 1949), Parts I & II, secs. 1-29.
15. *Hansard,* H. of C., Vol. 487 (1950-51), cols. 232-39, 1601-1715.
16. *National Health Service Act, 1952* [15 & 16 Geo. 6 & 1 Eliz. 2, Ch. 25] (London: Her Majesty's Stationery Office, 1952), pp. 1-4.
17. *Hansard,* H. of C., Vol. 499 (1951-52), col. 1782.
18. *National Health Service Act, 1946,* Part I.
19. *Report on Co-operation Between Hospital, Local Authority and General Practitioner Services* (London: Her Majesty's Stationery Office, 1952), p. 29; "Centralization in the Hospital Services: The Need for a Change of Policy," *The Lancet,* November 14, 1953, p. 1035.
20. *National Health Service Act, 1946,* First Schedule; Self, p. 24.
21. Dr. A. Talbot Rogers, "Some Administrative Problems of the General Practitioners," in Lesser, pp. 27-30; *Some Administrative Problems of the Health Services* (London: The Institute of Public Administration, 1951), pp. 13-14.
22. "Guillebaud Report," p. 152; *Report of the London Executive Council, 1955-56* (London: London Executive Council, 1956), pp. 5-8.
23. *Report of the London Executive Council, 1959-60,* pp. 7, 23, 34, 37, 40, 49.
24. *The National Health Service Act in Great Britain: A Review of the First Year's Working,* p. 75; "Guillebaud Report," pp. 152-53.
25. "Guillebaud Report," pp. 154-56.
26. *Ibid.,* p. 65.
27. *Ibid.,* pp. 66-67; Vincent Collings, "The Functions of a Regional Hospital Board," in Lesser, pp. 43-46; *Voluntary Service and the State: A Study of the Needs of the Hospital Service,* pp. 34-42.

28. *Voluntary Service and the State: A Study of the Needs of the Hospital Service*, pp. 62-63; "Guillebaud Report," p. 68.

29. *The National Health Service Act in Great Britain: A Review of the First Year's Working*, pp. 72-75.

30. *Ibid.*, p. 77.

31. Giles, pp. 220-34; "Guillebaud Report," pp. 227-33; *Hospitals and the State: Hospital Organization and Administration Under the National Health Service*, "Background and Blueprint" (London: The Acton Society Trust, 1955), pp. 30-31.

32. *Manchester Guardian*, November 7, 12, 21, 25, 1957, and January 3, April 15, August 16, 1958; *Brit. Med. J., Suppl.*, August 23, 1958, pp. 126-27.

33. "Annual Report of the Council," *Brit. Med J., Suppl.*, April 7, 1956, p. 174.

34. *Ibid.*, June 23, 1956, p. 395.

35. Self, pp. 24-25; "Guillebaud Report," p. 95; *Voluntary Service and the State: A Study of the Needs of the Hospital Service*, pp. 38, 42; *Brit. Med. J.*, December 12, 1959, p. 1344; *The National Health Service Act in Great Britain: A Review of the First Year's Working*, p. 69.

36. T. F. Fox, "Professional Freedom," *The Lancet*, July 28, 1951, p. 171.

37. *National Health Service Act, 1946*, Third Schedule; *Voluntary Service and the State: A Study of the Needs of the Hospital Service*, p. 65.

38. *Voluntary Service and the State: A Study of the Needs of the Hospital Service*, pp. 36-37.

39. "Guillebaud Report," pp. 95-97.

40. "Annual Report of the Council," *Brit. Med. J., Suppl.*, April 13, 1957, p. 172.

41. *Voluntary Service and the State: A Study of the Needs of the Hospital Service*, pp. 48-50.

42. "Guillebaud Report," pp. 88-89.

43. Dr. Donald Mcl. Johnson, "Can Medicine Be Divorced From Politics?," *Fellowship For Freedom in Medicine*, January, 1957, p. 30.

44. *Manchester Guardian*, April 2, 1957.

45. *Fellowship For Freedom in Medicine*, January, 1957, p. 2.

46. *Brit. Med. J., Suppl.*, April 7, 1956, p. 134.

47. "Proceedings of the Special Representative Meeting," *Brit. Med. J., Suppl.*, May 11, 1957, pp. 249-56.

48. *Brit. Med. J.*, April 6, 1957, p. 811; April 13, 1957, p. 873.

49. *Brit. Med. J., Suppl.*, May 11, 1957, pp. 256, 260.

50. "Annual Report of the Council," *Brit. Med. J., Suppl.*, April 7, 1956, pp. 120-21.

51. *Ibid.*, pp. 125-26; "Proceedings of the Annual Representative Meeting," *Brit. Med. J., Suppl.*, July 14, 1956, p. 35.

52. *Manchester Guardian*, April 4, 1955.

53. "Guillebaud Report," 61-62; *Hospitals and the State . . . Background and Blueprint*, pp. 29-30.

54. Johnson, p. 29.

55. "Annual Report of the Council," *Brit. Med. J., Suppl.*, April 7, 1956, p. 134; "Proceedings of the Annual Representative Meeting," *Brit. Med. J., Suppl.*, July 14, 1956, pp. 10-11.

56. "Guillebaud Report," p. 61.

57. *Report of the Committee on General Practice Within the National Health Service* ["Cohen Report"] (London: Her Majesty's Stationery Office, 1954), p. 8.

58. "Guillebaud Report," pp. 242-43.

59. *Report on Co-operation Between Hospital, Local Authority and General Practitioner Services*, p. 30.

CHAPTER V

1. Roberts, p. 14.

2. *Hansard*, H. of C., Vol. 461 (1949), col. 536.

3. Quoted in *Medical World Newsletter*, August, 1957, p. 5.

4. Roberts, pp. 14-18, 131, 133-42.

5. *The Times* (London), October 7, November 16, 1949.

6. Ross, p. 314; Roberts, pp. 11-13; Brian Abel-Smith and Richard M. Titmuss, *The Cost of the National Health Service in England and Wales* (London: Cambridge University Press, 1956), p. 2.

7. Abel-Smith and Titmuss, pp. 24, 45; *Report of the Ministry of Health, 1952,* Part I, p. 3.

8. *Ibid.*

9. "Memorandum Submitted by the Joint Emergency Committee of the Optical Profession to the Committee of Enquiry Into the Cost of the National Health Service, November, 1953," pp. 5-7.

10. "Guillebaud Report," p. 176; *The Times* (London), May 20, 1949, and April 28, 1950.

11. *The Times* (London), October 8, 1948; *Report of the Ministry of Health, 1953,* Part I, p. 98.

12. *The Times* (London), October 8, 1948.

13. *Ibid.,* November 16, 1949.

14. *Hansard,* H. of C., Vol. 472 (1950), cols. 937-38.

15. *Civil Estimates for the Year Ending 31st March, 1956, Class V* (London: Her Majesty's Stationery Office, 1955), pp. 55 ff.; Abel-Smith and Titmuss, pp. 2-3.

16. *National Health Service Note* [Mimeographed] (London: Ministry of Health, March, 1954).

17. *Report of the Ministry of Health, 1953,* Part I, p. 154, and *1958,* p. 5; *Civil Estimates for the Year Ending 31st March, 1958, Class V,* pp. 58-59; Abel-Smith and Titmuss, p. 45.

18. *The Times* (London), Nov. 7, 1949; *The Pharmaceutical Journal,* Vol. 109 (1949), 419, and Vol. 177 (1956), 353-54.

19. *Manchester Guardian,* Oct. 26, 1956.

20. *Hansard,* H. of C., Vol. 499 (1951-52), col. 1782; *N.H.S. Note, No. 12,* January, 1955, p. 2.

21. *The New Statesman and Nation,* Vol. 40 (1952), 144.

22. "Guillebaud Report," p. 195.

23. *Brit. Med. J., Suppl.,* May 31, 1958, p. 287; *Manchester Guardian,* April 11, 1957.

24. *Manchester Guardian,* February 26, 1958; *Interim Report of the Committee on Cost of Prescribing* ["Hinchliffe Interim Report"] (London: Her Majesty's Stationery Office, 1958), p. 3.

25. *Report of the Ministry of Health, 1952,* Part I, pp. 3, 173, *1956,* pp. 79, 208, and *1957,* pp. 83 ff.; *Manchester Guardian,* November 30, 1956, and November 28, 1957.

26. *Manchester Guardian,* October 26, 1956; *Report of the Ministry of Health, 1956,* Part I, p. 82; *The Pharmaceutical Journal,* Vol. 177 (1956), 387.

27. *The Pharmaceutical Journal,* Vol. 177 (1956), 353-54, 383; *Manchester Guardian,* October 26, 1956.

28. *Manchester Guardian,* November 23, 1956; *Brit. Med. J., Suppl.,* November 17, 1956, pp. 189-90.

29. *Brit. Med. J.,* March 22, 1958, p. 719; *Civil Estimates for the Year Ending 31st March, 1961, Class V,* pp. 79, 88; *N. H. S. Note: Summary of Main Figures in England and Wales, 1949-59,* p. 1.

30. *Final Report of the Committee on Cost of Prescribing* ["Hinchliffe Report"] (London: Her Majesty's Stationery Office, 1959), pp. 35, 87-91.

31. Abel-Smith and Titmuss, pp. 43-45; "Guillebaud Report," pp. 185-86; *Report of the Ministry of Health, 1952,* Part I, p. 3, *1954,* pp. 1-4, *1956,* p. 75, *1959,* p. 97, and *1960,* p. 86.

32. "Memorandum Submitted by the Joint Emergency Committee of the Optical Profession, 1953," pp. 8-10.

33. "Guillebaud Report," p. 194.

34. Abel-Smith and Titmuss, pp. 44-45.

35. *Ibid.*, p. 43; *Report of the Ministry of Health, 1952*, Part I, pp. 3, 69, *1953*, pp. 1-3, *1954*, p. 1-4, *1956*, pp. 2-4, 75, and *1958*, pp. 80-82; *Civil Estimates for the Year Ending 31st March, 1961, Class V*, pp. 80, 89.

36. Abel-Smith and Titmuss, p. 41: *Report of the Ministry of Health, 1952*, Part I, pp. 170-71, *1956*, pp. 202-3, *1958*, pp. 107 ff., and *1960*, p. 229.

37. "Guillebaud Report," pp. 192-93.

38. *Report of the Ministry of Health, 1952*, Part I, pp. 1-3, *1954*, pp. 1-4, *1956*, pp. 1-4, 202-3, and *1960*, p. 229; *Civil Estimates for the Year Ending 31st March, 1961, Class V*, pp. 64, 79, 89.

39. "Guillebaud Report," pp. 190-91.

40. *The Times* (London), February 2, 1961.

41. Abel-Smith and Titmuss, pp. 35-36; *Report of the Ministry of Health, 1952*, Part I, p. 3, and *1958*, pp. 1-7; *Civil Estimates for the Year Ending 31st March, 1957, Class V*, pp. 57 ff., and *1961*, pp. 64 ff.

42. *Civil Estimates for the Year Ending 31st March, 1954, Class V*, pp. 51 ff., *1957*, pp. 57 ff., and *1958*, pp. 58 ff.; Abel-Smith and Titmuss, p. 35; *Report of the Ministry of Health, 1959*, Part I, pp. 1-5.

43. *Civil Estimates for the Year Ending 31st March, 1961, Class V*, p. 64; *Report of the Ministry of Health, 1952*, Part I, p. 3, *1956*, p. 4, *1959*, pp. 2-4, and *1960*, p. 7.

44. *Report of the Ministry of Health, 1952*, Part I, p. 3, *1956*, p. 4, *1958*, p. 18, *1959*, p. 21, and *1960*, p. 23; *Civil Estimates for the Year Ending 31st March, 1961, Class V*, p. 64; *Brit. Med. J.*, November 21, 1959, p. 1108.

45. *Manchester Guardian*, June 17, July 3, 15, December 7, 1957; "Draft Definitive Policy Statement, No. 2, 1955," pp. 13-14.

46. *Manchester Guardian*, November 14, 1956.

47. *Civil Estimates for the Year Ending 31st March, 1958, Class V*, pp. 88-89; *1960*, pp. 88, 100-1; *1961*, pp. 104-5.

48. *Sixth Report From the Select Committee on Estimates, Session 1956-57: Running Costs of Hospitals* (London: Her Majesty's Stationery Office, 1957), p. v.

49. *N. H. S. Note: Summary of Main Figures in England and Wales, 1949-60*, pp. 6, 20.

50. *Report of the Ministry of Health, 1952*, Part I, pp. 1-3, *1956*, pp. 2-4, *1958*, pp. 1-6, and *1960*, p. 7; *Civil Estimates for the Year Ending 31st March, 1961, Class V*, pp. 64 ff.; *Preliminary Estimates of National Income and Expenditure, 1951-56* (London: Her Majesty's Stationery Office, 1957), p. 7, and *1953-58*, p. 7.

51. *Manchester Guardian*, February 20, March 20, November 7, 1957; *Hansard*, H. of C., Vol. 567 (1956-57), cols. 230 ff.

52. *Hansard*, H. of C., Vol. 569 (1957), cols, 590 ff., and Vol. 571 (1957), cols. 1502 ff.; *Manchester Guardian*, May 3, 21, July 18, 1957; *Brit. Med. J.*, May 18, 1957, p. 1189.

53. *Hansard*, H. of C., Vol. 582 (1958), cols. 1043-44.

54. *Ibid.*, Vol. 582 (1958), cols. 1217-18.

55. *Ibid.*, cols. 1185 ff.; *Manchester Guardian*, February 26, 1958.

56. *The Times* (London), February 6, 1961.

57. *Hansard*, H. of C., Vol. 513 (1952-53), cols. 1230-31.

58. "Guillebaud Report," pp. 9-10.

59. *Ibid.*, pp. 239-40, 269.

60. Abel-Smith and Titmuss, pp. 69-70, 159-60, 164-65.

61. *A Critical Examination of the Guillebaud Report on the Cost of the National Health Service* (London: Fellowship For Freedom in Medicine, 1957), pp. 1 ff.

62. January 26, 1956.

63. February 4, 1956, p. 353.

64. February 4, 1956, p. 115.

65. Vol. 100 (1956), 86.

66. February 4, 1956, p. 279.

67. *Hansard*, H. of C., Vol. 552 (1955-56), cols. 845 ff.

68. *Ibid.*, Vol. 571 (1957), col. 1504; *Brit. Med. J.*, November 28, 1959, pp. 1189-

90, and *Suppl.*, April 12, 1958, pp. 149-50; *Medical World Newsletter*, April, 1961, p. 3 (Table reproduced from *Hansard*, February 8, 1961, cols. 65-66).
69. *Medical World Newsletter*, October, 1961, p. 2.

CHAPTER VI

1. *Address by R. H. Turton, Minister of Health, at the Ninth Annual Conference of the Executive Councils' Association (England) held in London on the 18th and 19th October, 1956* (West Cliff, Preston: Executive Councils' Association [England], n.d.), p. 6.
2. "Cohen Report," pp. 2-3.
3. "Spens Report on Remuneration of General Practitioners," pp. 8 ff.
4. *N. H. S. Note: How the Doctor is Paid*, March, 1953, pp. 1-4; Ross, pp. 225-28.
5. Ross, pp. 28-29; *Report of the Working Party of Representatives of the General Medical Services Committee of the B. M. A. and Health Department* (London: British Medical Association, 1952), p. 2.
6. *The Danckwerts Award and the Working Party's Findings on the Future Distribution of the Central Pool* (London: British Medical Association, 1952), pp. 1-3.
7. *Ibid.*, pp. 3-8; *Report of the Working Party of Representatives*, pp. 2-8.
8. *Brit. Med. J., Suppl.*, May 3, 1958, pp. 226-27; *Superannuation Scheme for Those Engaged in the National Health Service in England and Wales: An Explanation* (London: Her Majesty's Stationery Office, 1952), pp. 16-17; *Medical World Newsletter*, January, 1958, pp. 5-9.
9. "Annual Report of the Council," *Brit. Med. J., Suppl.*, April 19, 1958, p. 162; April 25, 1959, p. 192.
10. *Medical World Newsletter*, February, 1958, pp. 1, 3, 5.
11. *Ibid.*, November, 1957, pp. 7-11.
12. *Royal Commission on Doctors' and Dentists' Remuneration, Minutes of Evidence*, 5-6 (London: Her Majesty's Stationery Office, 1958-59), pp. 282-83.
13. "Proceedings of the Annual Representative Meeting," *Brit. Med. J., Suppl.*, July 20, 1957, pp. 41-42.
14. *N. H. S. Note, No. 2A: How the Doctor is Paid*, January, 1961, pp. 1-3; *Brit. Med. J., Suppl.*, August 27, 1960, p. 81.
15. *Brit. Med. J., Suppl.*, June 11, 1955, p. 280; April 13, 1957, p. 164; April 19, 1958, p. 178.
16. "A Postal Inquiry Among 12,879 General Practitioner Principals, July, 1951," *Brit. Med. J., Suppl.*, September 26, 1953, p. 127.
17. Social Surveys [Gallup Poll], Ltd., "National Health Service Enquiry, June, 1956," p. 2.
18. J. H. F. Brotherston and Ann Cartwright, "The Attitudes of General Practitioners Toward Alternative Systems of Remuneration," *Brit. Med. J., Suppl.*, October 17, 1959, pp. 119-24.
19. *Towards a Reformed Health Service* (London: Fellowship For Freedom in Medicine, 1957), pp. 3 ff.
20. *Brit. Med. J., Suppl.*, May 3, 1958, p. 221.
21. *Royal Commission on Doctors' and Dentists' Remuneration, Minutes of Evidence*, 5-6, p. 291.
22. *Manchester Guardian*, March 31, April 8, 1958.
23. *Ibid.*, June 29, 1954.
24. *The Economist*, Vol. 183 (1957), 676-79.
25. *Medical World Newsletter*, September, 1955, pp. 7, 9; *Manchester Guardian*, January 25, 1958.
26. *Royal Commission on Doctors' and Dentists' Remuneration, Minutes of Evidence*, 3-4, p. 165; 9, pp. 445-56.
27. "Proceedings of the Annual Representative Meeting," *Brit. Med. J., Suppl.*, July 26, 1958, pp. 91-92.
28. *Royal Commission on Doctors' and Dentists' Remuneration, Minutes of Evidence*, 23, pp. 1282-83.

29. "The Newsam Report on Family Doctors' Services in the National Health Service" ["Newsam Report"], *Brit. Med. J., Suppl.,* January 17, 1959, pp. 15-17.

30. Stephen Taylor, *Good General Practice* (London: Oxford University Press, 1954), p. 29.

31. "Cohen Report," p. 30.

32. "The Committee's Report" ["Walker Report"], *Brit. Med. J., Suppl.,* September 26, 1953, p. 134.

33. *Manchester Guardian,* March 12, 1957.

34. *Brit. Med. J., Suppl.,* February 11, 1956, pp. 41-42, July 14, 1956, pp. 27-28, and July 28, 1956, pp. 75-76; *The Economist,* Vol. 182 (1957), 11.

35. *Manchester Guardian,* July 17, October 19, 1956; *Brit. Med. J., Suppl.,* October 27, 1956, p. 167.

36. *Brit. Med. J., Suppl.,* July 21, 1956, p. 145.

37. *Manchester Guardian,* December 6, 28, 29, 1956.

38. *The Times* (London), August 9, 1956.

39. *Royal Commission on Doctors' and Dentists' Remuneration, Written Evidence,* I, pp. 43-44; *Manchester Guardian,* February 21, June 6, 1957.

40. *Manchester Guardian,* March 22, 1957; *Brit. Med. J., Suppl.,* March 23, 1957, pp. 125-26.

41. *Manchester Guardian,* March 30, April 1, 8, 15, 1957.

42. *Brit. Med. J., Suppl.,* April 13, 1957, p. 209.

43. *The Lancet,* Feb. 9, 1957, p. 323.

44. *Manchester Guardian,* April 2, 5, 11, 1957.

45. *The Lancet,* March 2, 1957, p. 462; March 30, 1957, pp. 673-74.

46. *Manchester Guardian,* April 8, 1957.

47. *Medical World Newsletter,* April, 1957, pp. 1, 3; May, 1957, pp. 1, 3.

48. *Manchester Guardian,* April 2, 1957.

49. *The New Statesman and Nation,* Vol. 53 (1953), 262, 561.

50. J. H. F. Brotherston, Ann Cartwright, and F. M. Martin, "Public Reaction to the Current Dispute Between the Medical Profession and the Government," *The Lancet,* May 11, 1957, p. 982.

51. *Manchester Guardian,* April 12, 20, May 2, 1957.

52. "Proceedings of the Special Representative Meeting," *Brit. Med. J., Suppl.,* May 11, 1957, pp. 255-56.

53. *Manchester Guardian,* June 13, 1957; *Brit. Med. J., Suppl.,* May 11, 1957, pp. 255-56.

54. *The Lancet,* March 30, 1957, p. 674.

55. *Brit. Med. J., Suppl.,* May 25, 1957, p. 292.

56. *Medical World Newsletter,* December, 1957, p. 16.

57. *Brit. Med. J., Suppl.,* September 27, 1958, p. 149.

58. "Newsam Report." *Brit. Med. J., Suppl.,* January 17, 1959, p. 19.

59. "Supplementary Annual Report of the Council," *Brit. Med. J., Suppl.,* May 30, 1959, pp. 234 ff.

60. "Annual Report of the Council, *Brit. Med. J., Suppl.,* April 11, 1959, p. 134.

61. *Royal Commission on Doctors' and Dentists' Remuneration, Minutes of Evidence,* 23, pp. 1224-27.

62. *The Lancet,* January 5, 1957, pp. 31-32.

63. "Proceedings of the Special Representative Meeting," *Brit. Med. J., Suppl.,* October 8, 1960, pp. 131 ff.

64. *Report of the Royal Commission on Doctors' and Dentists' Remuneration, 1957-1960* ["Pilkington Report"] (London: Her Majesty's Stationery Office, 1960), pp. 114-18.

65. "Report of the Joint Working Party on Remuneration of General Practitioners," *Brit. Med. J., Suppl.,* August 27, 1960, pp. 79-82; *N.H.S. Note, No. 2A: How the Family Doctor is Paid,* October, 1960, pp. 1-3.

66. "Pilkington Report," pp. 120-22, 144-50.

67. "Report of the Council," *Brit. Med. J., Suppl.,* August 27, 1960, pp. 71-72, 79; "Package Deal Completed," *Brit. Med. J.,* October 8, 1960, pp. 1075-76.

CHAPTER VII

1. W. E. Dornal, "The Work of the Medical Practices Committee," in Lesser, pp. 36-38; "Guillebaud Report," p. 158.

2. *Report of the Working Party of . . . the General Medical Services Committee of the B. M. A. and Health Department* (London: Her Majesty's Stationery Office, 1952), pp. 2-4; *N. H. S. Note, No. 2A: How the Doctor is Paid,* January, 1961, pp. 1-2.

3. *Report of the London Executive Council, 1955-56,* p. 13; *1957-58,* p. 4; *1958-59,* p. 15.

4. *The Times* (London), September 9, 1949.

5. *Brit. Med. J., Suppl.,* June 11, 1955, p. 280.

6. *Report of the London Executive Council, 1957-58,* p. 16.

7. *Report of the Ministry of Health, 1953,* Part I, pp. 58-59, 240, *1958,* pp. 93, 315-16, 318, and *1960,* pp. 217-18; *Address by Iain Macleod, Minister of Health, at the Seventh Annual Conference of the Executive Councils' Association (England) held at Southport on the 14th and 15th October, 1954,* p. 3; *Brit. Med. J., Suppl.,* August 27, 1960, p. 81.

8. Dornal, p. 37; *Some Administrative Problems of the Health Services* (London: The Institute of Public Administration, 1951), pp. 7-8; "Cohen Report," p. 28; *Report of the Ministry of Health, 1953,* Part I, pp. 61-62, *1958,* p. 100, and *1959,* p. 77.

9. *Report of the Ministry of Health, 1954,* Part I, p. 66, *1955,* p. 61, *1956,* p. 61, *1957,* p. 63, and *1958,* p. 100; *The National Health Service (General Medical and Pharmaceutical Services) Regulations, 1954* (London: Her Majesty's Stationery Office, 1954), pp. 6-7; *Brit. Med. J., Suppl.,* June 7, 1958, p. 309.

10. *Manchester Guardian,* April 10, 1957; *N. H. S. Note,* December 31, 1952.

11. *Record of the Proceedings at the Tenth Annual Meeting of the Executive Councils' Association* (England) (West Cliff, Preston: Executive Councils' Association [England], 1957), pp. 92-95.

12. "Annual Report of the Council," *Brit. Med. J., Suppl.,* April 13, 1957, p. 164.

13. "Cohen Report," p. 28

14. *N. H. S. Note on N. H. S. Act, 1946; Memorandum of Evidence Submitted to the Committee of Enquiry Into the Costs of the N. H. S.* (London: Fellowship For Freedom in Medicine, 1954), p. 18.

15. "Proceedings of the Annual Representative Meeting," *Brit. Med. J., Suppl.,* July 10, 1954, pp. 38-44.

16. *Manchester Guardian,* July 5, 6, 1954.

17. "Proceedings of the Annual Representative Meeting," *Brit. Med. J., Suppl.,* July 21, 1956, p. 61.

18. Fox, p. 172.

19. *Brit. Med. J., Suppl.,* July 11, 1955, p. 281; *Medical World Newsletter,* December, 1957, p. 26.

20. *The Times* (London), April 25, 1957.

21. "Annual Report of the Council," *Brit. Med. J., Suppl.,* April 13, 1957, pp. 164-65; *Medical World Newsletter,* October, 1956, pp. 11, 13.

22. "Cohen Report," p. 26.

23. "Preliminary Memorandum of Evidence to the Royal Commission on Doctors' and Dentists' Remuneration," *Brit. Med. J., Suppl.,* November 23, 1957, p. 172.

24. *Brit. Med. J., Suppl.,* April 19, 1958, p. 193; "Cohen Report," p. 28.

25. *Brit. Med. J.,* September 6, 1958, p. 612.

26. *Brit. Med. J., Suppl.,* April 19, 1958, p. 193, and June 14, 1958, p. 339; L. S. Potter, "Entry Into General Medical Practice," *Brit. Med. J., Suppl.,* October 4, 1958, pp. 153-55; "Proceedings of the Council," *Brit. Med. J., Suppl.,* April 4, 1959, p. 126.

27. *Brit. Med. J., Suppl.,* June 21, 1958, p. 353; *Report of the Ministry of Health, 1956,* Part I, p. 54, *1957,* p. 59, *1958,* p. 96, and *1960,* p. 222.

28. *Royal Commission on Doctors' and Dentists' Remuneration, Minutes of Evidence,* 3-4, p. 118; *Report of the Ministry of Health, 1958,* Part I, p. 102, and *1960,* p. 60.

29. *Report of the Ministry of Health, 1958,* Part I, pp. 101-2, 106, *1954,* pp. 62, 69, *1955,* pp. 57-58, 64, and *1959,* pp. 79, 84; *Accounts, 1956-57: Summarised Accounts of Regional Hospital Boards, Boards of Governors of Teaching Hospitals, Hospital Management Committees, Executive Councils, etc.* (London: Her Majesty's Stationery Office, 1958), p. 36; *Report of the London Executive Council, 1954-55,* p. 20; *N. H. S. Note, No. 2A: How the Doctor is Paid,* January, 1961, p. 3; *Brit. Med. J., Suppl.,* April 19, 1958, p. 163, and February 7, 1959, p. 46.

30. *Brit. Med. J., Suppl.,* April 19, 1958, p. 193; May 3, 1958, p. 224; April 4, 1959, p. 126.

31. "Cohen Report," pp. 62-63; *Accounts, 1956-57,* p. 36; *Report of the Ministry of Health, 1953,* Part I, p. 68, *1956,* p. 62, *1957,* p. 67, *1958,* p. 310, and *1959,* pp. 79, 84; *N. H. S. Note, No. 2A: How the Doctor is Paid,* October, 1960, p. 3.

32. "Walker Report," *Brit. Med. J., Suppl.,* September 26, 1953, p. 144.

33. "Cohen Report," pp. 25-26.

34. *Brit. Med. J., Suppl.,* June 11, 1958, p. 278.

35. *Ibid.,* June 11, 1955, p. 279.

36. *Royal Commission on Doctors' and Dentists' Remuneration, Minutes of Evidence,* 3-4, pp. 116-17.

37. *Ibid., Written Evidence,* I, p. 46; *Brit. Med. J., Suppl.,* May 3, 1958, p. 223, and August 15, 1959, pp. 25-26.

38. *Brit. Med. J., Suppl.,* April 19, 1958, p. 193; Taylor, pp. 21-23; *Royal Commission on Doctors' and Dentists' Remuneration, Minutes of Evidence,* 3-4, p. 118, and *Written Evidence,* I, pp. 96, 98; "Cohen Report," p. 25; *Report of the Ministry of Health, 1958,* Part I, pp. 96, 310, 314, and *1959,* pp. 75, 255.

39. *Report of the Ministry of Health, 1958,* Part I, pp. 97-98, 310-11; *1960,* pp. 3, 59-60.

40. Taylor, pp. 91-92, 107-11; *Royal Commission on Doctors' and Dentists' Remuneration, Minutes of Evidence,* 3-4, pp. 115-16, and 9, p. 407.

41. *Medical World Newsletter,* August, 1957, p. 1.

42. *Ibid.,* pp. 1, 3; *Royal Commission on Doctors' and Dentists' Remuneration, Minutes of Evidence,* 3-4, pp. 115-17.

43. "Cohen Report," p. 27.

44. Taylor, p. 90.

45. "Cohen Report," pp. 10-12.

46. *Report of the Ministry of Health, 1955,* Part I, p. 51.

47. *Ibid., 1954,* pp. 61-62; *1959,* pp. 75-76; *1960,* p. 62.

48. "Health Centres: Interim Report by the Council of the B. M. A., July, 1948," *Brit. Med. J., Suppl.,* September 11, 1948, pp. 113-17.

49. *The Times* (London), September 10, 1949.

50. Rogers, p. 33.

51. "Cohen Report," pp. 19-21; "Guillebaud Report," pp. 207-8; J. A. Scott, "The Contribution of the Health Centre to the Public Health," *The Journal of the Royal Institute of Public Health and Hygiene,* XVI (1953), 188-89.

52. "A Postal Inquiry Among G. P. Principals," *Brit. Med. J., Suppl.,* September 26, 1953, p. 125; Stephen J. Hadfield, "A Field Survey of General Practice, 1951-52," *Brit. Med. J.,* September 26, 1953, p. 702.

53. *Brit. Med. J.,* July 26, 1958, p. 253, and December 19, 1959, pp. 1412-13; *The Guardian,* May 18, 1960; *Medical World Newsletter,* October, 1960, pp. 11-14; *Report of the Ministry of Health, 1958,* Part I, pp. 187-89.

54. "Cohen Report," pp. 59-60; "Report on Health Centres," *Medical World Newsletter,* October, 1956, pp. 4-10.

55. *Medical World Newsletter,* October, 1956, pp. 4-5; Scott, pp. 195-96.

56. *N. H. S. Note, No. 2,* September 16, 1952, pp. 1-2; *Manchester Guardian,* June 29, 1954.

57. Stephen Taylor, "The Health Centres of Harlow: An Essay in Cooperation," *The Lancet,* October 22, 1955, p. 868.

58. "Guillebaud Report," p. 208; *Brit. Med. J., Suppl.,* January 18, 1958, p. 20; *Manchester Guardian,* June 10, 1954, September, 28, 1956.

59. "Guillebaud Report," pp. 207-10.

60. Harold S. Diehl *et al.*, "British Medical Education and the National Health Service," *The Journal of the American Medical Association*, Vol. 143 (1950), 1495; *The Lancet*, June 22, 1957, pp. 1285-86.

61. *Manchester Guardian*, June 6, 1958; *Brit. Med. J., Suppl.*, May 10, 1958, p. 231; "State Expenditure on Universities in Great Britain," *Nature*, Vol. 170 (1952), 171-72; *Royal Commission on Doctors' and Dentists' Remuneration, Minutes of Evidence*, 14-15, pp. 765-67.

62. Diehl *et al.*, pp. 1493-95.

63. *Manchester Guardian*, December 18, 1954.

64. *Ibid.*, July 5, October 16, 1954; "Cohen Report," pp. 29-30.

65. *Brit. Med. J., Suppl.*, November 16, 1957, p. 152.

66. *Report of the Committee to Consider the Future Numbers of Medical Practitioners and the Appropriate Intake of Medical Students* ["Willink Report"] (London: Her Majesty's Stationery Office, 1957), pp. 2, 8-10, 13 ff., 31-33.

67. *Ibid.*, pp. 5-6, 25-30.

68. *Royal Commission on Doctors' and Dentists' Remuneration, Minutes of Evidence*, 14-15, pp. 730-31; 23, pp. 1295-96.

69. "Pilkington Report," p. 53.

70. *Royal Commission on Doctors' and Dentists' Remuneration, Minutes of Evidence*, 14-15, pp. 730-31; 23, pp. 1295-96.

CHAPTER VIII

1. Taylor, *Good General Practice*, pp. 134-44, 487-88.

2. *Ibid.*, pp. 123-32; "Walker Report," *Brit. Med. J., Suppl.*, September 26, 1953, pp. 142-43.

3. Taylor, *Good General Practice*, pp. 138-45.

4. Richard M. Titmuss, *Essays on 'The Welfare State'* (London: George Allen and Unwin, Ltd., 1958), p. 180; *Medical World Newsletter*, March, 1959, p. 3; *Brit. Med. J., Suppl.*, April 13, 1957, p. 166.

5. *Brit. Med. J., Suppl.*, June 23, 1956, p. 396.

6. *Ibid.*, June 11, 1955, p. 278, July 20, 1957, p. 41, and April 10, 1958, p. 165; *Report of the Ministry of Health, 1952*, Part I, p. 54, *1959*, p. 80, and *1960*, p. 63.

7. "Willink Report," p. 18; *Brit. Med. J.*, September 6, 1958, p. 622.

8. Hadfield, pp. 704-5; "Walker Report," *Brit. Med. J., Suppl.*, September 26, 1953, p. 138.

9. *Brit. Med. J.*, September 6, 1958, p. 622; November 29, 1958, p. 1350; November 26, 1960, p. 1593.

10. Taylor, *Good General Practice*, pp. 34 ff.

11. *Ibid.*, pp. 8-9.

12. Hadfield, p. 700.

13. "Cohen Report," pp. 23-24.

14. *Brit. Med. J., Suppl.*, May 28, 1955, p. 259.

15. *Ibid.*, April 28, 1956, pp. 229-30; *Report of the Ministry of Health, 1958*, Part I, p. 99.

16. *Brit. Med. J., Suppl.*, October 8, 1955, p. 82.

17. *Ibid.*, July 14, 1956, p. 29, and April 13, 1957, p. 166; "Guillebaud Report," pp. 170-71; *Report of the London Executive Council, 1958-59*, p. 30, and *1959-60*, p. 33.

18. *Report of the London Executive Council, 1959-60*, p. 32, *1955-56*, pp. 30-31, and *1956-57*, p. 30; *Manchester Guardian*, March 19, 1957.

19. *The Times* (London), March 16, 1956.

20. *Ibid.*, July 7, 1958; *The Guardian*, August 26, 1959; *Brit. Med. J.*, April 5, 1958, pp. 836-37; *Report of the Ministry of Health, 1959*, Part I, p. 181.

21. *Medical World Newsletter*, August, 1955, p. 6.

22. *Manchester Guardian*, April 18, 1958.

23. *Ibid.*, March 19, 1957, and October 25, 1956; *The Times* (London), March 16, 1956.

24. "Proceedings of the Annual Representative Meeting," *Brit. Med. J., Suppl.*, July 14, 1956, p. 39.

25. J. P. W. Mallalieu, "The Good Samaritans," *The New Statesman and Nation*, Vol. 52 (1956), 513-14.

26. Brotherston, Cartwright, and Martin, p. 984.

27. Rogers, p. 33.

28. Lord Moran, "Lessons From the Past," *Brit. Med. J., Suppl.*, July 5, 1958, p. 5.

29. "Guillebaud Report," p. 165; "Cohen Report," p. 5; Hadfield, p. 689.

30. Hadfield, p. 695.

31. *Brit. Med. J., Suppl.*, June 11, 1955, p. 280; July 14, 1956, p. 34.

32. *Report of the Ministry of Health, 1955*, Part I, p. 51; *1958*, p. 46.

33. "Walker Report," *Brit. Med. J., Suppl.*, September 26, 1953, p. 146.

34. *Ibid.*, p. 150; Hadfield, p. 698; Social Surveys, p. 1.

35. "Cohen Report," p. 43; Taylor, *Good General Practice*, p. 364.

36. *Report of the London Executive Council, 1958-59*, p. 17.

37. Hadfield, p. 692.

38. *Brit. Med. J., Suppl.*, June 11, 1955, p. 281; April 7, 1956, p. 124; April 13, 1957, p. 166.

39. *Medical World Newsletter*, December, 1957, p. 13; "Cohen Report," p. 33.

40. *The N.H.S. . . . Regulations, 1954*, pp. 21-22; "Report of the Medical Practices Committee," January, 1953, p. 6; *Report of the Ministry of Health, 1958*, Part I, p. 148, *1959*, p. 81, and *1960*, p. 102; Hadfield, p. 692.

41. *Memorandum on the Maternity Services Submitted to the Cranbrook Committee of Enquiry* (London: Fellowship For Freedom in Medicine, 1957), p. 2; Social Surveys, p. 1.

42. "Cohen Report," p. 32; "Walker Report," *Brit. Med. J., Suppl.*, September 26, 1953, p. 139.

43. *Report of the Ministry of Health, 1960*, Part I, p. 183.

44. "Guillebaud Report," p. 212.

45. *Report of the Maternity Services Committee* ["Cranbrook Report"] (London: Her Majesty's Stationery Office, 1959), pp. 49 ff.

46. *Medical World Newsletter*, April, 1959, pp. 15, 17; *Brit. Med. J.*, February 21, 1959, pp. 491-92.

47. *Manchester Guardian*, August 6, 1959.

48. Hadfield, p. 689; "Willink Report," pp. 19-21.

49. Taylor, *Good General Practice*, p. 146.

50. *Some Administrative Problems of the Health Services* (London: The Institute of Public Administration, 1951), p. 17.

51. "Walker Report," *Brit. Med. J., Suppl.*, September 26, 1953, p. 137.

52. R. Scott Stevenson, "Socialized Medicine in England," *Laryngoscope*, Vol. 62 (1952), 827.

53. Paul F. Gemmill, "An American Report on the National Health Service," *Brit. Med. J., Suppl.*, July 5, 1958, p. 18.

54. *Brit. Med. J., Suppl.*, July 19, 1958, p. 86.

55. "Annual Report of the Council," *Brit. Med. J., Suppl.*, April 11, 1959, p. 138.

56. John Fry, "A Year of General Practice: A Study in Morbidity," *Brit. Med. J.*, August 2, 1952, p. 249.

57. "Cohen Report," p. 37; E. Maurice Backett, J. A. Heady, and J. C. G. Evans, "Studies of a General Practice, II, The Doctor's Job in an Urban Area," *Brit. Med. J.*, January 16, 1954, p. 113; *General Practitioners' Records: An Analysis of the Clinical Records of Some General Practices During the Period April, 1952 to March, 1954* ("General Register Office Studies on Medical and Population Statistics," No. 9 [London: Her Majesty's Stationery Office, 1956]), p. 79.

58. Hadfield, p. 701; Taylor, *Good General Practice*, pp. 150-52; *Medical World Newsletter*, August, 1955, p. 5; Social Surveys, p. 2.

Notes 491

59. *The N.H.S. . . . Regulations, 1954*, pp. 17-18, and *1956*, pp. 16-17; *Report of the Ministry of Health, 1953*, Part I, p. 67, *1955*, p. 59, *1957*, p. 69, *1959*, p. 109, and *1960*, p. 72.
60. "Hinchliffe Interim Report," pp. 4-10.
61. *Ibid.*, p. 3.
62. *Manchester Guardian*, October 7, 1954.
63. "Cohen Report," p. 35.
64. *The Lancet*, June 8, 1957, p. 1194; *Fellowship For Freedom in Medicine*, February, 1958, pp. 26-27; *Manchester Guardian*, December 12, 1957, and January 16, 1959; *Brit. Med. J.*, December 5, 1959, p. 1265.
65. *Brit. Med. J.*, February 27, 1960, p. 658, and November 19, 1960, p. 1531, and *Suppl.*, July 19, 1958, p. 46, and December 26, 1959, p. 205; "Proceedings of the Council," *Brit. Med. J.*, *Suppl.*, December 27, 1958, p. 271; "Proceedings of the Annual Representative Meeting," *Brit. Med. J.*, *Suppl.*, August 29, 1959, p. 61, January 3, 1959, p. 3, and December 13, 1958, pp. 253-54.
66. Stevenson, p. 826.
67. P. G. Gray and Ann Cartwright, "Choosing and Changing Doctors," *The Lancet*, December 19, 1953, p. 1308.
68. "Willink Report," p. 12.
69. Hadfield, pp. 699-70; "A Postal Inquiry Among G. P. Principals," *Brit. Med. J.*, *Suppl.*, September 26, 1953, p. 113.
70. Taylor, *Good General Practice*, pp. 70-72.

CHAPTER IX

1. Fox, p. 171.
2. *Royal Commission on Doctors' and Dentists' Remuneration, Minutes of Evidence*, 5-6, p. 276.
3. *Medical World Newsletter*, May, 1959, p. 5.
4. *Members One of Another: Labour's Policy for Health* (London: Labor Party, 1959), p. 8.
5. "Newsam Report," *Brit. Med. J.*, *Suppl.*, January 17, 1959, p. 18.
6. *Brit. Med. J.*, July 5, 1958, p. 3.
7. *Ibid.*, November 12, 1955, p. 119.
8. "Newsam Report," *Brit. Med. J.*, *Suppl.*, January 17, 1959, p. 15.
9. *The N. H. S. . . . Regulations, 1954*, pp. 18-19, and *1956*, p. 3; "Cohen Report," p. 13; Titmuss, p. 139.
10. Gray and Cartwright, p. 1308.
11. "Willink Report," p. 5; Taylor, *Good General Practice*, p. 50; *Report of the Ministry of Health, 1953*, Part I, p. 6.
12. D. Reid Ross, "N. H. S. in Factory Town: A Survey of the Demand for Medical Care in an Industrial Community," *Medical World*, Vol. 78 (1953), 128-29.
13. "Cohen Report," p. 13.
14. Taylor, *Good General Practice*, pp. 8-9.
15. Hadfield, pp. 686-88.
16. Taylor, *Good General Practice*, pp. 65-66.
17. *Ibid.*, p. 188; "Walker Report," *Brit. Med. J.*, *Suppl.*, September 26, 1953, p. 141.
18. *Manchester Guardian*, October 27, 1954; *Brit. Med. J.*, April 16, 1960, p. 1215; John T. Baldwin, "Appointment System in General Practice," *Brit. Med. J.*, *Suppl.*, January 9, 1960, pp. 9-11.
19. Gemmill, p. 19.
20. Backett *et al.*, p. 114.
21. A. Bradford Hill, "The Doctor's Day and Pay: Some Sampling Inquiries Into the Pre-War Status," *Journal of the Royal Statistical Society*, CXIV (1951), 1.
22. Gray and Cartwright, p. 1308.
23. Fry, p. 250.
24. *General Practitioners' Records*, pp. 73-74.
25. Alistair Mair and George B. Mair, "Facts of Importance to the Organization

of a National Health Service From a Five Year Study of a General Practice," *Brit. Med. J., Suppl.,* June 20, 1959, p. 282.

26. Taylor, *Good General Practice,* p. 61.

27. J. H. F. Brotherston, Ann Cartwright *et al.,* "Night Calls: Their Frequency and Nature in One General Practice," *Brit. Med. J.,* November 28, 1959, pp. 1169-72.

28. D. Reid Ross, p. 126; Mair and Mair, p. 282.

29. *General Practitioners' Records,* p. 75; Backett *et al.,* p. 110.

30. Taylor, *Good General Practice,* p. 465.

31. *Royal Commission on Doctors' and Dentists' Remuneration, Minutes of Evidence,* 14-15, p. 701; Mair and Mair, p. 283.

32. Taylor, *Good General Practice,* pp. 67-70.

33. Titmuss, p. 176.

34. Hadfield, p. 688.

35. Taylor, *Good General Practice,* pp. 263-70.

36. *Ibid.,* pp. 306 ff.; "Walker Report," *Brit. Med. J., Suppl.,* September 26, 1953, p. 148; *Report of the Ministry of Health, 1952,* Part I, pp. 20-21, and *1955,* pp. 27-28; "Cohen Report," p. 42.

37. "Newsam Report," *Brit. Med. J., Suppl.,* Jan. 17, 1959, p. 14.

38. "Cohen Report," pp. 4-5.

39. Hadfield, p. 697.

40. Fry, p. 249; *General Practitioners' Records,* p. 77.

41. Hadfield, p. 695.

42. *Memorandum of Evidence Submitted to the Committee of Enquiry Into the Costs of the National Health Service,* p. 7.

43. *Brit. Med. J.,* July 19, 1952, p. 55.

44. Hadfield, p. 703.

45. "Walker Report," *Brit. Med. J., Suppl.,* September 26, 1953, p. 150.

46. Gemmill, pp. 18-19.

47. Norman Morris and Desmond O'Neill, "Out-Patient Gynaecology," *Brit. Med. J.,* May 3, 1958, pp. 1036-39.

48. P. Nestitz, "A Series of 1,817 Patients Seen in a Casualty Department," *Brit. Med. J.,* November 9, 1957, p. 1108.

49. *Ibid.,* p. 1109; *Manchester Guardian,* June 14, 1957.

50. *Medical World Newsletter,* November, 1955, pp. 9, 11; Social Surveys, p. 3.

51. Taylor, *Good General Practice,* pp. 84-85.

52. "Cohen Report," pp. 37-38.

53. "The Reform of the National Health Service: First Interim Report of the Council," *Brit. Med. J., Suppl.,* October 13, 1951, p. 147; *Brit. Med. J., Suppl.,* April 7, 1956, p. 134.

54. "Newsam Report," *Brit. Med. J., Suppl.,* January 17, 1959, pp. 18, 20.

55. *N.H.S. (Service Committees and Tribunal) Regulations, 1956,* pp. 4 ff.

56. *Report of the Committee on Administrative Tribunals and Enquiries* ["Franks Report"] (London: Her Majesty's Stationery Office, 1957), pp. 44-47.

57. *British Dental Journal,* Vol. 104 (1958), 371; *Manchester Guardian,* March 13, December 4, 22, 1958; *Tribunals and Inquiries Bill,* pp. 1 ff.; *Brit. Med. J., Suppl.,* May 24, 1958, p. 261.

58. *Brit. Med. J.,* November 6, 1954, p. 1114; *Report of the Ministry of Health, 1952, Part I,* p. 178, *1954,* p. 208, *1956,* p. 209, *1957,* pp. 223-24, *1958,* pp. 327-28, *1959,* pp. 268, 270, and *1960,* p. 237.

59. *Manchester Guardian,* March 25, 1954; June 28, August 8, 1956; March 4, 28, June 13, October 11, 1957.

60. *Brit. Med. J., Suppl.,* November 24, 1956, p. 195.

61. *Brit. Med. J.,* July 14, 1956, pp. 57-61.

62. "Newsam Report," *Brit. Med. J., Suppl.,* January 17, 1959, p. 19.

63. R. S. Ferguson, "The Doctor-Patient Relationship and 'Functional' Illness," *The Practitioner,* Vol. 176 (1956), 656-62.

64. *The Middle Class Way of Life* [Correspondence reprinted from the *Manchester Guardian*] (Manchester: *Manchester Guardian,* 1954), pp. 1-28.

65. *The Spectator,* Vol. 181 (1948), 144; *Fellowship For Freedom in Medicine,* July, 1950, p. 21.

66. "A Postal Inquiry Among G. P. Principals," *Brit. Med. J., Suppl.,* September 26, 1953, p. 113; Hadfield, p. 699.

67. "Walker Report," *Brit. Med. J., Suppl.,* September 26, 1953, pp. 134-36.

68. "Cohen Report," p. 13; "Guillebaud Report," p. 165.

69. H. Guy Dain, "The National Health Service After Ten Years," *Brit. Med. J., Suppl.,* July 5, 1958, pp. 1-3.

70. *Manchester Guardian,* July 24, 1958.

71. Gemmill, p. 19.

72. Stevenson, p. 826.

73. *Ibid.,* p. 829; Hadfield, pp. 691, 699, 704; "Walker Report," *Brit. Med. J., Suppl.,* September 26, 1953, p. 151.

74. "Newsam Report," *Brit. Med. J., Suppl.,* January 17, 1959, pp. 14, 18.

75. C. P. D. Grant, "Youth Looks at General Practice," *Brit. Med. J.,* April 30, 1955, p. 1051.

76. D. Reid Ross, pp. 129-30.

77. Brotherston, Cartwright, and Martin, p. 984.

78. Gemmill, pp. 20-21.

CHAPTER X

1. *Hansard,* H. of C., Vol. 592 (1958), cols. 1403-4.

2. "Guillebaud Report," pp. 99-100.

3. *Sixth Report From the Select Committee on Estimates, 1956-57: Running Costs of Hospitals,* pp. 17, 21, 59.

4. *Ibid.,* pp. 324-25; *Hospitals and the State: Hospital Organization and Administration Under the National Health Service,* "Creative Leadership in a State Service" (London: The Acton Society Trust, 1959), pp. 5-6.

5. *Sixth Report From the Select Committee on Estimates, 1956-57: Running Costs of Hospitals,* pp. 5-6, 230-31, 325-26, 331, 352; "Guillebaud Report," pp. 106-08.

6. *Hospitals and the State . . . Creative Leadership in a State Service,* pp. 11-13, 47-48.

7. *Ibid.,* pp. 9-11; *Hospitals and the State: Hospital Organization and Administration Under the National Health Service,* "The Central Control of the Service" (London: The Acton Society Trust, 1958), pp. 47-51.

8. *Hospitals and the State . . . The Central Control of the Service,* pp. 52-58.

9. *Sixth Report From the Select Committee on Estimates, 1956-57: Running Costs of Hospitals,* pp. v-xviii.

10. *Fifth Special Report From the Select Committee on Estimates, 1958-59: Running Costs of Hospitals,* pp. iii-ix.

11. *Hospitals and the State . . . The Central Control of the Service,* pp. 61-66.

12. *Hansard,* H. of C., Vol. 592 (1958), cols. 1390 ff.

13. *Hansard,* H. of L., Vol. 210 (1958), cols. 447 ff.

14. *National Health Service Act, 1946,* Part II, sec. 13.

15. *Hospitals and the State . . . The Central Control of the Service,* pp. 10 ff., 70-71.

16. *Ibid.,* pp. 30-32.

17. *Ibid.,* pp. 34-41; *National Health Service Act, 1946,* Part VI, sec. 57; *Sixth Report From the Select Committee on Estimates, 1956-57: Running Costs of Hospitals,* pp. 30-31.

18. *Hospitals and the State . . . The Central Control of the Service,* pp. 41-42.

19. *Sixth Report From the Select Committee on Estimates, 1956-57: Running Costs of Hospitals,* p. 50; "Guillebaud Report," pp. 68-69.

20. "Guillebaud Report," p. 79; *Hospitals and the State: Hospital Organization and Administration Under the National Health Service,* "Groups, Regions and Committees, Part II, Regional Hospital Boards" (London: The Acton Society Trust, 1957), pp. 30-35.

21. *Hansard*, H. of C., Vol. 552 (1955-56), col. 849.

22. *Fifth Special Report From the Select Committee on Estimates, 1958-59: Running Costs of Hospitals*, p. v.

23. Sir George Schuster, "Creative Leadership in a State Service," in *Hospitals and the State . . . Creative Leadership in a State Service*, pp. 34-36.

24. *Hospitals and the State . . . The Central Control of the Service*, pp. 20-21; "Guillebaud Report," pp. 67, 89-90, 304.

25. *Brit. Med. J., Suppl.*, July 20, 1957, p. 44; June 11, 1955, p. 280; April 7, 1956, p. 132; April 11, 1959, pp. 141-42.

26. *Manchester Guardian*, September 4, 1957.

27. *Voluntary Service and the State: A Study of the Needs of the Hospital Service*, p. 125.

28. *Hospitals and the State . . . Groups, Regions and Committees*, Part II, pp. 6-7, 13-15.

29. *Ibid.*, pp. 3-4, 8-13, 27; "Guillebaud Report," pp. 67, 80; *The Lancet*, Nov. 14, 1953, p. 1038.

30. *Report of the Committee on the Internal Administration of Hospitals* ["Bradbeer Report"] (London: Her Majesty's Stationery Office, 1954), p. 1; *Hospitals and the State . . . Background and Blueprint*, pp. 24-25; *N.H.S. Note: Summary of Main Current Figures*, August, 1960, p. 2.

31. "Annual Report of the Council," *Brit. Med. J., Suppl.*, April 13, 1957, p. 172; May 24, 1958, p. 264.

32. *Voluntary Service and the State: A Study of the Needs of the Hospital Service*, p. 125.

33. *Sixth Report From the Select Committee on Estimates, 1956-57: Running Costs of Hospitals*, pp. 71, 75, 100, 201, 226-27, 403.

34. *Voluntary Service and the State: A Study of the Needs of the Hospital Service*, pp. 42 ff., 121-24; "Guillebaud Report," pp. 80-81, 253; *Hospitals and the State: Hospital Organization Under the National Health Service*, "Groups, Regions and Committees, Part I, Hospital Management Committees" (London: The Acton Society Trust, 1957), pp. 8-9.

35. *Sixth Report From the Select Committee on Estimates, 1956-57: Running Costs of Hospitals*, pp. xvii, 106-07, 229; *Fifth Special Report From the Select Committee on Estimates, 1958-59: Running Costs of Hospitals*, p. vi.

36. *Fifth Special Report From the Select Committee on Estimates*, pp. iii-iv, 1-2, 6.

37. *Sixth Report From the Select Committee on Estimates, 1956-57: Running Costs of Hospitals*, pp. 101, 107, 205, 228-29.

38. "Guillebaud Report," pp. 80-81.

39. "Bradbeer Report," p. 8; *Hospitals and the State . . . Groups, Regions and Committees*, Part II, pp. 9 ff.

40. *Hospitals and the State . . . Groups, Regions and Committees*, Part II, pp. 15-16; *Report on the Grading Structure of Administrative and Clerical Staff in the Hospital Service* ["Noel Hall Report"] (London: Her Majesty's Stationery Office, 1957), pp. 4-8: "Bradbeer Report," pp. 9 ff., 50-54.

41. "Proceedings of the Annual Representative Meeting," *Brit. Med. J., Suppl.*, June 18, 1955, p. 291; "Annual Report of the Council," *Brit. Med. J., Suppl.*, April 7, 1956, p. 160, and April 13, 1957, p. 173.

42. "Bradbeer Report," pp. 18-20.

43. "Annual Report of the Council," *Brit. Med. J., Suppl.*, April 7, 1956, p. 160.

44. "Guillebaud Report," pp. 146-47.

45. *Sixth Report From the Select Committee on Estimates, 1956-57: Running Costs of Hospitals*, pp. 144, 227; *Brit. Med. J., Suppl.*, April 13, 1957, p. 173, and April 7, 1956, p. 163; "Bradbeer Report," pp. 38-39.

46. "Bradbeer Report," pp. 7, 16 ff.; "Guillebaud Report," p. 145.

47. "Bradbeer Report," pp. 41-47.

48. *Ibid.*, pp. 4-5, 67-68, 84; "Guillebaud Report," pp. 91-93; *Sixth Report From*

the Select Committee on Estimates, 1956-57: Running Costs of Hospitals, pp. 71-72, 142-43, 203, 227.

49. *Hospitals and the State: Hospital Organization and Administration Under the National Health Service,* "The Impact of the Change" (London: The Acton Society Trust, 1956), pp. 4, 45; *Voluntary Service and the State: A Study of the Needs of the Hospital Service,* pp. 60-61.

50. "Bradbeer Report," pp. 67-68; "Guillebaud Report," pp. 93-94.

51. "Guillebaud Report," p. 94; "Noel Hall Report," pp. 32-37; "Bradbeer Report," pp. 55-57.

52. *Hospitals and the State . . . The Impact of the Change,* pp. 18-25.

53. *Ibid.,* pp. 3-18, 27-34.

54. *Hospitals and the State . . . Background and Blueprint,* pp. 21-22; *Hospitals and the State . . . Groups, Regions and Committees, Part II,* pp. 37-38.

55. *Voluntary Service and the State: A Study of the Needs of the Hospital Service,* p. 125.

56. L. W. Wilding, "The London Story," *The London Hospital Illustrated,* III, No. 6 (1955), 10.

57. Abel-Smith and Titmuss, p. 28; *Civil Estimates for the Year Ending 31st March, 1960, Class V,* pp. 100-1; *Sixth Report From the Select Committee on Estimates, 1956-57: Running Costs of Hospitals,* pp. xiii, 259.

58. "Guillebaud Report," pp. 72-75.

59. *Hospitals and the State . . . Groups, Regions and Committees, Part II,* pp. 41-44.

60. *Sixth Report From the Select Committee on Estimates, 1956-57: Running Costs of Hospitals,* pp. 26-27, 187, 189, 266; "Guillebaud Report," p. 75.

61. *Hospitals and the State . . . Groups, Regions and Committees, Part II,* p. 42.

62. *Hansard,* H. of C., Vol. 592 (1958), col. 1409.

63. *Hansard,* H. of L., Vol. 210 (1958), cols. 449-50.

64. "Guillebaud Report," p. 253.

65. *Ibid.,* pp. 139-41.

66. *Report of the Ministry of Health, 1957,* Part I, p. 41; *Sixth Report From the Select Committee on Estimates, 1956-57: Running Costs of Hospitals,* pp. 335-37.

67. *Annual Report of King Edward's Hospital Fund for London, 1957,* pp. 7, 39-41.

68. *Report of the Ministry of Health, 1956,* Part I, p. 36, and *1957,* p. 41; *Manchester Guardian,* December 22, 1956.

69. "Noel Hall Report," pp. 1, 8-12, 19-31, 58-59.

70. *Fifth Special Report From the Select Committee on Estimates, 1958-59: Running Costs of Hospitals,* pp. iii-iv, 4-5.

71. *Ibid.,* p. iv; *Brit. Med. J., Suppl.,* August 23, 1958, pp. 126-27; *Manchester Guardian,* August 16, 1958.

72. "Noel Hall Report," pp. 41-42.

73. *Sixth Report From the Select Committee on Estimates, 1956-57: Running Costs of Hospitals,* p. v.

74. *Hospitals and the State . . . Creative Leadership in a State Service,* pp. 14 ff.

75. Schuster, pp. 29 ff.

CHAPTER XI

1. *Report of the Working Party on Hospital Costing* (London: Her Majesty's Stationery Office, 1955), pp. 3 ff.

2. *Accounts 1957-58,* pp. iii-iv.

3. *Report of the Ministry of Health, 1955,* Part I, pp. 42-44.

4. *Ibid.,* pp. 33-34; *1954,* p. 34.

5. *Report of the Ministry of Health, 1954,* Part I, p. 40; *1955,* p. 39; *1957,* pp. 43-44; *1958,* pp. 41-43; *1959,* pp. 33-34.

6. Schuster, pp. 51-54; *Manchester Guardian,* February 7, 1958.

7. *Final Report of the Committee on Hospital Supplies* (London: Her Majesty's Stationery Office, 1958), pp. 5 ff., 33-35.

8. *Interim Report of the Committee on Hospital Supplies* (London: Her Majesty's Stationery Office, 1957), pp. 4-5; *Accounts 1955-56,* pp. iii-iv.

9. *Final Report of the Committee on Hospital Supplies,* pp. 47-49.

10. *Sixth Report From the Select Committee on Estimates, 1956-57: Running Costs of Hospitals,* pp. 391-92.

11. *Fifth Special Report From the Select Committee on Estimates, 1958-59: Running Costs of Hospitals,* pp. 16-17.

12. *Report of the Ministry of Health, 1954,* Part I, pp. 30-31, *1956,* p. 33; *Accounts 1954-55,* pp. iii-iv, and *1958-59,* p. 4.

13. *Hospital Endowments Fund Account, 1958-59* (London: Her Majesty's Stationery Office, 1960), pp. 4-11; *Sixth Report From the Select Committee on Estimates, 1956-57: Running Costs of Hospitals,* pp. 3, 19-20; "Guillebaud Report," pp. 133-35.

14. *Brit. Med. J., Suppl.,* November 29, 1958, p. 228.

15. "Guillebaud Report," pp. 66, 148-50.

16. *N.H.S. Note,* August 14, 1948, p. 3, and July 15, 1959, p. 3; *Report of the Ministry of Health, 1953-1960,* Part I, Appendix.

17. *National Health Service (Pay-Bed Accommodation in Hospitals, etc.) Regulations, 1953,* No. 420 (London: Her Majesty's Stationery Office, 1953), pp. 2-11; *N.H.S. Note,* September 9, 1958, p. 3.

18. Warren Postbridge, "The Private Patient," *The Spectator,* Vol. 185 (1950), 457.

19. *Hansard,* H. of C., Vol. 592 (1958), col. 1404.

20. *The New Statesman and Nation,* Vol. 48 (1954), 426; *The Guardian,* August 26, 1959.

21. *Manchester Guardian,* October 7, 1954.

22. This charge was doubled in 1961.

23. *N.H.S. Note,* August 14, 1958, p. 3, and July 15, 1959, p. 3; *Report of the Ministry of Health, 1958, 1959,* Part I, Appendix; *Sixth Report From the Select Committee on Estimates, 1956-57: Running Costs of Hospitals,* p. 7.

24. A. N. Dixon, "What Future For Private Practice and Private Beds," in "N.H.S. Supplement," *The Times* (London), July 7, 1958, p. xxi; Information in letters to the author from E. R. Watkins, Branch Secretary of the B.U.P.A., May 24, 1956, and April 14, 1958; Interview with E. R. Watkins, April 24, 1954; *Annual Report and Statement of Accounts of the B.U.P.A. for the Year Ended June 30, 1959* (Oxford: The British United Provident Association, 1959), pp. 1-9.

25. *The General Practitioner Scheme* (Oxford: The British United Provident Association, 1959). By the middle of 1960, only 12,000 persons were covered by the scheme.

26. *Fellowship For Freedom in Medicine* November, 1958, pp. 5-10; August, 1956, pp. 15-16; February, 1959, p. 1.

27. *Hansard,* H. of C., Vol. 592 (1958), cols. 1414, 1392-93.

28. *Ibid.,* H. of L., Vol. 210 (1958), col. 448.

29. *Hospital Bed Occupancy: A Report of the First Group Set up by the Hospital Administrative Staff College* (London: King Edward's Hospital Fund for London, 1954), pp. 13-14; *The Lancet,* June 1, 1957, p. 1133; *Report of the Ministry of Health, 1960,* Part I, pp. 180, 182.

30. *Report of the Ministry of Health, 1957,* Part I, pp. 14-17; *1958,* p. 8; *1959,* p. 16.

31. *Ibid., 1960,* pp. 20, 182-83.

32. *Ibid., 1956,* pp. 8-9.

33. Hadfield, p. 695.

34. Robert Logan and Gordon Forsyth, "Health Service Achievements," *Manchester Guardian,* August 6, 1958.

35. *Annual Report of King Edward's Hospital Fund for London, 1956,* p. 27; *1957,* p. 22; *1958,* pp. 22-23; *Manchester Guardian,* November 16, 1956.

36. *Report of the Minister of Health, 1960,* Part I, pp. 178, 192-93, 194-95.
37. G. E. Godber, "Health Services, Past, Present and Future," *The Lancet,* July 5, 1958, pp. 2-6.
38. *Report of the Ministry of Health, 1954,* Part I, p. 8; *1955,* p. 8; *1957,* pp. 17-18.
39. *Ibid., 1954,* p. 8; *1958,* p. 14; *1959,* pp. 218-19; *1960,* p. 170.
40. *Report of the Nuffield Provincial Hospitals Trust, 1955-58,* pp. 12-13; *The Guardian,* June 15, 1960; Leslie F. Brown, "Hospitals For Today and Tomorrow," *Brit. Med. J., Suppl.,* April 4, 1959, p. 119.
41. *Report of the Ministry of Health, 1954,* Part I, p. 148; *1957,* p. 160.
42. *Sixth Report From the Select Committee on Estimates, 1956-57: Running Costs of Hospitals,* p. 62.
43. "N.H.S. Supplement," *The Times* (London), July 7, 1958, p. xxiii; *Manchester Guardian,* May 1, 11, 1959; *Report of the Ministry of Health, 1955,* Part I, pp. 19-21, *1957,* Part I, pp. 27-28, *1957,* Part II, pp. 105-6, and *1959,* Part I, p. 30.
44. *Sixth Report From the Select Committee on Estimates, 1956-57: Running Costs of Hospitals,* pp. 62, 195.
45. *The Times* (London), "N H S Supplement," July 7, 1958, p. xxi; *N.H.S. Note,* July 15, 1959, p. 4; *Report of the Ministry of Health, 1952,* Part I, p. 140, *1957,* Part I, pp. 29-30, 176, *1957,* Part II, pp. 97-100, *1958,* Part I, p. 37, *1959,* Part I, p. 32, and *1960,* Part I, p. 48.
46. *Report of the Ministry of Health, 1953,* Part I, p. 23, *1954,* p. 19, *1957,* pp. 29, 120, *1958,* pp. 34-35, and *1959,* pp. 31, 162; *N.H.S. Note,* Aug. 14, 1958, p. 5.
47. *Hansard,* H. of C., Vol. 592 (1958), col. 1405.
48. *Report of the Ministry of Health, 1957,* Part I, pp. 29, 122-23, 194; *1957,* Part II, pp. 227-28; *1958,* Part I, pp. 34-35, 304-5; *1959,* Part I, p. 248; *1960,* Part I, p. 203.
49. *Civil Estimates for the Year Ending 31st March, 1960, Class V,* pp. 108, 112; Sir Harold Himsworth, "New Pattern of Research," in "N.H.S. Supplement," *The Times* (London), July 7, 1958, p. vii.
50. *Civil Estimates For the Year Ending 31st March, 1960, Class V,* pp. 64-67; *Report of the Ministry of Health, 1953,* Part I, pp. 29-30, and *1957,* pp. 34-35.
51. G. S. Wilson, "Team Attack on Epidemics," in "N.H.S. Supplement," *The Times* (London), July 7, 1958, p. xxii; *Medical World Newsletter,* May, 1960, p. 15.
52. The Wellcome Trust was established in 1936 to foster research in veterinary and medical science.
53. Diehl *et al.,* p. 1493.
54. *The Washington Post and Times Herald,* September 24, 1958.
55. *Brit. Med. J.,* February 21, 1959, p. 117; May 16, 1959, p. 1307.
56. *The London Hospital Illustrated,* Vol. III, No. 8 (1957), 8.
57. *Voluntary Service and the State: A Study of the Needs of the Hospital Service,* pp. 90-91; *Report of the Ministry of Health, 1956,* Part I, p. 28; *Convalescent Treatment: Report of a Working Party* (London: Her Majesty's Stationery Office, 1959), pp. 6 ff.
58. *Convalescent Treatment: Report of a Working Party,* pp. 35-40; *Annual Report of King Edward's Hospital Fund for London, 1955,* pp. 20-21, *1956,* pp. 24-25, and *1958,* pp. 19-21.
59. *Report of the Committee of Inquiry on the Rehabilitation, Training and Resettlement of Disabled Persons* ["Piercey Report"] (London: Her Majesty's Stationery Office, 1956), pp. 2-3, 8-13, 110-11; *Report of the Ministry of Health, 1952,* Part I, pp. 132, 139, *1957,* p. 161, 170, *1959,* pp. 215, 227, and *1960,* pp. 179, 190.
60. "Piercey Report," pp. 1 ff., 14-20.
61. "Cranbrook Report," pp. 17-20, 26, 106-8.
62. *Report of the Ministry of Health, 1952,* Part I, pp. 130-31; *1959,* pp. 218-19; *1960,* pp. 182-83.
63. "Cranbrook Report," pp. 40 ff., 64, 84-88.
64. *Ibid.,* pp. 20-24, 29-32; *Report of the Ministry of Health, 1959,* Part I, p. 219; *Manchester Guardian,* November 8, December 12, 1958, and April 8, 1959.

65. *N.H.S. Note: Summary of Main Figures, 1949-1958,* p. 4; "Cranbrook Report," pp. 32-34.

66. "Cranbrook Report," pp. 65-66.

67. *Manchester Guardian,* May 13, 1959.

68. "Cranbrook Report," p. 66.

69. *Report on Confidential Enquiries Into Maternal Deaths in England and Wales, 1952-1954* (London: Her Majesty's Stationery Office, 1957), pp. 43-48.

70. "Cranbrook Report," pp. 11-13.

71. "Guillebaud Report," pp. 216-17; *Report of the Ministry of Health, 1952,* Part I, p. 131, *1959,* pp. 216, 218, 220, and *1960,* p. 182.

72. C. A. Boucher, *Survey of Services Available to the Chronic Sick and Elderly, 1954-1955* (London: Her Majesty's Stationery Office, 1957), pp. 8-11.

73. *Annual Report of King Edward's Hospital Fund for London, 1958,* pp. 23-24.

74. Boucher, pp. 13, 19; *Report of the Ministry of Health, 1955,* Part I, p. 25.

75. *Annual Report of King Edward's Hospital for London, 1958,* p. 24.

76. *Report of the Ministry of Health, 1955,* Part I, p. 74, *1957,* p. 33, and *1959,* pp. 36, 218; Boucher, p. 22; Lord Amulree, "Looking After the Old and the Sick," in "N.H.S. Supplement," *The Times* (London), July 7, 1958, p. xiii.

77. H. Droller, "A Geriatric Out-Patient Department," *The Lancet,* October 4, 1958, pp. 739-40.

78. *Report of the Ministry of Health, 1957,* Part I, p. 33; Boucher, p. 16.

79. J. DeLargg, "Six Weeks In: Six Weeks Out—A Geriatric Hospital Scheme for Rehabilitating the Aged and Relieving Their Relatives," *The Lancet,* February 23, 1957, pp. 418-19.

80. *Report of the Ministry of Health, 1953,* Part I, p. 29; *Annual Report of King Edward's Hospital Fund for London, 1952,* p. 19, *1956,* pp. 22-23, and *1957,* p. 18.

81. *Brit. Med. J.,* September 20, 1958, p. 741.

82. *Report of the Ministry of Health, 1955,* Part I, p. 26, *1957,* pp. 172-73, and *1958,* pp. 282-83; Boucher, pp. 24-29.

83. *Manchester Guardian,* October 25, 1957.

84. *Report of the Ministry of Health, 1960,* Part I, p. 205.

85. A. Lawrence Abel and Walpole Lewin, "Report on Hospital Building," *Brit. Med. J., Suppl.,* April 4, 1959, p. 110; *Report of the Ministry of Health, 1958,* Part I, pp. 18-19.

86. *Report of the Ministry of Health, 1958,* Part I, pp. vii, 18; *Brit. Med. J.,* November 14, 1959, p. 1028, and November 21, 1959, p. 1108.

87. Abel and Lewin, pp. 110-12.

88. "Proceedings of the Annual Representative Meeting," *Brit. Med. J., Suppl.,* September 5, 1959, pp. 70-71.

89. *The Guardian,* August 26, September 12, 1959.

90. Brown, pp. 118-22; G. E. Godber, "The Physician's Part in Hospital Planning," *Brit. Med. J., Suppl.,* April 4, 1959, pp. 115-18; John Fry, "A General Practitioner's Views on Hospital Planning," *Brit. Med. J., Suppl.,* April 4, 1959, pp. 124-26; Thomas McKeoun, "Fundamental Problems of Hospital Planning," *Brit. Med. J., Suppl.,* April 4, 1959, pp. 122-24.

CHAPTER XII

1. T. Atkin, "The Lotus-Eaters, or Stress, Neurosis and Tranquillizers," *Brit. Med. J.,* December 26, 1959, p. 1477.

2. *Report of the Working Party on Social Workers in the Local Authority Health and Welfare Services* ["Younghusband Report"] (London: Her Majesty's Stationery Office, 1959), p. 56; *Report of the Royal Commission on the Law Relating to Mental Illness and Mental Deficiency, 1954-1957* ["Newcastle Report"] (London: Her Majesty's Stationery Office, 1957), pp. 309-10.

3. "Bradbeer Report," p. 34.

4. *Report of the Ministry of Health, 1958,* Part I, pp. 22-23; "Newcastle Report," pp. 16-17, 205-6.

5. "Newcastle Report," pp. 16 ff.; *N.H.S. Note, No. 11*, December, 1956, pp. 1-2.

6. G. M. Carstairs and J. K. Wing, "Attitudes of the General Public to Mental Illness," *Brit. Med. J.*, September 6, 1958, p. 594.

7. *Annual Report of the Board of Control to the Lord Chancellor for the Year 1958* (London: Her Majesty's Stationery Office, 1959), pp. 3-4; *Report of the Ministry of Health, 1958*, Part I, pp. 23-28, 275, 292, *1958*, Part II, pp. 123-124, *1959*, Part I, p. 24, 236, and *1959*, Part II, pp. 127-29.

8. *Report of the Ministry of Health, 1952*, Part I, pp. 131, 139, *1958*, pp. 278-83, *1959*, p. 219, and *1960*, pp. 188, 192-93; *N.H.S. Note: Summary of Main Figures, 1949-60*, pp. 7-8.

9. *Report of the Ministry of Health, 1958*, Part I, pp. 27, 275.

10. *Ibid.*, pp. 24-25; *1958*, Part II, p. 123; *1959*, Part I, p. 26.

11. *Report of the Nuffield Provincial Hospitals Trust, 1955-58*, pp. 31-32; Nesta M. Roberts, "Treatment of Mentally Ill: Keeping Patients Out of Hospital," *Manchester Guardian*, June 11, 1959.

12. *Manchester Guardian*, November 10, 1956, and March 11, 1958; *The Guardian*, November 25, 1959; Alexander Kennedy, "Provisions for the Mentally Ill," in "N.H.S. Supplement," *The Times* (London), July 7, 1958, p. xiii; *Report of the Ministry of Health, 1953*, Part I, p. 14, and *1959*, p. 27; *Annual Report of King Edward's Hospital Fund for London, 1955*, pp. 8-11.

13. *Annual Report of King Edward's Hospital Fund for London, 1955*, pp. 45-46; *Manchester Guardian*, September 17, 1956; *The Economist*, Vol. 181 (1956), 869; *Report of the Ministry of Health, 1958*, Part I, p. 27.

14. *Report of the Ministry of Health, 1958*, Part I, pp. 23-24, and *1959*, Part II, pp. 136-42; By a Medical Officer, "Therapeutic Community," *Manchester Guardian*, June 12, 1956, and January 28, 29, 1959; *The Guardian*, November 25, 1959; *Brit. Med. J.*, November 8, 1958, pp. 1150-51.

15. *Hansard*, H. of C., Vol. 592 (1958), col. 1479.

16. David Sherret, "Impact of New Methods of Treatment in a Provincial Mental Hospital," *Brit. Med. J.*, April 26, 1958, pp. 994-96. Although it took place in Scotland, this experiment is no different from others in England, but it points up more graphically what can be achieved in 18 months.

17. *Manchester Guardian*, September 12, 1956; *Report of the Ministry of Health, 1958*, Part I, p. 29, and *1959*, Part II, pp. 131-34, 140-42.

18. "Newcastle Report," pp. 213-14.

19. *Report of the Ministry of Health, 1958*, Part II, pp. 124-25; *1959*, p. 131.

20. *Ibid.*, *1957*, pp. 223-26.

21. *The Lancet*, April 12, 1958, p. 791.

22. *Report of the Nuffield Provincial Hospitals Trust, 1955-58*, pp. 27-35.

23. *Annual Report of King Edward's Hospital Fund for London, 1957*, pp. 11-13, and *1958*, pp. 16-19; *Report of the Ministry of Health, 1958*, Part I, pp. 26-27.

24. *Report of the Ministry of Health, 1958*, Part II, pp. 125-26; *Medical World Newsletter*, May, 1959, p. 21; *Manchester Guardian*, August 22, 1959; *The Guardian*, October 3, 1959; *Report of the Central Health Services Council, 1956*, p. 11.

25. *Report of the Central Health Services Council, 1956*, p. 8.

26. *Report of the Ministry of Health, 1958*, Part II, p. 127; *Manchester Guardian*, April 15, 1958, and June 12, 1959.

27. *Manchester Guardian*, June 11, 1959; *Report of the Ministry of Health, 1958*, Part II, pp. 126-27.

28. *Report of the Ministry of Health, 1958*, Part II, p. 130, *1959*, Part II, pp. 140-41, *1958*, Part I, pp. 171-72, and *1960*, Part I, p. 2; "Newcastle Report," pp. 219-20, 226.

29. *Report of the Ministry of Health, 1958*, Part I, pp. 172, 281, and Part II, p. 128; *Manchester Guardian*, June 12, 1959.

30. "Newcastle Report," pp. 214-18; *Report of the Ministry of Health, 1958*, Part I, p. 174, and Part II, pp. 238-40.

31. *Manchester Guardian*, January 27, 1959; *Brit. Med. J.*, February 14, 1959, p. 448.

32. *Report of the Ministry of Health, 1955,* Part I, pp. 17, 31-32, and *1958,* pp. 172-73; "Younghusband Report," pp. 303-6.

33. "Newcastle Report," pp. 16-20.

34. *Manchester Guardian,* May 6, 1959; *N.H.S. Note, 11A: Mental Services,* October, 1959, p. 3.

35. *N.H.S. Note, 11A: Mental Services,* October, 1959, pp. 3-4.

36. "Newcastle Report," pp. 7 ff.

37. *Brit. Med. J.,* December 20, 1958, p. 1540; *Manchester Guardian,* May 2, 20, 1957, July 9, November 2, December 17, 1957, May 2, 1958, and April 28, 1959.

38. *Manchester Guardian,* January 17, 1958; *Brit. Med. J.,* January 3, 1959, p. 57; *N.H.S. Note, 11A: Mental Health Services,* October, 1959, pp. 3-4; *Report of the Ministry of Health, 1958,* Part I, p. 29.

39. *Mental Health Act, 1959* [7 & 8 Eliz. 2, Ch. 72] (London: Her Majesty's Stationery Office, 1959), pp. 1-3, 12-13, 15 ff., 102.

CHAPTER XIII

1. *Report of the Ministry of Health, 1958,* Part I, pp. 43-45.

2. *Ibid.,* pp. 43-44; *Sixth Report From the Select Committee on Estimates, 1956-57: Running Costs of Hospitals,* p. 385.

3. *Royal Commission on Doctors' and Dentists' Remuneration, Minutes of Evidence,* 21, p. 1096, and *Written Evidence,* I, pp. 19-20; "Pilkington Report," p. 72; *Brit. Med. J., Suppl.,* April 11, 1959, p. 144.

4. *Sixth Report From the Select Committee on Estimates, 1956-57: Running Costs of Hospitals,* p. 386; *Report of the Ministry of Health, 1958,* Part I, p. 44; *Brit. Med. J.,* January 3, 1959, p. 57.

5. Fry, pp. 124-25; *The Lancet,* June 1, 1957, p. 1135; *Hansard,* H. of C., Vol. 592 (1958), col. 1485; *Sixth Report From the Select Committee on Estimates, 1956-57: Running Costs of Hospitals,* pp. 290-91, 328-29.

6. *Sixth Report From the Select Committee on Estimates, 1956-57: Running Costs of Hospitals,* pp. xiv, 219, 268, 291, 394-97; "Walker Report," *Brit. Med. J., Suppl.,* September 26, 1953, pp. 146-47.

7. *Fifth Special Report From the Select Committee on Estimates, 1958-59: Running Costs of Hospitals,* pp. vii, 8-9; *Sixth Report From the Select Committee on Estimates, 1956-57: Running Costs of Hospitals,* p. 348.

8. *Report of the Ministry of Health, 1960,* Part I, pp. 182, 184.

9. Fry, "A General Practitioner's Views of Hospital Planning," *Brit. Med. J., Suppl.,* April 4, 1959, p. 124.

10. D. Reid Ross, p. 131.

11. *Report of the Ministry of Health, 1958,* Part I, pp. 17-18; *1960,* p. 188.

12. Charles R. McCash, "Plastic Surgery in the N.H.S.," *Medical World,* October, 1957, pp. 303-14.

13. *National Health Service: The Development of Consultant Services* (London: His Majesty's Stationery Office, 1950), pp. 20-21; *Memorandum to the Committee of Inquiry Into the Cost of the N.H.S.* (London: British Dental Association, 1953), pp. 8-9; *Report of the Ministry of Health, 1958,* Part II, pp. 169-70, *1959,* Part I, p. 222, and *1959,* Part II, pp. 187-88.

14. Bruce Cardew and H. M. C. Macaulay, "Are Our Hospital Casualty Services Adequate to Our Present Needs?," *Medical World Newsletter,* February, 1957, pp. 4-5.

15. "Guillebaud Report," p. 173; *Sixth Report From the Select Committee on Estimates, 1956-57: Running Costs of Hospitals,* p. xvi; D. Reid Ross, p. 131.

16. G. E. Godber, "The Scope For Home Care in the National Health Service," *The Practitioner,* Vol. 177 (1956), 5-6.

17. *Report of the Ministry of Health, 1954,* Part I, pp. 27-28, and *1956,* p. 30; "Annual Report of the Council," *Brit. Med. J., Suppl.,* April 7, 1956, p. 132; *Manchester Guardian,* June 11, 1955.

18. *Out-Patient Waiting Time* (London: Her Majesty's Stationery Office, 1958), pp. 3-9.

19. *Chest Clinics* (London: Her Majesty's Stationery Office, 1959), pp. 4-8.

20. *Report of the Ministry of Health, 1955*, Part I, p. 30; *Manchester Guardian*, February 3, 1958.

21. *Brit. Med. J.*, July 12, 1958, p. 112.

22. Ffrangcon Roberts, *The Cost of Health*, pp. 171-72.

23. *Royal Commission on Doctors' and Dentists' Remuneration, Minutes of Evidence*, 16-17, p. 870; *Brit. Med. J., Suppl.*, January 4, 1958, pp. 6-7.

24. H. G. McGregor, "Training of Consultants Under the N.H.S.: A Survey Made in the S.E. Metropolitan Region," *Brit. Med. J., Suppl.*, October 20, 1956, pp. 159-60.

25. "Pilkington Report," pp. 88-91; *Royal Commission on Doctors' and Dentists' Remuneration, Minutes of Evidence*, 14-15, p. 708; *Report of the Ministry of Health, 1958*, Part I, pp. 57-58.

26. *Brit. Med. J., Suppl.*, January 25, 1958, p. 29; *Manchester Guardian*, January 18, 21, 23, 25, February 7, 1958; "Pilkington Report," p. 56.

27. "Pilkington Report," pp. 84-95; *Royal Commission on Doctors' and Dentists' Remuneration, Minutes of Evidence*, 14-15, p. 708, and *Written Evidence*, I, pp. 2-4; *Report of the Ministry of Health, 1958*, Part I, p. 277; *The Lancet*, June 1, 1957, p. 1135.

28. "Willink Report," pp. 14-15.

29. *The Times* (London), October 7, 1958; *Manchester Guardian*, February 3, 1958; *The Guardian*, February 2, 1960; *Brit. Med. J., Suppl.*, May 10, 1958, p. 244.

30. *Report of the Ministry of Health, 1958*, Part I, pp. 58-59, and *1960*, pp. 29-30; "Pilkington Report," pp. 58, 86.

31. *Brit. Med. J.*, May 16, 1959, p. 1308, and *Suppl.*, June 6, 1959, p. 257; *Manchester Guardian*, May 27, 1959.

32. *Manchester Guardian*, December 14, 1957, December 8, 1958, and March 6, May 5, 8, 21, 27, 1959; *Brit. Med. J.*, March 14, 1959, pp. 702-3, 727, May 23, 1959, pp. 1355-56, June 6, 1959, p. 1465, and *Suppl.*, April 11, 1959, p. 143.

33. *Report of the Ministry of Health, 1959*, Part I, p. 221; *Royal Commission on Doctors' and Dentists' Remuneration, Minutes of Evidence*, 21, pp. 1133-34, and *Written Evidence*, I, pp. 24-25.

34. *Brit. Med. J., Suppl.*, June 14, 1958, p. 312; *N.H.S. Note, No. 12A*, January, 1959, pp. 1-6; "Pilkington Report," pp. 60, 69-70.

35. Abel-Smith and Titmuss, pp. 125-28.

36. *Hansard*, H. of C., Vol. 592 (1958), col. 1483.

37. *Ibid.*, col. 1554; *The New Statesman and Nation*, Vol. 46 (1953), p. 812; "Pilkington Report," p. 70; "Guillebaud Report," pp. 142-43.

38. "Guillebaud Report," p. 144; "Pilkington Report," pp. 70-72.

39. "Pilkington Report," pp. 61-62, 71; *Brit. Med. J., Suppl.*, January 4, 1958, p. 8; "Guillebaud Report," p. 143.

40. *Report of the Inter-Departmental Committee on the Remuneration of Consultants and Specialists* ["Spens Report on the Remuneration of Consultants"] (London: His Majesty's Stationery Office, 1948), pp. 1 ff.

41. *Royal Commission on Doctors' and Dentists' Remuneration, Written Evidence*, I, pp. 10-11, 66.

42. *Manchester Guardian*, April 17, 1957, and December 24, 1958; *Brit. Med J., Suppl.*, February 13, 1960, p. 49, and April 23, 1960, pp. 232-38.

43. "Pilkington Report," pp. 30, 40, 54.

44. *Ibid.*, pp. 69 ff., 102-3, 138-39.

45. *Royal Commission on Doctors' and Dentists' Remuneration, Minutes of Evidence*, 2, p. 63, and 21, p. 1099; *Medical World Newsletter*, January, 1958, p. 7; *Superannuation Scheme for Those Engaged in the N.H.S.*, 1952, pp. 5-6; *Brit. Med. J., Suppl.*, May 3, 1958, pp. 226-27.

46. "Pilkington Report," pp. 73-78; *Report of the Ministry of Health, 1960*, Part I, p. 144; *Brit. Med. J.*, February 21, 1959, pp. 517-18, and April 16, 1960, p. 1215.

47. *Brit. Med. J.*, July 12, 1958, p. 112.

48. "Proceedings of the Annual Representative Meeting," *Brit. Med. J., Suppl.*, July 20, 1957, p. 49.

49. *Ibid.*, January 4, 1958, p. 8; "Pilkington Report," pp. 81-82.

50. "Pilkington Report," p. 81; "Proceedings of the Annual Representative Meeting," *Brit. Med. J., Suppl.*, July 20, 1957, pp. 48-49; "Annual Report of the Council," *Brit. Med. J., Suppl.*, April 13, 1957, p. 175.

51. *Civil Estimates for the Year Ending 31st March, 1961, Class V*, p. 106; *Report of the Ministry of Health, 1958*, Part I, pp. 288-89, and *1959*, pp. 234-35.

52. "Annual Report of the Council," *Brit. Med. J., Suppl.*, April 13, 1957, p. 173, and April 11, 1959, p. 145; *The Guardian*, December 16, 1959; *Civil Estimates for the Year Ending 31st March, 1961, Class V*, pp. 107-9.

53. Sir Zachary Cope, "Ancillary Services," in "N.H.S. Supplement," *The Times* (London), July 7, 1958, p. xxii; *Brit. Med. J.*, December 5, 1959, p. 1264; June 4, 1960, p. 1745; *Medical World Newsletter*, January, 1960, pp. 13, 15; *Report of the Ministry of Health, 1960*, Part I, pp. 134-35.

54. *N.H.S. Note: Summary of Main Figures in England and Wales, 1949-1958*, pp. 3-5.

55. *Accounts 1958-59*, pp. 15-16, 29-30.

56. *Report of the Ministry of Health, 1958*, Part I, pp. 60, 64-68.

57. *Ibid.*, pp. 69-70; *Annual Report of King Edward's Hospital Fund for London, 1958*, pp. 31-32.

58. *The Work of Nurses in Hospital Wards: Report of a Job-Analysis* (London: The Nuffield Provincial Hospitals Trust, 1954), pp. 35-37, 151-53.

59. *Report of the Central Health Services Council, 1958*, pp. 4-5.

60. *Report of the Ministry of Health, 1958*, Part I, p. 60, *1958*, Part II, p. 184, and *1960*, Part I, p. 268; *Manchester Guardian*, December 12, 1958.

61. *Civil Estimates for the Year Ending 31st March, 1962, Class V*, p. 108.

62. *The Guardian*, April 26, May 7, 10, 1960.

63. *Brit. Med. J.*, Sept. 7, 1957, pp. 586-87; *Report of the Ministry of Health, 1958*, Part I, p. 60, *1958*, Part II, p. 182, *1959*, Part I, p. 47, and *1960*, Part I, p. 194; *Report by the Standing Nursing Advisory Committee on the Position of the Enrolled Assistant Nurse Within the National Health Service* (London: Her Majesty's Stationery Office, 1954), pp. 3-4.

64. *Report of the Ministry of Health, 1958*, Part I, pp. 68-69, and Part II, pp. 175-76, 182, 187; *Manchester Guardian*, March 4, 1957; Muriel M. Edwards, "Prestige and Popularity of Nursing," in "N.H.S. Supplement," *The Times* (London), July 7, 1958, pp. viii-ix.

65. *Annual Report of King Edward's Hospital Fund for London, 1956*, pp. 35-38, and *1958*, pp. 35-38; *Report of the Ministry of Health, 1958*, Part II, p. 176.

66. *Report of the Ministry of Health, 1958*, Part II, p. 183.

67. Stephen J. Hadfield, *Law and Ethics For Doctors* (London: Eyre and Spottiswoode, 1958), pp. 116 ff.; T. Lloyd Hughes, "Medico-Legal Problems Arising in the National Health Service," *Medico-Legal Journal*, Vol. 21 (1953), 18-21; A. E. Telling, "Professional Freedom and Responsibility Under the National Health Service," *The Lancet*, August 4, 1956, pp. 242-44.

68. "Proceedings of the Annual Representative Meeting," *Brit. Med. J., Suppl.*, July 14, 1956, pp. 48-49; *Manchester Guardian*, June 18, 1956.

69. *Report of the Ministry of Health, 1954*, Part I, pp. 29-30; Hughes, pp. 22-23.

70. Hadfield, p. 120; Rose Heilbron, "When is a Doctor Negligent?," *Brit. Med. J.*, December 28, 1957, pp. 1540-41.

71. *Brit. Med. J.*, August 16, 1958, p. 456; November 29, 1958, p. 1363.

72. *Ibid.*, December 27, 1958, p. 1599; *Report of the Ministry of Health, 1954*, Part I, p. 29.

73. Titmuss, *Essays on 'The Welfare State'*, pp. 122-32.

74. "Guillebaud Report," p. 240; *Annual Report of King Edward's Hospital Fund for London, 1957*, p. 5.

75. *Annual Report of King Edward's Hospital Fund for London, 1956*, p. 20.

76. *Manchester Guardian,* October 5, 1956.
77. *The Reception and Welfare of In-Patients in Hospitals* (London: Her Majesty's Stationery Office, 1953), pp. 1 ff.
78. *Report of the Ministry of Health, 1954,* Part I, pp. 25-26.
79. *Ibid., 1953,* Part I, p. 31, and *1956,* p. 33; Titmuss, p. 121; *Annual Report of King Edward's Hospital Fund for London, 1955,* p. 45, and *1956,* pp. 52-57.
80. *Annual Report of King Edward's Hospital Fund for London, 1958,* p. 14; Cecily Statham, "Noise and the Patient in Hospital," *Brit. Med. J.,* December 5, 1959, pp. 1247-48, and December 26, 1959, p. 1492; *Manchester Guardian,* June 12, 1959; *Report of the Ministry of Health, 1954,* Part I, p. 25; *The Reception and Welfare of In-Patients in Hospitals,* p. 19.
81. *The Welfare of Children in Hospital* ["Platt Report"] (London: Her Majesty's Stationery Office, 1959), pp. 1 ff.; *Brit. Med. J.,* January 17, 1959, pp. 166-69; *Report of the Ministry of Health, 1960,* Part I, p. 50.
82. *Manchester Guardian,* September 13, 1956.
83. *Ibid.,* April 19, 1955; *Voluntary Service and the State: A Study of the Needs of the Hospital Service,* pp. 72-73; "Guillebaud Report," p. 135.
84. "Guillebaud Report," pp. 135-36; *Report of the Ministry of Health, 1955,* Part I, pp. 31-32; Sir John Wolfenden, "The Contribution of Voluntary Service," in "N.H.S. Supplement," *The Times* (London), July 7, 1958, p. xix; *Annual Report of King Edward's Hospital Fund for London, 1954,* pp. 5-7, and *1956,* p. 18.
85. Abel-Smith and Titmuss, pp. 149-52.
86. *The Guardian,* April 8, 1960; *Manchester Guardian,* July 9, 1959.
87. *The New Statesman and Nation,* Vol. 43 (1952), 5; Vol. 50 (1955), 327.
88. *Manchester Guardian,* August 9, November 5, 1958.
89. *Ibid.,* January 11, 1958.
90. *Ibid.,* October 8, 1954.

CHAPTER XIV

1. "Guillebaud Report," pp. 199-200.
2. Kenneth H. Cowan, *Report of the Medical Officer of Health* [of the Administrative County of Essex], *1952* (Chelmsford: John Dutton, Ltd., 1953), pp. 62-67.
3. George G. Stewart, *The Essex County Health Handbook* (Cheltenham and London: Edward J. Burrow and Co., 1956), p. 46; "Guillebaud Report," p. 198.
4. *Brit. Med. J., Suppl.,* April 25, 1959, p. 190.
5. *Brit. Med. J.,* June 20, 1959, pp. 1581-82.
6. *N.H.S. Note: Expenditure for 1958-59,* February, 1959, p. 4; *Report of the Ministry of Health, 1958,* Part I, p. 200, *1959,* p. 150, and *1960,* p. 251.
7. *Report of the Ministry of Health, 1959,* Part I, pp. 144-45, *1958,* pp. 189-91, and *1960,* pp. 108, 250; *N.H.S. Note: Summary of Main Figures, 1949-60,* pp. 17-18.
8. *Ambulance Services Costing Return, 1951-1952* (London: Her Majesty's Stationery Office, 1953), pp. 1 ff.; *Report of the Ministry of Health, 1955,* Part I, p. 106.
9. *Report of the Ministry of Health, 1958,* Part I, pp. 190-99, *1959,* pp. 144-45, and *1960,* pp. 108, 250; *N.H.S. Note,* April 9, 1956; Stewart, pp. 33-34; "N.H.S. Supplement," *The Times* (London), July 7, 1958, p. xxiii.
10. Mestitz, p. 1109.
11. "Guillebaud Report," pp. 219-23; *Report of the Ministry of Health, 1958,* Part I, pp. 193-94.
12. *Report of the Ministry of Health, 1958,* Part I, pp. 163-67, *1955,* p. 95, *1959,* pp. 133-34, and *1960,* p. 249; C. Metcalfe Brown, "The Domiciliary Services Available to the Family Doctor," *The Practitioner,* Vol. 177 (1956), 48-49; *An Inquiry Into Health Visiting* ["Jameson Report"] (London: Her Majesty's Stationery Office, 1956), pp. 1-6, 103 ff., 134.
13. "Jameson Report," pp. 103-5; Stewart, pp. 30-31.
14. "Jameson Report," pp. 105-15; "Younghusband Report," p. 95.
15. *Report of the Ministry of Health, 1958,* Part I, p. 165; "Jameson Report," pp. 131-39.

16. "Jameson Report," pp. 144-56.

17. *Manchester Guardian,* October 10, 1959.

18. "Proceedings of the Annual Representative Meeting," *Brit. Med. J., Suppl.,* July 14, 1956, p. 22, and July 20, 1957, p. 33.

19. "Jameson Report," pp. 15-18, 36-38.

20. *Report of the Ministry of Health, 1958,* Part I, p. 156, *1959,* p. 127, and *1960,* p. 247.

21. *Brit. Med. J., Suppl.,* December 12, 1959, p. 192; *The Guardian,* November 2, 1959, and April 26, 1960.

22. *The Guardian,* January 22, 1960; *Report of the Ministry of Health, 1958,* Part I, pp. 156-59, *1959,* p. 125, and *1960,* p. 105.

23. *Report of the Ministry of Health, 1953,* Part I, pp. 124-25, *1956,* pp. 91-92, and *1958,* pp. 157-58, 160; *Manchester Guardian,* August 15, 1957; Stewart, p. 32.

24. Stewart, pp. 36-37; *Report of the Ministry of Health, 1953,* Part I, p. 127, *1958,* pp. 160-61, *1959,* pp. 129-30, 162, and *1960,* pp. 105-7, 248; "Younghusband Report," pp. 57-58, 128, 130-31.

25. "Younghusband Report," pp. 129-31, 162-63; *Manchester Guardian,* August 17, 1956; *Report of the Ministry of Health, 1953,* Part I, p. 129, *1955,* pp. 92-93, 100, *1958,* pp. 162-63, and *1959,* pp. 129-30.

26. *Report of the Ministry of Health, 1953,* Part I, pp. 109-11, *1956,* p. 87, *1958,* pp. 146-48, *1959,* pp. 121-22, and *1960,* pp. 101-2.

27. *Ibid., 1958,* p. 149, and *1959,* p. 273; *N.H.S. Note: Summary of Main Figures, 1949-60,* pp. 11-12

28. "Guillebaud Report," p. 213; "Cranbrook Report," pp. 44-45.

29. "Cranbrook Report," pp. 40-43; *Report of the Ministry of Health, 1959,* Part I, p. 122, and *1960,* p. 102.

30. *Report of the Ministry of Health, 1958,* Part I, p. 149; *N.H.S. Note: Summary of Main Figures, 1949-60,* pp. 11-12.

31. "Cranbrook Report," pp. 44-45.

32. *Report of the Ministry of Health, 1958,* Part I, pp. 149-50, *1959,* pp. 121, 274, and *1960,* pp. 101, 244.

33. J. T. A. George, C. R. Lowe, and Thomas McKeoun, "An Examination of the Work of Local Authority Child Welfare Clinics," *The Lancet,* January 8, 1953, pp. 88-92.

34. Effective June 1, 1961, orange juice, cod liver oil, and vitamin tablets were made subject to a charge sufficient to recover cost.

35. *Report of the Joint Sub-Committee on Welfare Foods* (London: Her Majesty's Stationery Office, 1957), pp. 5-6, 23-24.

36. *Report of the Ministry of Health, 1956,* Part I, pp. 88, 143-44, *1957,* pp. 144-47, *1958,* pp. 150, 255-58, and *1959,* pp. 121, 196-200.

37. *Manchester Guardian,* April 21, 1958.

38. "Cranbrook Report," pp. 45-56; *The Times* (London), February 6, 1961; *Report of the Ministry of Health, 1952,* Part I, pp. 83-84, *1953,* pp. 118-20, *1955,* p. 168, *1958,* pp. 151-53, and *1959,* p. 121.

39. *Report of the Ministry of Health, 1953,* Part I, pp. 120-22, *1955,* pp. 89-90, *1958,* pp. 153-55, *1959,* pp. 125-26, and *1960,* pp. 104, 246-47; *N.H.S. Note: Summary of Main Figures, 1949-59,* p. 6.

40. "Health of the School Children," *Nature,* Vol. 170 (1952), 111; *Manchester Guardian,* January 20, 1959; Stewart, pp. 27-28; J. A. H. Lee, "The Effectiveness of Routine Examination of School Children," *Brit. Med. J.,* March 8, 1958, pp. 575-76; "Annual Report of the Council," *Brit. Med. J., Suppl.,* April 7, 1956, pp. 136-37.

41. "Guillebaud Report," pp. 202-7.

42. G. L. C. Elliston, "A Better Health Service," *The Spectator,* Vol. 190 (1953), 409.

43. *Manchester Guardian,* May 29, 1958.

44. "Draft Definitive Policy Statement, No. 2, 1955," pp. 1-2.

45. "Annual Report of the Council," *Brit. Med. J., Suppl.,* April 13, 1957, pp. 170-71.

46. *Manchester Guardian*, April 3, 1957.

47. *The Guardian*, March 25, 1960; *Report of the Ministry of Health, 1958*, Part I, pp. 177-81, 334-35.

48. *Report of the Ministry of Health, 1958*, Part I, pp. 169-70; *1959*, pp. 137-38.

49. *Ibid., 1958*, pp. 175-76, *1959*, pp. 141-43, and *1960*, p. 240; *Report of the Central Health Services Council, 1955*, pp. 27-28, and *1956*, pp. 2, 12-13; *The Registrar General's Quarterly Return for England and Wales: Births, Deaths and Marriages, etc.: Quarter ended 31st December, 1959* (London: Her Majesty's Stationery Office, 1960), p. 14.

50. *Medical World Newsletter*, June, 1959, p. 26; *Hansard*, H. of C., Vol. 596 (1958), cols. 23-24; *Manchester Guardian*, April 22, May 2, 1958, and April 28, 29, 1959; *The Guardian*, January 2, 1960; *Brit. Med. J.*, April 26, 1958, pp. 1010-11, May 10, 1958, pp. 1114-15, 1117-18, May 16, 1959, p. 1307, April 9, 1960, p. 1141, and May 14, 1960, p. 1513.

51. *Report of the Central Health Services Council, 1955*, pp. 29-30, and *1956*, p. 3; *Report of the Ministry of Health, 1958*, Part I, pp. 181, 186, *1958*, Part II, p. 113, and *1960*, Part I, p. 99.

52. Malcolm Donaldson, "Early Diagnosis of Cancer: A Psychological Problem," *The Lancet*, October 11, 1958, p. 790; Jean Atken-Swan and Ralson Paterson, "Assessment of the Results of Five Years of Cancer Education," *Brit. Med. J.*, March 14, 1959, pp. 708-12; *Manchester Guardian*, January 25, April 27, 1957.

53. *Report of the Ministry of Health, 1958*, Part I, pp. 181-83, 185, 334-35, and *1959*, p. 139; *Medical World Newsletter*, June, 1959, p. 23.

54. *Report of the Ministry of Health, 1958*, Part I, pp. 167-68, 238, and *1959*, p. 137; *The Registrar General's Quarterly Return for England and Wales: Births, Deaths and Marriages, etc.: Quarter Ended 31st December, 1959*, p. 24.

55. Routledge and Kegan Paul, *The Family Life of Old People: An Inquiry in East London*, quoted in *Manchester Guardian*, October 28, 1957.

56. "Younghusband Report," pp. 60, 134-35; *Residential Accommodation For Old People, Homes for the More Infirm* [Circular] (London: Her Majesty's Stationery Office, 1955), pp. 1-2; *Report of the Ministry of Health, 1955*, Part I, p. 133, *1958*, pp. 238-41, *1959*, pp. 183-85, and *1960*, pp. 110-12.

57. *The Guardian*, April 2, 1960.

58. *Report of the Committee on the Economic and Financial Problems of the Provision for Old Age* ["Phillips Report"] (London: Her Majesty's Stationery Office, 1954), p. 72; *Manchester Guardian*, October 17, 1958; *The Guardian*, January 20, March 21, 1960; *Report of the Ministry of Health, 1958*, Part I, p. 247, and *1959*, pp. 184, 192-93.

59. *Report of the Ministry of Health, 1956*, Part I, p. 140, and *1959*, p. 193; "Younghusband Report," p. 60; *Manchester Guardian*, September 13, 1957.

60. *Manchester Guardian*, February 7, May 10, July 4, 1957, April 18, 1958, and September 1, 1959; Boucher, p. 41; *Report of the Ministry of Health, 1959*, Part I, p. 193.

61. *Report of the Ministry of Health, 1960*, Part I, p. 98; *Medical World Newsletter*, May, 1959, p. 7, and May, 1960, p. 19; *Brit. Med. J.*, March 7, 1959, p. 655, May 9, 1959, p. 1250, and *Suppl.*, August 30, 1958, p. 129, and May 30, 1959, p. 230; Boucher, pp. 44-45.

62. A. Elliott, "The Family Help and Night Attendant Services in Kent," *The Practitioner*, Vol. 177 (1956), 38.

63. H. D. Chalke, "The Aged in Their Own Homes: A Further Study," *Brit. Med. J.*, September 21, 1957, pp. 694-96.

64. *Hansard*, H. of C., Vol. 578 (1957), cols. 1460 ff.

65. *Report on Co-operation Between Hospital, Local Authority and General Practitioner Services*, pp. 8-15, 31-32.

66. *Ibid.*, pp. 20-24.

67. "Guillebaud Report," pp. 236-38.

68. "Cohen Report," pp. 45-46.

CHAPTER XV

1. *Report of the Committee on Recruitment to the Dental Profession* ["McNair Report"] (London: Her Majesty's Stationery Office, 1956), p. 5.

2. *Ibid.*, pp. 5-6, 25-27; "Pilkington Report," pp. 125, 129, 264; Stewart, pp. 16-17; *National Health Service (General Dental Services) Regulations, 1954,* No. 742 (London: Her Majesty's Stationery Office, 1954), pp. 4 ff.; *N.H.S. Note, No. 5: The Dental Services,* November, 1952, pp. 1-3.

3. "McNair Report," pp. 47-48; *Manchester Guardian,* February 7, 1958; *Report of the Ministry of Health, 1956,* Part I, pp. 72-73, *1958,* pp. 116-17, and *1959,* pp. 86, 94; "Guillebaud Report," p. 177.

4. "Guillebaud Report," pp. 183-84; "McNair Report," pp. 48-49.

5. *British Dental Journal,* Vol. 104 (1958), 331, and Vol. 108 (1960), 39, 65; *Report of the Ministry of Health, 1956,* Part I, pp. 65-66, and *1959,* p. 93.

6. *Report of the London Executive Council, 1954-55,* p. 25; *1959-60,* p. 34.

7. *Report of the Ministry of Health, 1959,* Part I, p. 93; *National Health Service (Service Committees and Tribunal) Regulations,* No. 1077 (London: Her Majesty's Stationery Office, 1956), p. 23.

8. *National Health Service (Service Committees and Tribunal) Regulations, 1956,* No. 1077, pp. 4 ff.; *Report of the Ministry of Health, 1952,* Part I, p. 178, *1953,* p. 107, *1954,* p. 208, *1956,* p. 209, *1959,* pp. 117, 268, and *1960,* p. 237.

9. *The Times* (London), September 28, 1949, p. 6.

10. *Manchester Guardian,* June 22, 1954.

11. *Ibid.,* August 22, 1956; *The Times* (London), July 4, 1949.

12. *Manchester Guardian,* September 12, 1957, and January 3, September 26, 1958; *The Guardian,* September 25, 1959.

13. *Manchester Guardian,* March 28, 1957.

14. *Report of the Ministry of Health, 1959,* Part I, p. 268.

15. *N.H.S. Note: Summary of Main Figures, 1949-60,* pp. 3-4.

16. *Report of the Ministry of Health, 1953,* Part I, p. 82, *1956,* p. 217, and *1959,* pp. 91-92, 265; *British Dental Journal,* Vol. 108 (1960), 136.

17. *Final Report of the Inter-Departmental Committee on Dentistry* ["Teviot Report"] (London: His Majesty's Stationery Office, 1946), pp. 4-8, 11-12.

18. *Memorandum to the Committee of Enquiry Into the Shortage of Recruits to the Dental Profession* (London: British Dental Association, 1955), pp. 4-6; *Report of the Ministry of Health, 1953,* Part I, pp. 83-84.

19. "McNair Report," pp. 10-24, 28-34.

20. *British Dental Journal,* Vol. 104 (1958), 331-32, and Vol. 105 (1958), 219-20; *Report of the Ministry of Health, 1956,* Part I, p. 70, *1958,* p. 115, and *1959,* p. 92; *Manchester Guardian,* March 9, 1957; *Hansard,* H. of C., Vol. 596 (1958), col. 19.

21. *Hansard,* H. of C., Vol. 596 (1958), col. 64; *British Dental Journal,* Vol. 104 (1958), 292, Vol. 105 (1958), 219-20, and Vol. 108 (1960), 271, 365, 379; *The Guardian,* November 10, 1959.

22. *Memorandum to the Committee of Enquiry Into the Shortage of Recruits to the Dental Profession,* p. 5.

23. *British Dental Journal,* Vol. 104 (1958), 292, and Vol. 108 (1960), 94, 403; *Report of the Ministry of Health, 1959,* Part I, p. 95.

24. *Report of the Ministry of Health, 1955,* Part I, p. 65.

25. "Teviot Report," p. 37; "McNair Report," pp. 35-36; "Guillebaud Report," pp. 182-83.

26. *Memorandum to the Committee of Enquiry Into the Cost of the National Health Service,* p. 7.

27. "From an Address of the Minister of Health to the Executive Councils' Association at Torquay, October 8, 1953," pp. 1-2; *British Dental Journal,* Vol. 104 (1958), 408, and Vol. 108 (1960), 401.

28. *Report of the Central Health Services Council, 1954,* p. 14; *Report of the Ministry of Health, 1955,* Part I, p. 72, *1958,* p. 109, and *1960,* p. 232.

29. *British Dental Journal,* Vol. 107 (1959), 48, 74; Vol. 108 (1960), 137.

30. *Address by Iain N. Macleod, Minister of Health, at the Seventh Annual Conference of the Executive Councils' Association held at Southport on the 14th and 15th October, 1954,* pp. 6-7.

31. *Royal Commission on Doctors' and Dentists' Remuneration: Minutes of Evidence,* 12-13, pp. 581-82, 635; 8, pp. 372-73.

32. "Spens Report on Remuneration of General Dental Practitioners," pp. 4-11.

33. *Royal Commission on Doctors' and Dentists' Remuneration, Minutes of Evidence,* 12-13, pp. 598-604, and *Written Evidence,* I, pp. 50-53; *British Dental Journal,* Vol. 87 (1949), 15, and Vol. 104 (1958), 321-22; "Guillebaud Report," p. 176; *The Times* (London), December 6, 1948, and May 20, 1949.

34. *The Times* (London), May 20, 1949.

35. Letter from S. Donald Cox, Assistant Secretary of the B.D.A., *The New Statesman and Nation,* Vol. 37 (1949), 613.

36. *Report of the Working Party on the Chairside Times Taken in Carrying Out Treatment by General Dental Practitioners in England, Wales and Scotland* ["Penman Report"] (London: His Majesty's Stationery Office, 1949) pp. 5 ff.

37. *British Dental Journal,* Vol. 98 (1955), 329; *Manchester Guardian,* April 18, 23, 1955; *Royal Commission on Doctors' and Dentists' Remuneration, Written Evidence,* I, pp. 53-54, and *Minutes of Evidence,* 12-13, pp. 604-10.

38. *Royal Commission on Doctors' and Dentists' Remuneration, Minutes of Evidence,* 12-13, p. 599.

39. *British Dental Journal,* Vol. 102 (1957), 317, 361; *Manchester Guardian,* February 22, 1957.

40. "Pilkington Report," pp. 44, 54, 127-28, 132.

41. *Ibid.,* pp. 134-37.

42. *Ibid.,* p. 132; *British Dental Journal,* Vol. 108 (1960), 171, 233-39, 357, and Vol. 109 (1960), 105; *Report of the Ministry of Health, 1960,* Part I, p. 5.

43. *Report of the London Executive Council, 1959-60,* p. 35; *Report of the Ministry of Health, 1959,* Part, I, p. 261, and *1960,* p. 230.

44. *Report of the Ministry of Health, 1959,* Part I, pp. 86-87, 91, 259, 263-64; *1960,* pp. 77-82, 226-31.

45. *Ibid., 1958,* Part II, pp. 164-67.

46. May Mellanby, W. J. Martin, and David Barnes, "Teeth of 5-Year-Old London School Children (1957) With a Comparison of the Results Obtained From 1929 to 1957," *Brit. Med. J.,* December 13, 1958, pp. 1441-43.

47. A. T. Wynne, "The School Dental Service: Are Statistics Vital?," *British Dental Journal,* October 6, 1959, p. 169; *Manchester Guardian,* May 4, 1957.

48. *Manchester Guardian,* August 21, 1957, and November 26, 1959; *Hansard,* H. of C., Vol. 596 (1958), col. 22; *British Dental Journal,* Vol. 104 (1958), 381-82, and Vol. 107 (1959), 77, 175-78, 325-66.

49. *British Dental Journal,* Vol. 108 (1960), 136, 316-17; *Report of the Ministry of Health, 1955,* Part I, pp. 74-75, and *1958,* Part II, pp. 167-69; *Report of the Central Health Services Council, 1955,* pp. 11 ff.; *Medical World Newsletter,* October, 1958, pp. 1-2; "Proceedings of the Annual Representative Meeting," *Brit. Med. J., Suppl.,* June 25, 1960, p. 395.

50. D. Reid Ross, pp. 133-34.

CHAPTER XVI

1. *National Health Service Act, 1946,* Part IV, sec. 41.

2. Giles, pp. 68-76; *N.H.S. Note: The Supplementary Ophthalmic Services,* November, 1956, p. 1.

3. Giles, pp. 55-56; "Memorandum Submitted by the Joint Emergency Committee of the Optical Profession to the Committee of Enquiry into the Cost of the N.H.S., November, 1953," pp. 13-17; Information in a letter to the author from G. H. Giles, August 10, 1956.

4. "Guillebaud Report," pp. 187-88.

5. *N.H.S. Note: Summary of Main Figures, 1949-59*, p. 2; *Brit. Med. J.*, March 5, 1960, p. 736.

6. "Memorandum Submitted by the Joint Emergency Committee of the Optical Profession," pp. 2-3; Giles, pp. 22-24, 29, 30-33.

7. *Report of the Ministry of Health, 1958*, Part I, p. 119, *1959*, p. 97, and *1960*, pp. 86, 233; *The Times* (London), February 6, 1961.

8. The terms "optician" and "optometrist" are used interchangeably.

9. Abel-Smith and Titmuss, p. 162.

10. D. Reid Ross, p. 134.

11. Stewart, pp. 15-16; "Guillebaud Report," pp. 184-85; Giles, pp. 91-93; *National Health Service (Supplementary Ophthalmic Services) Regulations, 1948*, No. 1273 (London: Her Majesty's Stationery Office, 1948), and *1956*, No. 1078.

12. *The Guardian*, February 23, March 4, 8, 18, 1960; *N.H.S. Note: The Supplementary Ophthalmic Services*, November, 1956, pp. 1-2; *Report of the Central Health Services Council, 1957*, p. 9; *Report of the Ministry of Health, 1957*, Part I, p. 81, *1959*, p. 98, and *1960*, pp. 86-88, 234-36.

13. *Report of the Ministry of Health, 1955*, Part I, p. 220, *1958*, p. 327, *1959*, pp. 98, 268, and *1960*, p. 237; Giles, pp. 188-91.

14. *Brit. Med. J.*, March 5, 1960, pp. 736-37; *The Guardian*, February 23, 1960.

15. "Memorandum Submitted by the Joint Emergency Committee of the Optical Profession," pp. 4-7.

16. *Brit. Med. J., Suppl.*, February 7, 1959, p. 47; *Report of the Ministry of Health, 1959*, Part I, pp. 98-99.

17. *Statement Specifying the Fees and Charges for the Testing of Sight and the Supply or Repair of Glasses, Revised as From December 1, 1959* (London: Her Majesty's Stationery Office, 1959), pp. 2-3.

18. *Report of the Ministry of Health, 1960*, Part I, p. 236.

19. "Ten Years of Eye Services: A Survey," *The Dioptric News*, XIII (1958), 385, 387-89.

CHAPTER XVII

1. "Hinchliffe Report," pp. 37-39.

2. *The Pharmaceutical Journal*, Vol. 107 (1948), 431, and Vol. 119 (1954), 215; *The National Health Service Act in Great Britain: A Review of the First Year's Working*, pp. 87-88; *Report of the Ministry of Health, 1958*, Part I, p. 124; Sir Hugh Linstead, "18,000 Pharmacists Kept Busy," in "N.H.S. Supplement," *The Times* (London), July 7, 1958, p. xviii.

3. *N.H.S. Note: Summary of Main Figures, 1949-60*, pp. 1-2.

4. *National Health Service (General Medical and Pharmaceutical Services) Regulations, 1954*, No. 669, pp. 14 ff.; *N.H.S. Note: The Pharmaceutical Services*, 1956; *Report of the London Executive Council, 1959-60*, pp. 16, 37.

5. Linstead, p. xviii; *The Pharmaceutical Journal*, Vol. 119 (1954), 215.

6. *The Pharmaceutical Journal*, Vol. 107 (1948), 260, and Vol. 109 (1949), 243; *Report of the Ministry of Health, 1954*, Part I, pp. 82-83, *1955*, p. 83, and *1956*, p. 83.

7. *Report of the Ministry of Health, 1958*, Part I, p. 125, and *1959*, pp. 105-6.

8. "Hinchliffe Report," pp. 8, 57-63; "Guillebaud Report," pp. 165-66.

9. "Hinchliffe Report," pp. 107-8.

10. J. P. Martin, *Social Aspects of Prescribing* (London: William Heinemann, Ltd., 1957), pp. 105-15.

11. *N.H.S. Note: Summary of the Main Figures, 1949-59*, p. 1; *Report of the Ministry of Health, 1959*, Part I, p. 104; "Hinchliffe Report," pp. 2-3, 31-32.

12. "Hinchliffe Report," pp. 13-15, 84; *Report of the Ministry of Health, 1956*, Part I, p. 84.

13. "Guillebaud Report," pp. 159-61, 166-67; "Hinchliffe Report," p. 14; "Hinchliffe Interim Report," p. 8.

14. *Report of the Ministry of Health, 1959*, Part I, p. 112; *Report of the London Executive Council, 1959-60*, pp. 38-39.

15. "Hinchliffe Report," p. 14.

16. *Report of the Ministry of Health, 1960,* Part I, p. 225.

17. *Civil Estimates for the Year Ending 31st March, 1961, Class V,* p. 64; *N.H.S. Note: Summary of Main Current Figures,* August, 1960, pp. 1-2; *N.H.S. Note: N.H.S. Expenditures for 1949-50,* pp. 1, 4; *Hansard,* H. of C., Vol. 569 (1957), cols. 1011-41, and Vol. 583 (1958), cols. 1192-94; "Hinchliffe Report," pp. 24-40.

18. "Hinchliffe Report," pp. 15-17; *Report of the Central Health Services Council, 1958,* pp. 9-10, and *1959,* p. 3; *Report of the Standing Joint Committee on Classification of Proprietary Preparations* (London: Her Majesty's Stationery Office, 1959), pp. 3-5.

19. "Hinchliffe Report," pp. 17-18.

20. *Report of the Standing Joint Committee on Classification of Proprietary Preparations* (1960), pp. 4-10; *Brit. Med. J., Suppl.,* September 10, 1960, p. 103.

21. *Brit. Med. J., Suppl.,* September 6, 1958, p. 601, and November 22, 1958, pp. 1250-52; "Hinchliffe Report," pp. 18-19, 50-52.

22. *Report of the Ministry of Health, 1959,* Part I, p. 112, and *1960,* p. 70; "Hinchliffe Interim Report," p. 6; *Brit. Med. J., Suppl.,* April 9, 1960, p. 200.

23. "Hinchliffe Report," pp. 41-48.

24. *Sixth Report From the Select Committee on Estimates, 1956-57: Running Costs of Hospitals,* pp. xiv-xv; *Fifth Special Report From the Select Committee on Estimates, 1958-59: Running Costs of Hospitals,* pp. viii-ix.

25. "Hinchliffe Report," pp. 53-56, 90-92.

26. *Report of the Ministry of Health, 1959,* Part I, p. 115; *The Guardian,* February 6, 1960; *Brit. Med. J., Suppl.,* January 30, 1960, p. 35.

27. "Proceedings of the Annual Representative Meeting," *Brit. Med. J., Suppl.,* July 20, 1957, p. 43; "Annual Report of the Council," *Brit. Med. J., Suppl.,* April 19, 1958, p. 165, and May 24, 1958, p. 262; Audrey Z. Baker, "The Pharmaceutical House and the Doctor," *Brit. Med. J.,* November 1, 1958, p. 1097.

28. "Hinchliffe Report," pp. 22, 65; *Report of the Ministry of Health, 1958,* Part I, p. 136.

29. *Brit. Med. J.,* May 16, 1959, p. 1290, and *Suppl.,* April 11, 1959, p. 137.

30. "Hinchliffe Report," pp. 65-68.

31. *Report of the Ministry of Health, 1959,* Part I, pp. 106-7.

32. *Ibid., 1955,* Part I, pp. 82-83; "Guillebaud Report," pp. 168-69.

33. *Special Report and First, Second and Third Reports From the Committee of Public Accounts, Session 1956-57* (London: Her Majesty's Stationery Office, 1957), pp. 568-76; *Manchester Guardian,* April 9, 1957.

34. *Report of the Ministry of Health, 1960,* Part I, p. 75; *Brit. Med. J.,* March 22, 1958, p. 719, and *Suppl.,* February 6, 1960, pp. 41-42; T. H. Manners Kerfoot, "Role of the Pharmaceutical Industry," in "N.H.S. Supplement," *The Times* (London), July 7, 1958, p. v; *The Guardian,* April 26, 1960; "Hinchliffe Report," p. 64.

35. "Hinchliffe Report," pp. 64-65, 70-80; *The Guardian,* April 26, 1960; C. W. Guillebaud, "Cost of the Service—and the Nation's Drug Bill," in "N.H.S. Supplement," *The Times* (London), July 7, 1958, p. v; "Guillebaud Report," p. 169.

36. "Hinchliffe Report," pp. 81-83, 100-1; *Report of the Ministry of Health, 1960,* Part I, pp. 70-71.

37. *Report of the Ministry of Health, 1959,* Part I, p. 115; *1960,* p. 71.

38. "Hinchliffe Report," pp. 39-40.

CHAPTER XVIII

1. *Hansard,* H. of C., Vol. 592 (1958), col. 1429.

2. July 4, 1958.

3. Brian Abel-Smith, "After Ten Years," *New Statesman,* XVI (1958), 37-38.

4. *Spectator,* Vol. 201 (1958), 88-89.

5. "N.H.S. Supplement," *The Times* (London), July 7, 1958, p. ii.

6. *Hansard,* H. of C., Vol. 592 (1958), col. 1450.

7. Aneurin Bevan, *In Place of Fear,* p. 95.

8. Letter from John Fry, *The Observer,* July 6, 1958.

9. Richard M. Titmuss, *Essays on 'The Welfare State',* p. 155.

10. *Medical World Newsletter,* January, 1957, p. 15.

11. *Annual Report of King Edward's Hospital Fund for London, 1954,* p. 5.

12. June 29, 1958.

13. *Brit. Med. J.,* November 26, 1960, p. 1584.

14. *Manchester Guardian,* October 2, 1958 (Statement made by Dr. Bruce Cardew, General Secretary of the Medical Practitioners' Union).

15. *Brit. Med. J., Suppl.,* November 5, 1960, p. 182.

16. *Brit. Med. J.,* November 19, 1960, p. 1511; *Report of the Ministry of Health, 1959,* Part II, pp. 25 ff.

17. July 7, 1958.

18. "N.H.S. Supplement," *The Times* (London), July 7, 1958, p. ii.

19. *The Practitioner,* Vol. 181 (1958), 1-2.

20. *U.S. News and World Report,* April 12, 1957, p. 66.

21. D. Reid Ross, p. 136.

22. Gemmill, p. 21.

23. "Newsam Report," *Brit. Med. J., Suppl.,* January 17, 1959, p. 19.

APPENDIX

Appendix

TABLE 1
Total Cost and Sources of Finance for the National Health Service in England and Wales, 1949-50 and 1959-60
(Millions of £/$)

COST OF SERVICES			SOURCES OF FINANCE		
Services	1948-50	1959-60	Sources	1949-50	1959-60
Hospital and Specialist	£213 ($ 596) 53%	£415 ($1,160) 57%	Exchequer	£305 ($ 855) 76%	£495 ($1,386) 68%
General Medical	£ 42.5 ($ 116) 10.5%	£ 66 ($ 185) 9%	Partly Exchequer and Partly Local Rates	—	£ 62 ($ 174) 8%
Pharmaceutical	£ 31.5 ($ 88) 8%	£ 76 ($ 213) 10.5%	National Health Insurance	£ 36 ($ 100) 9%	£ 99 ($ 277) 14%
General Dental	£ 42.5 ($ 119) 10.5%	£ 50 ($ 140) 7%	Superannuation Contribution	£ 20.5 ($ 57) 5%	£ 35 ($ 98) 5%
Supplementary Ophthalmic	£ 22 ($ 61) 5.5%	£ 15 ($ 42) 2%	Payments by Persons Using the Service	£ 20 ($ 56) 5%	£ 34 ($ 95) 5%
Local Health Authority	£ 28.5 ($ 80) 7%	£ 68 ($ 190) 9.5%	Rates	£ 14 ($ 40) 4%	—
All others	£ 22.5 ($ 63) 5.5%	£ 36 ($ 100) 5%	All others	£ 6.5 ($ 18) 1%	—
Total	£402 ($1,125)	£726 ($2,033)	Totals	£402 ($1,125)	£726 ($2,033)

(Figures have been rounded)

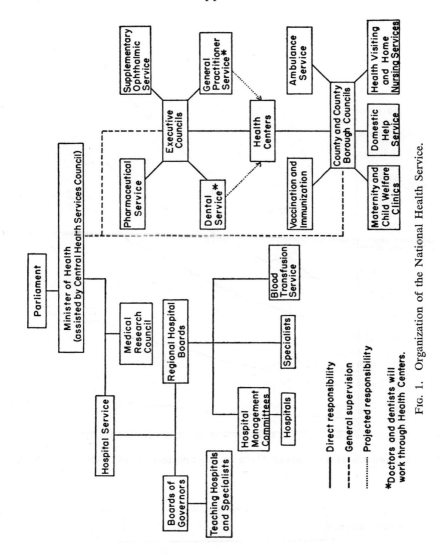

FIG. 1. Organization of the National Health Service.

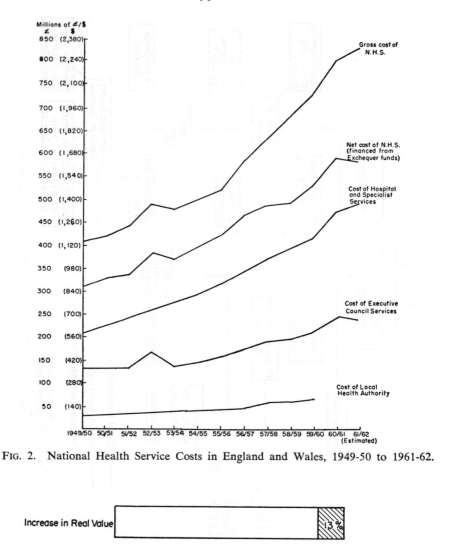

Fɪɢ. 2. National Health Service Costs in England and Wales, 1949-50 to 1961-62.

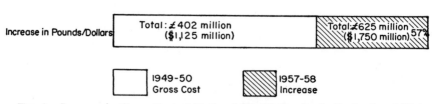

Fɪɢ. 3. Increase in Gross Cost of National Health Service in England and Wales for 1957-58 over that of 1949-50 in Pounds/Dollars and in Real Value.

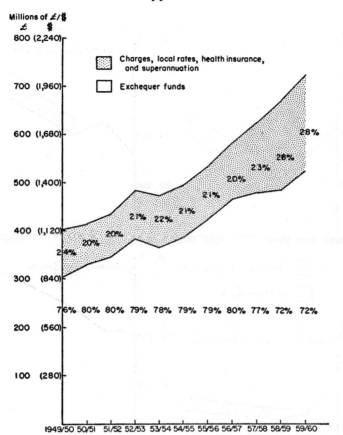

FIG. 4. Amount and Percentage of Exchequer and Non-Exchequer Funds Used to Finance the National Health Service in England and Wales, 1949-50 to 1959-60.

The gross cost as percentage of the gross national product for Great Britain (as determined in the *British Medical Journal, Supplement,* April 12, 1958, p. 150, and the *British Medical Journal,* November 28, 1959, pp. 1188-89, and in *Hansard,* H. of C., February 8, 1961, cols. 65-66) was:

1949-50	3.96%	1954-55	3.51%
1950-51	3.96%	1955-56	3.56%
1951-52	3.77%	1956-57	3.62%
1952-53	3.90%	1957-58	3.71%
1953-54	3.56%	1958-59	3.49%
		1959-60	3.60%

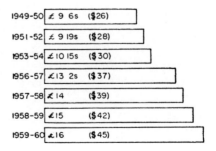

FIG. 5. Gross Cost Per Capita for the National Health Service in England and Wales.

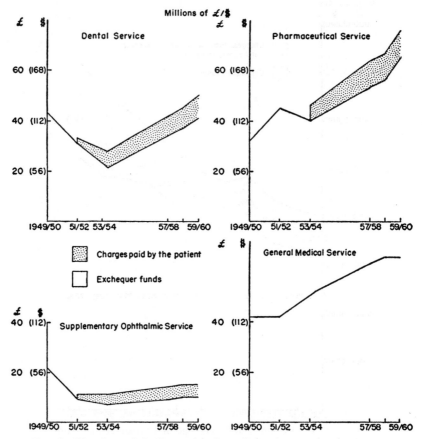

FIG. 6. The Cost of the Executive Council Services for England and Wales during Certain Representative Years, Showing the Proportion Paid by the Patients and the Exchequer.

BIBLIOGRAPHY

Bibliography

Books and Pamphlets Not Published by the Government

Abel-Smith, Brian, and Titmuss, Richard M. *The Cost of the National Health Service in England and Wales.* London: Cambridge University Press, 1956.

Adams, G. F., McQuilty, F. M., and Flint, M. Y. *Rehabilitation of the Elderly Invalid at Home.* London: The Nuffield Provincial Hospitals Trust, 1957.

Address by Iain N. Macleod, Minister of Health, at the Fifth Annual Conference of the Executive Councils' Association (England) held at Scarborough on the 2nd and 3rd October, 1952. West Cliff, Preston: Executive Councils' Association (England), n.d.

Address by Iain N. Macleod, Minister of Health, at the Seventh Annual Conference of the Executive Councils' Association (England) held at Southport on the 14th and 15th October, 1954. West Cliff, Preston. Executive Councils' Association (England), n.d.

Address by R. H. Turton, Minister of Health, at the Ninth Annual Conference of the Executive Councils' Association (England) held in London on the 18th and 19th October, 1956. West Cliff, Preston: Executive Councils' Association (England), n.d.

Address by Sir Reginald Taaffe Sharpe, Chairman of the National Health Service Tribunal for England and Wales, at the Eighth Annual Conference of the Executive Councils' Association (England) held at Brighton on the 20th and 21st October, 1955. West Cliff, Preston: Executive Councils' Association (England), n.d.

Annual Report and Statement of Accounts of the British United Provident Association for the Year Ended June 30, 1959. Oxford: The British United Provident Association, 1959.

Annual Report of King Edward's Hospital Fund for London, 1952 [and subsequent years to 1960]. London: King Edward's Hospital Fund for London, 1952-60.

Annual Report of the London Executive Council (National Health Service) For the Year April 1, 1950 to March 31, 1951 [and subsequent years to 1961]. London: London Executive Council, 1951-61.

Balint, Michael. *The Doctor, His Patient and the Illness.* New York: International Universities Press, Inc., 1957.

Bevan, Aneurin. *In Place of Fear.* New York: Simon and Schuster, 1952.

The British Dental Association. London: British Dental Association, 1952.

The British United Provident Association. Oxford: The British United Provident Association, 1960.

A Charter For Health. London: George Allen and Unwin, Ltd., 1946.

Cox, Alfred. "General Practice Fifty Years Ago: Some Reminiscences," *Fifty Years of Medicine: A Symposium.* London: British Medical Association, 1950.

A Critical Examination of the Guillebaud Report on the Cost of the National Health Service. London: Fellowship For Freedom in Medicine, 1957.

Eckstein, Harry. *The English Health Service: Its Origins, Structure and Achievements.* Cambridge, Mass.: Harvard University Press, 1958.

Family Practitioner Services. Rev. ed. West Cliff, Preston: Executive Councils' Association (England), 1958.

Ferguson, T., and MacPhail, A. N. *Hospital and Community.* London: Oxford University Press, 1954.

Gemmill, Paul F. *Britain's Search For Health.* Philadelphia: University of Pennsylvania Press, 1960.

A General Medical Service For the Nation. London: British Medical Association, 1938.

Giles, G. H. *The Ophthalmic Services Under the National Health Service Acts, 1946-1952.* London: Hammond, Hammond and Co., Ltd., 1952.

Hadfield, Stephen J. *Law and Ethics For Doctors.* London: Eyre and Spottiswoode, 1958.

Health in the Home and At Work: Report of the Haldane Society-Socialist Medical Association Joint Conference on Health, Safety and Welfare. London: Today and Tomorrow Publications, Ltd., 1954.

Herbert, S. Mervyn. *Britain's Health.* Harmondsworth, Middlesex: Penguin Books, Ltd., 1939.

Hill, Charles, and Woodcock, John. *The National Health Service.* London: Christopher Johnson, 1949.

Hobman, D. L. *The Welfare State.* London: John Murray, 1953.

Hospital Bed Occupancy: A Report of the First Group Set Up by the Hospital Administrative Staff College. London: King Edward's Hospital Fund for London, 1954.

Hospitals and the State: Hospital Organization and Administration Under the National Health Service. ("Background and Blueprint," No. 1; "The Impact of the Change," No. 2; "Groups, Regions and Committees, Part I, Hospital Management Committees," No. 3; "Part II, Regional Hospital Boards," No. 4; "The Central Control of the Service," No. 5; "Creative Leadership in a State Service," No. 6.) London: The Acton Society Trust, 1955-59.

Leff, Samuel. *The Health of the People.* London: Victor Gollangz, 1950.
Lesser, Henry (ed.). *The Health Services: Some of Their Practical Problems.* London: George Allen and Unwin, Ltd., 1951.
Levy, Hermann. *National Health Insurance: A Critical Study.* London: Cambridge University Press, 1944.
The London Hospital Medical College and Dental School, University of London, 1953-54. Catalogue. London: University of London, 1953.
The London Hospital: 216th Annual Report, 1956-57. London: London Hospital, 1957.
Mackintosh, James. *The Nation's Health.* London: The Pilot Press, Ltd., 1944.
Martin, J. P. *Social Aspects of Prescribing.* London: William Heinemann, Ltd., 1957.
The Medical Surrender: An Account of the Events Leading Up to the Acceptance by the Medical Profession in Great Britain of the National Health Service Act. London: Fellowship For Freedom in Medicine, 1951.
Members One of Another: Labour's Policy For Health. London: Labor Party, 1959.
Memorandum of Evidence Submitted to the Central Health Services Council Committee on General Practice. London: Fellowship For Freedom in Medicine, 1952.
Memorandum of Evidence Submitted to the Committee of Enquiry Into the Costs of the National Health Service. London: Fellowship For Freedom in Medicine, 1954.
Memorandum on the Maternity Services Submitted to the Cranbrook Committee of Enquiry. London: Fellowship For Freedom in Medicine, 1957.
Memorandum to the Committee of Enquiry Into the Cost of the National Health Service. London: British Dental Association, 1953.
Memorandum to the Committee of Enquiry Into the Shortage of Recruits to the Dental Profession. London: British Dental Association, 1955.
Memorandum to the Royal Commission on the Remuneration of National Health Service Doctors and Dentists. London: British Dental Association, 1957.
The Middle Class Way of Life. Correspondence reprinted from the *Manchester Guardian.* Manchester: *Manchester Guardian,* 1954.
Murray, D. Stark. *Health For All.* London: Victor Gollangz, Ltd., 1942.
The National Health Service Act in Great Britain: A Review of the First Year's Working. London: *The Practitioner,* 1949.
1954 Constitution and Rules of the Socialist Medical Association. London: Socialist Medical Association, 1954.
1960 Report and News Summary. London: The British United Provident Association, 1960.
The Nuffield Provincial Hospitals Trust: Fourth Report, 1955-1958. London: The Nuffield Provincial Hospitals Trust, 1958.

The Nuffield Provincial Hospitals Trust: Third Report, 1951-1955. London: The Nuffield Provincial Hospitals Trust, 1955.

The Policy of the Socialist Medical Association. Reprinted from *Socialist Medical Association Bulletin 114,* n.d. London: Socialist Medical Association, n.d.

The Preservation of Private Practice: Drugs For Private Patients. Broadsheet, No. 7. London: Fellowship For Freedom in Medicine, 1956.

Private Treatment in Illness. London: The British United Provident Association, n.d.

Problems of the Chronic Sick, the Aged and Infirm: A Challenge to the Nation. London: Socialist Medical Association, n.d.

Proceedings of the Annual Meeting of the British Medical Association, 1948. London: Butterworth and Co., 1948.

Proceedings of the Annual Meeting of the British Medical Association, 1949. London: Butterworth and Co., 1950.

Record of Proceedings at the Annual Meeting of the Executive Councils' Association (England). West Cliff, Preston: Executive Councils' Association (England), 1957-60.

Recovery Homes: A Report of an Inquiry into the Working of Recovery Homes and Their Value to the Hospital Service. London: King Edward's Hospital Fund for London, 1954.

Report of a Special Committee of the British Medical Association on the Care and Treatment of the Elderly and Infirm. London: British Medical Association, 1949.

Report of Sub-Committee on Amendments to the National Health Service Act. London: Fellowship For Freedom in Medicine, 1949.

Report of the Central Medical Services Committee on the Danckwerts Award and the Working Party's Findings on the Future Distribution of the Central Pool. London: British Medical Association, 1952.

Roberts, Ffrangcon. *The Cost of Health.* London: Turnstile Press, 1952.

Ross, James Sterling. *The National Health Service in Great Britain: An Historical and Descriptive Study.* London: Oxford University Press, 1952.

Scott, J. A., Cooper, D. J. B., and Seuffert, S. (eds.). *The National Health Service Acts, 1946 and 1948.* London: Eyre and Spottiswoode, 1950.

Some Administrative Problems of the Health Services. London: The Institute of Public Administration, 1951.

Spence, James, Walton, W. S., Miller, F. J. W., and Court, S. D. M. *A Thousand Families in Newcastle Upon Tyne: An Approach to the Study of Health and Illness in Children.* London: Oxford University Press, 1954.

Taylor, Stephen. *Good General Practice.* London: Oxford University Press, 1954.

Titmuss, Richard M. *Essays on 'The Welfare State.'* London: George Allen and Unwin, Ltd., 1958.

Towards a Reformed Health Service. London: Fellowship For Freedom in Medicine, 1957.

Twenty-Fifth Anniversary Commemoration Brochure. London: Socialist Medical Association, 1957.

Voluntary Service and the State: A Study of the Needs of the Hospital Service. London: George Barber and Son, Ltd., 1952.

Webb, Robert K. *The New Britain.* ("Headline Series," No. 114.) New York: Foreign Policy Association, 1955.

The Work of Nurses in Hospital Wards: Report of a Job-Analysis. London: The Nuffield Provincial Hospitals Trust, 1954.

Government Reports and Other Official Printed Material

Accounts 1954-55 [and succeeding years to 1960]: *Summarised Accounts of Regional Hospital Boards, Boards of Governors of Teaching Hospitals, Hospital Management Committees, Executive Councils, etc.* London: Her Majesty's Stationery Office, 1956-61.

Ambulance Services Costing Return, 1951-1952. London: Her Majesty's Stationery Office, 1953.

Annual Report of the Board of Control to the Lord Chancellor for the Year 1953 [and succeeding years to 1959]. London: Her Majesty's Stationery Office, 1954-1960.

Beveridge, Sir William. *Social Insurance and Allied Services* ["Beveridge Report"]. American ed. New York: The Macmillan Co., 1942.

Boucher, C. A. *Survey of Services Available to the Chronic Sick and Elderly, 1954-1955.* ("Ministry of Health Reports on Public Health and Medical Subjects," No. 98.) London: Her Majesty's Stationery Office, 1957.

Britain: An Official Handbook. London: Her Majesty's Stationery Office, 1959.

Carling, Sir Ernest Rock, and McIntosh, T. S. *Hospital Survey: The Hospital Services of the North-Western Area.* London: His Majesty's Stationery Office, 1945.

Chest Clinics ("Hospital Organization and Management Service Reports," No. 3.) London: Her Majesty's Stationery Office, 1959.

Choice of Careers: Dentistry. London: Her Majesty's Stationery Office, 1959.

Civil Estimates for the Year Ending 31st March, 1955, Class V: Health, Housing and Local Government [and subsequent years to 1962]. London: Her Majesty's Stationery Office, 1954-61.

Classification of Proprietary Preparations: Report of the Standing Joint Committee. London: Her Majesty's Stationery Office, 1959.

Clinical Research in Relation to the National Health Service. London: Her Majesty's Stationery Office, 1953.

Convalescent Treatment: Report of a Working Party. London: Her Majesty's Stationery Office, 1959.

Cope, V. Zachary, Gill, W. J., Griffiths, Arthur, and Kelly, G. C. *Hospital Survey: The Hospital Services of the South-Western Area.* London: His Majesty's Stationery Office, 1945.

Cowan, Kenneth H. *The Essex County Handbook*. Chelmsford: Edward J. Burrow and Co., 1953.

————. *Report of the Medical Officer of Health* [of the Administrative County of Essex], *1952*. Chelmsford: John Dutton, Ltd., 1953.

Current Medical Research: A Report of the Articles in the Report of the Medical Research Council for the Year 1956-57. London: Her Majesty's Stationery Office, 1958.

The Development of Consultant Services. London: His Majesty's Stationery Office, 1950.

Distribution of Remuneration Among General Practitioners. London: Her Majesty's Stationery Office, 1952.

Eason, Sir Herbert, Clark, R. Veitch, and Harper, W. H. *Hospital Survey: The Hospital Services of the Yorkshire Area*. London: His Majesty's Stationery Office, 1945.

Economic Survey, 1960. London: Her Majesty's Stationery Office, 1960.

Fifth Special Report From the Select Committee on Estimates, Session 1958-59: Running Costs of Hospitals. London: Her Majesty's Stationery Office, 1959.

50 Facts About Britain's Economy. London: Central Office of Information, 1959.

Final Report of the Committee on Cost of Prescribing ["Hinchliffe Report"]. London: Her Majesty's Stationery Office, 1959.

Final Report of the Committee on Hospital Supplies. London: Her Majesty's Stationery Office, 1958.

Final Report of the Inter-Departmental Committee on Dentistry ["Teviot Report"]. London: His Majesty's Stationery Office, 1946.

Flatlets For Old People. London: Her Majesty's Stationery Office, 1958.

Fourth Special Report From the Select Committee on Estimates, Session 1957-58. London: Her Majesty's Stationery Office, 1958.

General Practitioners' Records: An Analysis of the Clinical Records of Some General Practices During the Period April, 1952 to March, 1954. ("General Register Office Studies on Medical and Population Statistics," No. 9.) London: Her Majesty's Stationery Office, 1956.

General Register Office. *Births, Deaths and Marriages, Infectious Diseases, Weather and Population Estimates*. London: Her Majesty's Stationery Office, 1956 to First Quarter, 1960.

General Register Office. *Matters of Life and Death*. London: Her Majesty's Stationery Office, 1956.

Gray, A. M. H., and Topping, A. *Hospital Survey: The Hospital Services of London and Surrounding Area*. London: His Majesty's Stationery Office, 1945.

Hansard, House of Commons.

Hansard, House of Lords.

Health Services in Britain ("Central Office of Information Reference Pamphlet.") London: Her Majesty's Stationery Office, 1957.

Hospital Costing Returns, Year Ended 31st March, 1956. London: Her Majesty's Stationery Office, 1956.

Hospital Costing Returns, Year Ended 31st March, 1957. London: Her Majesty's Stationery Office, 1957.

Hospital Costing Returns, Year Ended 31st March, 1958. (*Hospitals Which Operated the Main Scheme,* Vol. I; *Hospitals Which Operated the Alternative Scheme,* Vol. II.) London: Her Majesty's Stationery Office, 1958-59.

Hospital Endowments Fund Account, 1954-55 [and succeeding years to 1960]. London: Her Majesty's Stationery Office, 1955-60.

Hunter, John B., Clark, R. Veitch, and Hart, Ernest. *Hospital Survey: The Hospital Services of the West Midlands Area.* London: His Majesty's Stationery Office, 1945.

An Inquiry Into Health Visiting: Report of a Working Party on the Field Work, Training and Recruitment of Health Visitors ["Jameson Report"]. London: Her Majesty's Stationery Office, 1956.

Interim Report of the Committee on Cost of Prescribing ["Hinchliffe Interim Report"]. London: Her Majesty's Stationery Office, 1958.

Interim Report of the Committee on Hospital Supplies. London: Her Majesty's Stationery Office, 1957.

Interim Report on the Future Provision of Medical and Allied Services ["Dawson Report"]. London: His Majesty's Stationery Office, 1920.

Jones, A. Trevor, Nixon, J. A., and Picken, R. M. F. *Hospital Survey: The Hospital Services of South Wales and Monmouthshire.* London: His Majesty's Stationery Office, 1945.

Lett, Sir Hugh, and Quine, A. E. *Hospital Survey: The Hospital Services of the North-Eastern Area.* London: His Majesty's Stationery Office, 1946.

Logan, W. P. D., and Cushion, A. A. *Morbidity Statistics from General Practice,* Vol. I ("General Register Office Studies on Medical and Population Statistics," No. 14.) London: Her Majesty's Stationery Office, 1958.

Maternity Benefits. (Leaflet N.I. 17A.) London: Ministry of Pensions and National Insurance, 1958.

Mental Health Act, 1959 (7 & 8 Eliz. 2, Ch. 72). London: Her Majesty's Stationery Office, 1959.

Midwives Act, 1951 (14 & 15 Geo. 6, Ch. 53). London: His Majesty's Stationery Office, 1951.

National Health Service Act, 1946 (9 & 10 Geo. 6, Ch. 81). London: His Majesty's Stationery Office, 1946.

National Health Service (Amendment) Act, 1949 (12, 13, & 14 Geo. 6, Ch. 93). London: His Majesty's Stationery Office, 1949.

National Health Service Act, 1951 (14 & 15 Geo. 6, Ch. 31). London: His Majesty's Stationery Office, 1951.

National Health Service Act, 1952 (15 & 16 Geo. 6 & 1 Eliz. 2, Ch. 25). London: Her Majesty's Stationery Office, 1952.

National Health Service Bill: Summary of the Proposed New Service. London: His Majesty's Stationery Office, 1946.

National Health Service Notes. Mimeographed. London: Ministry of Health, 1952-60.

No. 1: Explanatory Note, February, 1959, pp. 1-6.

No. 2: The General Medical Services, September, 1960, pp. 1-2.

No. 4: The Supplementary Ophthalmic Services, May, 1961, pp. 1-2.

No. 5: The Dental Services, November, 1952, pp. 1-3; May, 1961, pp. 1-3.

No. 9: Maternity Services Provided Under the National Health Service, November, 1958, pp. 1-4.

No. 10: Comparison of the Position Before and After the Introduction of the National Health Service, May, 1961, pp. 1-2.

No. 11A: Mental Health Services, October, 1959, pp. 1-4; *No. 11,* February, 1961, pp. 1-4.

No. 12: Hospital and Specialist Services, January, 1957, pp. 1-6.

No. 12A: Pay of Hospital Medical Staff, October, 1955, pp. 1-7; January, 1959, pp. 1-7; October, 1960, pp. 1-7.

A Guide to the Ophthalmic Service to Be Set Up Under the National Health Service Act, n.d., pp. 1-4.

How the Doctor Is Paid, March, 1953, pp. 1-4; *No. 2,* January, 1959, pp. 1-4; *No. 2A,* October, 1960, pp. 1-5; *No. 2A,* January, 1961, pp. 1-5.

Misconceptions About the National Health Service, September, 1959, pp. 1-2.

National Health Service Expenditures For 1949/50 [and succeeding years to 1959/60], 1950-61; *Estimated Expenditures for 1960/61 and 1961/62,* 1961.

A Short Survey of Health Services Available Before the Introduction of the National Health Service, March, 1953, pp. 1-4.

Summary of Main Current Figures in England and Wales, October, 1958, pp. 1-6; July, 1959, pp. 1-7; August, 1960, pp. 1-7.

Summary of Main Figures in England and Wales, 1949-1959, pp. 1-7; *1949-1960,* pp. 1-20.

A National Health Service ("White Paper"). London: His Majesty's Stationery Office, 1944.

The National Health Service (General Dental Services) Regulations, 1954. No. 742. London: Her Majesty's Stationery Office, 1954.

The National Health Service (General Dental Services) Amended Regulations, 1957. No. 229. London: Her Majesty's Stationery Office, 1957.

The National Health Service (General Medical and Pharmaceutical Services) Regulations, 1954. No. 669. London: Her Majesty's Stationery Office, 1954.

The National Health Service (General Medical and Pharmaceutical Services) Amended Regulations, 1956. Nos. 1076 and 1745. London: Her Majesty's Stationery Office, 1956.

The National Health Service (Pay-Bed Accommodation in Hospitals, etc.)

Regulations, 1953. No. 420. London: Her Majesty's Stationery Office, 1953.

The National Health Service (Service Committees and Tribunal) Regulations, 1948. 1956. London: His [Her] Majesty's Stationery Office, 1948; 1956.

The National Health Service (Superannuation) Regulations, 1955. No. 1084. London: Her Majesty's Stationery Office, 1955.

The National Health Service (Superannuation) Amended Regulations, 1957. No. 788. London: Her Majesty's Stationery Office, 1957.

The National Health Service (Supplementary Ophthalmic Services) Regulations, 1948. 1956. No. 1272; No. 1078. London: His [Her] Majesty's Stationery Office, 1948; 1956.

Nurses Act, 1949 (12 & 13 Geo. 6, Ch. 73). London: His Majesty's Stationery Office, 1949.

On the State of the Public Health During Six Years of War. London: His Majesty's Stationery Office, 1946.

Operating Theatre Suites. ("Hospital Building Bulletin.") London: Her Majesty's Stationery Office, 1957.

Organization and Management of Domestic Work in Hospitals. ("Hospital O and M Service Report," No. 4.) London: Her Majesty's Stationery Office, 1960.

Out-Patient Waiting Time. ("Hospital O and M Service Report," No. 1.) London: Her Majesty's Stationery Office, 1958.

Parsons, L. G., Fryers, S. Clayton, and Godber, G. E. *Hospital Survey: The Hospital Services of the Sheffield and East Midlands Area*. London: His Majesty's Stationery Office, 1945.

Pharmacy Act, 1953 (1 & 2 Eliz. 2, Ch. 19). London: Her Majesty's Stationery Office, 1953.

Pharmacy Act, 1954 (2 & 3 Eliz. 2, Ch. 61). London: Her Majesty's Stationery Office, 1954.

Preliminary Estimates of National Income and Expenditure, 1948 to 1953. 1954 to 1959. London: Her Majesty's Stationery Office, 1954; 1960.

The Reception and Welfare of In-Patients in Hospitals. London: Her Majesty's Stationery Office, 1953.

The Registrar General's Statistical Review of England and Wales For the Two Years 1952-1953: Supplement on Mental Health. London: Her Majesty's Stationery Office, 1958.

The Registrar General's Statistical Review of England and Wales For the Year 1957. Part I. London: Her Majesty's Stationery Office, 1958.

Report by the Government Actuary on the National Health Service Superannuation Scheme, 1948-1955. London: Her Majesty's Stationery Office, 1959.

Report by the Standing Nursing Advisory Committee on the Position of the Enrolled Assistant Nurse Within the National Health Service. London: Her Majesty's Stationery Office, 1954.

Report of the Central Health Services Council for the Year Ended Decem-

ber 31st, 1954 (and succeeding years to and including 1960). London: Her Majesty's Stationery Office, 1955 to 1961.

Report of the Committee of Enquiry Into the Cost of the National Health Service ("Guillebaud Report"). London: Her Majesty's Stationery Office, 1956.

Report of the Committee of Inquiry on the Rehabilitation, Training and Resettlement of Disabled Persons ("Piercey Report"). London: Her Majesty's Stationery Office, 1956.

Report of the Committee on Administrative Tribunals and Enquiries ("Franks Report"). London: Her Majesty's Stationery Office, 1957.

Report of the Committee on General Practice Within the National Health Service ("Cohen Report"). London: Her Majesty's Stationery Office, 1954.

Report of the Committee on Recruitment to the Dental Profession ("McNair Report"). London: Her Majesty's Stationery Office, 1956.

Report of the Committee on the Economic and Financial Problems of the Provision for Old Age ("Phillips Report"). London: Her Majesty's Stationery Office, 1954.

Report of the Committee on the Internal Administration of Hospitals ("Bradbeer Report"). London: Her Majesty's Stationery Office, 1954.

Report of the Committee to Consider the Future Numbers of Medical Practitioners and the Appropriate Intake of Medical Students ("Willink Report"). London: Her Majesty's Stationery Office, 1957.

Report of the Inter-Departmental Committee on the Remuneration of Consultants and Specialists ("Spens Report on the Remuneration of Consultants"). London: His Majesty's Stationery Office, 1948.

Report of the Inter-Departmental Committee on the Remuneration of General Dental Practitioners ("Spens Report on the Remuneration of General Dental Practitioners"). London: His Majesty's Stationery Office, 1948.

Report of the Inter-Departmental Committee on the Remuneration of General Practitioners ("Spens Report on Remuneration of General Practitioners"). London: His Majesty's Stationery Office, 1946.

Report of the Joint Committee on Prescribing. London: Her Majesty's Stationery Office, 1954.

Report of the Joint Sub-Committee on Welfare Foods. London: Her Majesty's Stationery Office, 1957.

Report of the Joint Working Party on the Medical Staffing Structure in the Hospital Service ("Platt Report"). London: Her Majesty's Stationery Office, 1961.

Report of the Maternity Services Committee ("Cranbrook Report"). London: Her Majesty's Stationery Office, 1959.

Report of the Medical Research Council for the Year 1954-1955.. 1956-1957. London: Her Majesty's Stationery Office, 1956; 1958.

Report of the Ministry of Health For the Year Ended December 31, 1952 (and subsequent years to 1960). Parts I and II. London: Her Majesty's Stationery Office, 1953-61.

Report of the Ministry of Health For the Year Ended March 31, 1946. London: His Majesty's Stationery Office, 1946.

Report of the Royal Commission on Doctors' and Dentists' Remuneration, 1957-1960 ("Pilkington Report"). London: Her Majesty's Stationery Office, 1960.

Report of the Royal Commission on the Law Relating to Mental Illness and Mental Deficiency, 1954-1957. London: Her Majesty's Stationery Office, 1957.

Report of the Sub-Committee on the Hospital Pharmaceutical Service. London: Her Majesty's Stationery Office, 1955.

Report of the Working Party on Hospital Costing. London: Her Majesty's Stationery Office, 1955.

Report of the Working Party on Midwives. London: His Majesty's Stationery Office, 1949.

Report of the Working Party on Social Workers in the Local Authority Health and Welfare Services ("Younghusband Report"). London: Her Majesty's Stationery Office, 1959.

Report of the Working Party on the Chairside Times Taken in Carrying Out Treatment by General Dental Practitioners in England, Wales and Scotland ("Penman Report"). London: His Majesty's Stationery Office, 1949.

Report of the Working Party on the Recruitment and Training of Nurses. London: His Majesty's Stationery Office, 1947.

Report on Confidential Enquiries Into Maternal Deaths in England and Wales, 1952-1954. ("Reports on Public Health and Medical Subjects," No. 97.). London: Her Majesty's Stationery Office, 1957.

Report on Co-operation Between Hospital, Local Authority and General Practitioner Services. London: Her Majesty's Stationery Office, 1952.

Report on Definition of Drugs. London: Her Majesty's Stationery Office, 1960.

Report on the Grading Structure of Administrative and Clerical Staff in the Hospital Service ("Noel Hall Report"). London: Her Majesty's Stationery Office, 1957.

Residential Accommodation For Old People, Homes For the More Infirm. (Ministry of Health circular for County Councils and County-Borough Councils.) London: Her Majesty's Stationery Office, 1955.

Royal Commission on Doctors' and Dentists' Remuneration: Minutes of Evidence. 1-23. London: Her Majesty Stationery Office, 1958-59.

Royal Commission on Doctors' and Dentists' Remuneration, 1957-1960: Supplement to Report. London: Her Majesty's Stationery Office, 1960.

Royal Commission on Doctors' and Dentists' Remuneration: Written Evidence. I. London: Her Majesty's Stationery Office, 1957.

Savage, Sir William, Frankau, Sir Claude, and Gibson, Sir Basil. *Hospital Survey: The Hospital Services of the Eastern Area.* London. His Majesty's Stationery Office, 1945.

Sixth Report From the Select Committee on Estimates Together With the Minutes of the Evidence Taken Before the Sub-Committee D and Ap-

pendices, Session 1956-57: Running Costs of Hospitals. London: Her Majesty's Stationery Office, 1957.

Special Report and First, Second and Third Reports From the Committee of Public Accounts, Session 1956-57. London: Her Majesty's Stationery Office, 1957.

Statement Specifying the Fees and Charges for the Testing of Sight and the Supply or Repair of Glasses, Revised as From December 1, 1959. London: Her Majesty's Stationery Office, 1959.

Stewart, George G. *The Essex County Health Handbook: The Health Services in the County of Essex.* Cheltenham and London: Edward J. Burrow and Co., 1956.

Superannuation Scheme for Those Engaged in the National Health Service in England and Wales: An Explanation. London: Her Majesty's Stationery Office, 1952.

Titmuss, Richard M. *History of the Second World War: Problems of Social Policy.* London: His Majesty's Stationery Office, 1950.

The Welfare of Children in Hospital: Report of the Committee ("Platt Report"). London: Her Majesty's Stationery Office, 1959.

Articles in Newspapers and Periodicals

Abel, A. Lawrence, and Lewin, Walpole. "Report on Hospital Building," *British Medical Journal, Supplement,* April 4, 1959, pp. 109-12.

Allison, V. D. "Hospital Central Sterile Supply Departments," *British Medical Journal,* September 10, 1960, pp. 772-78.

"Alternative Medical Services: Report By General Medical Services Committee," *British Medical Journal, Supplement,* May 30, 1959, pp. 234-42.

"Annual Report of the Council of the British Medical Association," *British Medical Journal, Supplement,* April 7, 1956, April 13, 1957, April 19, 1958, April 11, 1959, and March 19, 1960.

Atkin, T. "The Lotus-Eaters, or Stress, Neurosis and Tranquillizers," *British Medical Journal,* December 26, 1959, pp. 1477-80.

Bach, H. E., *et al.* "The Health Centres of Harlow—The Second Phase," *The Lancet,* November 15, 1958, pp. 1055-60.

Backett, E. Maurice, Heady, J. A., and Evans, J. C. G. "Studies of a General Practice, II, The Doctor's Job in an Urban Area," *British Medical Journal,* January 16, 1954, pp. 109-15.

Baker, Dr. Dudley M. "Family Doctor or Hospital?," *Fellowship For Freedom in Medicine,* October, 1956, pp. 13-15.

Baldwin, John T. "Appointment System in General Practice," *British Medical Journal, Supplement,* January 9, 1960, pp. 9-11.

Beveridge, (William) Lord. "The Role of the Individual in Health Service," *British Medical Journal,* December 11, 1954, pp. 1371-73.

Boland, E. R. "Administration of Medicine," *British Medical Journal,* July 3, 1948, pp. 9-19.

Breach, Dr. A. C. E. "Whitley Councils and the Health Service," *Fellowship For Freedom in Medicine,* October, 1956, pp. 13-15.

Brotherston, J. H. F., and Cartwright, Ann. "The Attitudes of General Practitioners Toward Alternative Systems of Remuneration," *British Medical Journal, Supplement,* October 17, 1959, pp. 119-24.

Brotherston, J. H. F., Cartwright, Ann, and Martin, F. M. "Public Reaction to the Current Dispute Between the Medical Profession and the Government," *The Lancet,* May 11, 1957, pp. 981-85.

Brotherston, J. H. F., Cartwright, Ann, *et al.* "Night Calls: Their Frequency and Nature in One General Practice," *British Medical Journal,* November 28, 1959, pp. 1169-72.

Brown, C. Metcalfe. "The Domiciliary Services Available to the Family Doctor," *The Practitioner,* Vol. 177 (1956), 48-53.

"By a Special Correspondent." "Cost of the Health Service," *British Medical Journal, Supplement,* April 12, 1958, pp. 149-51.

Calder, Ritchie. "Doctors' Parliament," *The New Statesman and Nation,* Vol. 37 (1949), 665-66.

Cardew, Bruce, and Macaulay, H. M. C. "Are Our Hospital Casualty Services Adequate to Our Present Needs?," *Medical World Newsletter,* February, 1957, pp. 4-5.

Carstairs, G. M., and Wing, J. K. "Attitudes of the General Public to Mental Illness," *British Medical Journal,* September 6, 1958, pp. 594-97.

"Centralization in the Hospital Services: The Need For a Change of Policy," *The Lancet,* November 14, 1953, pp. 1035-39.

"Chairman's Address at the Annual General Meeting, 1956," *Fellowship For Freedom in Medicine,* January, 1957, pp. 7-10.

Chalke, H. D. "The Aged in Their Own Homes: A Further Study," *British Medical Journal,* September 21, 1957, pp. 694-96.

Collings, Joseph S. "General Practice in England Today, A Reconnaissance," *The Lancet,* March 25, 1950, pp. 555-85.

Colwell, Catherine, and Post, Felix. "Community Needs of Elderly Psychiatric Patients," *British Medical Journal,* August 22, 1959, pp. 214-17.

"The [Walker] Committee's Report," *British Medical Journal, Supplement,* September 26, 1953, pp. 131-55.

Constad, Dr. Victor. "The Price of Public Ignorance," *Fellowship For Freedom in Medicine,* July, 1950, pp. 20-23.

Daley, Sir Allen. "The Place of the Hospital in a National Health Service," *British Medical Journal,* July 25, 1953, pp. 163-70; August 1, 1953, pp. 243-50.

Davies, J. O. F., and Lewin, Walpole. "Observations on Hospital Planning," *British Medical Journal,* September 10, 1960, pp. 763-68.

Davies, Richard Llewelyn. "Architectural Problems of New Hospitals," *British Medical Journal,* September 10, 1960, pp. 768-72.

Davis, H. "National Health Service and Pharmacy," *The Pharmaceutical Journal,* Vol. 119 (1954), 215-19.

Davison, Sir Ronald. "Health Means Test?," *The Spectator,* Vol. 188 (1952), 739.

De Largg, J. "Six Weeks In; Six Weeks Out: A Geriatric Hospital Scheme for Rehabilitating the Aged and Relieving Their Relatives," *The Lancet,* February 23, 1957, pp. 418-19.

Diehl, Harold S., *et al.* "British Medical Education and the National Health Service: A Report to the Trustees of the American Medical Association," *The Journal of the American Medical Association,* Vol. 143 (1950), 1492-1501.

"Disciplinary Procedure Within the National Health Service," *Fellowship For Freedom in Medicine,* October, 1951, pp. 9-14.

Donaldson, Malcolm. "Early Diagnosis of Cancer: A Psychological Problem," *The Lancet,* October 11, 1958, pp. 790-91.

Droller, H. "A Geriatric Out-Patient Department," *The Lancet,* October 4, 1958, pp. 739-41.

Eckstein, Harry H. "The Politics of the British Medical Association," *The Political Quarterly,* XXVI (1955), 345-59.

Elliott, A. "The Family Help and Night Attendant Services in Kent," *The Practitioner,* Vol. 177 (1956), 38-47.

Elliston, G. L. C. "A Better Health Service," *The Spectator,* Vol. 190 (1953), 409-10.

"Evidence to the Royal Commission: Hospital Medical Staff," *Medical World Newsletter,* June, 1958, pp. 5-17.

"An Examination of the Whitley Council Machinery," *British Medical Journal, Supplement,* April 7, 1956, pp. 169-75.

Farrer-Brown, Leslie. "Hospitals For To-Day and To-morrow," *British Medical Journal, Supplement,* April 4, 1959, pp. 118-22.

Ferguson, R. S. "The Doctor-Patient Relationship and 'Functional' Illness," *The Practitioner,* Vol. 176 (1956), 656-62.

Flavus. "Hospital Diary," *The New Statesman and Nation,* Vol. 43 (1952), 5-6.

Fox, T. F. "Professional Freedom," *The Lancet,* July 21, 1951, pp. 115-19; July 28, 1951, pp. 171-75.

Fry, John. "Care of the Elderly in General Practice: A Socio-Medical Reassessment," *British Medical Journal,* September 21, 1957, pp. 666-70.

⸺. "The Family Doctor," *Twentieth Century,* CLXIV (1958), 51-61.

⸺. "A General Practitioner's Views on Hospital Planning," *British Medical Journal, Supplement,* April 4, 1959, pp. 124-26.

⸺. "Why Patients Go to Hospital," *British Medical Journal,* December 12, 1959, pp. 1322-27.

⸺. "A Year of General Practice: A Study in Morbidity," *British Medical Journal,* August 2, 1952, pp. 249-52.

Gemmill, Paul F. "An American Report on the National Health Service," *British Medical Journal, Supplement,* July 5, 1958, pp. 17-21.

"A General Practitioner." "Three Months of N.H.S.," *The Spectator,* Vol. 181 (1948), 425-26.

"General Practitioner Observer." "The Future of General Practice: I,

Great Expectations; II, The Patient's Viewpoint; III, The General Practitioner Today; IV, The Pay Problem; V, The GP's Premises; VI, Abuse by the Patient; VII, Obstetrics; VIII, Research," *Medical World Newsletter,* June, 1955, July, 1955, August, 1955, September, 1955, October, 1955, November, 1955, December, 1955, and January, 1956.

George, J. T. A., Lowe, C. R., and McKeoun, Thomas. "An Examination of the Work of Local Authority Child Welfare Clinics," *The Lancet,* January 10, 1953, pp. 88-92.

Gilbert, John W. "The Public Dental Service of England and Wales," *International Dental Journal,* II (1951-52), 496-516.

Godber, G. E. "Health Services, Past, Present, and Future," *The Lancet,* July 5, 1958, pp. 1-6.

———. "The Physician's Part in Hospital Planning," *British Medical Journal, Supplement,* April 4, 1959, pp. 115-18.

———. "The Scope For Home Care in the National Health Service," *The Practitioner,* Vol. 177 (1956), 5-9.

Goodfellow, Dr. D. R. "Reflections on Leaving General Practice in England," *Fellowship For Freedom in Medicine,* August, 1949, pp. 11-14.

Grant, C. P. D. "Youth Looks at General Practice," *British Medical Journal,* April 30, 1955, pp. 1049-51.

Gray, P. G., and Cartwright, Ann. "Choosing and Changing Doctors," *The Lancet,* December 19, 1953, pp. 1308-9.

Hadfield, Stephen J. "A Field Survey of General Practice, 1951-52," *British Medical Journal,* September 26, 1953, pp. 683-706.

Harper, James. "Out-Patient Adult Psychiatric Clinics," *British Medical Journal,* February 7, 1959, pp. 357-60.

Hastings, Somerville. "Hospitals Today: A Criticism," *Medical World Newsletter,* August, 1958, pp. 5-9.

Haynes, Alfred H. "Five Years of Welfare State," *Fortnightly,* Vol. 180 (1953), 21-25.

"Health Centres: Interim Report by the Council of the B.M.A., July, 1948," *British Medical Journal, Supplement,* September 11, 1948, pp. 107-17.

"Health Centres: Report of the Medical Practitioners' Union," *The Medical World,* March 18, 1949, pp. 109-15.

"The Health Service and the Doctor," *Medical World Newsletter,* May, 1957, pp. 4-11.

Heilbron, Rose. "When is a Doctor Negligent?," *British Medical Journal,* December 28, 1957, pp. 1540-41.

Hill, A. Bradford, "The Doctor's Day and Pay: Some Sampling Inquiries Into the Pre-War Status," *Journal of the Royal Statistical Society,* CXIV (1951), 1-34.

Hilson, D. "Integration of General Practitioners Within the Hospital Service: Preliminary Report on a Pilot Scheme," *British Medical Journal, Supplement,* December 12, 1959, pp. 187-90.

Hindle, Thomas. "Original Communications," *British Dental Journal,* Vol. 96 (1954), 233-35.

Howard, Miles. "Ten Years On," *The Spectator,* Vol. 201 (1958), 88-89.

Hughes, T. Lloyd. "Medico-Legal Problems Arising in the National Health Service," *Medico-Legal Journal,* Vol. 21 (1953), 17-33.

Hunt, J. H. "The Scope and Development of General Practice in Relation to Other Branches of Medicine: A Constructive Review," *The Lancet,* October 1, 1955, pp. 681-86.

Inch, R. S. "The Pharmaceutical Industry," *British Medical Journal,* October 4, 1958, pp. 846-49.

Joad, C. E. M. "On Doctors," *The New Statesman and Nation,* Vol. 45 (1953), 255-56.

Johnson, Dr. Donald Mcl. "Can Medicine Be Divorced From Politics?," *Fellowship For Freedom in Medicine,* January, 1957, pp. 29-31.

Joules, Horace. "The Progress of the National Health Service," *The British Medical Student's Journal,* Vol. 4 (1949), 17-18.

Lee, Dr. Terence. "The General Practitioner and the National Health Service," *Fellowship For Freedom in Medicine,* December, 1949, pp. 15-19.

Lee, J. A. H. "The Effectiveness of Routine Examination of School Children," *British Medical Journal,* March 8, 1958, pp. 573-76.

"The Legal Liability of the Hospital Doctor," *Fellowship For Freedom in Medicine,* October, 1956, pp. 9-11.

Lloyd, Major Sir Guy. "The Layman's Point of View," *Fellowship For Freedom in Medicine,* December, 1954, pp. 15-18.

"Loss of Trained Nursing Staff From Hospitals," *The Lancet,* August 14, 1948, pp. 266-68.

Lowe, C. R., and McKeoun, Thomas. "A Scheme For the Care of the Aged and Chronic Sick," *British Medical Journal,* July 26, 1952, pp. 207-10.

McCash, Charles R. "Plastic Surgery in the N.H.S.," *Medical World,* October, 1957, pp. 309-14.

McGregor, H. G. "Training of Consultants Under the N.H.S.: A Survey Made in the S. E. Metropolitan Region," *British Medical Journal, Supplement,* October 20, 1956, pp. 159-60.

McKeoun, Thomas. "Fundamental Problems in Hospital Planning," *British Medical Journal, Supplement,* April 4, 1959, pp. 122-24.

MacMillan, Duncan. "Community Treatment of Mental Illness," *The Lancet,* July 26, 1958, pp. 201-4.

Macrae, J. M. "Original Communications," *British Dental Journal,* Vol. 87 (1949), 1-4.

Mair, Alistair, and Mair, George B. "Facts of Importance to the Organization of a National Health Service From a Five Year Study of a General Practice," *British Medical Journal, Supplement,* June 20, 1959, pp. 282-84.

Mallalieu, J. P. W. "The Good Samaritans," *The New Statesman and Nation,* Vol. 52 (1956), 513-14.

"Medical Planning Commission Draft Interim Report," *British Medical Journal,* June 20, 1942, pp. 743-53.

"Medical Planning Research Interim General Report," *The Lancet,* November 21, 1942, pp. 599-622.

"A Medical Specialist." "Private Practice and the Health Service," *The New Statesman and Nation,* Vol. 46 (1953), 812.

Mellanby, May, Martin, W. J., and Barnes, David. "Teeth of 5-Year-Old London School Children (1957) With a Comparison of the Results Obtained From 1929 to 1957," *British Medical Journal,* December 13, 1958, pp. 1441-43.

"Memorandum of Evidence to the Royal Commission on Doctors' and Dentists' Remuneration," *British Medical Journal, Supplement,* November 23, 1957, pp. 157-73.

"Memorandum of the Central Consultants and Specialists Committee on the Report of the Bradbeer Committee on the Internal Administration of Hospitals," *British Medical Journal, Supplement,* April 7, 1956, pp. 160-65.

Mestitz, P. "A Series of 1,817 Patients Seen in a Casualty Department," *British Medical Journal,* November 9, 1957, pp. 1108-9.

Moran, Lord. "Lessons From the Past," *British Medical Journal, Supplement,* July 5, 1958, pp. 3-5.

Morison, Dr. C. Rutherford. "The Future of Obstetrics Under the N.H.S.," *Fellowship For Freedom in Medicine,* June, 1952, pp. 7-12.

Morris, David. "Experiment in Liaison," *Woman Health Officer,* XXVIII (1955), 283-87.

Morris, Norman, and O'Neill, Desmond. "Out-Patient Gynaecology," *British Medical Journal,* May 3, 1958, pp. 1036-39.

Murley, R. S. "Patient and Doctor," *Fellowship For Freedom in Medicine,* June, 1954, pp. 18-23.

"National Health Service Supplement," *The Times* (London), July 7, 1958.

"The Newsam Report on Family Doctors' Services in the National Health Service," *British Medical Journal, Supplement,* January 17, 1959, pp. 11-21.

Ogilvie, Sir Heneage. "Mr. Stassen's Granny," *The Spectator,* Vol. 184 (1950), 333.

Pemberton, John. "Illness in General Practice," *British Medical Journal,* February 19, 1949, pp. 306-8.

Pickering, G. W. "The Function of a Teaching Hospital," *The Lancet,* January 5, 1957, pp. 1-2.

"Porritt Committee's Questionary Seeking Views on Medical Services," *British Medical Journal, Supplement,* November 5, 1960, pp. 181-83.

"A Postal Inquiry Among 12,879 General Practitioner Principals, July, 1951," *British Medical Journal, Supplement,* September 26, 1953, pp. 105-31.

Postbridge, Warren. "The Private Patient," *The Spectator,* Vol. 185 (1950), 457-58.

Potter, L. S. "Entry Into General Medical Practice," *British Medical Journal, Supplement,* October 4, 1958, pp. 153-55.

"Private Practice Today: Nine GPs. Report on Their Recent Experience," *Fellowship For Freedom in Medicine,* May, 1954, pp. 5-13.

"Proceedings of the Annual Conference of Representatives of Local Medical Committees," *British Medical Journal, Supplement,* May 28, 1960, pp. 304-13; June 4, 1960, pp. 336-45.

"The Reform of the National Health Service: First Interim Report of the Council," *British Medical Journal, Supplement,* October 13, 1951, pp. 141-48.

"Relationship Between the Medical Profession and the State in the National Health Service," *British Medical Journal, Supplement,* April 23, 1960, pp. 239-41.

"Report of the Proceedings of the Annual General Meeting of the Fellowship," *Fellowship For Freedom in Medicine,* December, 1951, pp. 5-12; January, 1957, pp. 11-16.

"Report on Health Centres by the London Local Medical Committee," *Medical World Newsletter,* October, 1956, pp. 4-10.

Roberts, Ffrangcon. "Where Are We Going? Medicine in a Planned Economy," *British Medical Journal,* March 13, 1948, pp. 485-89.

Rogers, A. Talbot. "A Family Doctor's Report on Socialized Medicine," *The Progressive,* Vol. 21 (1957), 18-20.

———. "Health Centre Prospects," *The Spectator,* Vol. 181 (1948), 363-64.

Ross, D. Reid. "N.H.S. in Factory Town: A Survey of the Demand For Medical Care in an Industrial Community," *Medical World,* February, 1953, pp. 125-38.

Roth, Martin. "Problems of An Ageing Population," *British Medical Journal,* April 23, 1960, pp. 1226-30.

Sampson, Edward. "Dentistry and Demand," *The Spectator,* Vol. 173 (1944), 75-76.

Sanderson, Allendale. "Five Years of the National Health Service," *Twentieth Century,* CLIV (1953), 120-26.

Scott, J. A. "The Contribution of the Health Centre to the Public Health," *The Journal of the Royal Institute of Public Health and Hygiene,* XVI (1953), 186-96.

Sheldon, J. H. "Problems of An Ageing Population," *British Medical Journal,* April 23, 1960, pp. 1223-26.

Sherret, David. "Impact of New Methods of Treatment in a Provincial Mental Hospital," *British Medical Journal,* April 26, 1958, pp. 994-96.

Speller, R. S. "Whitleyism: The Formation and Work of the Administrative and Clerical Staffs Council of the Whitley Councils for the Health Services," *The Hospital,* Vol. 47 (1951), 867-75.

Statham, Cecily. "Noise and the Patient in Hospital: A Personal Investigation," *British Medical Journal,* December 5, 1959, pp. 1247-48.

Stevenson, R. Scott. "Socialized Medicine in England," *Laryngoscope,* Vol. 62 (1952), 813-45.

Swift, George. "Postgraduate Education For the General Practitioner," *British Medical Journal,* September 6, 1958, pp. 580-83.

Taylor, (Stephen) Lord. "Hospitals of the Future," *British Medical Journal,* September 10, 1960, pp. 752-58.

Taylor, Stephen. "The Health Centres of Harlow: An Essay in Co-operation," *The Lancet,* October 22, 1955, pp. 863-70.

Telling, A. E. "Professional Freedom and Responsibility Under the National Health Service," *The Lancet,* August 4, 1956, pp. 242-44.

Thomson, Sir Arthur. "History and Development of Teaching Hospitals in England," *British Medical Journal,* September 10, 1960, pp. 749-51.

Webley, Laurence. "Property Transactions Between Practitioners and the National Health Service Act," *Medical World Newsletter,* October, 1956, pp. 11-13.

Wilding, L. W. "The London Story," *The London Hospital Illustrated,* III, No. 6 (1955), 8-10.

Woodhouse, Dr. Barbara. "Payment For Service Rendered. Is it Desirable? Is it Feasible?," *Fellowship For Freedom in Medicine,* March, 1955, pp. 23-26.

Wright, Catherine H., and Roberts, Llewelyn. "The Place of the Home-Help Service in the Care of the Aged," *The Lancet,* February 1, 1958, pp. 254-56.

Miscellaneous Material

"Ambulance Services: Minister's Suggestions For Economies." Statement by the Minister of Health, April 9, 1956, pp. 1-2.

"By a Doctor." "Points About the National Health Service, 1948-1952." January, 1953.

"The Doctors' Pay Claim." Statement by the Ministry of Health, April, 1957, pp. 1-4.

"Draft Definitive Policy Statement, No. 2 (Revised), December, 1955." Socialist Medical Association.

"From an Address of the Minister of Health to the Executive Councils' Association at Torquay, October 8, 1953."

"Memorandum Submitted by the Joint Emergency Committee of the Optical Profession to the Committee of Enquiry Into the Cost of the National Health Service, November, 1953."

"Report of the Medical Practices Committee." January, 1953, pp. 1-8.

Social Surveys [Gallup Poll], Ltd. "National Health Service Enquiry, June, 1956."

INDEX

Index

Abel, A. Lawrence, and Lewin, Walpole, on hospital construction, 302

Abel-Smith, Brian, and Titmuss, Richard M., on efficiency in the hospital service, 265

Abuses, in Health Service, 75, 80, 100; in prescribing, 104, 108

Acton Society Trust, on administration of three types of hospitals, 256-58; on separate status of teaching hospitals, 259-60; mentioned, 249, 255, 265, 462

Administration of Health Service, by national board or corporation, 30, 31, 97; by government department, 30, 34; as proposed by White Paper, 34-35; opposition to proposed central control, 38; fear of "bureaucratic" control, 39; policy favored by Aneurin Bevan, 42; lack of effective co-operation between the divisions of the Service, 82-83; avoidance of too much centralization, 83-84; use of voluntary boards and committees, 84; part played by professions, 90-91, 223; subordination of doctors to lay administrators, 91-92; use of circulars, 93. *See also* Administrative machinery of Health Service

Administrative machinery of Health Service, evolutionary character of, 83; sentiment favorable toward, 98. *See also* Executive Councils, Hospital administration, Hospital house committees, Hospital management committees, Local health authorities, Minister of Health, Ministry of Health, Regional hospital boards

Advisory Council for Management Efficiency, 271

Aged, care of, 76; cost of medical care for, 101, 120-21; income of, 389; desire to remain in the community, 389; institutional accommodations for, 389-90; small homes for, 390, 470; special one-bedroom flats for, 390-91; board-ing out in private homes, 391; voluntary help for, 391-92; dependence upon domiciliary services, 391-94; recreational facilities for, 392; chiropody service for, 392, 470; meals on wheels for, 392, 470; use of domestic help for, 393; popular interest in the problem of, 393-94

Aged sick, care of by health visitors, 370, 371; care of by home nurses, 372, 373; assistance from domestic help, 374, 393. *See also* Chronic illness

Almoners, 14, 76, 291-92, 298, 300, 346, 355, 464

Ambulance service, before 1948, 18; cost of, 366; efficiency of, 367, 368-69, 468-69; character of, 367-68; mentioned, 15, 19, 21, 83, 88, 100, 105, 364, 365, 449

Amendment Act of 1949, 81, 106

Amendment Act of 1951, reasons for adoption of, 81-82; provisions of, 82, 106

Amendment Act of 1952, 82, 107

Amenity beds, 105, 113, 278

American politician, makes a cursory appraisal of the Health Service, 78-79

Anesthetics, 329, 335, 345

Approved Societies, 9, 10, 11, 12, 43

Assistantship, terms and conditions of, 164, 208

Association of British Pharmaceutical Industry, 444, 445

Association of Chief Financial Officers, 240

Association of Executive Councils, 85-86

Association of Hospital Management Committees, 240

Atlee, Clement, 41

Backett, E. Maurice *et al.*, on rate of home visiting, 213; mentioned, 180

Bevan, Aneurin, consults with profes-

ment, 252, 253; on the cost of private beds, 276; on health education, 283; on advertising drugs, 444; influence in controlling the Health Service, 453. *See also* Medical profession

British Medical Guild, 141, 143

British Medical Journal, maligns new law, 48-49; on professional standards, 53; letters from angry doctors, 55; on rejection of new service, 56-57; on publicity pressuring doctors, 60; on acceptance of Health Service, 54-65; predicts confusion in new service, 73; on early operation of Service, 75; on politics in the Health Service, 95; on prescription charge, 109-10; on Guillebaud Report, 121-22; on Cohen Report, 126; on rejection of the Spens principle, 141; on Cranbrook Report, 197

British National Formulary, 201, 439, 441, 442, 443

British Pharmaceutical Codex, 442

British Pharmacopoeia, 441

British Red Cross, 18, 321, 360, 367, 392, 454

British Transport Commission, 92, 97

British United Provident Association, private hospital insurance, 278-79; general practitioner scheme, 279

Brotherston, Dr. J. H. F., *et al.,* on night calls, 213; on quality of medical care, 231; mentioned, 180-81

Bureaucratic controls, 223, 224, 225, 452

Cancer, treatment of, 21; research in, 288; educating public about, 387; mentioned, 18. *See also* Lung cancer

Capitation and loading fees, 128, 130, 133-34, 148, 150

Care and after-care of the sick, 83, 366, 388-89

Casualty department, 329, 331, 368

Cave Report, on hospitals, 14-15; dire predictions of prove groundless, 356

Central Health Services Council, character of, 84; standing committees of, 240; on co-operation among the divisions of the Health Service, 395; mentioned, 34, 88, 90, 119, 272, 318, 385, 424, 448, 453

Central Pool, 128, 129, 130, 131-32, 133, 150, 188, 203

Chancellor of the Exchequer, imposes ceiling on funds for Health Service, 104

Charges, permitted by Amendment Act of 1949, 81; permitted by Amendment

Act of 1951, 81-82; permitted by Amendment Act of 1952, 82; exemptions from, 82, 104, 107, 113; reasons for, 104; at inception of Service, 105; in 1951, 106; in 1952, 106-8; in 1956, 109-10; in 1961, 113; in dental service, 416-17; in ophthalmic service, 424-25; for drugs, 431, 432

Charity, comment of a doctor on its elimination by the new service, 65

Chest clinics, 332

Child welfare, milk program for school children, 4; child welfare clinics, 364, 377-78, 469; health of children, 369, 469; mortality rate, 472-73. *See also* Day nurseries, Dental service, Mental hospitals, Preventive medicine, School medical program, Supplementary ophthalmic service, Welfare Foods Scheme

Chiropodists, 346, 347, 466

Chiropody, 298, 299, 382, 392

Chronic illness, treatment of in the 1940's, 19; role of local authorities, 296; waiting list for geriatric beds, 297; geriatric outpatient departments, 297, 298-99; utilization of beds for, 297-98; geriatric units for inpatients, 298; day hospitals for, 299; Social Rehabilitation Units for, 299; short-stay convalescent homes for, 299; lack of sufficient hospital staff for, 300; need of new hospitals for, 300-1; cost of geriatric inpatients, 301; long-stay annexes, 315; care for chronic sick, 388, 469-70; mentioned, 101, 206, 241, 281, 351

Churchill, Sir Winston, affirms government support for a national health service, 23-24; on Conservative Party support for Health Service, 80; on the rising costs of the Service, 100; mentioned, 41

Circulars, nature and purpose of, 93; use of by Ministry of Health, 93, 242

Clinical freedom, under the National Health Insurance, 28; for dentists, 70; for specialists, 336, 467; for opticians, 426; for general practitioners, 206-7, 207-9, 223, 225, 229, 230, 435, 452, 460; mentioned, 34, 38, 40, 61, 91, 353

Clinical Research Board, 464

Cohen, Sir Henry, 126

Cohen Report, on system of administration, 98; on importance of general practitioner service, 124; on capitation method of remuneration, 139; on filling a vacancy, 157; on trainee program, 163; on abuses of partnerships, 167;